D1474360

ENCYCLOPEDIA OF

# stem cell research

ENCYCLOPEDIA OF

# stem cell research

VOLUME 1

GENERAL EDITORS

CLIVE N. SVENDSEN AND ALLISON D. EBERT

University of Wisconsin, Madison

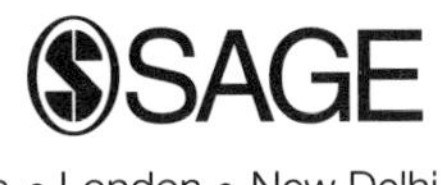

Los Angeles • London • New Delhi • Singapore

A SAGE Reference Publication

*For information:*

SAGE Publications, Inc.
2455 Teller Road
Thousand Oaks, California 91320
E-mail: order@sagepub.com

SAGE Publications Ltd.
1 Oliver's Yard
55 City Road
London EC1Y 1SP
United Kingdom

SAGE Publications India Pvt. Ltd.
B 1/I 1 Mohan Cooperative Industrial Area
Mathura Road, New Delhi 110 044
India

SAGE Publications Asia-Pacific Pte. Ltd.
33 Pekin Street #02-01
Far East Square
Singapore 048763

*About the covers:*

Volume 1: Microscopic 5x view of a colony of undifferentiated human embryonic stem cells being studied at the University of Wisconsin. Volume 2: Microscopic 10x view of a colony of undifferentiated human embryonic stem cells. Copyright University of Wisconsin Board of Regents.

*Library of Congress Cataloging-in-Publication Data*

Encyclopedia of stem cell research / Clive N. Svendsen, Allison D.Ebert, general editors.
p. ; cm.
Includes bibliographical references and index.
ISBN 978-1-4129-5908-7 (cloth)
1. Stem cells--Encyclopedias. I. Svendsen, Clive. II. Ebert, Allison.
[DNLM: 1. Stem Cells--Encyclopedias--English. 2. Stem Cell Transplantation--Encyclopedias--English. QU 13 E565 2008]
QH588.S83E53 2008
616'.02774--dc22 2008022785

08 09 10 11 12 10 9 8 7 6 5 4 3 2 1

GOLSON BOOKS, LTD.
President and Editor: J. Geoffrey Golson
Creative Director: Mary Jo Scibetta
Managing Editors: Susan Moskowitz, Joseph K. Golson
Copyeditor: Anne Hicks
Layout Editors: Kenneth W. Heller, Oona Hyla Patrick
Proofreaders: Joyce H-S Li, Barbara Paris
Indexer: J S Editorial

SAGE REFERENCE
Vice President and Publisher: Rolf A. Janke
Project Editor: Tracy Buyan
Cover Production: Janet Foulger
Marketing Manager: Amberlyn Erzinger
Editorial Assistant: Michele Thompson
Reference Systems Manager: Leticia Gutierrez

Photo credits are on page 902.

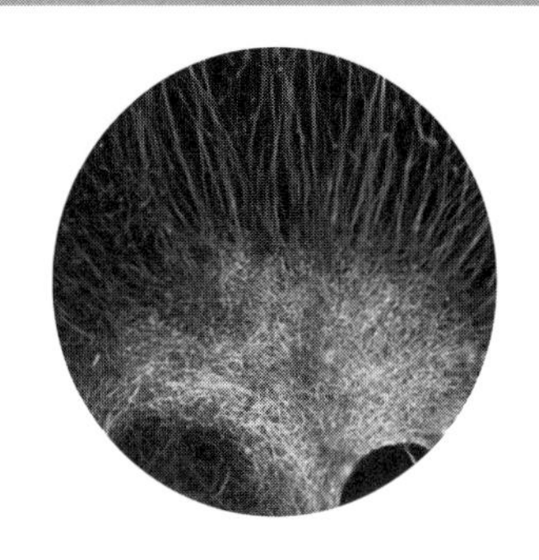

# CONTENTS

# About the General Editors

## CLIVE N. SVENDSEN, Ph.D.

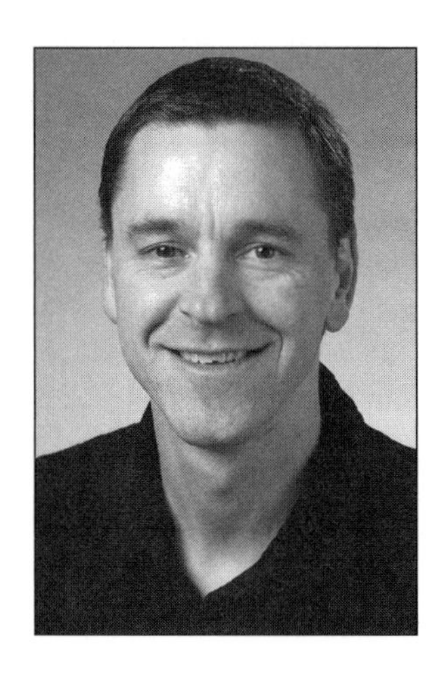

Clive N. Svendsen was fascinated with neuroscience while working both in Cambridge, England (University of Cambridge), and Cambridge, Massachusetts (Harvard University), throughout the 1980s.

He received his Ph.D. from the University of Cambridge (Jesus College) in 1992 and established a research team at the Cambridge Center for Brain Repair. In 2000 he moved to back to the United States and is currently professor of neurology and anatomy at the University of Wisconsin, Madison, Director of the NIH-funded Stem Cell Training Program and Co-Director of the Wisconsin Stem Cell and Regenerative Medicine Center. He has published over 100 scientific papers and his main interests are in stem cell biology and neuroscience. His research goals are to develop novel ways to treat neurological illness using stem cells. One approach is to isolate stem cells from patients with specific neurological diseases. These can be used to understand some of the mechanisms that lead to neurons dying in these diseases.

## ALLISON D. EBERT, Ph.D.

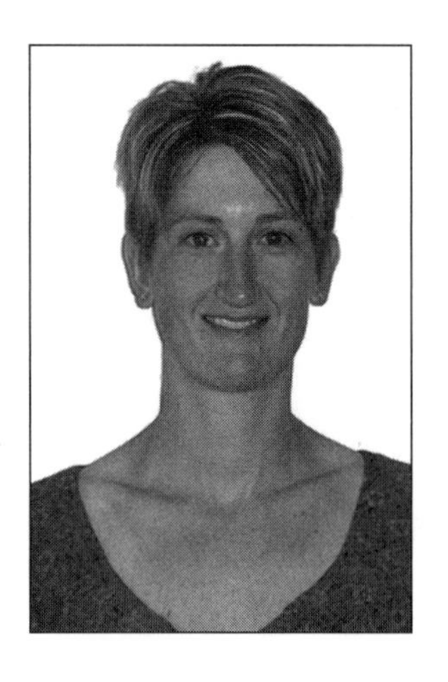

Allison D. Ebert received undergraduate degrees in chemistry and psychology in 1999 from Indiana University in Bloomington, Indiana. She then went to Northwestern University in Chicago, Illinois, where she received a Ph.D. in neuroscience in 2005, specializing in neurobiology. While at Northwestern, she studied the molecular mechanism of neuronal death in models of Parkinson's disease and tested gene therapy techniques designed to halt the progression of the disease.

Wanting to continue studying possible therapies for neurodegenerative disorders, she moved to the University of Wisconsin, Madison, as a postdoctoral fellow and currently as an Assistant Scientist in Dr. Clive Svendsen's lab in the Stem Cell Research Program.

Her research interests include using stem cells in vitro to study the molecular processes of neurodegenerative diseases and in vivo as a cell-based drug delivery system in models of Parkinson's and Huntington's diseases.

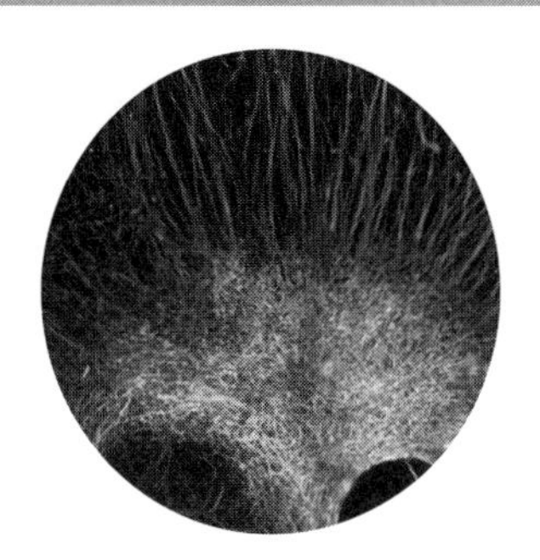

# Introduction

**WHAT IS A** stem cell? We have a basic working definition, but the way we observe a stem cell function in a dish may not represent how it functions in a living organism. Only this is clear: Stem cells are the engine room of multicelluar organisms for both plants and animals. They live in cave-like "niches," surrounded by intricate signals that allow them to divide—either to make more of themselves (self-renew), or to produce a progeny that can go on to make a specific type of tissue. They can often be plucked from this environment and placed in a nutrient broth at body temperature and encouraged to divide, although the niche is generally lost and their characteristics often change.

Historically, the discovery of the microscope by Hans and Zacharias Janssen in 1590 paved the way toward modern stem cell biology. Before this time, the composition of animals and plants was a complete mystery. But with the microscope, cells were finally revealed by Robert Hook in 1655. He surely must have shouted "Eureka!" as he first stared at the strange, hollow, roomlike structures that made up cork! Interestingly, there was a long gap until animal cells were first described by Theodor Schwann in 1839. In 1855, Rudolph Virchow, a great German pathologist, explained the idea that all living things come from other living cells, and thus paved the way for our current definition of stem cells. Around this time, scientists started to take an interest in teratology, or as they described the field "the study of malformations or monstrosities." These were, in fact, the first descriptions of embryonic carcinoma cells, which are primitive stem cells that can make all types of body tissue (hair, bone, and brain along with others) within a single "monstrous" mass. This must have been both frightening and intriguing for 19th-century scientists. But it was E. D. Wilson in his classic textbook *The Cell in Development and Inheritance* who first coined the phrase *stem cell* in 1896 and this term stuck.

Fast forward to the 1950s and perhaps the biggest surge in stem cell science was initiated when bone marrow was first transplanted into irradiated mice and shown to reconstitute the stem cell population. The term *hematopoietic stem cell* was coined and this area of biology dominated the stem cell field for many years, and is still the only proven area of stem cell use in clinical trials. While stem cells were then found in the skin, gut, and other tissues, their characterization always lagged behind the hematopoeitic stem cells that expressed a range of convenient cell surface markers that could be used to sort them. Also, in other tissues, the stem cells were often buried very deep and difficult to remove and isolate. This led to the search for a "universal" type of stem cell, which was eventually isolated and characterized from mouse embryos by Martin Evans, who was awarded the Nobel Prize for Medicine in 2007. These embryonic stem cells from the mouse could divide endlessly in culture, while maintaining the potential to create every tissue in the body.

In 1998, Dr. James Thomson isolated similar cells from human embryos and opened up a Pandora's box of ethical issues along with a fascinating new source of human cells. A year before in 1997, Dr. Ian Wilmut had shown that adult mammalian cells retained all of the genes necessary to produce a whole animal by cloning Dolly the sheep from an adult mammary gland tissue. The adult cell had been reprogrammed back to an embryonic state in the egg. In 2007, Dr. James Thomson in the United States and Dr. Yamanaka in Japan simultaneously discovered that if you took adult human cells they too could be reprogrammed back to an embryonic state by overexpressing powerful stem cell genes. These so-called induced pluripotent stem (iPS) cells were not derived from live embryos and could be generated from any patient, thus removing both the ethical and immunological issues at one time. While some issues remain with iPS cells, they represent the future for cell therapy.

Today, stem cells have taken on an almost mystical quality. Perhaps this is because some stem cells are the master organizers of all living multicellular organisms, giving rise to every tissue in the body. Maybe it is because it is now possible to cure some diseases of the blood system through transplanting adult stem cells into the circulation. Maybe it is due to the fact that many different types of resident stem cell might one day be transplanted from carefully grown cultures or activated within the body to replace diseased tissues leading to cures for the incurable. The stem cell mystique may lie in simply gaining insights into the origins of human development and ailments such as cancer, or being able to model complex diseases of humans and screen novel drugs. Above and beyond the science, there remains an undercurrent of moral and ethical issues associated with creating cell lines through the destruction of living embryos, which perhaps may now be deflated due to iPS cells. However, controversies, breakthroughs, and frustration will continue to swirl in eternal storms through this rapidly moving area of research. But what does the average person make of all this, and how can an interested scholar probe this vast sea of information?

## THE ENCYCLOPEDIA

In this wave of advances, and with extensive information available over the internet, you may ask why an *Encyclopedia of Stem Cell Research* is required. Surely, it will be out of date quickly! To this we reply that all of history requires punctuation points. This encyclopedia provides a source for experts to consider what is known and not known; a chance for the public, schools, colleges, and researchers to have access to a synthesis of this broad area in two volumes; for those in regions of the globe where widespread internet is still a distant dream, a chance to educate and enlighten; a chance to learn about who is doing the research and where it is being done; and finally, a chance to understand the basic concepts from A to Z in stem cell biology in simple, clear articles and learn about the politics, ethics, and challenges everyone in the field is currently facing. Of course, the encyclopedia cannot cover all aspects of stem cell biology, but we sincerely hope it will provide a stepping stone to more detailed investigation on a chosen topic.

For stem cell researchers, particularly the novice, the literature is scattered with a patchwork of terminology that clouds all efforts to characterize the stem cell world into neat descriptive words—"stem cell," "progenitor cell," and "precursor" are often used interchangeably. Further complexity comes when comparing embryonic and adult cells, cells in different tissues, and cells from different species. The combinations are endless. For this encyclopedia, the focus is on describing the different types of stem cell that have been reported so far and trying, where possible, to explain for each age, tissue and species what is know about the biology of the cells and their history. We do not attempt to come up with a new terminology, but simply explain what the different areas of this field consider to be stem cells and work from there.

We apologize in advance if your favorite researcher has not been included, or a country with interesting stem cell biology has been left out. This is simply a result of space and time. But we do hope to have captured at least a strong flavor of stem cell biology as it stands today and to have provided the reader with a reference manual to probe the mysteries of the field.

## THE FUTURE

Many professionals are involved in stem cells. Engineers are developing new environments in which to grow stem cells; statisticians are producing new algorithms to detect genomic changes as stem cells divide and differentiate; chemists are designing new drugs to modulate stem cell biology; ethicists are debating the meaning of embryonic life; and politicians are working out how stem cells may get them more (or less) votes. While stem cells are exciting alone, they are also clearly fueling the traditional areas of developmental biology and emerging field of regenerative medicine.

It is good to be a stem cell biologist these days. California recently announced $3 billion over 10 years to fund stem cell research, and other states are also stepping up to the plate and funding this science. In some ways, this flow of private and state money has been enhanced by President George W. Bush's refusal to allow federal funding to be used to generate new embryonic stem cell lines from excess human embryos in IVF clinics.

However, there is also a bigger groundswell of support for stem cell research in general. The public feels that eventually stem cells will save lives, not destroy them. Whether this will happen remains to be seen. Stem cells are not miracle cells. Treatments will require robust clinical trials carried out under blinded conditions.

Many of us wait patiently for the first FDA-approved trials in the United States or other well-designed trials in the rest of the world. While seemingly very slow, they are coming. And then we will see.

Clive N. Svendsen and Allison D. Ebert
General Editors

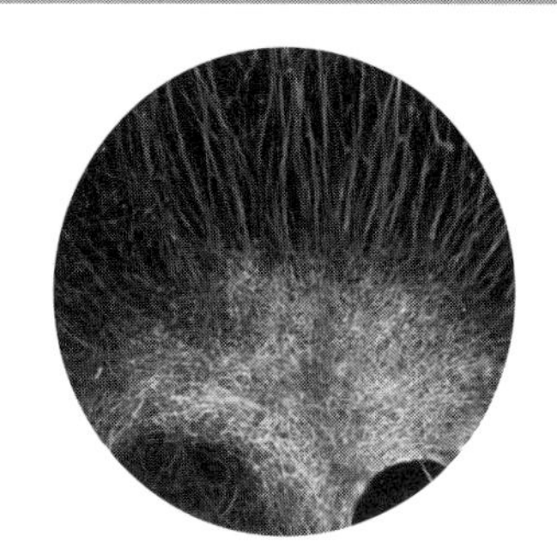

# Reader's Guide

This list is provided to assist readers in finding articles related by category or theme.

**COUNTRIES**



**DISEASES**



**ETHICS**



**HISTORY AND TECHNOLOGY**



**INDUSTRY**

**INSTITUTIONS**

Albert Einstein College of Medicine
Baylor College of Medicine
Bonn University
Burnham Institute
Caltech
Cambridge University
Case Western Reserve University/
Cleveland Clinic
Children's Hospital, Boston
Columbia University
Coriell Institute
Duke University
Genetics Policy Institute
Harvard University
Indiana University
Johns Hopkins University
Kyoto University
Massachusetts General Hospital
Massachusetts Institute of Technology
Mayo Clinic
McMaster University
Mount Sinai School of Medicine
National Academy of Science
Northwestern University
Oregon Health & Science University
Ottawa Health Research Institute
Oxford University
Princeton University
Reeve-Irvine Research Center
Robarts Research Institute
Rockefeller University
Rutgers University
Salk Institute
Scripps Research Institute
Sloan-Kettering Institute
Stanford University
Stowers Institute
University of California, Berkeley
University of California, Davis
University of California, Los Angeles
University of California, San Diego
University of California, San Francisco
University of Connecticut
University of Georgia
University of Miami
University of Michigan
University of Minnesota
University of North Carolina,
Chapel Hill
University of Pittsburgh
University of Southern California
University of Texas Heath Science
Center at Houston
University of Toronto
University of Washington/
Hutchinson Cancer Center
University of Wisconsin, Madison
Vanderbilt of University
Wake Forest University
Weill-Cornell Medical College
Whitehead Institute
Yale University

**LEGAL ISSUES**

Federal Government Policies
Funding for IVF
International Laws
National Stem Cell Bank
*Roe v. Wade*

**ORGANIZATIONS**

American Association for the
Advancement of Science
Australian Stem Cell Centre
California Institute for
Regenerative Medicine
Canadian Stem Cell Network
China Stem Cell News
Christopher Reeve Foundation
Community of Stem Cell Scientists
Danish Stem Cell Research Center
East of England Stem Cell Network
European Consortium for Stem Cell
Research—EuroStemCell
International Society for
Stem Cell Research
International Stem Cell Forum
Japan Human Cell Society
Lasker Foundation
Medical Research Council UK
Stem Cell Initiative

**PEOPLE**



**POLITICS**



**RELIGION**



**STATES**

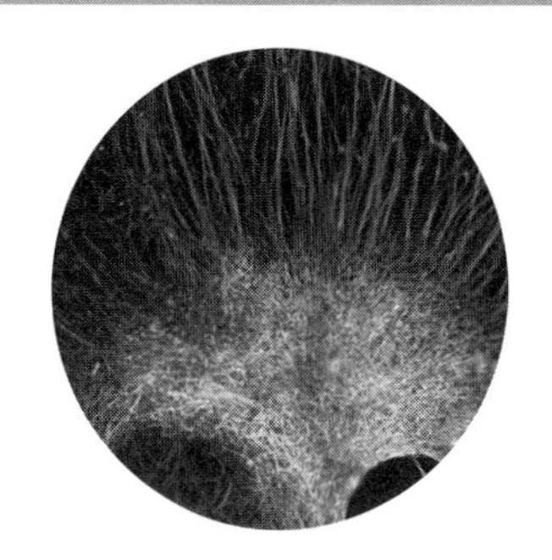

# List of Articles

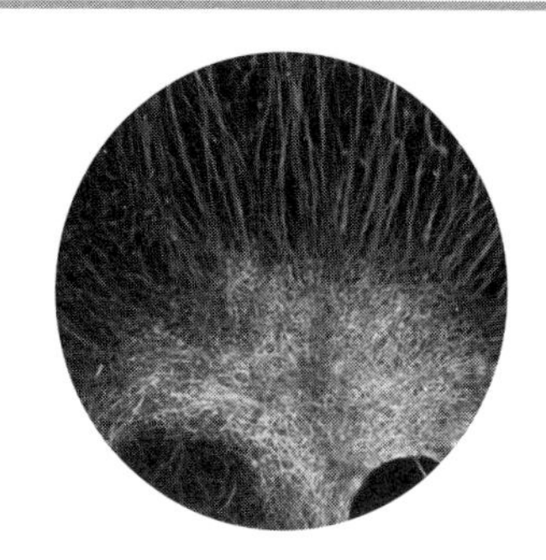

# List of Contributors

Alexander, Caroline M.
*University of Wisconsin, Madison*

Arabski, Jessica
*Georgetown University*

Arshad, Sameen
*National University of Science and Technology Pakistan*

Asad, Sana Fatima
*National University of Science and Technology Pakistan*

Baig, Madiha Anwar
*National University of Science and Technology Pakistan*

Bala, Poonam
*University of Delhi India*

Barnhill, John
*Independent Scholar*

Billal, Muhammad
*National University of Science and Technology Pakistan*

Blau, Helen
*Stanford University*

Boslaugh, Sarah
*BJC HealthCare*

Byun, John
*Independent Scholar*

Cheema, Faisal Habib
*Columbia University Medical Center*

Chen, Steven T.
*Johns Hopkins University School of Medicine*

Chen, Susanna N.
*Western University of Health Sciences*

Corfield, Justin
*Geelong Grammar School, Australia*

Crabbe, Annelies
*Katholieke Universiteit Leuven*
*Belgium*

Davidson, Michele R.
*George Mason University*

Destro, Anna Maria
*Eastern Piedmont University School of Medicine*
*Italy*

Eversole, Theodore W.
*Independent Scholar*

Firdous, Mamoona
*Columbia University Medical Center*

Giakoumopoulos, Maria
*University of Wisconsin, Madison*

Herrera, Fernando
*University of California, San Diego*

Imtiaz, Anam
*National University of Science and Technology*
*Pakistan*

Ireton, Renee C.
*University of Washington*

Kaushik, Anjan P.
*University of Virginia School of Medicine*

Khaleeq, Tahawur Abbas
*National University of Science and Technology*
*Pakistan*

Khan, Faris
*Columbia University Medical Center*

Khan, G. Ishaq
*Dow University of Health Sciences*

Khan, Quratulain
*National University of Science and Technology*
*Pakistan*

Knoll, Benjamin
*University of Iowa*

Kte'pi, Bill
*Independent Scholar*

Kulczycki, Andrzej
*University of Alabama, Birmingham*

Kuo, John S.
*University of Wisconsin*

Meisner, Lorraine F.
*University of Wisconsin*

Michaud, Lyn
*Independent Scholar*

Michon, Heather K.
*Independent Scholar*

Miller, Cathie G.
*Henry Ford Health System*

Noubissi Kamdem, Felicite
*University of Wisconsin*

Ogle, Brenda M.
*University of Wisconsin, Madison*

Padula, Alessandra
*Università degli Studi di L'Aquila, Italy*

Pandit, Rahul
*St. Petersburg State Medical Academy*
*Russia*

Pang, Priscilla
*Case Western Reserve University*

Pinato, David James
*Eastern Piedmont University School of Medicine*
*Italy*

Quadri, S. A. Qader
*Dow University of Health Sciences*

Rahman, Wasiq
*Columbia University Medical Center*

Rameshwar, Pranela
*University of Medicine and Dentistry of New Jersey*

Rao, Muhammad Zeeshan Afzal
*Columbia University Medical Center*

Raval, Amish
*University of Wisconsin*

Raza, Aun
*National University of Science and Technology Pakistan*

Rehen, Stevens K.
*Universidade Federal do Rio de Janeiro, Brazil*

Richards, Misty Charissa
*Albany Medical College*

Salem, Aliasger K.
*University of Iowa*

Salguero, Mario
*University of Wisconsin, Madison*

Schwindt, Telma Tiemi
*Universidade Federal de São Paulo Brazil*

Sebley, Caroline M.
*Kansas City University of Medicine and Biosciences*

Shahverdian, Devin Edwin
*Maricopa Integrated Health System*

Shi, Daniel Xudong
*University of Wisconsin, Madison*

Singh, Azara
*Christian Medical College India*

Slack, Jonathan
*University of Minnesota*

Stacpoole, Sybil R. L.
*University of Cambridge*

Stacy, Robert
*Independent Scholar*

Steenblock, David A.
*Personalized Regenerative Medicine*

Steindler, Dennis
*University of Florida*

Suzuki, Masatoshi
*University of Wisconsin, Madison*

Tamada, Yosuke
*University of Wisconsin, Madison*

Tariq, Areej
*National University of Science and Technology Pakistan*

Vanderby, Ray
*University of Wisconsin, Madison*

Vescovi, Angelo L.
*University of Milan Bicocca Italy*

Vyas, Krishna Subhash
*University of Kentucky*

Walsh, John
*Shinawatra University, Thailand*

Waskey, Andrew Jackson
*Dalton State College*

Wilnise, Jasmin
*State University of New York*

Winograd, Claudia
*University of Illinois, Urbana-Champaign*

Wu, Charlene
*Johns Hopkins University*

Yi, Ling Ka
*University of Wisconsin, Madison*

Yoohanna, Jennifer
*University of California, Los Angeles*

Zafar, Atif
*Dow University of Health Sciences*

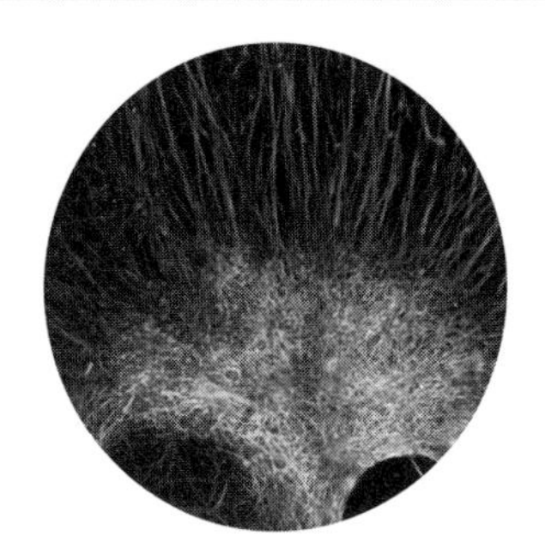

# Chronology

**June 1, 1909:** Alexander Maximow presents a lecture at the Hematological Society of Berlin introducing the concept of stem cells as the common ancestors of cellular elements in the blood.

**1959:** First successful use of stem cell transplants in humans, in three separate studies all involving hematopoietic stem cells (HSCs). E. D. Thomas and colleagues use syngeneic grafts from identical twins to treat two leukemia patients, George Mathé and colleagues perform allogeneic (from a separate individual who is not an identical twin) bone marrow transplants on five patients accidentally exposed to irradiation, and McGovern and colleagues treat a leukemia patient with autologous (from the patient) bone marrow cells.

**1963:** E. A. McCullough and colleagues prove that stem cells exist in the bone marrow of mice and that HSCs have the key properties of self-renewal and could become any type of blood cell.

**June 1966:** R. J. Cole, R. G. Edwards, and J. Paul isolate embryonic stem cells (ESCs) from the preimplantation blastocysts of rabbits.

**1968:** First successful use of bone marrow transplantation to treat patients with leukemia or hereditary immunodeficiency: success due to presence of HSCs in the marrow graft, which can reconstitute blood and immune systems after myeloablation.

**1974:** Congress imposes moratorium on federal funding for clinical research on embryonic tissue and embryos, which remains in place until 1993.

**1981:** *Nature* announces that two research groups, working independently, successfully derived embryonic stem cells from the inner cell mass cells of the blastocyst in mice; one group is led by Martin Evans at the University of Cambridge (UK), the other by Gail Martin at the University of California, San Francisco.

**1987:** Peter Hollands demonstrates the first therapeutic in vivo (in a living animal) use of ESCs: injection of ESCs restores lost bone marrow stem cells in lethally irradiated mice.

**1988:** Bone Marrow Donors Worldwide, a collaborative network of stem cell donor registries and cord blood banks, founded in Leiden (the Netherlands) to facilitate sharing of HLA phenotype and other information to physicians of patients who need a hematopoietic stem cell transplant.

**1992:** Y. Matsui and colleagues announce successful isolation of mouse embryonic germ cells, which have properties similar to embryonic stem cells.

**January 1993:** Newly elected president Bill Clinton instructs Donna Shalala, Secretary of the U.S. Department of Health and Human Services, to remove the ban on embryonic research.

**1995:** Congress bans federal funding for research on embryos, but leaves it unclear whether this ban applies to cells already derived from an embryo.

**November 1995:** James A. Thomson and colleagues at the University of Wisconsin derive the first non-human primate embryonic stem cells, from rhesus monkeys, suggesting that embryonic stem cells could also be derived from humans.

**November 5 and 10, 1998:** James A. Thomson at the University of Wisconsin, and John D. Gearhart at Johns Hopkins University report almost simultaneously that they have successfully isolated human embryonic stem cells (hESCs). Despite the therapeutic potential of hESCs, which can become any type of cell in the human body and thus offer hope for currently intractable conditions such as Parkinson's disease and spinal cord injury, the announcement is not without controversy due to the origins of the cells used in the research. Thomson's team worked with cells from human embryos created in vitro ("in glass," i.e., in the laboratory) while Gearhart's team obtained their stem cells from human fetal primordial germ cells.

**August 2000:** The National Institutes of Health (NIH) legal department advices that NIH may fund research on cells derived from blastocysts, but may not fund the derivation of the cells themselves (which may be performed by private companies).

**December 2000:** Mouse experiments by Timothy Brazelton and colleagues at Stanford University discover that HSCs can transform themselves to neuronal cells, demonstrating a plasticity (ability to become other types of cells than blood cells) which could have important therapeutic implications). This research has been challenged on several grounds but research continues because of the ready availability of HSCs (every person could serve as their own donor, making hESCs unnecessary).

**July 2001:** The Jones Institute, a private infertility clinic in Norfolk, Virginia, announces that it has created embryos from donated gametes (reproductive cells).

**August 9, 2001:** President George W. Bush, in a speech on prime-time national television, announces federal research funding will be available for the first time for hESC research, but that such research would be limited to the estimated 60 preexisting stem cell lines.

**November 2001:** NIH invites proposals for stem cell research and releases a list of 74 acceptable stem cell lines; many of the lines are not suitable for human trials because they have been grown in mouse media.

**November 25, 2001:** Advanced Cell Technology, a private company in Worcester, Massachusetts, announces that it has cloned human embryos from adult cells, creating cells that are a perfect genetic match for the donor.

**2002:** The United Kingdom announces that stem cell research is a scientific priority and allocates an additional £40 million to support stem cell research.

**January 2003:** Nine funding agencies form the International Stem Cell Forum (ISCF) to encourage international collaboration and promote increased funding for stem cell research; as of January 2004,14 agencies from 13 countries have joined the ISCF.

**2004:** Annual Report of the International Bone Marrow Transplant Registry reports that over 27,000 patients annually are treated by blood stem cell transplantation, for various cancers, hereditary diseases, and bone marrow failure

**March 2004:** Hwang Woo-Suk and colleagues at Seoul National University announces in the prestigious journal *Science* that he successfully cloned patent-specific stem cells suing somatic nuclear transfer. Because the embryos were cloned in order to produce stem cells, rather than for reproduction, this reported success reopens the debate about therapeutic cloning (cloning cells for the purpose of treating human disease). Hwang's previous research had been in genetically modified livestock, and he claimed to have successfully cloned two cows in 1999, although he provided no scientific data to back up this claim.

**June 25, 2004:** New Jersey becomes the first state to fund stem cell research, as legislators create the Stem Cell Institute of New Jersey and allocate it $9.5 million in state funding.

**November 2, 2004:** Partly as a response to federal research funding restrictions, California becomes the second state to allocate funding for stem cell research, as voters approve Proposition 71. This bill creates the California Institute for Regenerative Medicine, which is allocated $3 billion in taxpayer funding over 10 years.

**January 1, 2005:** Connecticut Governor M. Jodi Rell announces that she will recommend that the state budget include a special fund to support stem cell research in Connecticut. The state budget, passed in June, includes $100 million to support stem cell research over 10 years.

**May 23, 2005:** The Starr Foundation announces awards of $50 million to support stem cell research at Weill Medical College of Cornell University, Rockefeller University, and Memorial Sloan-Kettering Cancer, all in New York City.

**May 31, 2005:** The State of Connecticut Stem Cell Advisory Committee allocates $19.78 million in stem cell research funds to researchers from Yale, Wesleyan, and the University of Connecticut. These are the first grants from Connecticut's Stem Cell Research Fund, which was created in 2005 and is charged with allocating approximately $100 million to support stem cell research by the year 2015.

**June 2005:** Hwang Woo-Suk and colleagues publish an article in *Science* claiming that they have created 11 human embryos from somatic cells from different donors. He claims to have developed a more efficient process that uses fewer eggs to create more hESCs.

**July 13, 2005:** Illinois Governor Rod Blagojevich issues an executive order which creates the Illinois Regenerative Institute for Stem Cell Research, which will award $10 million in state funds to support stem cell research. This makes Illinois the fourth state, and the first midwestern state, to allocate public funds to stem cell research.

**August 18, 2005:** Colin McGuckin, Nico Forraz and colleagues at Kingston University (UK) announce discovery of cord-blood-derived embryonic-like stem cells (CBEs), which appear to be more versatile than adult stem cells found in bone marrow, although less versatile than hESCs. This discovery could skirt ethical objections to hESC research with cells derived from embryos, because umbilical cord blood can be acquired without destruction of human life.

**September 19, 2005:** Brian Cummings, Aileen Anderson and colleagues at the University of California, Irvine, announce that they successfully used adult neural stem cells to repair spinal cord damage in mice. The mice receiving neural stem cells showed improvement in coordination and walking ability, suggesting the research may lead to therapies to aid humans with spinal cord injuries.

**September 21, 2005:** Floridians for Stem Cell Research and Cures, Inc., an advocacy group for stem cell research, propose a ballot initiative requiring the state of Florida to spend $200 million in state funds over the next 10 years in support of stem cell research. On September 23, Citizens for Science and Ethics, Inc., a group opposing stem cell research, files a petition which would amend Florida's state constitution to prohibit embryonic stem cell research.

**November 2005:** Gerald Schatten a former colleague of Hwang Woo-Suk now at the University of Pennsylvania, announces there were ethical irregularities in Hwang's procurement of oocyte (egg) donations used in his research. Roh Sung-il, a close collaborator, announces at a press conference on November 21 that oocyte donors had been paid $1,400 each for their eggs. On November 24, Hwang announces that he will resign from his post due to the scandal.

**December 16, 2005:** New Jersey becomes the first state to allocate public funds for hESC research, as a state commission grants $5 million awarded to 17 research projects, most located at the University of Medicine and Dentistry of New Jersey, Rutgers University, and Princeton University.

**December 29, 2005:** In South Korea, a Seoul National University investigation of Hwang's scientific work concludes that all 11 stem cell lines claimed in his 2005 published paper were fabricated.

**2006 (calendar year):** Over 1,100 articles on ESC research are published, a nearly 10-fold increase from 140 in 1997.

**January 11, 2006:** *Science* retracts both of Hwang's papers due to scientific misconduct and fraud. On January 12, Hwang holds a press conference to apologize but does not take responsibility for the fraud claiming that members of his scientific team sabotaged his work.

**April 2006:** Maryland allocates $15 million in state funding for ESC research, beginning in July 2006, through passage of the Stem Cell Research Act.

**May 12, 2006:** South Korea indicts scientist Hwang Woo-suk on charges of fraud, embezzlement, and bioethics violations. Three of his collaborators are also charged with fraud.

**June 21, 2006:** Florida Governor Jeb Bush, speaking at the annual biotechnology Industry Organization meeting, announces his disapproval of hESC research. Bush further announces that no stem cell research will be performed at any Florida university, nor at the Scripps Research Institute in Palm Beach.

**July 2006:** ES Cell International in Singapore becomes the first company to commercially produce hESCs that are suitable for clinical trials; vials of stems cells are offered for sale on the internet for $6,000.

**July 18, 2006:** Senate Majority Leader Bill Frist (R-TN) publishes an editorial in the *Washington Post* announcing his support of federal funding of stem cell research, in opposition to President Bush's policy. Frist also announces that he sees no contradiction between stem cell research and his pro-life beliefs.

**July 19, 2006:** President Bush vetoes a bill, passed by the House in 2005 and the Senate in July 2006, that would expand federal funding for hESC research.

**August 23, 2006:** Scientists from the private company Advanced Cell Technology announce they have developed a technique which allows them to remove a single cell from an embryo. The embryo is not harmed in the process and the cell can then be grown in the lab, circumventing ethical objections to hESC research which requires the destruction of embryos.

**November 7, 2006:** Missouri voters pass Amendment 2, a constitutional amendment that states that any hESC research or treatment allowed by the federal government will also be allowed in Missouri. The narrow victory (51%–49%) galvanizes opposition to the bill, much of which is centered on their contention that it would allow human cloning.

**November 28, 2006:** In the wake of the Hwang Woo-Suk scandal, a panel lead by John I. Brauman recommends changes in the procedures used to review papers submitted for publication in *Science*. The changes recommended include flagging high-visibility papers for further review, requiring authors to specify their individual contributions to a paper, and online publication of more of the raw data on which papers are based.

**January 7, 2007:** Dr. Anthony Atala of Wake Forest University and colleagues from Wake Forest and Harvard Universities report the discovery of amniotic–fluid-derived stem cells (AFS), which seem to hold similar promise to hESCs. The researchers reported that AFS could be extracted without harm to mother or child, thus avoiding some of the moral controversies regarding hESCs.

**February 28, 2007:** Governor Chet Culver of Iowa signs the "Iowa Stem Cell Research and Cures Initiative," a bill which ensures that Iowa researchers will be allowed to conduct stem cell research and that Iowa patients will have access to stem cures and therapies. The bill also prohibits human cloning.

**March 31, 2007:** New York passes a budget for the fiscal year 2008 that includes an appropriation of $100 million for stem cell and regenerative medicine research. The funds will be distributed through the Empire State Stem Cell Trust, which will be funded at $50 million per year for 10 years after the initial appropriation of $100 million.

**April 11, 2007:** Richard K. Burt and colleagues report success in treating type 1 diabetics in Brazil with stem cells taken from their own blood. The experimental procedure, reported in the *Journal of the American Medical Association*, has allowed the diabetics to stop taking insulin for as long as three years.

**May 30, 2007:** California Governor Arnold Schwarzenegger and Canada's Premier of Ontario Dalton McGuinty announce an agreement between Canada's International Regulome Consortium and the Stem Cell Center at the University of California, Berkeley, to coordinate research. McGuinty also announced the creation of the Cancer Stem Cell Consortium, which will coordinate and fund cancer stem cell research, and announced an initial donation of $30 million Canadian to the consortium from the Ontario Institute of Cancer Research.

**June 6, 2007:** Rudolf Jaenisch and colleagues at the Whitehead Institute, affiliated with the Massachusetts Institute of Technology in Boston, announce in *Nature* that they have succeeded in manipulating mature mouse stem cells so they have the properties of ESCs. In the same issue of *Nature*, Shinya Yamanaka and colleagues at Kyoto University announce that they have developed a method to reprogram stem cells in mice back to the embryonic state, so they may then develop into different body cells similarly to hESCs. If this technique is adaptable to human cells, it would allow researchers to bypass most of the controversy involved with the use of hESCs derived from human embryos.

**June 20, 2007:** President Bush vetoes legislation that would have allowed federal funding for ESC research using cells from embryos from fertility clinics that would be destroyed anyway. At the same time, Bush issues an executive order encouraging federal financial support of research aimed at creating stem cells without destroying embryos. The veto places him in opposition to most American voters and many members of the Republican Party. In response to the Bush veto, Democratic presidential candidates Hillary Clinton and Barack Obama pledge to support federal funding for hESC studies if elected.

**August 3, 2007:** Kitai Kim, George G. Daley and colleagues and Children's Hospital, Boston, report in the journal *Cell Stem Cell* that Hwang Woo-Suk, the discredited Korean researcher, did have one significant research result which appears to be genuine.

The Children's researchers determined that Hwang's purposed ESCs were produced by parthenogenesis (virgin birth) from unfertilized eggs, a result since achieved by other researchers as well.

**November 6, 2007:** New Jersey voters reject a ballot measure which would have allowed the state to borrow $450 million to fund for stem cell research. Defeat of the initiative is attributed to the state's worsening fiscal condition and a vocal alliance of conservatives, antiabortion activists, and representatives of the Catholic Church who oppose stem cell research.

**November 14, 2007:** Shoukhrat Mitalipov and colleagues at the Oregon Health and Science University's national Primate Research Center announce in *Nature* that they have successfully derived ESCs by reprogramming genetic material from the skin cells of rhesus macaque monkeys.

**November 20, 2007:** The journals *Cell* and *Science* report on discoveries by two independent teams of scientists that reprogram human skin cells to have the characteristics of hESCs. One team is led by Shinya Yamanaka; the other is led by James Thomson of the University of Wisconsin, Madison.

**2008:** Rudolf Jaenisch and colleagues correct sickle cell anemia in mice using iPS cells.

**January 14, 2008:** Doris Taylor and colleagues at the University of Minnesota report success in creating a beating rat heart by injecting cells from newborn rats into the values and outer structure from a dead rat heart.

**February 20, 2008:** Scientists at Novocell, a private biotechnology company located in San Diego, announce that they have successfully used hESCs to control diabetes in mice whose own insulin-producing cells had been destroyed.

Sarah Boslaugh
BJC HealthCare

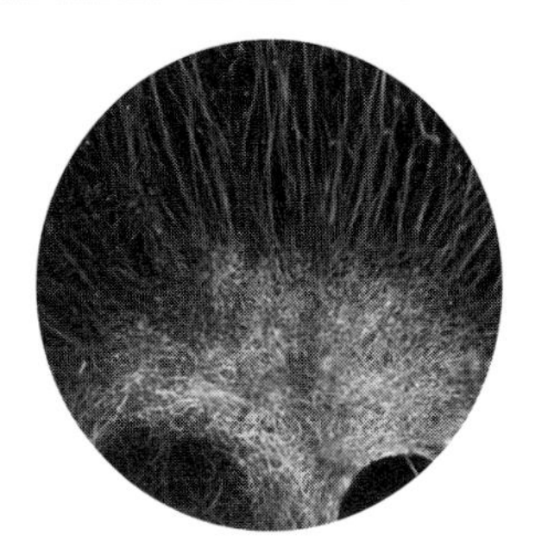

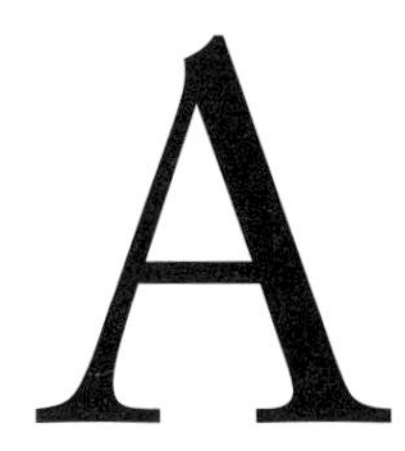

## Aastrom Biosciences, Inc.

**AASTROM IS A** regenerative medicine company developing autologous cell products for the repair or regeneration of multiple human tissues, based on its proprietary tissue repair cell (TRC) technology. Aastrom is a private biotechnology company based out of Ann Arbor, Michigan, with a board of directors composed of individuals with broad experience at both large public and private biotech and pharmaceutical companies.

Aastrom's TRCs are a proprietary mixture of bone marrow–derived adult stem and progenitor cells produced using patented single-pass perfusion technology in the Aastrom Replicell system. The clinical procedure begins with the collection of a small sample of bone marrow from the patient's hip in an outpatient setting. TRCs are then produced in the automated Replicell system over a 12-day period. It has been demonstrated in the laboratory that TRCs are able to develop into different types of tissue lineages in response to inductive signals, including blood, bone, cartilage, adipose, and vascular tubules.

In previous clinical trials, TRCs have been shown to be safe and reliable in regenerating certain normal healthy bone marrow tissues. TRC-based products have been used in over 250 patients and are currently in clinical trials for bone regeneration (osteonecrosis of the femoral head and long bone fractures) and vascular regeneration (critical limb ischemia applications). The company is also developing programs to address cardiac and neural regeneration indications. TRC-based products have received Orphan Drug Designation from the U.S. Food and Drug Administration for use in the treatment of osteonecrosis of the femoral head and the treatment of dilated cardiomyopathy, a severe chronic disease of the heart. In addition to using TRC technology in regulated clinical trials, certain non-U.S. regions allow autologous cell products to be used in patient treatments without further registration or marketing authorization. This enables Aastrom to gain experience through the limited treatment of patients to support the development of its clinical trial strategy. Current clinical programs focus on bone, cardiac, vascular, and neural repair and regeneration.

RESTORE-CLI, a phase IIb prospective, controlled, randomized, double-blind, multicenter clinical trial to treat patients suffering from peripheral arterial disease is currently underway. Aastrom has applied its TRC technology to treat critical limb ischemia (CLI) to determine whether vascular repair cells (VRCs) can safely treat patients with peripheral arterial disease–induced critical limb ischemia and reduce the incidence of major amputations in the treated limbs. The primary objective of the clinical trial is to assess the safety of the TRC-based product in CLI patients. Secondary objectives include assessing amputation rates, wound closure and blood flow in the affected limbs, patient quality of life, and the reduction of pain and analgesic use.

Interim results from the first 13 patients treated in a multiarm phase I/II single-center clinical trial to evaluate the safety of VRCs and normal bone marrow cells in the treatment of chronic diabetic foot wounds associated with CLI were presented at the 2nd Congress of the German Society for Stem Cell Research in Wurzburg, Germany. These results reflect treatment experience from four diabetic patients with ischemia-related chronic tissue ulcers who were treated with Aastrom VRCs, a cell mixture derived from the patient's bone marrow that is processed using TRC technology to generate large numbers of predominantly mesenchymal stem and early progenitor cells; seven patients who were treated with normal bone marrow cells; and two standard-of-care patients, who received no cells. All patients received standard wound care as described by the American Diabetes Association.

Twelve months posttreatment, all patients in the interim analysis who were treated with VRCs reported no major amputations, no cell-related adverse events, and healing of all open wounds. Of the seven patients treated with normal bone marrow cells, five reported results similar to the VRC-treated patients 12 months posttreatment, one reported similar results to the VRC-treated patients 18 months posttreatment, and one patient received a major amputation. Of the two standard-of-care patients, one patient received a major amputation and one patient experienced no improvement in wound healing after 12 months.

A second oral presentation by Ulrich Noth, M.D., of the Orthopaedic Institute, Konig-Ludwig-Haus, University of Wurzburg, Germany, discussed clinical results involving the first use of Aastrom bone repair cells to treat patients suffering from osteonecrosis of the femoral head. Osteonecrosis of the femoral head involves the death of cells in the bone and marrow within the femur head and in many cases leads to total hip replacement. Dr. Noth presented data from four patients. All patients tolerated the procedure well; have reported a reduction in hip pain with no signs of disease progression, as determined by magnetic resonance imaging and X-ray; and were back to work within six months after treatment. In addition, no cell-related adverse events were observed, and none of these patients have required hip replacement surgery.

These data demonstrate, for the first time, that Aastrom's cell products may have a beneficial long-term effect in two key indications: critical limb ischemia and osteonecrosis of the femoral head. Although still in their early stages, these results lend substantial scientific support to the clinical development program focused on autologous stem cell products for regenerative medicine.

**SEE ALSO:** Bone Diseases; Cells, Sources of; Diabetes; Stem Cell Companies.

**BIBLIOGRAPHY.** Aastrom Biosciences, www.aastrom.com (cited November 2007); PR Newswire, www.prnewswire.com (cited November 2007); Prohost Biotechnology, www.prohostbiotech.com (cited November 2007).

Fernando Herrera
University of California, San Diego

# Advocacy

**ADVOCACY FOR STEM** cells, in its broadest sense, means people getting together to discuss how the scientific and clinical potential of the cells can be moved forward. Advocates for stem cell research are often associated with an interest in a specific disease for which stem cells may offer some hope. Many of the debates have centered on embryonic stem cell research where the ethical issues associated with the isolation of embryonic stem cells pitch religious groups against patient advocates. Because adult stem cell research does not involve the destruction of embryos there is little opposition to this research—although advocacy is always useful to push a field forward.

Debates on stem cell research have been carried by governmental agencies, politicians, interest groups, clergy, religious organizations, scientists, businesses, and individuals. These have included pro-life advocates, bioethicists, the papacy, patient advocate groups, and even U.S. President George W. Bush. The main areas of stem cell advocacy have been scientific, ethical, political, commercial, and personal. Issues generated in each of these areas have attracted different advocates.

## ORGANIZATIONS

Physicians hope to someday have new therapies that can mitigate or even cure diseases that today are incurable or at best managed—the new field of "regenerative medicine." There are a large number of voluntary associations representing people with a variety of specific health issues (for example, the Michael J. Fox Foundation for Parkinson's Disease), or are more general, such as the American Association of Retired Persons (AARP). They have either touted stem cells as the ultimate cure, or expressed concerns over the dangers posed by as-of-yet unknown risks of the use of stem cells in treatments. For example, embryonic stem cells implanted in humans last a lifetime and may pose cancer risks or have other unintended consequences.

Discussions by advocates in the media about stem cells garners much public interest, and their concerns may gain public hearing before health organizations such as the Food and Drug Administration, which ultimately gives permission for all medicines, including those made from stem cells, to be allowed on the market for patient use.

Among those individuals who have advocated a broad approach to stem cell research were the late Christopher Reeve and his wife Dana Reeve and Michael J. Fox. After his spinal cord injury in an equestrian event, Christopher Reeve created the Christopher Reeve Foundation (CDRF). The foundation is a charity that promotes spinal cord injury research, which includes stem cell research. It is also an advocate of the election of "pro-science" presidents of the United States who will give unqualified support to stem cell research. Michael J. Fox was diagnosed with Parkinson's disease in the late 1990s and started a foundation that supports the use of stem cells for the treatment of Parkinson's disease and funded many studies in the early part of 2000.

The Coalition for the Advancement of Medical Research (CAMR) is a coalition of over 100 organizations that lobby for stem cell research. The organizations in CAMR include colleges and universities, patient organizations, scientific societies, foundations, and other organizations. It lobbies Congress, the federal bureaucracy, and the president when a hearing can be obtained. CAMR is an advocate for embryonic as well as adult stem cell research. The Genetics Policy Institute (GPI) was founded by lawyer Bernard Seigal and spawned the powerful advocacy group known as the Pro-Cures Movement. These organizations are attempting to lobby the public to get interested in stem cell research through education and debate.

## POLITICIANS AND CORPORATIONS

For every pro–stem cell advocacy group there are also many politicians or other groups that are against stem cell research for moral or religious reasons. Political debates have been conducted by politicians in the United States in both state governments and in the federal government. They have in many cases taken positions that are strongly against stem cell research. For example, President George W. Bush made a decision that to be eligible for funding for research sponsored by the government of the United States, only stem cell lines already existing that were derived from embryonic stem cells could be used and no new ones could be created that would involve destroying embryos. In the partisan atmosphere of contemporary American politics it would have been impossible for any decision he made not to be controversial.

Members of the Democratic Party are usually more supportive of embryonic stem cell research than are Republicans. Their position has therefore pressed for adoption of legislation that is open to federal research. In contrast, some conservative supporters of Republican politicians fear that support of stem cell research can become a slippery slope that leads to removing all opposition to abortion, and even to the destruction of small children for research purposes as Peter Singer, an ethicist at Princeton University, advocates. Fiscal issues affect members of Congress who support funding stem cell research whether embryonic or not. Fiscal realities and the hopes for regenerative medicine often clash.

Corporate supporters of embryonic stem cell research often have financial motivations as their central goal. Patents on stem cell research have been issued that have later created suits over the use of proprietary stem cell lines. This can often cloud the true balance of what is right or wrong about stem cell research, and goes beyond simple advocacy. Conflicts of interest quickly arise when money and patents are involved.

**SEE ALSO:** Christopher Reeve Foundation; Ethics; Religion, Catholic; Religion, Christian; Religion, Protestant; Special Interest/Lobby Groups; Stem Cells, Bush Ruling.

**BIBLIOGRAPHY.** Janet T. Arnes. *Stem Cell Research: Issues and Bibliography* (Novinka Books, 2006); Kristen Renwick Monoe, Jerome S. Tobis, and Ronald B. Miller, eds., *Fundamentals of the Stem Cell Debate: The Scientific, Religious, Ethical and Political Issues* (Taylor & Francis, 2004); Michael Ruse and Christopher A. Pynes, eds., *The Stem Cell Controversy: Debating the Issues,* 2nd ed. (Prometheus Books, 2006); Brent Waters and Ronald Cole-Turner, eds., *God and the Embryo: Religious Voices on Stem Cells and Cloning* (Georgetown University Press, 2003).

Andrew J. Waskey
Dalton State College

# Alabama

**ALABAMA IS ONE** of 26 U.S. states with no legislation pertinent to stem cell research or cloning. Artur Davis, a congressman from Alabama's 7th district with plans to run for governor or senator in 2010, has a legislative record primarily focused on social and health issues. Though he has largely voted with the Democratic Party during his time in the House, some of the rare exceptions are bills related to abortion and cloning, when he takes the conservative position. He was the lead Democratic sponsor in 2005 of the Stem Cell Therapeutic and Research Act, a bill establishing a national cord blood bank, expanding the federal bone marrow stem cell program, and notably, establishing a data program to encourage doctors and patients to explore treatment options for their ailments. Davis's cosponsor was Chris Smith, a New Jersey Republican.

A popular position among Alabama moderates is that human embryonic stem cell research should be opposed, and other stem cell research should be augmented. These moderates contend that nonembryonic stem cells have not been sufficiently explored and that there is yet no reason to believe that embryonic stem cells offer significantly more treatment possibilities than nonembryonic ones do. Because human embryonic stem cell–derived treatments are still available thanks to private and state funding, increasing awareness of non–embryonic stem cell–derived treatments is important to this group. There is perhaps a poetic contrast in the recommendation of umbilical cord stem cell blood over embryonic stem cells. That said, in January 2007, Davis voted with the Democratic Party to expand the number of embryonic stem cell lines available for federal funded research.

Republican Jeff Sessions, the junior senator from Alabama, is considered one of the most conservative senators on the Hill. He has consistently voted against abortion, cloning, and human embryonic stem cell research. He voted in favor of the HOPE Stem Cell Research Act of 2007 to promote the derivation of pluripotent stem cell lines from naturally dead embryos (embryos that died of some cause not related to the research). He has repeatedly spoken out, in public and on the Senate floor, against embryonic stem cell research and has criticized its proponents for referring to limits on embryonic stem cell research as bans on stem cell research, when adult stem cells are still available. Senior Senator Richard Shelby, also a Republican, has not been as vocal as his colleague but has voted similarly on the pertinent issues.

The case of Carron Morrow was widely reported. A 58-year-old mother of two from Alabama, Morrow suffered a heart attack in 2006 while preparing for an outdoor party. In the aftermath of the attack, her heart was functioning at less than half the normal level, and she had difficulty walking without assistance. She was placed on a heart transplant list and, while waiting, agreed to join an adult stem cell therapeutic study at the Texas Heart Institute in Houston. On her birthday, October 16, 2006, surgeons removed bone marrow cells from her hip and, after cultivation, injected them into her heart. She recovered fully in less than a year, and her case has been used to underscore the efficacy of nonembryonic stem cells; Morrow herself declares that she's proof that adult stem cells "work far better."

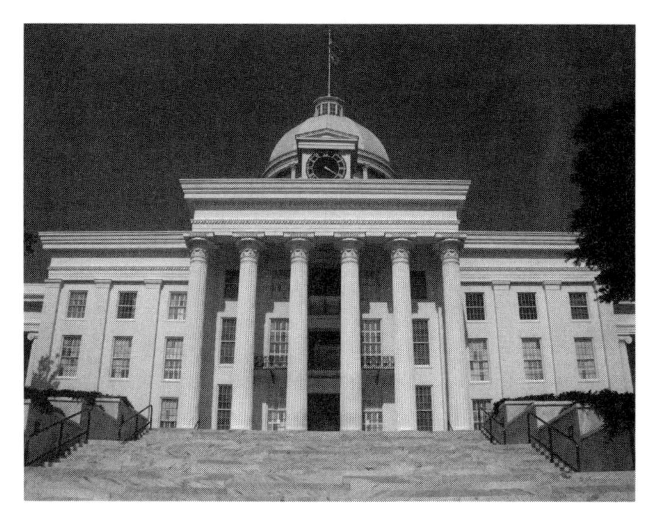

*Alabama is one of 26 U.S. states with no legislation related to stem cell research or cloning.*

## THE TUSKEGEE STUDY

A spectre often raised in Alabama in discussions of medical ethics is that of the Tuskegee Study of Untreated Syphilis in the Negro Male, which was conducted from 1932 to 1972. The study was conducted in Tuskegee, Alabama, on poor and mostly illiterate black men—generally sharecroppers—who, after being diagnosed with syphilis, were not informed of their diagnosis but simply told they had "bad blood" and offered meals, burial insurance, and trips to the clinic where the study was conducted. The study group was formed by the U.S. Public Health Service and blatantly disregarded any need for informed consent on the part of its participants. Rather, when consent was given, it was given in response to deceptive questions: patients might consent to a spinal tap when told it was a free treatment, for instance, with the implication being that it would be part of their cure. In fact, the doctors had no intention of curing them, though for the bulk of the period of the study they could have done so (penicillin had been adopted as an effective treatment in 1947, 15 years into the 40-year study). The men were simply observed until they died, and in the meantime, 40 of their wives became infected with the disease and 19 of their children were born with congenital syphilis. Famously, Dr. John Heller, the head of the study at the time when it came to public attention, defended its ethical incursions by arguing that the men in the study were not sick patients but "clinical material."

The story was brought to public attention when San Francisco Public Health Service employee Peter Buxtun complained about it to his superiors in 1966, but when nothing happened—in fact, the Centers for Disease Control affirmed that the study needed to continue until it was "complete" (at which point the subjects would be autopsied)—he went to the press. In 1972 a Congressional hearing determined that the study was medically unjustified and terminated it immediately. Lawsuits inevitably followed, along with medical and research legislation to rewrite the regulations governing interaction with human subjects in any scientific study.

The Tuskegee Study is often conjured up in Alabama's discussions of abortion, fetal tissue, cloning, and embryonic stem cell research. All of these things, in the conservative view, require the involvement of nonconsenting life—potential life, unborn life, or former life—treated as "clinical material." Although this is especially pertinent when cloning is the topic at hand because of the fears that clones would be treated as nonhuman and subjected to the sort of abuse the Tuskegee Study participants were, Senator Sessions and others also bring it up frequently in reference to the treatment of embryos in stem cell research.

Interestingly, in a 2002 poll conducted by Research America, 63 percent of Alabamans believed therapeutic cloning should be allowed (31 percent opposed it), but only 13 percent thought cloning should be legal if conducted for reproductive reasons (84 percent opposed it).

**SEE ALSO:** Blood; Cells, Adult; Cells, Embryonic; Cells, Umbilical; Federal Government Policies; Moral Status of Embryo.

**BIBLIOGRAPHY.** M. Bellomo, *The Stem Cell Divide: The Facts, the Fiction, and the Fear Driving the Greatest Scientific, Political and Religious Debate of Our Time* (American Management Association, 2006); C. B. Cohen, *Renewing the Stuff of Life: Stem Cells, Ethics, and Public Policy* (Oxford University Press, 2007); K. R. Monroe, R. Miller, and J. Tobis, eds., *Fundamentals of the Stem Cell Debate: The Scientific, Religious, Ethical, and Political Issues* (University of California Press, 2007); C. Vestal, "States Take Sides on Stem Cell Research," Stateline.org (January 31, 2008), www.stateline.org/live/details/story?contentId=276784 (cited January 2008).

Bill Kte'pi
Independent Scholar

# Albert Einstein College of Medicine

**THE ALBERT EINSTEIN** College of Medicine (AECOM) is a graduate school of Yeshiva University. It is a private medical school located in the Jack and Pearl Resnick Campus of Yeshiva University in the Morris Park neighborhood of the borough of the Bronx of New York City. AECOM also offers graduate biomedical degrees through the Sue Golding Graduate Division, in addition to the medical school. More than 200 faculty members perform biomedical research with an enrollment of nearly 400 graduate students. AECOM conducts research in basic biomedical science. The school receives more than $170 million annually in peer-reviewed grants from the National Institutes of Health. AECOM is affiliated with six hospitals: Montefiore Medical Center, Jack D. Weiler Hospital (a division of Montefiore Medical Center), Jacobi Medical Center, Bronx-Lebanon Hospital in the Bronx, Beth Israel Medical Center in downtown Manhattan, and Long Island Jewish Medical Center on Long Island.

Through its affiliation network, AECOM runs the largest postgraduate medical training program in the United States, offering over 150 residency programs to more than 2,500 physicians in training. The AECOM Department of Family and Social Medicine offers the Residency Program in Social Medicine (established in 1970), created to address the shortage of primary care clinicians trained to work in underserved communities.

The institute's primary biomedical research focus is on defining the regional localization and the biological properties of neural stem cells during embryonic and postnatal development and in the mature and the aging mammalian brain. Stem cells are also being used as "biological probes" to elucidate the pathogenesis of a spectrum of complex and poorly understood acquired and genetic nervous system disorders. In these prototypical disorders, distinct profiles of regional stem cells or their more lineage-restricted neuronal or glial progeny undergo irreversible cellular dysfunction and premature death or cellular transformation in response to acute or more chronic injury signals.

Further, the knowledge gained from these multidisciplinary studies is being channeled into the design of innovative genetic, epigenetic, and stem cell–associated regenerative therapies. Research scientists within the institute are in the process of defining the dynamic roles of environmental factors, cell–cell signaling pathways, and cell autonomous cues in promoting stem cell activation, expansion, lineage restriction, lineage commitment, cell cycle exit, and terminal differentiation. Institute investigators have identified specific transcription factor codes that endow the progeny of specific stem cell subpopulations with their unique cellular properties. These insights have already allowed institute scientists to "reprogram" specific regional stem and progenitor cell subpopulations both in vitro and in vivo to acquire the cellular properties of specific neuronal and glial subtypes. Specific complements of these discrete neural cell subtypes are invariably affected in different classes of neurological diseases including neurodegenerative diseases such as Alzheimer's disease, Parkinson's disease, Huntington's disease and motor neuron disease/amyotrophic lateral sclerosis, primary brain tumors, demyelinating and dysmyelinating disorders, stroke, HIV infection, epilepsy, diabetes mellitus and associated metabolic syndromes, and premature aging.

Other institute investigators have also used embryonic stem cells both to define the initial stages of neural induction and patterning of the neural tube that have previously been difficult to examine experimentally and as therapeutic reagents for those diseases of the nervous system in which multiple regional neuronal and glial subtypes are targeted. The overall aim of these studies is to identify innovative approaches to brain repair by activation of latent neural stem cell pools throughout the neuraxis to engage in selective regeneration of those cell types and neural network connections that have been compromised in specific disease states in the adult brain.

The ability to selectively activate, elaborate, and modulate these latent developmental programs to participate in selective neural regenerative responses within discrete temporal intervals and spatial domains will help to reestablish functional neural networks that preserve the integrity of previously acquired informational traces. More important, a better understanding of the pathogenesis of individual neurological disorders will allow institute scientists to more effectively and selectively employ these emerging neural regenerative strategies. These approaches include elucidation of the complex and modifiable epigenetic code regulating interrelated genome-wide transcriptional networks using innovative gene microarray and related molecular technologies that identify and target primary DNA modifications, changes in the combinatorial properties of the histone code, and precise alterations in the profiles and biological actions of multiple distinct classes of noncoding RNAs and other RNA-mediated pathogenic mechanisms.

These studies will ultimately allow institute investigators to develop effective strategies to augment the endogenous stem cell response to injury or to cell transformation by the use of novel therapeutic modalities that selectively enhance positive injury response cues (neuromodulatory cytokines and targeted transcription factors), concurrently promote the removal of inhibitory signals (inactivation of inflammatory cytokines and blockade of receptors that mediate inhibition of neurite outgrowth and axonal pathfinding by myelin and associated breakdown products), facilitate communications between the lesion site and the stem cell generative zones by enhancing the propagation of retrograde signals that establish morphogenetic gradients to enhance soluble factor signal transduction and also promote intimate cell–cell communications within functional compartments through the elaboration of selected classes of gap junction proteins (connexins) and other versatile intercellular signaling networks (e.g., Notch and integrin pathways), and facilitate genetic reprogramming of transformed cells to promote the reestablishment of the mature differentiated phenotype.

**SEE ALSO:** Amyotrophic Lateral Sclerosis; Huntington's Disease; Parkinson's Disease; Parkinson's Disease Foundation; Stroke.

**BIBLIOGRAPHY.** AECOM, www.aecom.yu.edu (cited November 2007); Department of Neuroscience, neuroscience.aecom.yu.edu (cited November 2007).

Fernando Herrera
University of California, San Diego

# Alvarez-Buylla, Arturo

**A LEADER IN** the field of neuroscience and stem cell–neurobiology research, Arturo Alvarez-Buylla has been involved in considerable research into the assembly of brains, brain tumors, and their repair as well as the ontogeny and the phylogeny of behavior. This work has covered not only developmental biology, developmental neuroscience, and neurobiology but also molecular and cellular neurobiology, as well as the field of plasticity. Dr. Alvarez-Buylla has himself been involved in designing a device for mounting tissue sections on histological slides, developing a digital stereotaxic apparatus for mice and songbirds, working on a computer-based mapping system for tissue sections, and developing fluorescent staining techniques.

Arturo Alvarez-Buylla completed his Bachelor of Science degree at Queen's University, Kingston, Canada, in 1978, and from 1981 to 1982 he studied at the Universidad Nacional Autónoma de Mexico (UNAM), in Coyoacán with an Undergraduate International Fellowship, remaining at the university until 1983, when he gained his license in Biomedical Research at UNAM, also gaining the university's Medal Gavino Barreda. While at UNAM, Dr. Alvarez-Buylla was involved in graduate courses at the university; he then went to Rockefeller University in New York, completing his doctoral thesis, "Radial Glia and the Migration of Young Neurons in the Adult Avian Brain," which was accepted in 1988.

For the next year, Dr. Alvarez-Buylla was involved in postdoctoral research at Rockefeller University, remaining at the university until 2000, working as an assistant professor from 1989 until 1991, as assistant professor and head of laboratory from 1991 until 1995, and as associate professor and head of laboratory from 1995 until 2000. It was when he was at Rockefeller University that Dr. Alvarez-Buylla was able to show that precursor cells were found in the same region in brains of both adult mice and birds. In 2002 he won the Robert L. Sinsheimer Award in Molecular Biology.

In 2001, Dr. Alvarez-Buylla moved to the Neurosurgery Research Department at the University of California, San Francisco, where he continued his research in neurosurgery, wining the Jacob Javits Award in 2000; two years later, he shared with Dr. R. McKay and Dr. S. Weiss the Neuronal Plasticity Prize from the Fondation IPSEN in France.

As he is involved in the production of many scholarly papers, Dr. Alvarez-Buylla's work has appeared in many journals including *Cell Tissue Research*, the *Journal of Comparative Neurology*, the *Journal of Neuroscience*, the *New England Journal of Medicine*, and *Science*. His most recent work has been on the extending of knowledge over the use and adaptability of neural cells in the adult mammalian brain and their use in generating new neurons and glia. It has seen a number of important breakthroughs in the field, first outlined in his article, with Florian T. Merkle, titled "Neural Stem Cells in Mammalian Development," published in *Current Opinion in Cell Biology* on October 11, 2006; in his article, with many collaborators, on "Postnatal Deletion of Numb/Numblike Reveals Repair and Remodeling Capacity in the Subventricular Neurogenic Niche," published in *Cell* on December 15, 2006; in another article, coauthored with Daniel A. Lim and Yin-Cheng Huang, "The Adult Neural Stem Cell Niche: Lessons for Future Neural Cell Replacement Strategies," published in *Neurosurgery Clinics of North America* on January 18, 2007; and in another article written with Florian T. Merkle and Zaman Mirzadeh, "Mosaic Organization of Neural Stem Cells in the Adult Brain," published in *Science* on July 5, 2007.

These articles led to his work with Rebecca Ihrie, which disproved the assumption made by many scientists by which neurons and glial cells were thought to have been derived from separate pools of progenitor cells and that no new neurons could be produced once development was complete. Dr. Alvarez-Buylla and Dr. Ihrie were able to show that classical neuroscience, which upheld the "no new neuron" concept, was untrue and that there was an ongoing adult neurogenesis that was then supported by a population of multipotent neural stem cells. This further allowed the researchers to show that adult neural stem cells were heavily influenced by their local microenvironment and, at the same time, also contributed extensively to the architecture of these germinal zones. The researchers were also able to show that there was significant heterogeneity existing within the populations of germinal zone astrocytes. Their results were published in a joint-authored paper, "Cells in the Astroglial Lineage Are Neural Stem Cells," published in *Cell and Tissue Research* on September 5, 2007. In turn, this work led to a recent article, coauthored with Erica L. Jackson, titled "Characterization of Adult Neural Stem Cells and Their Relation to Brain Tumors," published in *Cells Tissues Organs* in January 2008.

Dr. Alvarez-Buylla is a member of the Society for Neuroscience, the International Brain Research Organization, the Society for Biochemistry, the Academia de Ciencias de America Latina, and the International Society for Stem Cell Research.

**SEE ALSO:** Brain; Cells, Adult; University of California San Francisco.

**BIBLIOGRAPHY.** Lawrence K. Altman, "Research Dispels Myth that Brain in Adults Is Unable to Renew," *New York Times* (April 18, 1995); Sandra Blakeslee, "Researchers Find a Type of Stem Cell May Have the Ability to Repair the Brain," *New York Times* (December 18, 2001); Rebecca Ihrie and Arturo Alvarez-Buylla, "Cells in the Astroglial Lineage Are Neural Stem Cells," *Cell and Tissue Research* (v.331/1, 2008); Erica L. Jackson and Arturo Alvarez-Buylla, "Characterization of Adult Neural Stem Cells and Their Relation to Brain Tumors," *Cells Tissues Organs* (online, January 28, 2008); Daniel A. Lim, Yin-Cheng Huang, and Arturo Alvarez-Buylla, "The Adult Neural Stem Cell Niche: Lessons for Future Neural Cell Replacement Strategies," *Neurosurgery Clinics of North America* (v.18/1, 2007); Jason E. Long, et al., "Dix-Dependent and -Independent Regulation of Olfactory Bulb Interneuron Differentiation," *Journal of Neuroscience* (v.27/12, 2007); Florian T. Merkle and Arturo Alvarez-Buylla, "Neural Stem Cells in Mammalian Development," *Current Opinion in Cell Biology* (v.18/6, 2006); Florian T. Merkle, et al., "Cellular Composition and Cytoarchitecture of the Adult Human Subventricular Zone: A Niche of Neural Stem Cells," *Journal of Comparative Neurology* (v.494/3, 2006); N. Sanai, A. Alvarez-Buylla, and M. S. Berger, "Neural Stem Cells and the Origin of Gliomas," *New England Journal of Medicine* (v.353/8, 2005); *Who's Who in Science and Engineering 1996-1997* (Marquis Who's Who, 1996).

Justin Corfield
Geelong Grammar School

# American Association for the Advancement of Science

**THE AMERICAN ASSOCIATION** for the Advancement of Science (AAAS) is an international non-profit organization dedicated to advancing science around the world through education, leadership, and advocacy. In addition to organizing membership activities, AAAS publishes the journal *Science*, as well as many scientific newsletters, books, and reports, and spearheads programs that raise the bar of understanding for science worldwide. Membership in AAAS is open to all individuals who support the goals and objectives of the association and who are willing to contribute to the achievement of those goals and objectives. Founded in 1848, AAAS also serves many affiliated societies and academies of science, serving 10 million individuals.

*Science* has the largest paid circulation of any peer-reviewed general science journal in the world, with an estimated total readership of 1 million. AAAS has nearly 120,000 individual and institutional members and 262 affiliates, serving scientists in fields ranging from plant biology to dentistry. In addition to publishing *Science* and other science-related publications, hosting scientific conferences and meetings, and helping scientists advance their careers, AAAS undertakes numerous programs and activities that promote science to the public and monitor issues that affect the scientific community. AAAS established the Center for Science, Technology, and Congress in July 1994. Funded by

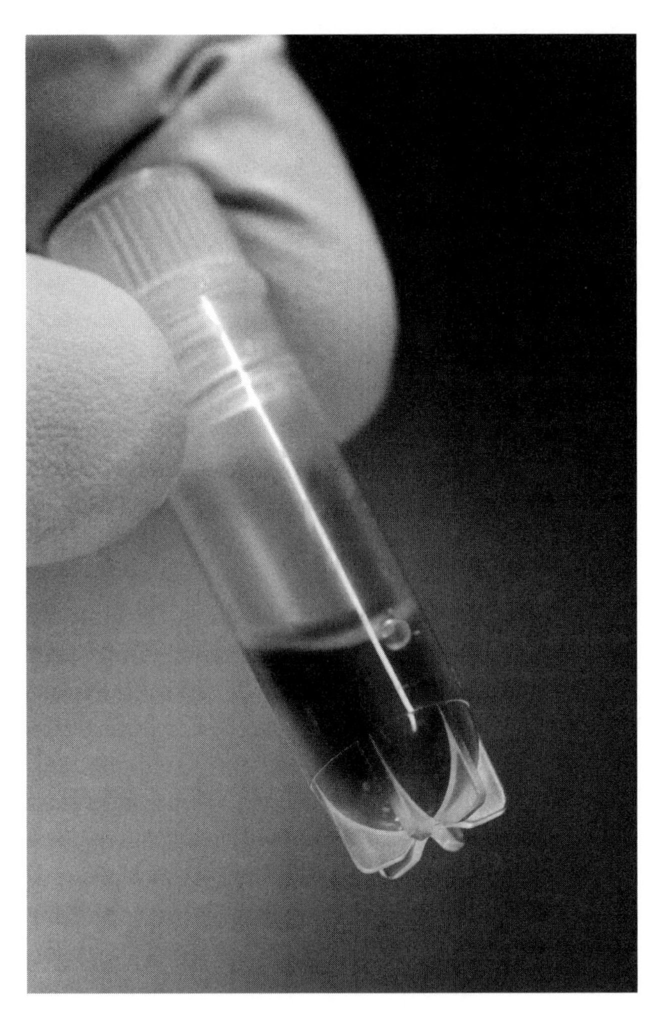

*The AAAS promotes dialogue on stem cell research, and with its affiliates it reaches over 10 million people.*

a grant from the Burroughs-Wellcome Fund, the center provides timely, objective information to Congress on current science and technology issues and assists the science and engineering community in understanding and working with Congress.

## AAAS AND STEM CELL RESEARCH

AAAS and the Institute for Civil Society (ICS) decided to undertake a study to propose recommendations for conducting stem cell research. To do so, they assembled a working group with broad expertise and diverse views to advise them and to assist with preparing a report. This study and the recommendations flowing from it were informed by the values of the members of this advisory group; the discussions that took place during a public meeting hosted by AAAS and ICS on August 25, 1999; and reports and recommendations of other groups in the United States and elsewhere that have reflected on the issues involved. These values include belief in the promotion of patient welfare and the social good, scientific freedom and responsibility, self determination, encouragement of civic discourse, public accountability of scientists and research institutions, and respect for diverse religious, philosophical, and secular belief systems.

AAAS and ICS recognize that there are varied social, political, ethical, and religious viewpoints to be considered in discussions about the scientific use of tissue from human embryos and fetuses. Scientists do not presume to know all the answers and ramifications of basic research in human stem cells. Therefore, it is important to promote continued dialogue among all segments of society concerning the implications of stem cell research, and AAAS and ICS are committed to fostering an ongoing educational process that informs such public dialogue.

The issue of stem cell research burst on the scientific scene in November 1998, when researchers first reported the isolation of human embryonic stem cells (hESCs). The discovery, made by Dr. James A. Thomson, a biologist at the University of Wisconsin, Madison, offered great promise for new ways of treating disease. The cells, which are derived from several-day-old embryos, can theoretically differentiate into virtually any type of human cell—from blood cells to skin cells. Scientists hope to find ways of using them to repair damaged tissue.

Dr. Thomson's breakthrough work was not eligible for funding from the U.S. National Institutes of Health (NIH)—the federal government's primary sponsor of biomedical research and the sponsor of some of his other research projects. Instead, he set up a separate lab to work on hESCs that was supported by private funding from the Geron Corporation of Menlo Park, California, and the Wisconsin Alumni Research Foundation.

The work was ineligible for public funding because of a ban placed by Congress on NIH-funded human embryo research. In 1995, Congress attached the ban to the bill appropriating funds for NIH. It has been retained in each successive appropriations bill (appropriations bills are passed annually), and until 2001, no public funding was ever provided for hESC research in the United States. Because of the great potential promised by Dr. Thomson's discovery, however, NIH sought legal counsel from the Department of Health and Human Services (HHS) on the application of the ban to hESC research. In January 1999, HHS concluded that scientists could use public funds for research on hESCs, with some restrictions on method of harvest. NIH thus began drafting guidelines governing funding for hESC studies.

Some opponents of hESC research argue that research on stem cells obtained from adults is just as promising and renders hESC research unnecessary. Most scientists, however, dispute this claim, citing great potential in the field of adult stem cells but several drawbacks compared with hESCs. Proponents of hESC research advocate funding for both fields.

In December 1999, NIH released draft guidelines allowing federally funded research on hESCs derived in the private sector and providing for stringent oversight of such research. The guidelines allowed research on cells derived only from embryos left over from fertility treatments and donated with the consent of the progenitors. In addition, if a fertility clinic were to profit from the sale of embryos used for stem cell derivation, research on those cells would not be allowed. After reviewing a flood of comments, NIH released final guidelines on August 25, 2000, and with the backing of President William J. Clinton, solicited applications for its first hESC research grants.

AAAS helps advance science education through a number of programs that focus on school curriculums, resources for educators, public education, scientific career advancement, and workforce training.

**SEE ALSO:** Cells, Embryonic; Clinical Trials (Adult Cells); Clinical Trials Worldwide; Congress: Votes and Amendments (Cloning/Embryos); United States.

**BIBLIOGRAPHY.** American Association for the Advancement of Science, www.aaas.org (cited November 2007); *Science Magazine*, www.sciencemag.org (cited November 2007).

Fernando Herrera
University of California, San Diego

# Amyotrophic Lateral Sclerosis

**AMYOTROPHIC LATERAL SCLEROSIS** (ALS), commonly known as Lou Gehrig's disease, is a neurological disease that affects the motor neurons. There is no definitive test for the diagnosis of ALS, so it is one of exclusion, relying on signs and symptoms that pertain to dysfunction in both upper motor neurons (UMNs) and lower motor neurons (LMNs). There is only one treatment regularly used for the treatment of ALS, but it is not a cure. In general, ALS is diagnosed later than other disease processes in part because of the vague symptoms it can generate and also the time it takes for the physician to rule out other causes. The ultimate cause of death in ALS patients is the loss of muscle strength to properly breathe. The potential for stem cell research in playing a role in ALS treatment lies in the possibility of regenerating dead or dying motor neurons in the hopes of regaining muscle function and control.

Most neurons in the human nervous system are made up of dendrites, a cell body, and axons. The dendrites are responsible for receiving information, the cell body for processing that information and for creating products to be exported—such as neurotransmitters, and the axon for transmitting that information to other cells through the synapse previously mentioned. Because the axons are covered in a layer of fat called myelin, they have a white color. For that reason, areas of the central nervous system that are made up predominantly by axons are termed *white matter*. The cell bodies lack this fatty layer, and so they are gray. This is where the term *gray matter* comes from.

The human nervous system can be conceptually separated into two different functional halves. The first is the sensory system, responsible for receiving information from the environment and sending this information to higher centers for processing, such as the cerebral cortex. The other half of the human nervous system is the motor system.

The motor pathways in the nervous system are responsible for sending information from the central nervous system, comprising primarily the brain and spinal cord, out to the target organs and muscles to cause a response. The information in this outflow tract is carried by two neurons arranged in series connected by a synapse in the anterior aspect of the spinal cord. The first of these neurons starts in the motor strip, the autonomic nervous system centers, or other higher-processing centers, and they send fibers to the anterior aspect, or ventral horn, of the spinal cord. This first neuron is conventionally termed the UMN. It is in the ventral (anterior) horn that the UMN synapses, or connects, with the lower motor neuron LMN, which carries information from the spinal cord outward to its target. ALS is a disease that primarily affects the motor half of the nervous system.

## PATHOLOGY OF ALS

In ALS, both the UMNs and the LMNs degenerate. The disease is characterized by the loss of motor neurons that are subsequently replaced by glia, or other supporting cells of the nervous system. On magnetic resonance imaging (MRI) of the brain, bilateral white matter changes can be appreciated. The spinal cord and the ventral roots of the LMNs atrophy and become smaller. Because the muscles that they usually innervate are receiving less of a signal, those muscles also become smaller and wasted, leading to an appearance termed *denervation atrophy*.

If one were to put the motor neurons from a patient with ALS under the microscope, a unique finding to ALS are Bunina bodies. These are eosinophilic, or pink, collections that contain a cysteine protease inhibitor, cystatin C. More commonly seen are intracellular inclusions in both the degenerating neurons and glia.

Although the appearance of motor neurons and the central nervous system in general have been elucidated by MRI and neuropathology, the definitive cause of ALS is unknown. Current research focuses on many different possibilities, with some pertaining to enzyme deficiencies, infectious etiologies, environmental factors, and a whole slew of other possibilities.

## SYMPTOMS AND TREATMENT

Because both the UMN and the LMN degenerate, both UMN signs and LMN signs are observed on clinical exam. Typically, UMN signs are problems you would foresee with the loss of the normal inhibitory input the UMNs usually have on the LMNs. That would lead one to see a hyperactive state in the musculature, which is indeed the case. Specific findings related to UMN degeneration include hyperreflexia (an exaggerated response to reflex testing), increased tone (an inability to relax certain muscle groups), and weakness.

As opposed to the UMN, the LMN provides an excitatory component to the muscle groups so that a loss of LMN health leads to a different set of signs and symptoms. LMN signs include fasciculations (twitching of isolated muscle groups), atrophy, and weakness. A combination of both UMN and LMN signs often leads a neurologist to consider ALS as the diagnosis, but not before exhausting other possible diagnoses, such as multiple sclerosis, myasthenia gravis, Eaton-Lambert syndrome, and others. For that reason, ALS is termed a diagnosis of exclusion.

The first drug ever approved by the U.S. Food and Drug Administration for the treatment of ALS is still used today. Riluzole was approved in 1995 and is manufactured by Sanofi-Aventis. Its exact mechanism of action in prolonging survival in ALS patients is unknown; however, the drug does have certain pharmacologic properties that could be the underlying source of its efficacy. Riluzole has been shown to decrease glutamate release, preventing any possible toxic effects to motor neurons that could have been caused by overexcitation—something that often involves glutamate. Trials with the drug have shown a median increase in survival time of three months. It should be stressed, however, that Riluzole is by no means a cure for ALS.

The potential for stem cell research lies in the ability to regenerate both UMNs and LMNs. What some researchers emphasize is the importance of understanding the underlying principles, such as the importance of timing and cell delivery, immune modulation, and the need for a multidisciplinary approach. With a better comprehension of these factors, the treatment of ALS has a better chance of being successful in patient care.

### EPIDEMIOLOGY

ALS can be classified as either sporadic or familial. The sporadic form accounts for about 90 percent of ALS patients, and the familial form makes up the other 10 percent. The disease is slightly more common in males, with a male-to-female ratio of approximately 1.3 to 1.5. The incidence of ALS increases with each decade of life, especially after the age of 40 years. Incidence reaches its peak at the age of 74 years and decreases after that point.

There are only two risk factors associated with the development of ALS. They are age and family history. Certain theories have been proposed, such as an increased risk in laborers engaged in heavy labor, repetitive muscle use, trauma, and electrical shock. A large, case–control study found that physical activity was not associated with ALS. However, they did find that increased leisure time physical activity is associated with an earlier age of onset in ALS patients.

There are certain areas of the world that show a high prevalence of ALS. Three regions in particular in the western Pacific include Guam, the Kii Peninsula of Japan, and West New Guinea. Of note, in these populations, ALS is often linked with parkinsonism and Alzheimer's disease.

**SEE ALSO:** Moral Status of Embryo; Multiple Sclerosis; Spinal Cord Injury; Stem-Like Cells, Human Brain; Stroke; Tissue Culture.

**BIBLIOGRAPHY.** A. C. Lepore and N. J. Maragakis, "Targeted Stem Cell Transplantation Strategies in ALS," *Neurochemistry International* (v.50/7–8, 2007); J. J. Veldink, S. Kalmijn, G. J. Groeneveld, et al., "Physical Activity and the Association with Sporadic ALS," *Neurology* (v.64, 2005); P. M. Worms, "The Epidemiology of Motor Neuron Diseases: A Review of Recent Studies," *Journal of the Neurological Sciences* (v.191, 2001).

Steven T. Chen
Johns Hopkins University School of Medicine

# Anversa, Piero

**PIERO ANVERSA IS** a distinguished investigator in the field of cardiovascular applications of stem cell research. His work contributed to a paradigm shift about cardiac physiology, strengthening the position that conceives of the heart as a self-renewing organ. He was born in Parma, Italy, in 1940. He gained his medical degree at the University of Parma in 1965, where he worked as assistant professor of pathology until 1980. In the early 1980s, he started his collaboration with the New York Medical College, where he was appointed professor of medicine in microbiology, immunology, and pathology. In 1985 Dr. Anversa permanently moved to United States, where he currently holds the office of director of the New York Medical College Cardiovascular Research Institute and vice chairman of the Department of Medicine.

Piero Anversa made a great effort to change the widespread conception of the heart as a terminally differentiated postmitotic organ, incapable of any sort of regeneration. One of the first observations that opened the way to such a deep revision of cardiac cellular homeostasis was the finding of male cells, endowed with a XY karyotype, in female hearts transplanted into male recipients. A deeper investigation of this heart chimerism phenomenon subsequently demonstrated a group of c-kit-positive cells, which can differentiate into myocytes, endothelial cells, and smooth muscle cells. This multipotent, clonogenic, and self-renewing cell population was proven to be a primitively cardiac sort of stem cell. Cardiac stem cells (CSCs) have been isolated from different species of mammalian hearts, including human ones. They are distributed into the myocardium along with supporting cells, forming stem cell niches. Such a peculiar microenvironment significantly interacts with CSCs, regulating their proliferative potential through junctional proteins and soluble mediators in a mostly unidentified manner. The origin of these stem cell pools has been a debated issue ever since the first observations of heart chimerism were made: A scrupulous analysis of mouse embryonic heart made by Eberhard and Jockusch provided the evidence that all resident CSCs are formed during embryonic life, whereas heart chimerism in sex-mismatched transplants can be explained by the migration of host cells from atrial remnants to the donor heart.

## REGENERATIVE CARDIOLOGY

Piero Anversa and his cardiovascular research team played a major role in regenerative cardiology not only in trying to figure out cardiac stem cell compartment features but also in attempting to translate such basic information regarding stem cell physiology into a novel and promising therapeutic strategy. The possibility of regenerating cardiac tissue through a cellular therapy has been first explored in mice by Dr. Anversa using lineage negative bone marrow cells (BMCs), a mixed population of cells composed of hematopoietic and mesenchymal stem cells, along with endothelial progenitors. In 2001 his team demonstrated that the injection of BMCs into infarcted myocardium can mend the ischemic lesion, and many following clinical trials performed on humans corroborated such beneficial effects, which have been interpreted as the consequence of a novel proliferation of myocytes and vascular structures mediated by BMCs' differentiation or the effect of a paracrine stimulation of CSCs mediated by the graft.

After the identification of CSCs, a new and better source for cellular therapy seemed to appear. In contrast to exogenous cells, CSCs should better carry out the regenerative task because they are physiologically involved in myocardial homeostasis. In addition, every exogenous cell type used (BMCs, skeletal myoblasts, embryonic myocytes, and endothelial cells), although capable of enhancing cardiac function, behaved as a passive graft acquiring a rather immature aspect and enhanced overall cardiac function modifying the biomechanical properties of the scarred portion of the heart. Embryonic stem cells, which have also been proposed as exogenous progenitor cells, have tumorigenic properties and would represent a heterologous source: Because they express HLA class I antigens in discrete quantities, they could induce an immune response. Myocardial regeneration has been demonstrated to happen in humans after infarction through the activation of resident CSCs, and the reason why such a phenomenon does not lead to a complete *restitutio ad integrum*, but to a scar formation, is one of the most challenging issues involving Dr. Anversa's research.

According to Dr. Anversa, enhancing such physiological regenerative properties could be the best regenerative approach suitable for ischemic and nonischemic heart failure. This goal may be achieved by isolating CSCs directly from the patient, expanding them to therapeutically employable quantities, and injecting them back to the diseased heart. The complex ex vivo stem cell harvesting process and the lack of expansion protocols are significant difficulties that will need to be solved before this therapy becomes available as a standard treatment. To restore cardiac function, CSCs need to migrate, divide, and differentiate properly; nevertheless, Dr. Anversa determined that the stem cell pool is modified by many factors such as age, gender, and myocardial overload. All these conditions induce CSCs to acquire a senescent phenotype, characterized by specific molecular alterations (e.g., telomere dysfunction), which could reduce their therapeutic potential if not corrected.

To increase myocardial regeneration, many improvements have currently been tested: Dr. Anversa proposed the use of bioengineered scaffolds loaded with CSCs, together with growth factors to promote a better interaction between CSCs and the surrounding environment. The New York Medical College Cardiovascular Research Team is presently collaborating with Louisville University on a myocardial regeneration phase I trial, which is going to assess the safety and the feasibility of intracoronary autologous CSC transplantation in patients with ischemic cardiomyopathy. More than 200 patients worldwide have already undergone such procedure with BMC infusion, and none reported any adverse events. From a clinical perspective, only comparative tests will be able to clarify in the future whether undifferentiated CSC transplant has a better clinical outcome than other kinds of techniques.

**SEE ALSO:** Cells, Embryonic; Clinical Trials Within U.S.: Heart Disease; Heart Attack; New York.

**BIBLIOGRAPHY.** Annarosa Leri, Jan Kajstura, and Piero Anversa, "Cardiac Stem Cells and Mechanisms of Myocardial Regeneration," *Physiological Reviews* (v.85, 2005).

David James Pinato
Eastern Piedmont University
School of Medicine

# Arizona

**ARIZONA IS A** state in the southwestern part of the continental United States. It was the 48th state to join the union, which it did in 1912. It is bordered to the south by the Mexican state of Sonora, to the east by New Mexico, and to the north by Utah. The Colorado River forms the western border, separating Arizona from California and Nevada. Much of the state is occupied by flat, hot deserts, but there are also large stands of evergreen trees and many lakes—man-made as well as natural—that lend variety to the topography and land cover of the state. Geographical features such as the Grand Canyon are internationally renowned. The state is the 6th largest in the country, with a total area of nearly 114,000 square miles, but its population of a little less than 6.5 million is the 16th largest in the country, which indicates a low population density, much of which is concentrated in the capital city, Phoenix, together with other large urban areas such as Mesa, Tucson, and Yuma. Bordering Mexico, the state is home to many migrants from that country, and there are various political issues related to migration—both legal and illegal—that are significant in Arizonan political discourse.

Arizona has tended to favor Republican politicians and policies in recent decades. The only Democratic candidate to have been endorsed by Arizona in more than four decades was Bill Clinton. However, a small number of public positions are filled by Democratic Party candidates. In this context, progressive policies such as stem cell research do not receive public or executive support, although debate is open and generally civil. In debates following President Bush's response to the 2006 Stem Cell Research Enhancement Act, for example, which he eventually vetoed, Arizona's senators were split. Republican Senator John McCain, who was subsequently a presidential candidate, supported the Senate majority position and claimed it represented a framework for ethical medical research. Republican Jon Kyl supported the president on one measure, and Democrat Jim Pederson took the opposite view. The senators were able to articulate positions that were coherent, rather than driven by monolithic ideology.

The result of this has been that Arizonan state law has yet to rule on the issue of research in stem cell areas. A Stem Cell Research Committee was formed and met in January 2006. The result of their deliberations was that no recommendations for legislative action were made. State law currently requires health professionals to inform pregnant patients about options surrounding umbilical cord blood donations and related stem cell issues. Research involving embryos or fetuses obtained as the result of abortions is prohibited, as is the process of somatic cell nuclear transfer of human cells. Academic researchers at tertiary-level educational institutions in the state tend to favor stem cell research, as might be expected, and have lent their voices for more freedom to act. Human interest stories in local and global media that illustrate that stem cell–based research is starting to lead to positive health outcomes that were previously impossible is also having a gradual effect on public opinion.

Private-sector firms, in contrast, continue medical research within the state, including the use of nonforbidden forms of stem cell activities. Scottsdale-based firm Medistem Laboratories Inc., for example, has announced research that uses cord blood transplants to try to stimulate new blood vessel creation, and hence tackle Critical Limb Ischemia (CLI). CLI is characterized by the narrowing and hardening of the arteries, which can lead to significant problems in the feet and leg areas. As many as 8–12 million people in the United States suffer from CLI, which would of course represent a potentially lucrative market for effective treatments, irrespective of the medical breakthrough that would be needed.

**SEE ALSO:** *Individual U.S. State Articles*; Biotechnology, History of; Clinical Trials Within U.S.: Batten Disease; Clinical Trials Within U.S.: Blind Process; Clinical Trials Within U.S.: Cancer; Clinical Trials Within U.S.: Heart Disease; Clinical Trials Within U.S.: Peripheral Vascular Disease; Clinical Trials Within U.S.: Skin Transplants (Burns); Clinical Trials Within U.S.: Spinal Cord Injury; Clinical Trials Within U.S.: Traumatic Brain Injury; Ethics; Federal Government Policies; Moral Status of Embryo; Special Interest/Lobby Groups; United States.

**BIBLIOGRAPHY.** "Medistem Labs Launches Pre-Clinical Cord Blood Research for Treatment of CLI," *Stem Cell Business News* (February 8, 2007), www.stemcell-researchnews.com (cited November 2007); Arizona State Senate, "Stem Cell Research," Issue Brief (October 2, 2007), www.azleg.state.az.us (cited November 2007); David R. Berman, *Arizona Politics and Government: The Quest for Autonomy, Democracy, and Development* (University of Nebraska Press, 1998); Paul Giblin, "Arizona's Senators Part Ways on Stem Cell Research," *Knight Ridder Tribune Business News* (July 19, 2006), p.1; Thomas E. Sheridan, *Arizona: A History* (University of Arizona Press, 1995).

John Walsh
Shinawatra International University

# Arkansas

**AFTER SCIENTISTS BASED** at the University of Wisconsin revealed that they had successfully harvested embryonic stem cells from human embryos, several states rapidly responded with either support or bans on related research. Arkansas is one of the states to ban such research. In 2003, Arkansas, along with North and South Dakota, completely banned all forms of cloning, even if related to stem cell research and therapies. Types of cloning include reproductive cloning as well as somatic cell nuclear transfer, which is also called therapeutic cloning.

Arkansas law prohibits research on an aborted live fetus but allows research on a fetus that was aborted and born dead. Cloned embryos are outlawed, as is the sale of a fetus or fetal material. Opponents of providing a monetary reward for the production of a source of embryonic stem cells warn that such a practice could lead to the forcing of a woman to produce and abort a fetus against her will or to unfairly entice a woman from a low socioeconomic status to do so to advance her position. Prohibition of monetary gain from fetuses or fetal materials protects both women and fetuses from exploitation.

Despite its restrictive laws regarding stem cell procurement, Arkansas nevertheless has a long track record of stem cell therapies. In fact, the Myeloma Institute for Research and Therapy at the University of Arkansas for Medical Sciences (UAMS) has performed thousands of blood stem cell transplants for multiple myeloma patients; the number of transplants that they have performed surpasses that of any other facility on the planet. The Myeloma Institute for Research and Therapy, as well as UAMS, is in Little Rock.

At the UAMS Winthrop P. Rockefeller Cancer Institute, the Cell Differentiation Program works to understand how cancerous and healthy cells develop and differentiate. This knowledge can then be applied to stem cell biology in an effort to guide the differentiation of these stem cells. A current major usage of stem cells in cancer therapies is the delivery of healthy blood stem cells to reconstitute a patient's immune system and blood cell population after chemotherapy, particularly for a myeloma. Stem cell therapy for multiple myeloma patients involves a high dose of chemotherapy to kill diseased blood cells, followed by a transfusion of healthy blood and blood stem cells.

Former Governor of Arkansas Mike Huckabee is in favor of research on currently existing stem cell lines, which most experts agree are too contaminated to continue to work on; however, he firmly opposes cloning. In early 2008 Governor Huckabee was a U.S. presidential candidate and hoped his conservative stance on stem cell research would aid his campaign.

**SEE ALSO:** *Individual U.S. State Articles*; Biotechnology, History of; Clinical Trials Within U.S.: Batten Disease; Clinical Trials Within U.S.: Blind Process; Clinical Trials Within U.S.: Cancer; Clinical Trials Within U.S.: Heart Disease; Clinical Trials Within U.S.: Peripheral Vascular Disease; Clinical Trials Within U.S.: Skin Transplants (Burns); Clinical Trials Within U.S.: Spinal Cord Injury; Clinical Trials Within U.S.: Traumatic Brain Injury; Ethics; Federal Government Policies; Moral Status of Embryo; Special Interest/Lobby Groups; United States.

**BIBLIOGRAPHY.** M. Bellomo, *The Stem Cell Divide: The Facts, the Fiction, and the Fear Driving the Greatest Scientific, Political and Religious Debate of Our Time* (American Management Association, 2006); C. B. Cohen, *Renewing the Stuff of Life: Stem Cells, Ethics, and Public Policy* (Oxford University Press, 2007); C. Fox, *Cell of Cells: The Global Race to Capture and Control the Stem Cell* (Norton, 2007); K. R. Monroe, R. Miller, and J. Tobis, eds., *Fundamentals of the Stem Cell Debate: The Scientific, Religious, Ethical, and Political Issues* (University of California Press, 2007); M. Ruse and C. A. Pynes, eds., *The Stem Cell Controversy: Debating the Issues* (Contemporary Issues) (Prometheus Books, 2006); C. Vestal, "States Take Sides on Stem Cell Research," *Stateline.org* (January 31, 2008), www.stateline.org (cited January 2008).

Claudia Winograd
University of Illinois, Urbana-Champaign

# Australia

**STEM CELL RESEARCH** in Australia dates back to the early 1990s, with an Australian researcher gaining a patent for deriving animal embryonic stem cells in 1992. Much of this early research was conducted by Dr. Alan Trounson from Monash University in Melbourne, Victoria. He had been part of the team that delivered the first in vitro fertilization baby in Australia in 1980, and during the late 1990s, he had been involved in work using human embryonic stem cells. In 2000 Dr. Trounson led a group of scientists from the Monash Institute of Reproduction and Development that was able to report work on developing nerve stem cells derived from embryonic stem cells. The success was reported on the front page of *Nature* magazine, and it received much international attention. It certainly helped focus research in Australia and overseas on the potential for more research into the use of stem cells, but it also sparked off much political debate about the efficacy of certain aspects of stem cell research.

In 2003 the Australian Stem Cell Center was founded as part of the National Biotechnology Centre of Excellence. Since then, the center has received about $100 million in funding, and although it is located at Monash University in the Monash Science, Technology, Research, and Innovation Precinct, it brings together research capabilities from not only Monash University but also the University of Adelaide (South Australia), the University of New South Wales (Sydney), the University of Queensland (Brisbane), the Peter MacCallum Cancer Centre (Melbourne), the Victor Chang Cardiac Research Institute (Sydney), the Murdoch Children's Research Institute (Melbourne), and the Howard Florey Institute of Experimental Physiology and Medicine (Melbourne).

The aim was to establish an integrated series of national research programs, and the result was that the Australian Stem Cell Center quickly built itself into one of the premier stem cell research organizations in the world. It brought together researchers focusing on embryonic and adult stem cells and was focused on using this research to help patients suffering from damaged cardiac tissue following heart attacks, for the regeneration of bone marrow for transplantation, and in the use of stem cells in work on combating lung diseases such as cystic fibrosis. Work on cardiac regeneration and hematology remains at the forefront of research in Australia.

## GOVERNMENT RESPONSE

Although there were few problems with mainstream stem cell research, the issue of the use of embryonic stem cells for therapeutic cloning research, by which human embryonic stem cells were created, used, and destroyed, became a major political issue. The federal government, uncertain about what to do, appointed John Lockhart to head a stem cell review committee to decide on the ethical issues that arose from the use of embryonic stem cells. John Stanley Lockhart, a former barrister who had been a judge of the Supreme Court of the Australian Capital Territory before becoming a member of the Appellate Body of the World Trade Organization in Geneva, Switzerland, heard from many bodies and individuals about the scientific merits of stem cell research, as well as the ethical and religious problems that arose. His report had to be submitted by December 19, 2005.

Initially, in 2002, the federal government of Prime Minister John Howard placed a ban, on the advice of Tony Abbott, Minister of Health, on the use of embryonic stem cells. Mr. Abbott spoke openly about his own religious convictions and the ethical problems that he felt might arise from an expansion of research into stem cells. This belief in increased regulation had seen the passing of the Human Embryos Act and the Prohibition of Human Cloning Act, both in 2002. The ban led to Senator Kay Patterson from the Liberal Party in Victoria (and also Minister of Health and Ageing from 1992 until 2003) launch a private member's bill to overturn the ban. The cosponsor of the bill was Mal Washer, a West Australian Liberal from the House of Representatives, and the bill had the support of several other politicians such as the former leader of the Democrat Party, Natasha Stott-Despoja.

With the bill being debated, the governing Liberal Party and the opposition Australian Labor Party both offered their members a "conscience" vote. The bill passed the Senate, and on December 6, 2006, it went for debate in the House of Representatives, where supporters and opponents were believed to have approximately equal numbers. In the debate on the use of embryonic stem cells, an amendment, essentially a procedural move to send the bill back to the Senate, was put to the vote. Both Prime Minister John Howard, described in the press as being "visibly pensive" and the opposition leader Kevin Rudd, declared their opposition to the bill—with Mr. Howard subsequently embracing Juliet Lockhart, the widow of John Lockhart (who died soon after completing the report), and Kevin Rudd speaking passionately about his late mother's battle with Parkinson's disease.

Three leading cabinet ministers opposed the bill—Peter Costello, the Treasurer and Deputy Prime Minister; Tony Abbott, the Minister of Health who had originally imposed the ban; and Kevin Andrew, the Minister of Workplace Relations. The bill was, however, supported by Dr. Brendan Nelson, a medical doctor and former national president of the Australian Medical Association, who was at that time Minister of Education, Science and Training (and later Defence Minister and Mr. Howard's successor as Liberal Party leader), and the amendment was rejected with a comfortable majority of 23; a vote on whether the motion should have a third reading passed by 82 to 62, leaving the motion itself to be passed without a division.

The parliamentary vote not only widened the amount of research that could be conducted on stem cells but also helped to concentrate public attention on the possible advances that could be made from the new medical techniques. This led to increased funding for the Australian Stem Cell Centre. There was also new promising research at the Neural Stem Cell Laboratory, part of the Queensland Brain Institute at the University of Queensland in Brisbane, where Dr. Rodney L. Rietze, a Pfizer Australia Senior Research Fellow, is Head of the Neural Stem Cells and Aging Laboratory.

The importance in the research using stem cells in Australia was demonstrated when Professor Stephen Livesey, the Chief Executive Officer of the Australian Stem Cell Centre, was given the George

W. Hyatt Memorial Award by the American Association of Tissue Banks to recognize his "outstanding contribution to scientific research in tissue engineering." This had led to the discovery and development by Professor Livesey of AlloDerm.

## AUSTRALIAN STEM CELL CENTRE

The Australian Stem Cell Centre (ASCC) is a major Australian collaborative initiative uniting many of the country's leading academic researchers with the biotechnology industry to develop innovative therapeutic products to treat a range of serious injuries and debilitating diseases. The ASCC commenced operation in 2003, in partnership with many leading Australian research institutes and universities. The principal objective of the ASCC is to integrate a national multi-institution research and discovery program to develop treatments for serious diseases through the application of stem cells and related technologies. A core role of the ASCC is to attract and secure commercial partners to advance outstanding research outcomes toward clinical trials initially, and eventually into the hands of medical practitioners for the benefit of their patients. Complementary to these goals, the ASCC proactively works to enhance the public's awareness and understanding of stem cell and regenerative research. The ASCC also provides educational opportunities to research students and postdoctoral research scientists, facilitating a growth in human resources with experience and links to international stem cell networks and institutes. The ASCC is committed to the highest scientific and commercial ethical principles. Commonwealth and state legislation draw clear boundaries regarding lawful and unlawful scientific practice relating to embryo research and cloning technology in Australia. The ASCC is Australia's Biotechnology Center of Excellence and has partnered with nine leading Australian universities and research institutions.

The center's principal objective is to integrate a national multi-institutional research and discovery program to develop treatments for serious disease through the application of stem cells and related technologies. The center is headquartered on the Monash University campus in Melbourne. The main administration and dedicated laboratories also are based in Melbourne. In addition, the center is establishing a second campus at the University of Queensland in Brisbane.

In 2002 the ASCC received a competitively awarded grant of $43.55 million from the Howard government's backing Australia's Ability, Biotechnology Centre of Excellence Program. To complement federal funding, the State Government of Victoria's Science Technology & Innovation program awarded the ASCC a further $10 million to support infrastructural elements of the Biotechnology Centre of Excellence. In May 2004, the prime minister announced a further $55 million grant under Backing Australia's Ability II to support the ASCC's activities from 2006 to 2011.

The ASCC's research and progress is closely monitored by several governmental agencies: the Australian Research Council; Australian government; Department of Industry, Tourism and Resources; state government of Victoria; and Department of Innovation, Industry, and Regional Development.

The ASCC currently has 16 research projects in progress across a range of four platform technologies combined with therapeutic programs in hematology and cardiac disease and a pilot program in respiratory disease. Hematology is currently the most comprehensive of these programs and in the very near term will make up several projects in multiple institutes and states. This program represents a cross-disciplinary, multi-institution approach to creating a new paradigm in the supply of blood products such as red blood cells and platelets. This effort is an innovative approach to the use of stem cell technologies based on world-class expertise in the ASCC. This program has the potential to place Australia at the forefront of cell-based therapeutics and may be the first widespread use of a product based on human embryonic stem cell technologies.

The ASCC is also investigating the use of therapeutics for congestive heart failure, which may offer benefits to an extremely large and growing patient population. Preventing or delaying the onset of heart failure using adult stem cells and related technologies is a highly competitive area of

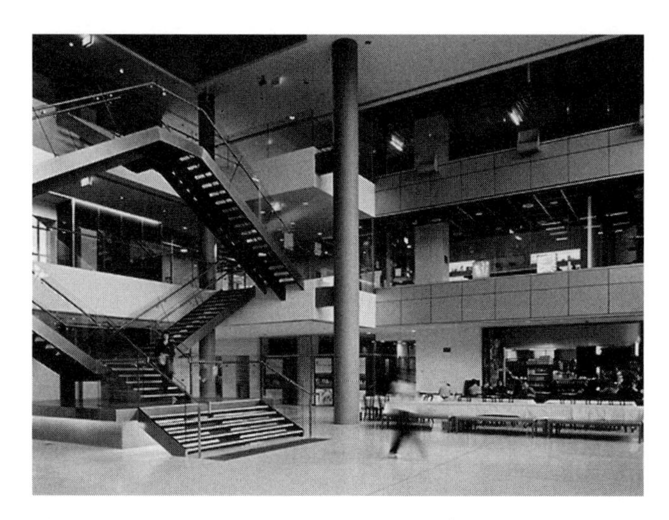

*The Australian Stem Cell Centre has won $100 million in funding and is one of the top stem cell centers in the world.*

stem cell research. The ASCC has specific expertise in the application of cardiac stem cell technology and is supporting adult stem cell projects with a direct application to cardiac disease, as well as platform technologies that may further affect the development of this focus.

ASCC Research Services, a division of the ASCC, provides important support to the Australian stem cell community, including adult and embryonic stem cell training; provision of boutique proteins that are required for stem cell growth, maintenance, and differentiation; derivation of new human embryonic stem cell lines and applications of proprietary in-house technologies for the creation of improved cells lines; and implementation of a flow cytometry facility.

It is anticipated that the center will enter into a number of collaborative arrangements with commercial partners to access certain technologies for use by the center's research scientists. The ASCC has a number of collaborative agreements with industry to advance specific aspects of stem cell research. These include agreements with the international company Stem Cell Sciences Ltd to derive, characterize, and distribute new human embryonic stem cell lines as a tool for academic researchers (to whom they will be provided unencumbered of intellectual property restrictions); with Singapore-based ES Cell International Pte Ltd for the commercialization of research outcomes at Monash University that are relevant to diabetes; with Australian biotechnology company Nephrogenix Pty Ltd for expertise relevant to the development of kidneys, blood, and cardiac tissue, which is closely aligned with the key areas of interest of the ASCC; and with U.S.-based company LifeCell Corporation to collaborate in the area of tissue repair.

This includes a license to use their proprietary acellular matrix technology in ASCC programs and the ability to collaborate in future development for products incorporating both LifeCell and ASCC technology.

**SEE ALSO:** Cells, Embryonic; International Laws.

**BIBLIOGRAPHY.** Australian Stem Cell Centre, www.stemcellcentre.edu.au (cited November 2007); Jane Bunce and Peter Veness, "Stem Cell Cloning Ban Overturned," AAP Press Release (December 6, 2006), www.news.com.au (cited January 2008); D. Cyranoski, "Australia Lifts Ban on Cloning," *Nature* (v.444/7121, 2006); A. McLennan, "Which Bank? A Guardian Model for Regulation of Embryonic Stem Cell Research in Australia," *Journal of Law and Medicine* (v.15/1, 2007); Katharine Murphy, "Howard, Russ Fail to Block Human Cloning Bill," *The Age* (December 7, 2006); A. H. Sinclair and P. R. Schofield, "Human Embryonic Stem Cell Research: An Australian Perspective," *Cell* (v.128/2, 2007).

Fernando Herrera
University of California, San Diego
Justin Corfield
Geelong Grammar School

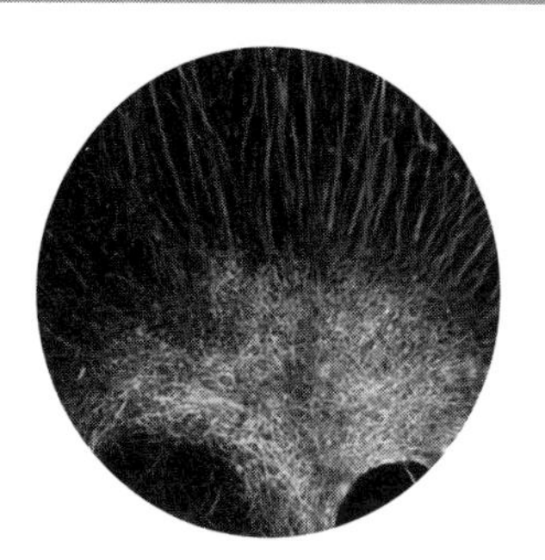

# B

## Batten Disease

**BATTEN DISEASE IS** a rare but fatal neurodegenerative disease that affects children and for which no treatment exists, other than possible future stem cell research treatments. The disease is named after the British physician Frederick Batten, who first identified and described the condition in 1903. It is also known as Spielmeyer-Vogt-Sjogren-Batten disease.

Batten disease manifests itself in children somewhere between the ages of 4 and 10 years. Early signs might include vision impairment, poor circulation, hyperventilation, reduced communicative ability, and behavioral changes. As a neurodegenerative disease, Batten disease causes the patient to progressively lose motor skills, communication skills, and brain functions. The results are distressing not just to the patients concerned but also to their carers. The disease is one of a set of conditions known as neuronal ceroid lipofuscinosis; there are approximately 400 patients suffering from it in the United States at any one time (some estimates put this number at 1,000). Batten disease is a genetically inherited disease that leads to a mutation in the patient that prevents the elimination of toxins from the brain. It also leads to a buildup of lipofuscins in the body, and these combinations of proteins and fats are the symptoms by which the disease is detected.

Since the 1990s, a team of scientists including Dean Hamer, working at the U.S. National Institutes of Health, have discovered certain elements of the X chromosome, resulting in the discovery of the genetic causes of Batten disease, among other conditions. In the years since, six genes have been discovered that are associated with the onset of the disease, although it has not yet been determined what functions most of these genes possess. However, the determination of the cause of the disease has led to an indication of how treatments could be created. These treatments are based on injecting genetic material directly into the affected area—the brain of an affected child.

In the last few years, several teams have been working with injecting fetal stem cell material into the brains of children with Batten disease, and there have been reports of positive outcomes, although it is too soon to determine whether a permanent cure is possible or whether the treatment is temporary in effect. Nevertheless, patients have responded well to the treatment, and certain motor skills and communication skills have been returned to them. Parents who are able to talk to their children after years of them being unable to speak find their quality of life to be greatly improved, irrespective of whether that improvement will be sustained permanently. Under current conditions, it should be evident by around 2010 whether the improvement in patients' health will be permanent. A company known as StemCells, Inc., based at Palo Alto, California, is one of the leaders in this area of research and has announced the successful completion of the first half of U.S. Food and Drug Administration–approved clinical trials of purified human neural cells. Qualified experts have found no safety issues associated with the low-level dosages so far employed, and higher dosages are subsequently to be used. The treatment is a proprietary preparation of human central nervous system stem cells (HuCNS-SC cells). The cost of the treatment is not known, but it is likely to be high. To avoid patients rejecting the foreign cells, the immune system must be suppressed to some extent, and it is in this area that most problems are anticipated to arise. However, tests show that this problem has been successfully negotiated within the trials conducted.

A further stream of research has been sparked by the detection of mature-onset Batten disease in a breed of dog known as the Tibetan Terrier, as well as some other breeds. Testing shows that perhaps 5 percent of these dogs may suffer from the disease. Dog owners and their associations have been working in partnership with patients and their carers in sharing information and jointly sponsoring and supporting research. It is hoped that new forms of treatment might, in due course, arise from this collaboration.

The source of most of the genetic material used to treat Batten disease is aborted fetuses, which are the main source of the stem cells required. The use of fetal cells is controversial on a number of grounds. There is a moral or ethical issue concerning the use of human genetic material per se, and the issue of using material from abortions continues to divide society. However, fetal cells are currently the only known source for the stem cells required, and the treatment relieves terrible suffering. In the future, alternative sources of stem cells might be identified, including, for example, children who have died from natural causes or as the victims of road traffic or other accidents. The use of organs from such sources is much more widely (although not universally) accepted in most societies. A further ethical issue concerns the use of children in medical experimentation. Although only children suffer from Batten disease, there is still the need to consider whether they are able to give informed consent to a new and unproven form of treatment, especially given the progressive damage to their brains. The basic principle that applies is that consent is provided on behalf of the children by their parents or other legally appointed guardian.

**SEE ALSO:** Cells, Neural; National Institutes of Health; StemCells, Inc.

**BIBLIOGRAPHY.** "StemCells Inc. Announces Important Milestone in Batten Disease Clinical Trial," *Business Wire* (June 18, 2007); Kristian Foden-Vencil, "Batten Disease Patients Benefit from Stem Cell Injections," Oregon Public Broadcasting (December 12, 2006); Ketzel Levine, "Batten Disease Unites Parents, Dog Owners," National Public Radio (June 20, 2006); Batten Disease Support and Research Association, www.bdsra.org (cited November 2007).

John Walsh
Shinawatra University

# Baylor College of Medicine

**BAYLOR COLLEGE OF MEDICINE** is a private medical school located in Houston, Texas, on the grounds of the Texas Medical Center. It has been consistently rated the top medical school in Texas and among the best in the United States. Its Graduate School of Biomedical Sciences is also highly rated. Baylor has become one of 63 American colleges with an endowment greater than $1 billion. In 2005 Baylor College of Medicine ranked 13th in terms of research funding from the U.S. National Institutes of Health (NIH), and its Graduate School of Biomedical Sciences ranked 22nd for best Ph.D. program in the biological sciences (2007). In addition, several individual departments earn particularly heavy NIH funding, receiving several Top Ten rankings by NIH in 2005

The Stem Cells and Regenerative Medicine Center (STaR Center) is housed at Baylor College of Medicine. The STaR Center focuses on three major areas of stem cell research: adult stem cells, embryonic stem cells, and cancer stem cells. Although embryonic stem cells capture most of the public's attention, the potential benefits of cancer stem cells are just as promising. The overall mission of the STaR Center is both to facilitate stem cell research of all types at Baylor College of Medicine and the clinical translation of such research into regenerative medicine.

The STaR Center was founded in 2005 and is directed by Dr. Margaret Goodell. Dr. Karen Hirschi serves as deputy director. The center comprises roughly 30 members overall, belonging to more than a dozen departments at Baylor, including molecular and cell biology, pediatrics, medicine, obstetrics/gynecology, and pathology. Dr. Goodell and her staff have worked with stem cell groups at Rice University, the University of Texas Health Science Center, and the University of Texas M. D. Anderson Cancer Center in the past and expect to collaborate more in the future. Dr. Goodell specializes in adult stem cells, specifically hematopoietic stem cells, which reside in bone marrow and give rise to new bloods cells over the course of a person's lifetime.

Fellow founder Dr. Karen Hirschi, deputy director at STaR and a member of the Center for Cell and Gene Therapy, focuses on vascular development and regeneration. Dr. Hirschi's primary interest is in understanding the events leading to blood vessel formation, as well as in elucidating regulators of vascular cell commitment and differentiation and modulators of vascular cell proliferation and migration during blood vessel assembly. Another focus of her laboratory is investigating the potential of adult and embryonic stem and progenitor cells to contribute to neovascularization in response to tissue injury and growth.

Dr. Thomas Zwaka, the third founder of the center as well as an assistant professor in the Center for Cell and Gene Therapy and department of molecular and cell biology at Baylor, focuses on embryonic stem cells. Dr. Goodell has been on the faculty at Baylor College of Medicine since 1997 and is a member of the Center for Cell and Gene Therapy, as well as the Departments of Pediatrics, Molecular & Human Genetics, and Immunology. Directing a laboratory of about 20 students and postdoctoral fellows, she has performed groundbreaking work on adult-derived stem cells. She is widely recognized as a leader in the field of stem cell biology and serves on the board of the International Society for Stem Cell Research and on the Education Committee for the American Society of Hematology. She is a frequent speaker at national and international conferences, a senior editor of the journal *Stem Cells*, and serves on several editorial boards and as a reviewer for a multiple journals and granting agencies. She is the recipient of a Leukemia and Lymphoma Society Scholar Award, and in 2004, she received the DeBakey Award for Excellence in Research at Baylor College of Medicine.

**SEE ALSO:** Cells, Embryonic; International Society for Stem Cell Research; National Institutes of Health.

**BIBLIOGRAPHY.** Baylor College of Medicine, www.bcm.edu (cited November 2007); International Society for Stem Cell Research, www.isscr.org (cited November 2007); *Stem Cell Research News*, www.stemcellresearchnews.com (cited November 2007).

Fernando A. Herrera
University of California, San Diego

# Belgium

**BELGIUM IS ONE** of the most active European countries when it comes to stem cell research whether from embryonic or from adult stem cells. Along with Finland, France, Portugal, Spain, Sweden, and the United Kingdom, Belgium is an enthusiastic backer for both encouraging and engaging in stem cell research.

The position of the Belgian system of stem cell research is complicated. Most of the research is conducted at the regional level instead of the national level. The Flanders Inter-University Institute for Biotechnology has united all of the Flemish Universities. It received a major portion of the financing from the government of Flanders for research. The research covers 40 percent of the research costs. From the funds grants are made to local, regional and to other organizations for research. In addition the funds are often used to support collaboration with industry, which often supplies its own funds for research projects. The French-speaking universities of Wallonia also engage in stem cell research, but because the research is often conducted as part of other research, it is not always clear what in the absence of labeling is stem cell research and what is not.

An important leader of stem cell research is Dr. Catherine Verfaillie who has recently returned after years of research at the University of Minnesota. She is heading the Belgium Institute for Stem Cell Research at the University of Leuven and is a leader in the use of adult stem cells.

Between 1994 and 2003 Belgium produced only 1¼ percent of the publications in the world on stem cell research. Belgian high-profile projects include research into the use of stem cells for the treatment of cancer, Alzheimer's, and Parkinson's disease. The patenting of stem cell research technology is low in Belgium. By 2007 only 12 stem cell patents had been granted. However, there is a long-standing practice of seeking patents in other countries, so Belgian patents are probably greater in number.

A recent research breakthrough in Belgium was the discovery of a way to clone human embryos from laboratory-matured eggs. The discovery is expected to produce new embryonic stem cell lines. The cloned embryos will be used to provide infertile couples with eggs and sperm. In Belgium, reproductive cloning is banned as it is in many other countries. However, therapeutic cloning is legal if certain guidelines are followed. In general, Belgium has a flexible policy with regard to stem cell research.

In April 2003 the Belgian Parliament adopted a bill that allows research on supernumerary embryos. The bill also allowed the creation of human embryos for research and somatic cell nuclear transfer. The new law made Belgium one of the most liberal countries in the world on human embryonic stem cell research.

**SEE ALSO:** European Consortium for Stem Cell Research—EuroStemCell; Verfaillie, Catherine.

**BIBLIOGRAPHY.** Davor Solter, et al., *Embryo Research in Pluralistic Europe* (Springer-Verlag, 2004); Geertrui Van Overwalle, *Study on the Patenting of Inventions Related to Human Stem Cell Research in Europe* (DANE Publishing, 2001).

Andrew J. Waskey
Dalton State College

# Biotechnology, History of

**THE 17TH CENTURY** is seen as the most propitious era for scientific intervention. The period is often described as the *century of genius*, for most scientific leaps began in this era and continued well into the 18th century, only to be regrouped retrospectively in the early part of the 20th century. The invention of the telescope, the thermometer, and the barometer benefitted those countries at war. In addition, however, the scientific and philosophical interests that emerged at the time also stimulated productive thoughts and aspirations that were expressed in the latter part of the century. The period, thus, was marked by a very successful scientific revolution.

In France, Western Europe, and England, the period between Galileo's first publications and Newton's *Principia* was characterized by changes that altered the development of new technologies. The granting of patents in Florence and England constituted an important chapter in the history of technological inventions. The terms *invention*, *inventor*, and *monopoly*, and legalizing them, became significant with regard to technology.

Development of the science of mechanics and power technology marked yet another phase in the development of technological innovations in later years. Although the need to devise improved technology was a prominent feature of this innovation, there was a concomitant improvement in the way new technology was put to practical use for the benefit of mankind. What was more important was how these new technologies fitted into the need of the society in terms of reliability, economic viability, and the felt need of the community at large.

Amid new technology, an important factor that influenced its practical application was the rise of a unanimous sense of reasoning and logic of progress. This led to the establishment of technological institutions that were directly supported by the state. France and Britain became active recipients of this institutional progress. Although, initially, the need to have such set-ups came from the army and civil services, it was not long before their relevance was recognized in making technology completely autonomous and open to the public. In England, advanced technology in terms of railroad networks and bridges reflected the rise of a specific technological profession—that of engineering. Gradually, moving into the 18th and 19th centuries, there is a continuous expansion of mining and textile industries that benefitted greatly from the new technologies.

It was not until the first half of the 19th century that science as a profession, per se, was organized on sound basis into a definite structure that also continued in later years. New scientific paradigms were created to cater to the needs of the expanding scientific horizons. Thus began new ideas of introducing electro-technology and of improved concepts of power. Much of the 19th century gave hope of successful technological progress. Some of these successes were used in war situations; for example, the invention of the Bessemer steel-making process by Henry Bessemer (1813–98). Bessemer invented new designs for heavy guns using new and cost-effective methods of manufacturing them.

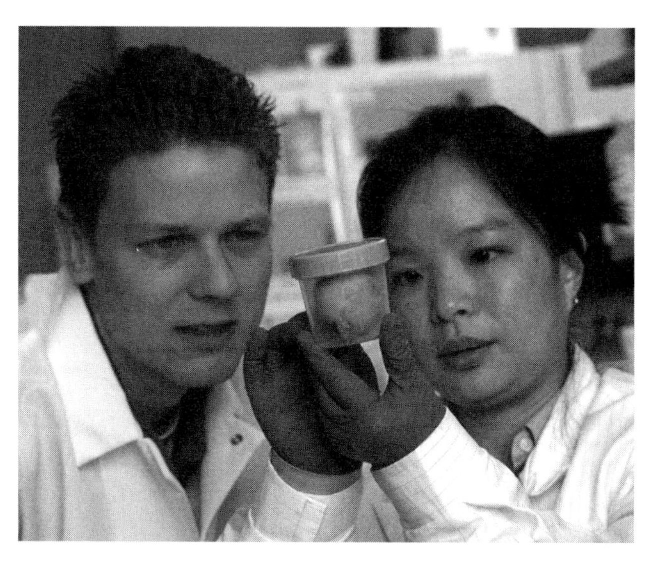

*In the past 30 years, Western scientists have used the term* biotechnology *to refer to laboratory-based techniques.*

With the systematization of science, it would seem imperative that medicine, which is so closely allied to the biological sciences, would be equally receptive. This was, however, not always the case. Medicine as a separate profession had its own trajectories, which were occasionally influenced directly by scientific and technological innovations. Pasteur's theory of disease brought in new perspectives on studying disease situations, and hence of practical medicine. The accumulated experience and research of previous years found expression in the second half of the 20th century, when new paradigms of scientific technology were formulated. This was technological revolution at its best. The evolutionary history of technology, thus, continued to be made up of technical innovations and newer processes of invention to address the changing needs of human society. George Basalla, on the contrary, sees the evolution of the history of technology in a different perspective. He believes that new technology emerges as a result of nature's superfluities.

The past few years have witnessed a sudden spur in research activities aiming to understand the development of the human body. Newer and more advanced technology has proven to be a major spur in the pace of such activities, and the new field that entails application of biological organisms to industry and medicine is called biotechnology. This field also encompasses a whole set of procedures for altering biological organisms in accordance with the needs of the community. Over the past three decades, biotechnology has been used by the Western scientific establishment to refer to laboratory-based techniques. Thus, although the new paradigms of science and its technological processes may offer promising potentials to the scientific community, they also warn us of the plausible dangers these may cause—dangers in terms of posing formidable challenges to the ethical values of mankind. Nevertheless, of late, more funds and efforts are being channeled into medical topics, focusing on newer biotechnologies that are the product of a plethora of discoveries over the past eight decades.

The rise of newer biotechnologies also reflects the engagement of the scientific community in unraveling the means by which technology could be applied to the benefit of humankind. On the significance of discoveries, Jonathan Morris believes that

> these discoveries have allowed scientists to become genetic engineers, enabling them to move genes from one living organism to another and change the proteins made by the new organism, whether it is a bacterium, plant, mouse, or even a human.

## NEW DIRECTIONS

Science and technology tend to have a symbiotic relationship in terms of mutual benefits accruing in both fields. On the one hand, although they both provide a means to alleviate human suffering, in terms of population increase, poverty, or health issues, they are also blamed for the evils of the modern world. Proponents of the latter view see an increasing propensity toward materialism and a decline in religious values and, hence, toward materialism. The truth, however, is that although the idea of materialism may be prone to criticism, it is a reflection on the developmental stage of a given society—a reflection on the felt need of the society at large. This means that no modern health and medical benefits can be accepted in isolation with the rest of the technological developments.

Given the gradual transition from chance or accidental discoveries to more specific and paradigm-oriented ones, it is not surprising that the world today seems overwhelmed by the emergence of stem cell research and stem cell therapeutics. The precursor to most stem cell technologies was probably provided by scientific curiosity about treating human diseases by altering the genetic constitution of human cells. It is a truism that stem cell research has ushered in an era in medical practice involving cell-based treatment of several diseases and illnesses. Despite the manifest functions of a rapidly developing technology and the recognized relevance of stem cell research in solving health problems, issues pertaining to the moral ethics of such research in a society cannot go amiss. In recent years, serious concerns have been expressed by the scientific community and the public about biotechnology and genetic engineering. Reflecting back in history, almost all societies have emphasized the relevance of ethics, contributing significantly to our understanding of morals and ethics. Plato was one of the first philosophers who advocated theories on ethics and morals.

The role played by stem cells in the development of the body is one of the most vibrant, yet controversial, areas in medical research. Although James Thomson and his colleagues devised new methods of maintaining human stem cells in culture, following the path breaking work by Leroy Stevens of naming of embryonic stem cells in 1970, Louis Pasteur is credited with establishing the scientific basis of biotechnology in the 19th century. His theory of the microbial origins of fermentation provided a new paradigm for science in later years.

But how does the scientific community convince society at large about the potential promises of the new form that medical practice has taken? The answer to this conundrum is not an easy one. However, it can be ascertained that because the Western medical profession was organized only retrospectively at the turn of the 20th century, it might be worthwhile studying the trajectories and compelling means by which humans have over the years realized the significance of newer technologies. While studying these technologies, surely, there are bound to be some less remarkable discoveries that were discarded during the process.

Historically speaking, advancement in scientific and medical knowledge has been concomitant with the need to reframe a new paradigm, and hence find new opportunities for proving this new paradigm. New discoveries often led to new inventions that would otherwise be seen as impossible. On the issue of scientific and technological progress, Francis Bacon identifies four major impediments to a smooth trajectory of these advancements. These include the idols of the Tribe, of the Den or Cave, of the Theater, and of the Marketplace. The Idols of the Tribe reflect the tendency to explain the phenomena in simplistic and general terms as a result of various psychological and physical constraints. The Idols of the Den have limitations imposed by the level of education of the scientific community. The Idols of the Theater tend to be strong in controlling the system as a result of the intellectual capabilities; they provide a base from where other thoughts emerge. Finally, the Idols of the Marketplace indicate various issues that emerge as a result of linguistic problems, and hence in limited human communication. As Donald Cardwell remarks, most importantly, the four ideals reflect the "limiting framework within which invention, creation and discovery are exercised."

On the issue of the role of technological discoveries, Cardwell writes,

> The complexity that characterizes major technological advances and the frequent dependence of invention on the intervention of outsiders imply that predicting the future course of technology with any degree of accuracy is practically impossible.

Francis Bacon is also credited with providing the first classification of scientific inventions and an international framework for the advancement of science, technology, and technological innovations that have an effect on mankind. He remarked that "the true and lawful goal of the sciences is none other than that human life be endowed with new discoveries and powers."

Hence, although the scientific community may continue to explore more advanced means of conquering disease conditions through newer technologies, it may still be hard to predict the effect and practical applications and the extent to which their limitations can be directed to absolute human benefit. Ironically, the rise of biotechnology opened up new vistas on the relationship between medical technology and society in terms of maintaining a balance between the quest for knowledge and human values. Nevertheless, ethical issues will always remain an integral part of the new paradigms in science, medicine, industry, and the society in which they are practiced.

To explore the potential effect of newer technologies, and to address social, legal, and ethical implications, the latest developments in biotechnology have made the participation of policy makers, the public, scientists, and physicians more imperative. Issues on government support and stipulations become central to this participation. As a major technological revolution of this century, biotechnologies have altered the way in which issues of health, disease, and environment are to be dealt with in relation to the society at large. Open debates and public discussions characterize this change.

## SOCIAL IMPLICATIONS

Although several legal, moral, and ethical issues have emerged as a result of the rapid pace of the development of biotechnologies, one area that looms large concerns the cloning of human beings, although to date no scientific rationale has come to the fore. One major concern, however, is the people's perception of the cloned individual and questions about identity and individuality, dignity, autonomy, and kinship ties in a social system. Francis Fukuyama's recent work, *Our Posthuman Future: Consequences of the Biotechnology Revolution*, reveals the trends in science, politics and philosophy, and medicine that may threaten to transform the very essence of human existence.

Issues of protecting human dignity and self-identity in relation to uses of human genetic materials have been taken up by an international ethics committee, the United Nations Educational, Scientific, and Cultural Organization (UNESCO). Gary E. McCuen discusses at length the role of the committee, called the UNESCO International Bioethics Committee; it set out its mandate of "preparation of an international instrument on the protection of the human genome," while addressing the legal, ethical, and social implications of the new technology. The cloning of an adult sheep called Dolly at the Roslin Institute in Scotland brought about a great deal of controversy on the moral ramifications of this success.

It also led to the identification of several potential medical applications for the technique by which the replica of an adult sheep was produced. The temporary ban on cloning in the late 1990s indicated that something that is morally incorrect is capable of becoming moral through public debate and discussions performed "before the new technology could be used." This, as Gary McCuen saw it,

> converted the grievous harms they now see into matters of preference and attitude, making moral truth the creature of public opinion and plebiscite. The moral arms of cloning are inherent in the concept itself, and in the fact that obtaining further information about harms and hazards depends upon the deliberate manufacture, manipulation, and destruction of human embryos.

In light of the above views, even a permanent ban on research activities is no sure way of preventing wrongful usage of the new technologies. Moral beliefs and values are relative to individual cultures, which limits the applicability of universal moral standards. This means that what is moral in one culture may not be considered so in another culture. Viewed using this perspective, stem cell research and newer biotechnologies also have different meanings assigned to them depending on the social milieu in which they are placed. Stated otherwise, with the rapid development of technoscience, along with its handmaiden field of genetics, the science–industrial complex, Steven Best and Douglas Kellner suggest:

> seems to rush toward a posthuman culture that unfolds in the increasingly intimate merging of technology and biology. The posthuman involves both new conceptions of the human in an age of information and communication, and new modes of existence as flesh merges with steel, circuitry, and genes from other species. Technoscience, thus, intensifies further translates research activities and experimentation into human cloning.

## THE FUTURE

Amid the ensuing controversies over biotechnology, technoscience, and stem cell research, as well as the various social and moral implications of these new disciplines, what remains to be seen is the way these disciplines are handled by the government with respect to people's rights and their perceptions of these rights. The plausible ramifications of these new technologies may be hard to predict, although it is almost certain that in the years to come, they would have taken care of a lot of health issues and maladies with which biomedicine perhaps may not have dealt in their entirety.

Perhaps there may still be several questions unanswered by the medical community: To what extent can a policy be developed that will reflect people's concern while at the same time developing new therapeutics for incurable diseases? How do physicians and theologians come to an amicable understanding of the effects of new technologies on society? Can biotechnology really transform our lives? In the past, the effect of technologies could not be predicted with exactitude, so people had to adjust after they were introduced. However, now people's participation is also considered to be equally important when informing them of the possible social effect of new technologies. As Jonathan Morris remarks:

> as biotechnology is one area that has aroused serious concerns over its applicability before authentication of experiments, what remains to be seen is the extent this is likely to draw state support only in the light of predictions that biotechnology can lead to miraculous medi-

cal treatments, and that humanity may benefit from these discoveries.

Despite the perceived social effect of specific new technologies, especially human cloning and stem cell research, the systematic investigations, trial experiments, and application of knowledge systems are worth an appraisal.

A final note on the emerging technologies and their relevance in contemporary societies. As indicated above, new technologies have been associated with complex ethical issues that are new to mankind. In view of this, it is important to note that the emerging trends in globalization have further necessitated a consideration of cultural aspects, and hence new challenges for ethical decisions, for decisions in one culture may have different consequences in another culture. Because culture entails a set of institutions, including religion, polity, beliefs, and values accumulated over several years, knowledge of these practices and institutions is imperative in matters of morals and ethics. As Thomas Budinger and Miriam Budinger put it, "there is a need to revisit the major moral, spiritual, and ideological theories in order to address the ethical problems with some accuracy."

**SEE ALSO:** Cells, Embryonic; Cloning; Thomson, James.

**BIBLIOGRAPHY.** George Basalla, *The Evolution of Technology* (Cambridge University Press, 1998); Steven Best and Douglas Kellner, *The Postmodern Adventure* (Guilford and Routledge, 2001); Thomas F. Budinger and Miriam D. Budinger, *Ethics of Emerging Technologies* (Wiley, 2006); Donald Cardwell, *The Norton History of Technology* (Norton, 1995); Francis Fukuyama, *Our Posthuman Future: Consequences of the Biotechnology Revolution* (Farrar, Straus and Giroux, 2002); Gary E. McGuen, *Cloning Science and Society: Ideas in Conflict* (Gary E. McCuen, 1998); Jonathan Morris, *The Ethics of Biotechnology: Biotechnology in the 21st Century* (Chelsea House, 2006); *Executive Summary: Biotechnology and Society in the 21st Century* (UNESCO, 1999).

Poonam Bala
University of Delhi

# Birth Dating of Cells by Retrovirus

**BIRTH DATING OF** cells is important to fully elucidate when a cell has been created, to determine what factors or conditions may have led to its conception. Birth dating has been applied within many cell constructs, though recent attention has focused on cells within the central nervous system. With the relatively recent discovery of neurogenesis, a process of creating functionally integrated neurons from progenitor cells, a plethora of innovative techniques to track the rate of cell birth have been developed.

Among some of the most widely used techniques for birth dating of cells are analyses based on the incorporation of nucleotide analogs during cell division, expression of specific markers during the maturation process, and genetic marking with retroviruses. The most robust and reliable results for birth dating are generated from nucleotide analogs and genetic marking by retrovirus, whereas the expression of specific markers has elicited relatively poor results. Birth dating of cells by retrovirus has stimulated a great deal of interest because of the ability to visualize tissue directly, as opposed to the nucleotide analog methodology, which requires tissue fixation and DNA denaturing. Though the retroviral method is invasive, many researchers feel that the pros outweigh the cons of this newly developed birth dating technique.

Within the paradigm of neurogenesis, it is extremely important to understand when a functional neuron has been created. This information is critical, as it allows researchers to focus on aspects of the microenvironment at a specific time point that led to the production of new cells. This essentially enables researchers to "rewind time" to reliably chart cell birth and development in a living system. As a consequence, important facts about neurogenesis can be collected, such as the region of the brain in which this process is occurring, particular factors/neurotransmitters that are present in the microenvironment at the appropriate time, genes that may be upregulated or downregulated, and so on. Birth dating of cells by retrovirus can provide all of these details in a living system, which has afforded the most convincing evidence thus far that newborn neurons in the adult mammalian central nervous system are in fact functional and physiologically active. The ability of a retrovirus to integrate into normally functioning tissue offers a tremendous advantage compared with other techniques.

To fully comprehend the use of a retrovirus to date the birth of a cell, one must understand the properties of a retrovirus. Retroviruses are enveloped viruses with an RNA genome that replicate via a DNA intermediate. Retroviruses rely on the enzyme reverse transcriptase to reverse transcribe its genome from RNA into DNA, which can then be integrated into the host's genome using the enzyme integrase. The virus then replicates as part of the host cell's DNA. Furthermore, there are many different subfamilies of retroviruses that each have different properties. For example, the oncovirus subfamily of retroviruses depends on host cell proliferation for completion of the viral life cycle, whereas the lentivirus subfamily replicates without this process. It is important for researchers to understand the intricacies of the retroviral vector they choose, as some vectors rely on the breakdown of the host cell's nuclear membrane for integration, whereas some possess the appropriate nuclear import abilities so that integration into the host cell's genome can occur at all times.

Analysis of cell birth based on genetic marking with retroviruses involves the expression of transgenes from retroviruses. Transgenes are genes that are taken from the genome of the retrovirus and introduced into the genome of the cell of interest. For this mechanism to take place, viral integration into the host genome must occur. Some retroviruses, such as the Muloney murine leukemia virus, lack nuclear import mechanisms, causing the retrovirus to limit viral integration to when the host nuclear membrane dissolves during mitosis. Ultimately, this allows such a retrovirus to serve as a sufficient marker of host cell division. Expression of a live reporter such as green fluorescent protein (GFP) allows direct visualization of fully functioning newborn cells. GFP fills the cell body of the neuron or cell of interest, making structural analysis an additional possibility. To appropriately label proliferating cells, a highly concentrated retroviral stock carrying the GFP transgene must be administered. Though retroviral labeling can be quite variable, there is usually a relatively high percentage of GFP cells expressed.

## PROS AND CONS

Birth dating of cells through use of a retrovirus has many pros and cons. In terms of benefits, this method has elicited some of the most robust results to date concerning analysis of adult neurogenesis in living creatures. It is a specific procedure that facilitates identification of the few newborn neurons surrounded by billions of preexisting neurons in the adult central nervous system. Retroviral dating of recently created cells also allows direct visualization and analysis of such cells through use of the GFP live reporter. This is a major benefit, as one can observe living cells functioning in their normal environment as opposed to requiring cells to be sacrificed and subsequently fixed. Furthermore, whole-cell morphology can be analyzed using this method. Although the nucleotide analog method of birth dating is limited to the nuclear region of the cell of interest, genetic marking by retrovirus can truly evaluate all aspects of the cell. Again, GFP facilitates this process, as it is a live reporter, in addition to serving as a protein that permeates the cell body of a neuron.

Although this method does possess many benefits, there are some significant disadvantages to its use. The first and most apparent disadvantage to this method involves the invasive stereotaxic injection into specific brain regions. Considering that the majority of mammalian neurogenesis occurs in three deep-set regions of the brain, the actual administration of the retrovirus into these regions is challenging. The three regions of interest are the subventricular zone of the lateral ventricles, the subgranular zone of the dentate gyrus in the hippocampus, and the more rostral olfactory bulbs.

A needle must directly penetrate these regions so that high doses of retrovirus may be administered in a deliberate and intentional manner. As a result, although the retrovirus itself may be specific, the likelihood of experimental error during direct administration is high. Finally, birth dating of cells by retrovirus presents a risk of infection in the host organism. Any direct penetration of the skull and brain tissue of a mammal presents immunological challenges that may affect the corresponding results of the experiment.

In summary, birth dating of cells by retrovirus has become a reliable and innovative method for investigating adult neurogenesis. Although researchers are satisfied with results obtained from this single-cell genetic technique thus far, future goals include combining small inhibitory RNA—a short sequence of RNA that can be used to silence gene expression—to generate even more specific results.

**SEE ALSO:** Brain; Cancer; Cells, Neural.

**BIBLIOGRAPHY.** Bruce Alberts, et al., *Molecular Biology of the Cell*, 4th ed. (Garland Science Publishers, 2002); Michael J. Aminoff, David A. Greenberg, and Roger P. Simon, *Clinical Neurology*, 6th ed. (Lange Medical Books/McGraw-Hill, 2005); Paul F. Lewis and Michael Emerman, "Passage through Mitosis Is Required for Oncoretroviruses but Not for the Human Immunodeficiency Virus," *Journal of Virology* (v.68/1, 1994); Guo-li Ming and Hongjun Song, "Adult Neurogenesis in the Mammalian Central Nervous System," *Annual Review of Neuroscience* (v.28, 2005); Henriette van Praag, et al., "Functional Neurogenesis in the Adult Hippocampus," *Nature* (v.415, 2002).

Misty C. Richards
Albany Medical College

# Blood

**RECENTLY, STEM CELLS** have gained a tremendous amount of attention. The scientific press emphasizes the particular values of embryonal stem cells, which presumably have true pluripotentiality. The lay press, in contrast, focuses on the discussion of topics such as the legal, moral, religious, and practical aspects of stem cell research, and particularly the indeterminate use of stem cells in the treatment of patients and the issue of harvesting embryonal stem cells. In the beginning, there was a concept that hematopoietic stem cells are only capable of producing blood cells, but now researchers have shown that hematopoietic stem cells may also show plasticity and mature into liver cells, bone cells, or new muscle cells (e.g., replacing injured myocardium). This article covers the physiology of blood, the role of stem cells, bloodborne diseases involving stem cells in bone marrow, and briefly reviews bone marrow transplantation.

## NORMAL BLOOD

The function of blood in body is nutritive, respiratory, excretory, body defense (immunity), and for the transportation of hormones, vitamins, and drugs. Normal blood is composed of different types of cells suspended in plasma, which makes up about 55 percent of total blood volume. The plasma mainly consists of a variety of chemical constituents dissolved in water and blood cells. In terms of categories of cells, there are red blood cells, platelets, basophils, eosinophils, neutrophils, monocytes, and lymphocytes. The chemicals are mainly proteins (e.g., albumin, globulin, and fibrinogen), vitamins (e.g., A, D, E, and K), hormones (e.g., steroid hormones), electrolytes (e.g., Na+, K+, and Ca++), organic molecules (e.g., urea, glucose, and lipids), and antibodies.

Half of blood volume is contributed by the red blood cell mass. Red cells contain hemoglobin, the protein that performs the function of binding oxygen from the lungs and delivering it to the tissues of the body. White blood cells, which include neutrophils and monocytes, also called phagocytes, have the ability to ingest fungi or bacteria and kill them. Whenever there is an infection in the body, these neutrophils and monocytes leave the blood vessels and move into the tissue spaces and start ingesting the invading bacteria or fungi,

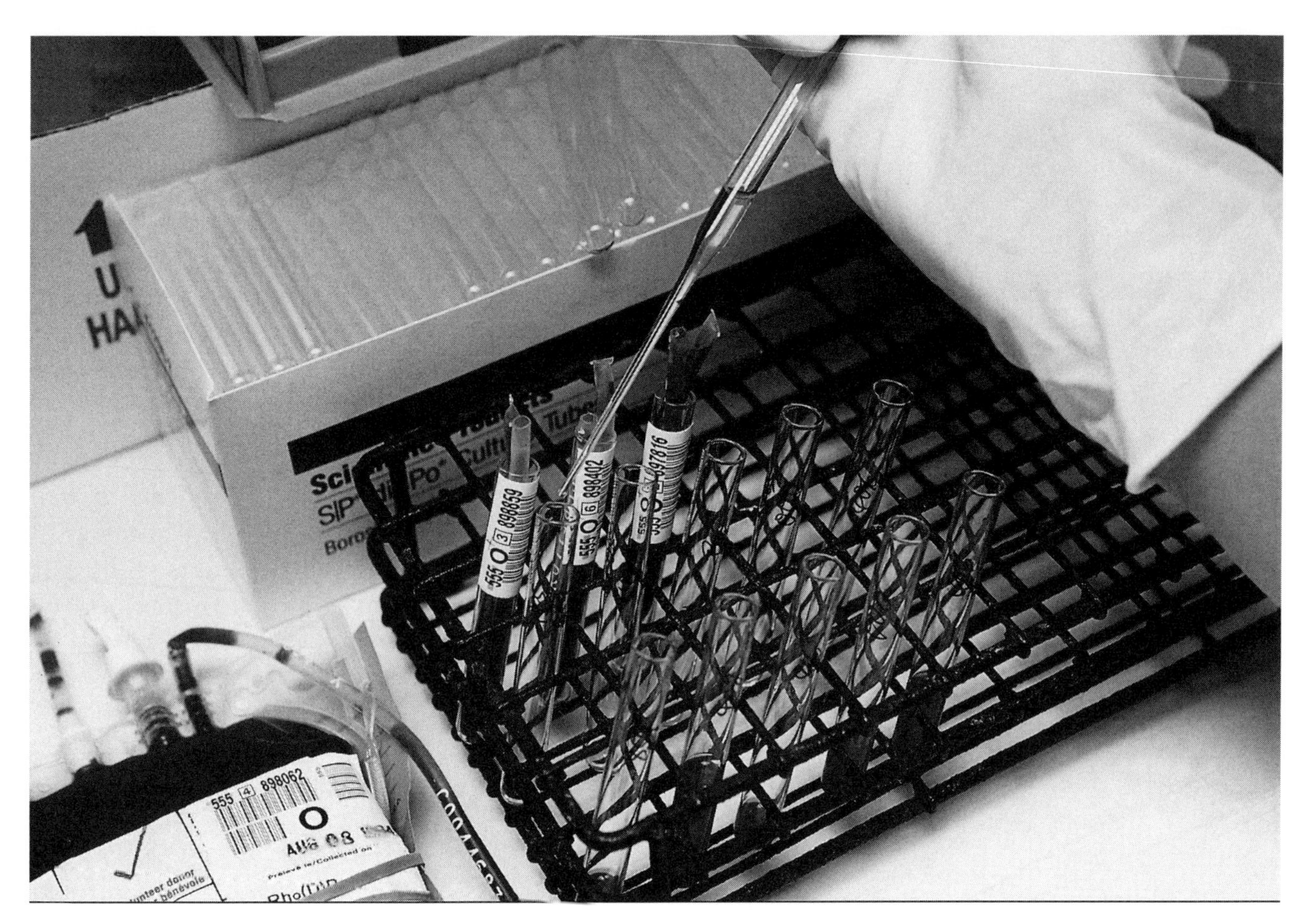

*Public and private umbilical cord blood banks are collecting and storing cord blood for use as an alternative source of hematopoietic stem cells, but more of these cells are still needed.*

thus protecting the body against infection. In allergic responses, eosinophils and basophils play an important role. One of the most important cell types in the line of defense of the body are lymphocytes (T cells, B cells, and natural killer cells), which are found in spleen, lymph nodes, lymphatic channels, and blood. Platelets, which are derivatives of special types of cells called megakaryocytes in the bone marrow, play a role in stopping bleeding when the body is injured. Whenever there is an insult to the vessel wall, platelets come in contact with the wall and both undergo a shape change and release substances that attract more platelets to the injury site, forming a plug by clumping together, making a clot. Gradually, the vessel wall heals at the site of the clot and comes back to its normal condition.

All bones have active marrow at birth. Bone marrow is a spongy tissue that occupies the central cavity of bone. Here all blood cells are formed. With the passage of time, as a person reaches adulthood, active bone marrow is restricted to only skull bones, hip and shoulder bones, ribs, breast bone, and the vertebrae, whereas the bones of the legs, feet, hands, and arms lack functioning marrow.

Hematopoiesis is the process of formation of new blood cells. All blood cells come from a single class of primitive mother cells called pluripotent stem cells. These stem cells then differentiate into specific blood cell types by a process called differentiation. They are tremendously important in body growth and development and in the repair of tissues. Stem cells have the ability to differentiate into any type of cells in the body, acquiring their characteristics and functioning like they do. Therefore, stem cells have great value in treating different medical conditions. Diseases such as leukemia, lymphoma, and other blood-related disorders have been treated by taking adult blood stem cells from the bone marrow of a donor, who could be either unrelated or a relative of the person.

There are two main types of stem cells: Embryonic stem cells have the characteristic of discriminating into more than 200 types of cells. Adult stem cells are capable of differentiating into varieties of a specific cell type, depending on the location they are found in the body. For example, blood stem cells are capable of giving rise to red blood cells, white blood cells, and platelets. The term *adult stem cells* is used because these cells are farther along the course of differentiation as compared with embryonic stem cells.

## UMBILICAL CORD BLOOD STEM CELLS

Umbilical cord blood stem cells can be taken out after birth from the umbilical cord. This blood is also enriched with hematopoietic stem cells similar to bone marrow. The use of cord blood as a source of stem cells has superiority, as umbilical cord blood is sufficient and easily available. Umbilical cord stem cells are also regarded as neonatal stem cells and are less mature as compared with the hematopoietic stem cells of adult bone marrow.

At this time, public and private cord blood banks are collecting and storing cord blood. In terms of the treatment of leukemia and other blood disorders, cord blood has recently gotten immense attention as an alternative source of hematopoietic stem cells. However, for the treatment of blood disorders in adults, the number of hematopoietic stem cells available is not adequate.

## APLASTIC ANEMIA

In aplastic anemia, there occurs a failure of hematopoiesis; the bone marrow appears empty, and the blood cell count falls to a great degree. The mechanism working behind aplastic anemia is now regarded as being immune mediated, in which there is active destruction of stem cells by lymphocytes. Because of this destruction, a reduction in all blood cell types occurs; this reduction is called pancytopenia. The affected types of blood cells are red cells, white blood cells, and platelets. This immune response can be initiated by number of factors such as exposure to chemicals and drugs, endogenous antigens produced by modified bone marrow, or viral infection.

Aplastic anemia can be efficaciously treated by immunosuppressive therapy or stem cell transplantation. Hematopoiesis can be restored by antithymocyte globulin (ATG) and drugs such as cyclosporine in about two thirds of patients. ATG comprises rabbit-derived antibodies that are infused in the patient's blood against human T cells in the prevention and treatment of acute rejection in therapy and organ transplantation in aplastic anemia. However, the improvement of the blood cell count is often inadequate, recurrent pancytopenia requires retreatment, and complications such as myelodysplasia have been reported in patients with the disease.

## ACUTE LEUKEMIAS

Acute leukemias are characteristically transformed cells that vary with respect to their immunologic, cytogenetic, and morphological properties. This type of cancer is rarely seen in people younger than 40 years and usually tends to occur around the age of 65 years. This disease is more common in men than women. Acute leukemias are divided into lymphoid and myeloid types by morphological and cytochemical criteria. According to researchers, there are variety of causes that scientist believe may contribute in this disease, but still the primary cause is unknown. Some of the factors involved include diet, interaction with the environment, exposure to ionizing radiation, medicines, and increased susceptibility.

In acute leukemias, the bone marrow starts developing abnormal cells. These cells have a characteristically faster growth rate than the normal healthy blood cells and begin to replace them. The body's immune system is badly damaged as a result of the lack of formation of new cells for fighting infections, and ultimately the bone marrow stops working adequately. These patients have an increased susceptibility to infections and, as a result of a depletion of healthy blood cells, tend to have a gain in risk for bleeding. There are a number of symptoms that could be found in patients with acute leukemias such as bleeding gums, bone pain or tenderness, skin rash, abnormal menstrual periods, and bleeding from the nose. The physical examination of such patients reveals a swollen spleen, liver, or lymph nodes. White blood cell count can be either normal or high or low, whereas the platelet count will be lower than normal values, and anemia is found when a complete blood count is performed. When bone marrow aspiration is carried out in such patients, many show leukemic cells.

## BONE MARROW TRANSPLANT

A bone marrow transplant is the process of replacing the bone marrow of a patient that is not working properly with healthy bone marrow. There are many circumstances that may involve bone marrow needing to be transplanted, such as hereditary immune deficiencies, hereditary metabolic diseases, hereditary blood diseases, and several types of cancer. Healthy bone marrow taken from a donor and transplanted into the person with the disease is called an allograft; if the marrow is taken from the same patient before chemotherapy or radiation therapy, it is called an autograft.

In conditions such as leukemia, to eliminate the cancer cells, high doses of chemotherapy may be needed. During this process, however, normal, healthy cells are destroyed as well as the diseased cells. In other cases in which there is abnormal blood cell production, these conditions can be corrected by healthy bone marrow transplantation, which restores the production of white blood cells, red blood cells, and platelets.

Once bone marrow is taken from the donor, it is filtered, treated, and either transplanted immediately or frozen and stored for future purpose. Then donor marrow is transfused into the patient through a vein, where it is naturally transmitted to the bone cavities, where it grows and replaces the old bone marrow. Stem cells, by using special medications, can be made to move from the bone marrow to the bloodstream and can be taken out through a special procedure called leukapheresis.

Before the transplantation, the donor's compatibility is tested to determine the tissue type or human leukocyte antigen type. Human cells contain specific proteins on their surface that differ in every individual. Similarly, leukocytes also have certain surface proteins. Therefore, human leukocyte antigen type can be determined by testing the leukocytes present in the blood sample of the patient and the donor. The body's immune system has the ability to identify these surface proteins, and the lymphocytes of the patient can start killing or rejecting the transplant.

The donor's immune cells also identify the patient's cells and start attacking them in turn. These reactions are common in nonidentical siblings, even though tissue typing has been carried out. If the donor or recipients are identical twins, the reactions do not happen. Therefore, to overcome this problem, the immune system of the recipient is suppressed before transplantation, and after transplantation, the donor's immune cells are suppressed.

Bone marrow transplant may be recommended in a number of conditions including leukemias (acute myelogenous, acute lymphoblastic, chronic myelogenous, chronic lymphocytic), lymphomas (non-Hodgkin's, Hodgkin's), plasma cell disorders (myeloma, amyloidosis), congenital disorders (immunodeficiencies, thalassemia, sickle cell anemia), and acquired bone marrow disorders (severe aplastic anemia, myelodysplastic syndrome, myeloproliferative disorders).

**SEE ALSO:** Birth Dating of Cells by Retrovirus; Bone Diseases; Bone Marrow Transplants; Cancer; Cells, Umbilical.

**BIBLIOGRAPHY.** The Century Foundation, www.tcf.org (cited December 2007); Health Library at Stanford, healthlibrary.stanford.edu (cited December 2007); University of Pennsylvania Health System, pennhealth.com (cited December 2007).

G. Ishaq Khan
Dow University of Health Sciences

# Bone Diseases

**BONE IS THE** main weight-bearing tissue of the body and functions to withstand mechanical forces several times the weight of the body. Despite the numerous shapes and sizes of the bones in the body, bone tissue is structurally and microscopically similar throughout. Bone tissue exists in two general forms: Cortical bone composes the shell of many of the long bones and has low porosity and high density and strength. Cancellous (or trabecular) bone is found at the ends of long bones or in low–weight bearing areas (such as the lower jaw) and is composed of microscopic interconnecting bony trabecula, giving macroscopically high porosity and low density.

Although bone tissue is generally thought of as a rigid structure, it contains both elastic and stiff components. The bone extracellular matrix is approximately 65 percent inorganic, mainly calcium and phosphate in the form of hydroxyapatite, and 35 percent organic matrix (osteoid), mainly collagen, which is a ropelike fiber. This general composition gives bone marked rigidity while retaining some elasticity, with the collagen fibers of the organic matrix providing high tensile strength to resist pulling forces and the inorganic mineral providing high compressive strength to resist crushing forces.

Contrary to the popular belief that bones are inert structures, bone tissue is remarkably active. Bone is constantly being remodeled to maintain optimal structure, which includes two parallel processes. Bone resorption, or breaking down of bone tissue, is carried out by the osteoclasts. Bone formation is carried out by the osteoblasts, which lay down new bone to replace the old. A small number of osteoblasts become entrenched in their own calcified matrix and become stationary osteocytes, which have recently been identified as playing a role in initiating and coordinating the remodeling process. Approximately 99 percent of calcium is also stored in the bones; this calcium is constantly being removed for use throughout the body, to be replaced later.

Within the hollow interior of the long bones and among the trabecula of cancellous bone lies the bone marrow. Bone marrow is separated into red and yellow marrow. Red marrow is the myeloid, or blood, portion of the marrow and is where most new red blood cells are produced. Yellow marrow is made mostly of fat cells but also contains multiple other types of stromal cells, including fibroblasts, osteoblasts, and blood vessel cells. Some of these cells play important roles in maintaining specific microenvironments within the marrow, such as the hematopoietic stem cell compartment, which provides the multipotent cells that form all types of blood cells. Bone marrow stromal cells, or mesenchymal stem cells, have also been isolated that have the ability to differentiate into bone, fat, and cartilage lineages. Cells with a similar differentiation ability, called pericytes, are localized in the bone marrow immediately adjacent to blood vessels.

## TYPES OF BONE DISEASES

Bone diseases often arise from the breakdown of one of the surprising number of homeostatic processes that bone performs. The most common bone diseases originate from disruption of the delicate balance of bone remodeling, leading to either excessive bone formation (osteopetrosis) or resorption (osteoporosis). Osteoporosis is clinically defined as a symptomatic, generalized decrease in bone mass.

Osteoporosis naturally begins after about age 40 years in both men and women and proceeds with about a 3–4 percent loss of bone mass per decade; it can also be accelerated by endogenous or exogenous factors, such as the withdrawal of estrogen in postmenopausal osteoporosis of women. Because of the reduction in bone mass, fractures become much more probable, mostly in the vertebrae and hip. Because of the weakening bone, these fractures often need to be fixated with rods or fracture plates, and if the break is severe enough, a joint replacement may be necessitated. Because of the progressing disease and the prevalence of osteoporosis in the elderly, a population that heals slowly, even these interventions often fail, leaving survivors seriously disabled. Osteoporosis has been diagnosed in about 10 million Americans, costing nearly $18 billion in medical expenses in 2002. The disease affects women, mainly postmenopausal, much more frequently than men, with about a 4:1 ratio of women to men.

Similar to osteoporosis, osteomalacia is a disease that weakens the bones. However, in osteomalacia, the bone remodeling process remains balanced, and the defect lies in the mineralization of the bone tissue. Osteomalacia has been linked to vitamin D deficiency, whether from external factors such as diet or internal problems such as digestive tract or kidney disorders, and can often be treated with vitamin D supplements. Osteopetrosis is opposite of these bone deteriorating diseases, swinging the bone remodeling process too far toward formation. Osteopetrosis is a much less common congenital condition characterized by defective osteoclast function that results in malformed bones that cannot resist average forces and break easily. The condition is rare, but it currently has no cure and can only be clinically managed by repairing the inevitable fractures. Paget's disease represents another imbalance of the bone remodeling process, in which resorbed bone is replaced by softer, more fragile bone. Although the mechanisms of Paget's disease are not understood, fracture risk increases as a result of poor bone quality.

Genetic abnormalities also underlie many bone diseases. Osteogenesis imperfecta (OI) occurs in about 1 in 20,000 people and is often called brittle bone disease. The disease arises from the aberrant production of type I collagen, the main elastic constituent of bone. People who suffer from OI produce either a poorer quality or a decreased quantity of collagen than normal, leading to weak bones that fracture easily. Fibrous dysplasia of bone is a disorder characterized by fibrous lesions that develop within bone, leading to weakened bone and increased pain, fracture, or deformity.

Similar to almost every other tissue in the body, bone is subject to cancerous growth of its cells, although to a lesser degree than other tissues, with malignant bone tumors being rare. Osteosarcomas are the most common primary malignant bone tumors, usually affecting children and young adults at locations of rapidly growing bone. Luckily, the prognosis is generally positive after removal of the osteosarcoma. However, because osteosarcomas can sometimes require removal of a large portion of bone, fixation devices such as fracture plates or even total joint replacements may be required to maintain proper load-bearing capabilities.

Infection is also not selective and can affect bone tissue, when it is termed *osteomyelitis*. Although normally resistant to this disease, bones become susceptible to infection after events such as surgery or trauma. Although generally treatable with antibiotics and minor surgery, infections sometimes require major resections of bone.

## CURRENT TREATMENT STRATEGIES

Most bone diseases progress slowly in degrading the skeletal system, and in general, treatment strategies reflect the stage of progression of the disease. The amount of invasiveness of the procedure required also increases as bone diseases progress, with early to midstage progressions of skeletal diseases often requiring only noninvasive methods to relieve symptoms, halt the progression of, or even reverse the disorder.

Osteoporosis is an example of a bone disease that is often preventable or treatable if caught early. Because osteoporosis usually occurs in postmenopausal women, many preventative measures such as increased exercise, weight loss, and calcium supplements are highly recommended to those at risk and help to prevent the beginning stages of bone loss. When decreased bone mass and increased risk of fracture is diagnosed, drug therapies are often prescribed that include bisphosphonates, estrogen/hormone therapy, and selective estrogen receptor modulators. Bisphosphonates act on the remodeling cycle of bone and decrease bone resorption while not affecting bone formation, with the long-term goal of increasing bone mass. Many of these drug approaches have also been attempted in other bone deteriorating diseases, such as OI, but have been less successful there.

If bone can no longer maintain its weight-bearing responsibilities and severely limits normal daily activity, such as in late-stage osteoporosis or after removal of large tumors, artificial materials must be implanted to replace or assist the defective skeletal structures. Current approaches in medicine at this point commonly dictate implantation of high-strength biomaterials such as metals or ceramics. The current gold standard is titanium implants, which combine high strength and excellent biocompatibility. Inside the body, titanium forms an extremely inert passivating layer that limits the immune response to only a short, acute response and allows titanium implants remarkable capacity for integration with host bone. The great success of titanium implants can be attributed to their predictable and long-term restoration of mechanical function, leading to an explosion of popularity in recent years. However, artificial implants such as titanium still have drawbacks, such as inadequate bone ingrowth and failure to maintain adequate peri-implant bone density because of osteolysis at the bone–implant interface, requiring painful revision surgeries.

## REGENERATIVE MEDICINE AND STEM CELL APPROACHES

Many of the drawbacks and failures of artificial implants can be attributed to the fact that they repair but do not regenerate damaged tissue. In this respect, the field of regenerative medicine has modeled many treatments after the natural development and regeneration of bone tissue.

Biomechanical factors have been known for many years to mediate bone growth and remodeling. This process is best exemplified by astronauts who spend long flights in weightless space, leading to widespread bone loss. Through currently unknown pathways, biomechanical forces stimulate osteoblastic deposition and calcification of bone, and lack of force leads to resorption. Through this feedback system, bone changes both its mass and morphology to develop the strength required as well as the optimal shape to satisfy its load-bearing requirements. The form, magnitude, and frequency of the mechanical load on bone have all been shown to affect the bone response. This is likely one reason why exercise is such a critical factor in preventing bone loss associated with osteoporosis. Simple mechanical stimulation such as that gained from standing on a vibrating platform has been shown to prevent postmenopausal bone loss in women. Less understood are other physical factors such as ultrasound that have shown to improve fracture healing and other forms of skeletal repair.

Chemical cues in the form of growth factors have also been applied in the regeneration of bone. The transforming growth factor (TGF) superfamily has been one of the most extensively studied in this respect. TGF 1 can stimulate cellular proliferation, chemotaxis, and collagen type I production in bone cells; its main role in bone repair seems to be stimulating initial osteoid production and recruiting and expanding the bone cell progenitor pool. Bone morphogenetic proteins (BMPs) can exert strong bone-forming effects by inducing differentiation of immature mesenchymal cells, as well as exhibiting chemotactic and proliferative effects. The powerful BMP2 also stimulates bone formation when injected into muscle tissue.

Outside of the TGF superfamily, the fibroblast growth factors are mitogenic growth factors and exert multiple effects on bone formation including expansion of progenitors and stimulation of angiogenesis (growth of new blood vessels), so that much-needed nutrients can reach newly forming bone. Angiogenic-specific growth factors such as vascular endothelial growth factor and platelet-derived growth factor also promote new vessel infiltration and exert mitogenic and chemotactic effects on bone and progenitor cells. Delivery of all of these growth factors has led to accelerated fracture or artificial implant healing and can even induce regeneration of critical size defects, which are injuries in bone that would never completely heal naturally. However, growth factors often degrade quickly in the body, so release systems such as polymers that provide constant growth factor levels over time are required for their efficient use.

Last, providing cellular help to damaged skeletal tissue is a promising avenue for successful regeneration. Originally, mature osteoblasts were tested for this approach and were successful in regenerating small defects in bone, but their limited proliferative potential prevented their use in repairing largely damaged bone. This restriction inspired the search for alternative pools of cells, leading to the discovery of many different pools of multipotent cells with bone-forming ability. Bone marrow stromal cells, or mesenchymal stem cells, can be isolated that retain a large proliferative potential as well as the ability to differentiate to bone, cartilage, and fat. These cells can form bone with high efficiency and have been successfully used in many studies to treat bone defects and diseases.

Multipotent pericytes that surround blood vessels in the bone marrow and multipotent fibroblast-like cells from fat tissue have also been isolated and exhibit the ability to form new bone tissue when correctly implanted. Taking an even farther step back in development, the mechanisms behind the differentiation of embryonic stem cells to bone cells is just beginning to be understood and may represent an almost infinite pool of renewable cells to treat bone disease.

The most exciting and promising approaches combine all of these strategies to grow mature bone tissue outside the body before implantation into diseased areas. Cells, growth factors, and mechanical stimulation are simultaneously placed into a tissue engineering scaffold, which is a biomaterial that provides structure and encourages the growth of bone tissue. Although much research still needs to be done to determine optimal combinations of cells, growth factors, mechanical stimulation, and biomaterials, tissue engineered scaffolds could potentially offer long-term regenerative cures for many bone diseases.

**SEE ALSO:** Blood; Bone Marrow Transplants; Cancer.

**BIBLIOGRAPHY.** E. F. McCarthy and F. J. Frassica, *Pathology of Bone and Joint Disorders* (W. B. Saunders, 1998); National Osteoporosis Foundation, www.nof.org (cited November 2007); National Institute of Arthritis and Musculoskeletal and Skin Diseases, National Institutes of Health, www.niams.nih.gov (cited November 2007); R. P. Lanza, R. Langer, and J. P. Vacanti, eds., *Principles of Tissue Engineering* (Academic Press, 2007).

Paul A. Clark
University of Wisconsin, Madison
John S. Kuo
University of Wisconsin, Madison

# Bone Marrow Transplants

**BONE MARROW IS** a spongy material that fills the bone cavities. It contains a network of blood vessels and fibers surrounded by fat and cells. At the time of birth, bone marrow can be found in all bones. When the person reaches adulthood, however, not all of the marrow is still functioning. Inactive bone marrow can be found in the bones of legs, feet, hands, and arms; functioning marrow is restricted to the bones of the skull, shoulders, ribs, hips, breastbone, and vertebrae. Bone marrow contains special type of cells—stem cells—that are producing different types of cells by the process of differentiation. This article discusses the fundamentals of bone marrow, stem cells, and the process involving in bone marrow transplantation.

Blood is composed of plasma and the blood cells. These blood cells come from a single class of primitive mother cells called stem cells. The process of formation of new blood cells is called hematopoiesis. Stem cells are performing the role of producing different types of blood cells (red blood cells, platelets, neutrophils, monocytes, eosinophils, basophils, and lymphocytes) by the process of differentiation. Blood cells are formed in the bone marrow, and when they are fully developed and capable of performing their role in the body, they leave the bone marrow and enter the blood stream.

There are two main types of stem cells: embryonic stem cells, which are capable of differentiating into different types of blood cells in the body, and adult stem cells, which can modify themselves according to the specific cell type, depending on the location of the body.

The cells involved in transplant can be removed from the body from three sources: from the umbilical cord after the birth of a baby, from the bone marrow, and from peripheral blood.

## BONE MARROW TRANSPLANT

The transplantation of bone marrow is a process involving the exchange of the diseased or inadequately functioning bone marrow of a patient with healthy and actively working marrow. In certain diseases such as leukemias or aplastic anemia, transplantation of bone marrow is a standard method of restoring the formation of new blood cells. There are a number of conditions for which bone marrow transplantation is needed. These conditions include lymphomas (Hodgkin's, non-Hodgkin's), plasma cell disorders (amyloidosis, myeloma), leukemias (acute myelogenous, acute lymphoblastic, chronic myelogenous, chronic lymphocytic), acquired bone marrow disorders (severe aplastic anemia, myelodysplastic syndrome, myeloproliferative disorders), and congenital disorders (sickle cell anemia, thalassemia, immunodeficiencies).

Regarding stem cell transplantation, which may be from bone marrow, peripheral blood, or cord blood, the patient's own stem cells can be used in what are called autologous transplants, or a matched donor, who could be either related or unrelated to the patient, can donate blood in what are called allogeneic transplants. In diseases such as leukemias, the transplantation of blood-forming (hematopoietic) stem cells is carried out to reestablish the body's own blood and immune cell production. Hematopoietic stem cells have the ability to differentiate into any of the three cell types: white blood cells, red blood cells, and platelets. Whenever bone marrow is taken from the donor, it is immediately filtered, treated, and transplanted or is frozen or stored for future use. This procedure is performed by transfusing the donor's marrow into the patient by means of a vein; the transplanted bone marrow is naturally transmitted to the bone cavities. After reaching the bone cavities, the new marrow starts to proliferate and replace the old marrow.

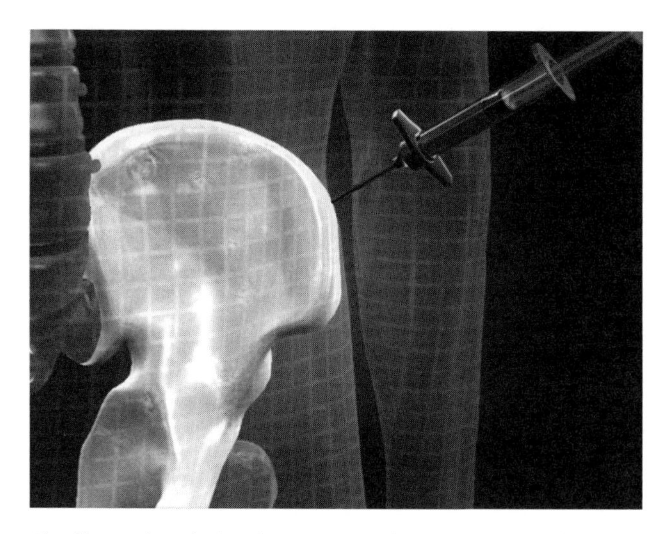

*The illustration depicts bone marrow being harvested from the hip bone, which contains active bone marrow even in adults.*

## PERIPHERAL BLOOD

Peripheral blood is also regarded as circulating blood. At this time, peripheral blood is considered to be the most important source for stem cell transplantation. Our bone marrow naturally releases peripheral blood stem cells in the circulating blood; these are blood-forming stem cells. Only a small number of the stem cells can be found in circulating blood. Therefore, to collect an adequate amount of stem cells from circulating blood, the donor is given medications that help more blood-forming stem cells to move out of the bone marrow.

There is a special procedure called *apheresis* that is carried out in which these cells are collected from the circulating blood. In this process, a needle is inserted in the vein of the donor, usually in the arm. A machine receives the donor's blood and removes the stem cells, and the rest of the blood is returned to the body of donor. Within a time period of two to three weeks, the donor's body naturally starts replacing the removed cells.

## CORD BLOOD STEM CELL TRANSPLANTATION

For stem cell transplantation, umbilical cord blood is a rich source, as are peripheral blood and bone marrow. Cord blood is taken from the placenta and umbilical cord after the birth of a baby, and the donated cord blood is stored and frozen for the future use. In certain blood diseases, the allogeneic transplants are preferred over the autologous transplants, because the donor's stem cells show better results in fighting against diseased cells as compared with the patient's own cord blood.

After transplantation comes a series of chemotherapy and radiation therapy treatments. These therapies generally have an effect on dividing cells. As cancer cells have the ability to divide more often then normal cells, chemotherapy and radiation therapy have specific effects on cancer cells. High doses of chemotherapeutic drugs and radiations are given that can cause severe damage to the bone marrow of the patient. Therefore, the patient is unable to produce the required blood cells for the body. In the case of leukemias or other diseases, destroying the bone marrow actually may be a planned part of the treatment. In any such situation, however, chemotherapy and radiation therapy help the patient in replacing damaged stem cells with healthy and functioning stem cells, which are capable of producing new blood cells.

## BONE MARROW TRANSPLANT PROCESS

Bone marrow transplant is challenging and is one of the most complicated treatment methods, needing a skilled and systematic approach by an entire bone marrow transplantation team and their nurse managers. Planning is the first and most important step in this procedure. There are series of tests and procedures for the screening and scheduling of the patient undergoing bone marrow transplantation. The tests and all other preparations are arranged according to the condition and medical history of the patient. These tests may include a physical examination; X-rays; computer-assisted tomography scans; a complete evaluation of the blood for any infection; an evaluation of the bone marrow; a lumbar puncture; a dental examination, as the treatment will likely cause the mouth to become sensitive and easily infected; blood tests to evaluate heart, lung, liver, kidney, and hormone function; and a psychological evaluation of the patient. These measures are necessary for determining the patient's eligibility for bone marrow transplant.

Cooperation between the patient and the physician is very important during bone marrow transplant. The patient is taught about all the important issues and potential risks involved in transplantation, and once the patient is ready to participate, a hospital consent form is signed by him or her, authorizing the procedure. Next, an intravenous catheter is placed in the large veins of chest for drawing blood samples, for providing the patient with antibiotics and nutritional support, for blood or blood products, and for the transplantation of new marrow. These catheters are capable of remaining in place for long periods in which one end is kept outside the chest and special attention is given to the catheter, keeping its end clean and free from infection. The patients also are educated about how to manage the catheter at their homes.

The length of the hospital stay of a patient depends on various factors such as how long it takes for the transplanted marrow to engraft and become capable of producing healthy blood cells, how much independence the patient is showing, the need for blood transfusion, caregiver attention and support for the patient, and the nutritional status of the patient. The goal of providing special care to the patient at the hospital is to avoid the adverse effects of high doses of chemotherapy or radiotherapy. These adverse effects are most likely to be immunosuppression; anemia; bleeding caused by the low number of platelets in the blood; damage to different organs, such as heart, kidney, liver, or lungs, which may lead to their malfunction; and nausea, vomiting, or a decreased appetite.

In hospital care, the most important issue is providing adequate care in an environment that is free of infectious agents, as the patient's own immune system is not able to fight against the infections. Therefore, it is very necessary for the hospital staff and visitors to go through preventive measures such as the use of masks, gowns, and thorough handwashing. Antibiotics, antiviral agents, antifungal agents, and immunoglobulin therapy are given to the patient for the prevention of infection. This special attention is continued until the destruction of the patient's own marrow and transplanted peripheral stem cells or until the marrow starts producing enough white blood cells to fight against the infection.

Transplant patients often begin developing anemia and thrombocytopenia and require blood transfusions from time to time. In addition, during chemotherapy, the gastrointestinal tract is badly affected, so it is necessary to prevent the patient from eating anything, allowing the gastrointestinal tract to heal. During this time, patients get all necessary nutrients by means of a catheter; this is known as total parenteral nutrition. Most of the patients stay in hospital for about one to two months. Once the patient has returned home, follow-up appointments are required occasionally for evaluation purposes. These follow-ups usually take from one to four days, in which tests are performed to evaluate how well the treatment is working.

**SEE ALSO:** Blood; Bone Diseases; Cancer; Cells, Umbilical; Cells, Sources of.

**BIBLIOGRAPHY.** Bone marrow transplants, www.bmt-infonet.org (cited December 2007); National Donor Marrow Program, www.marrow.org (cited December 2007); Bone Marrow Foundation, www.bonemarrow.org (cited December 2007); Bone marrow transplantation, www.nature.com/bmt (cited December 2007); Bone marrow—cancer information, www.medicinenet.com (cited December 2007).

G. Ishaq Khan
Dow University of Health Sciences

# Bonn University

**THE UNIVERSITY OF BONN**, also known as Bonn University, is located in Bonn, Germany. It is a public research university with international collaborations, and is called in German *Rheinische Friedrich-Wilhelms-Universität Bonn*. It is one of Germany's largest universities, boasting famous intellectuals among its alumni, including Friedrich Nietzsche and Karl Marx.

In 1818 Frederick William III of Prussia (Friedrich Wilhelm in German) founded a new institution at Bonn to provide a university for the Rhineland area of Germany. The old university at Bonn had been founded in 1777 but was shut down during the French occupation of the Rhineland. Frederick William wanted to open a nonsectarian university with schools of both Roman Catholic and Protestant theology. Additionally, the university was given schools of law, medicine, and philosophy.

A major research institute at Bonn University today is the German Reference Center for Ethics in the Life Sciences, tailored after the Georgetown University (Washington, D.C.) model of the National Reference Center for Bioethics Literature. It was founded on January 1, 1999, and designed by the Institute for Science and Ethics (Institut für Wissenschaft und Ethik).

Within the Faculty of Medicine, the Institute of Reconstructive Neurobiology, directed by Dr. Oliver Brüstle, has four research groups focused on stem cells. The mission of the institute is to develop "novel stem cell–based therapies for diseases of the central nervous system." For example, the Stem Cell Engineering Group, led by Dr. Frank Edenhofer, investigates the factors that determine whether a stem cell will self-renew or differentiate. Additionally, researchers in this

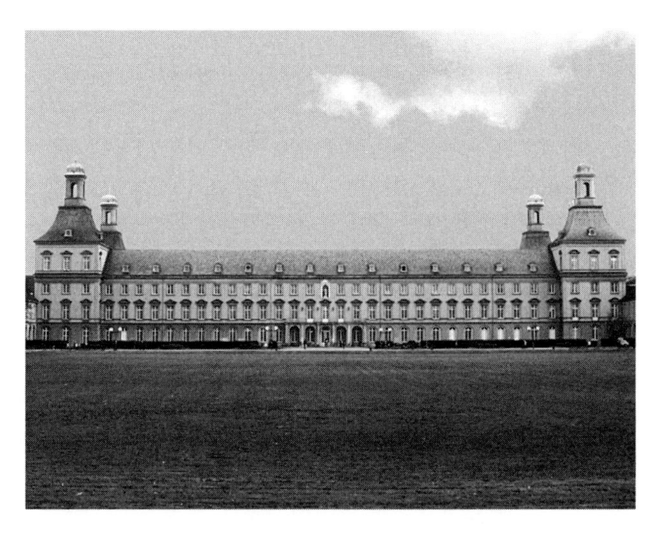

*At Bonn University, the Stem Cell Pathologies Group is investigating the link between stem cells and cancer.*

group work to understand how to direct a stem cell population to differentiate into specific neural cell lines and thus harness stem cells for therapeutic uses.

The Neural Regeneration Group, led by Dr. Harald Neumann, works to understand how microglia, or support cells in the brain, act as the brain's immune system; additional work focuses on guiding embryonic stem cell differentiation into microglia. This group was established in 2004. The Stem Cell Pathologies Group, led by Dr. Björn Scheffler, investigates the link between stem cells and cancer. Finally, the Neurodevelopmental Genetics Group, led by Dr. Sandra Blaess, studies the genetic cues in differentiation stem cells, and how these cues may go awry in diseases of aging.

The Institute of Reconstructive Neurobiology is a member of the European Consortium for Stem Cell Research (EuroStemCell) and the Stem Cell Network of North Rhine Westphalia Germany. It receives funding from public and private sources within Germany.

**SEE ALSO:** Brain; Cancer; Cells, Embryonic; Differentiation, In Vitro and In Vivo; European Consortium for Stem Cell Research—EuroStemCell; Germany; Stem Cell Network of North Rhine.

**BIBLIOGRAPHY.** M. Bellomo, *The Stem Cell Divide: The Facts, the Fiction, and the Fear Driving the Greatest Scientific, Political and Religious Debate of Our Time* (AMACOM/American Management Association, 2006); C. B. Cohen, *Renewing the Stuff of Life: Stem Cells, Ethics, and Public Policy* (Oxford University Press, 2007); C. Fox, *Cell of Cells: The Global Race to Capture and Control the Stem Cell* (Norton, 2007); K. R. Monroe, R. Miller, and J. Tobis, eds., *Fundamentals of the Stem Cell Debate: The Scientific, Religious, Ethical, and Political Issues* (University of California Press, 2007); M. Ruse and C. A. Pynes, eds., *The Stem Cell Controversy: Debating the Issues (Contemporary Issues)* (Prometheus Books, 2006).

Claudia Winograd
University of Illinois, Urbana-Champaign

# Brain

**FOR MANY YEARS** the accepted dogma of neuroscience was that there was no neurogenesis, or birth of new neurons, in the adult brain. A corollary of this dogma was therefore that the brain did not contain stem cells. This dogma was established by the father of neuroscience, Santiago Ramón y Cajal. Today, scientists accept the presence of stem cells in the adult brain as fact.

The first scientist to report adult neurogenesis was Fernando Nottebohm. Dr. Nottebohm saw new neurons in adult male canaries as they learned a new song in the spring. He was most likely not the first scientist to see adult neurogenesis, but he was the first to report it. Scientists had probably seen adult neurogenesis before, but refrained from reporting these findings—the view that there were no new neurons in the brain was accepted as fact and reporting data against this fact was a difficult action. Dr. Nottebohm's brave report established him as a regenerative neuroscientist, and he remains a leading expert today.

Modern scientists accept neurogenesis in the adult brain. Specifically, new neurons are believed to arise for the systems of olfaction and memory. For the olfactory bulb, new neurons arise in the subventricular zone of the brain, and reside there until needed. They then proceed through the rostral migratory stream and are incorporated into

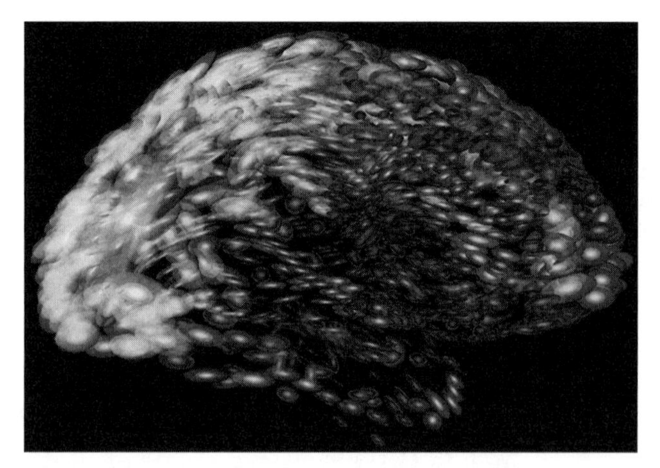

*Stem cell therapy has potential for treating people with neurodegenerative disorders.*

the olfactory bulb. In the hippocampus, the brain region associated with learning and memory, new neurons are formed to help establish new memories. Hippocampal neurons are born in the dendate gyrus region of the hippocampus. These neurons do not migrate, but rather remain in the dendate gyrus and are incorporated into this structure.

An additional important stem cell population in the brain is for glial cells, or the support cells of the brain. The glial cell population is constantly turning over, meaning old cells die off and new cells are generated to replace them. Glial cells absorb toxic materials in the brain, as well as support the neurons in metabolic processes. Therefore, it is important that they can die and be replaced by healthy glia. Because they are the constantly dividing cell population in the brain, glia are generally the cells involved in brain tumors; only about one percent of all brain tumors consist of pure neuronal elements. Rather, brain tumors are masses of glial overgrowth.

Numerous neurological disorders result from degeneration of neurons, including Alzheimer's disease, Parkinson's disease, Huntington's disease, multiple sclerosis, and amyotrophic lateral sclerosis. Often the cause of this degeneration is unknown; however, in some cases it can be due to improper support from glia. In the latter two diseases, the glial cells degrade and the supported neurons die as a result. Stem cell therapy may someday be a possibility for people with neurodegenerative disorders. Additionally, spinal cord injuries are incurable because the growth of new neurons is inhibited by endogenous factors in the spinal cord. Perhaps by better understanding these inhibitory factors, as well as learning how to guide differentiation of stem cells, scientists can use stem cells for spinal cord regenerative medicine.

Recently, a team of scientists at Johns Hopkins University in Baltimore, Maryland, mapped the distribution of astrocytes, a specialized type of glial cell, in the adult human brain. This study is critical for understanding brain stem cells because it is believed that astrocytes are the cells that support new neurons arising from neuronal stem cells. The map supports further study of the subventricular zone, which is precisely the region where new neurons are believed to reside as they await the signal to differentiate into specific neurons.

**SEE ALSO:** Amyotrophic Lateral Sclerosis; Bonn University; Cancer; Cells, Adult; Clinical Trials Outside U.S.: Amyotrophic Lateral Sclerosis; Clinical Trials Outside U.S.: Spinal Cord Injury; Clinical Trials Within U.S.: Spinal Cord Injury; Clinical Trials Within U.S.: Traumatic Brain Injury; Huntington's Disease; Johns Hopkins University; Multiple Sclerosis; Nottebohm, Fernando; Parkinson's Disease; Stem-Like Cells, Human Brain.

**BIBLIOGRAPHY.** P. Andersen, et al., eds., *The Hippocampus Book (Oxford Neuroscience Series)* (Oxford University Press, 2006); C. D. Davis and P. R. Sanberg, *Cell Therapy, Stem Cells and Brain Repair (Contemporary Neuroscience)* (Humana Press, 2006); F. H. Gage, G. Kempermann, and H. Song, *Adult Neurogenesis (Cold Spring Harbor Monograph)* (Cold Spring Harbor Laboratory Press, 2007); G. Kempermann, *Adult Neurogenesis: Stem Cells and Neuronal Development in the Adult Brain* (Oxford University Press, 2005); F. Nottebohm, "Neuronal Replacement in Adult Brain," *Brain Research Bulletin* (April 2002); F. Nottebohm, "The Road We Traveled: Discovery, Choreography, and Significance of Brain Replaceable Neurons," *Annals of the New York Academy of Sciences* (June 2004); P. Taupin, *Adult Neurogenesis and Neural Stem Cells in Mammals* (Nova Biomedical Books, 2007).

Claudia Winograd
University of Illinois, Urbana-Champaign

# Brazil

**BRAZIL IS THE** largest nation in Latin America, the fifth most populous in the world, and the eighth largest economy regarding purchasing power. Most famous for its Amazon Rainforest and natural resources, Brazil is now 17th in the world in the number of scientific indexed papers published. Stem cells from different sources have been studied in Brazil, and preclinical and clinical trials are under way. Although the news from this country is encouraging, the Brazilian stem cell community still faces many challenges, including the low number of scientists working in the field.

The Federative Republic of Brazil is the fifth largest country in the world, with 8,514,877 square kilometers (3,287,612 square miles), exceeded in size only by Russia, Canada, China, and the United States. Besides the Amazon rainforest, which covers most of its north territory, the country also comprises a wide range of tropical and subtropical landscapes, including plateaus, low mountains, savannas, and wetlands. Together, they nourish some of the world's greatest biodiversity.

Brazil is the largest nation in Latin America and the fifth most populous in the world. A recent census showed that the population, although growing less than predicted, reached 183,987,291 inhabitants in 2007. The population density is concentrated in a few large urban centers inland and along the 7,367 kilometers (4,600 miles) of coastline along the Atlantic Ocean. Brazil is a multicultural and multiethnic society. Europeans (mostly Portuguese, but also Italians and Germans), Africans, native South Americans, and Asians have all contributed to the formation of Brazilian history and culture. Catholicism is the predominant religion, and Brazil has the largest Roman Catholic population in the world. The country's official language is Portuguese.

Brazil has the world's eighth largest economy regarding purchasing power; however, it has one of the worst distributions of wealth in the planet: 10 percent of the people possess nearly half of the country's income, and the poorest 40 percent of the population receive less than one-tenth of the nation's total income.

## SCIENCE AND TECHNOLOGY INVESTMENT

With a few exceptions, Brazilian scientific publications are produced at the public universities and research institutes located in the southeast and south of Brazil. Those regions are responsible for most of the scientific articles from the nation, which equalled 0.23 percent of the world's total between 1994 and 2003. Cell biology, neuroscience, and molecular biology are examples of fields of study that are well developed in Brazil.

Brazil started to increase its investment in science 10–15 years ago. Technological research in Brazil is largely carried out in public universities and research institutes, all of which are primarily financed by the government. Expenses on science and technology were 0.91 percent of the gross domestic product in 2004, which yielded 7,047 patents granted worldwide in 2005. This investment policy placed Brazil 17th in scientific indexed papers published from 1999 to 2003, above its neighbors Argentina (29th), Chile (39th), and Mexico (27th). In November 2007, Brazil's President Luíz Inácio Lula da Silva announced about US$22 billion would be spent on science, technology, and innovation over the next three years—an investment never seen before in Brazil.

The study of stem cells is one of the areas in which Brazil is investing. The nation's equivalent of the U.S. National Science Foundation allocated US$5 million for basic stem cell research last year alone. Taking advantage of Brazil's tradition of cell biology research, several laboratories answered this call and started to study biology and the medical applications of both embryonic and adult stem cells.

## STEM CELL RESEARCH IN BRAZIL

Chagas' disease cardiomyopathy is caused by the parasite *Trypanosoma cruzi*, spread by *barbeiros* (kissing bugs), which are rife in poorer regions of Brazil. Mice infected with *T. cruzi* developed a heart muscle disease with histopathological and functional characteristics similar to those observed in humans. Chronically infected mice treated intravenously with bone marrow–derived adult stem cells (BMCs) obtained from normal litter mates showed a significant decrease in inflammation and fibrosis in their hearts.

These results in experimental models, when associated with others obtained on phase I–II clinical trials, encouraged a phase III clinical trial, which is being carried out by a network of 33 institutions and is sponsored by the Brazilian

Ministry of Health. This study, which intends to establish safety and efficacy, has four groups, with 300 patients in each disease: cardiomyopathy caused by Chagas' disease, acute and chronic ischemic heart, and dilated cardiomyopathy. The 1,200 patients studied received conventional therapy, but half of them also received autologous BMCs.

If these studies present clearly positive results, the Brazilian government has announced that this therapy will become available for free at the public hospitals. So far, the partial results, at least in chronic Chagasic cardiomyopathy, have been optimistic: treatment with BMCs improved cardiac function and patients' quality of life, and no adverse events could be related to the therapy so far.

Clinical trials using autologous BMCs for other diseases have been also carried out in Brazil. One example is a phase I clinical trial to test BMC treatment in acute stroke, the third leading cause of death in Brazil. BMCs from patients were collected and injected in their cerebral arteries. The preliminary results suggested that intraarterial injections of BMCs in stroke patients are safe and feasible. Another case report described the migration of autologous BMCs, previously labeled with Tc-99m-HMPAO, implanted into the brain after acute ischemic stroke. This method, intended to follow grafted stem cells within the brain, was shown to be feasible.

Another recent group of studies has shown potential for the use of autologous adult stem cells for the treatment of type 1 diabetes mellitus, an autoimmune disease caused by the destruction of cells that produce insulin. The strategy is to induce moderate immunosuppression by chemotherapy in newly diagnosed patients to prevent further loss of insulin-producing cells by autoimmune attacks. After this procedure, each patient receives transfusions with autologous hematopoietic stem cells. So far, the treatment seems to be safe, with 14 of 15 patients experiencing a transient loss of insulin dependence over 19 months.

Although promising, clinical trials with autologous bone marrow cells are controversial, given that the fate of such engrafted cells is still unknown. In the heart, for example, recent results indicate that improvements are not caused by the formation of new muscle cells by the injected blood cells. Actually, no one can determine whether the positive effects described here are the result of the replacement of damaged cells or dependent on factors released by BMC.

Umbilical cord blood stem cells can be used in transplants to treat a variety of pediatric disorders including leukemia, sickle cell disease, and metabolic disorders. In Brazil, 10 percent of the umbilical cord blood used in transplants has come from public blood banks. However, there is still a need for voluntary donors, forcing the search for material abroad and raising the costs of the procedure.

The BrasilCord Network–Public Network of Placentary and Umbilical Cord Blood Storage for Hematopoietic Stem-Cells Transplant was created by the Department of Health in 2004. Cord blood stem cell banks, located in strategic regions of the country, form the network. Using public resources, its storage capacity went from 3,000 to 10,000 umbilical cord blood bags. In addition to public banks, there are also several private banks operating in Brazil.

To date, there are approximately 50 public laboratories supported by the government that are working on stem cells. A few of these laboratories are dedicated to mouse embryonic stem cell research, both mouse and human neural stem cells, and human dental pulp stem cells, among others.

## HUMAN EMBRYONIC STEM CELLS

In 2005, the Brazilian House of Representatives approved the biosecurity law, which made it legal to work with human embryos stored for at least three years at in vitro fertilization clinics to derive human embryonic stem cells (hESs). In 2006, a religious former general attorney appealed to the Brazilian Supreme Court to repeal article five of the biosecurity law, which allowed scientists to use hESs for research. The Brazilian Supreme Court is currently deciding whether it will allow the continuation of the research using these cells. Meanwhile, Brazilian scientists have been working with hES lines donated from institutions abroad.

Despite the achievements described here, the future of stem cell research in Brazil faces several challenges. Problems are still to be solved, including the bureaucracy needed to import scientific reagents necessary for research, federal policies to reabsorb and integrate the knowledge and experience gained by young scientists trained abroad, and improving the infrastructure of the laboratories. However, the future of stem cells in Brazil is bright, and it is not foreseen that such challenges will hinder the continuing improvement and international recognition of Brazilian science.

**SEE ALSO:** Cells, Adult; Cells, Embryonic; Clinical Trials Worldwide; EC Cell Isolation; Experimental Models; Heart.

**BIBLIOGRAPHY.** P. L. Correa, et al., *Clinical Nuclear Medicine* (v.32/11, 2007); I. Kerkisa, et al., "Isolation and Characterization of a Population of Immature Dental Pulp Stem Cells Expressing OCT-4 and Other Embryonic Stem Cell Markers," *Cells Tissues Organs* (v.184, 2006); Marcelo Leite, "Stem Cell Research in Brazil: A Difficult Launch," *Cell* (v.124, 2006); "Brazil," *Encyclopedia Britannica Online*, www.britannica.com (cited November 2007); Luisa Massarani, "Stem Cell Research Fund Launched in Brazil," *Science and Development Network*, www.scidev.net (cited November 2007); R. Mendez-Otero, et al., "Potential Roles of Bone Marrow Stem Cells in Stroke Therapy," *Regenerative Medicine* (v.2/4, 2007); A. Packer and R. Meneghini, "Articles with Authors Affiliated to Brazilian Institutions Published from 1994 to 2003 with 100 or More Citations: I—The Weight of International Collaboration and the Role of the Networks," *Anais da Academia Brasileira de Ciências* (v.78/4, 2006); M. Soares, et al., "Cellular Therapy in Chagas' Disease: Potential Applications in Patients with Chronic Cardiomyopathy," *Regenerative Medicine* (v.2/3, 2007); Marcia L. Triunfol, "Latin American Science Moves into the Spotlight," *Cell* (v.131, 2007); B. Tura, et al., "Multicenter Randomized Trial of Cell Therapy in Cardiopathies—MiHeart Study," *Trials* (v.8, 2007); J. C. Voltarelli, et al., "Autologous Nonmyeloablative Hematopoietic Stem Cell Transplantation in Newly Diagnosed Type 1 Diabetes Mellitus," *JAMA* (v.297/14, 2007).

Helena Lobo Borges
Universidade Federal do Rio de Janeiro
Stevens Kastrup Rehen
Universidade Federal do Rio de Janeiro

# BrdU/Thymidine

**IF STEM CELLS** are to be introduced into a tissue as a therapeutic mechanism to stimulate the repair of damaged tissue, or in a preliminary study to see merely where they go, scientists must have a way of monitoring what becomes of the stem cells postinjection. One way is to mark the DNA with a chemical that would remain in the DNA for generations of cell divisions. A marker of choice—until recent warnings—has been BrdU, a thymidine analog.

Deoxyribonucleic acid, or DNA, carries the genetic information of an organism, in most every cell (red blood cells do not contain nuclei and therefore do not carry DNA). DNA is made up of four nucleotide bases that contain nitrogenous rings: deoxyadenosine, deoxycytidine, deoxyguanosine, and thymidine. *Deoxy* does not need to be included in the name of thymidine because thymidine is not found in ribonucleic acid (RNA), which contains adenosine, cytidine, and guanosine, but in lieu of thymidine, it carries an analog, uridine. BrdU is short for 5-bromo-2-deoxyuridine, a modified deoxyuridine that is quite similar structurally to thymidine and therefore can incorporate into replicating DNA. The process of supplying a dividing cell with BrdU that it will then incorporate into new DNA is called BrdU labeling. BrdU has a bromine in its nitrogenous ring, which can be detected by an antibody to BrdU in histological stains.

The purpose of BrdU-labeling DNA is that BrdU incorporates into DNA that is actively replicating, replacing some of the thymidine that would normally be incorporated. BrdU is not naturally found in cells—it must be added by the researcher. Thus, any cell undergoing cell division, and therefore DNA replication, at the time of BrdU addition will take up BrdU into its DNA, and subsequent cells resulting from cell division of this first cell will also have BrdU in their DNA, although if BrdU is not reintroduced, the BrdU concentration per cell will be diluted by approximately one-half with every cell division.

Scientists can label stem cells with BrdU and introduce these labeled stem cells into new tissue. After a period of time, the tissue can be stained histologically for the presence of BrdU in tissue cells. Any cell that has BrdU in its DNA is presumed to have derived from the initial stem cells injected. If the laboratory has a high level of technology with sensitive equipment, scientists can trace a stem cell through several generations of division, thus determining the end fate of the injected stem cells and their progeny.

Recently, Dr. Catherine Verfaillie, who was at the University of Minnesota at the time, warned that stem cells injected into tissues could die and release their BrdU into the surrounding space. Neighboring cells could then take up this BrdU and label their DNA, confounding results that expect all BrdU-labeled cells to have arisen from the injected, labeled stem cells.

Some scientists agree, but others argue that this effect does not occur. In addition, in tissues such as the brain, where mature neurons do not divide and thus should not take up free BrdU, these neurons might still incorporate BrdU if an injury triggers novel DNA synthesis, even if not in preparation for cell division. This effect was observed by Dr. Pasko Rakic of Yale University in New Haven, Connecticut.

Another line of research uses BrdU labeling to provide evidence for an "immortal DNA strand" in adult stem cells. Adult stem cells divide into two cells—another stem cell and a daughter cell that can differentiate into specific cell types. When DNA is replicated before cell division, such that each of the two resulting cells receives an equal copy of the DNA, the allotment is random; that is, which one of the two copies of each gene is segregated into which of the two resultant cells is arbitrary. The immortal DNA strand hypothesis states that to avoid random DNA mutations that inevitably occur during DNA replication and cell division, tainting stem cell DNA, adult stem cells do not randomly distribute their DNA into the two resultant cells. Rather, there is one strand per chromatid that is always kept in the stem cell population.

Some scientists use BrdU to label the adult stem cell DNA and show that this label is not diluted from the stem cell after several generations of cell division, indicating that the adult stem cell has retained an immortal DNA strand. Evidence has been seen in multiple stem cell types ranging from plant root tips to murine neural stem cells. This hypothesis was first proposed in 1975 by (Hugh) John Cairns.

**SEE ALSO:** Belgium; Lineages; MRI Tracking; University of Minnesota; Verfaillie, Catherine; Yale University.

**BIBLIOGRAPHY.** C.-Y. Kuan, "Hypoxia-Ischemia Induces DNA Synthesis without Cell Proliferation in Dying Neurons in Adult Rodent Brain," *Journal of Neuroscience* (v.24/47, 2004); J. R. Merok, et al., "Cosegregation of Chromosomes Containing Immortal DNA Strands in Cells that Cycle with Asymmetric Cell Kinetics," *Cancer Research* (v.62/23, 2002); H. Pearson, "Stem-Cell Tagging Shows Flaws," *Nature* (v.439, 2006).

Claudia Winograd
University of Illinois, Urbana-Champaign

# Burnham Institute

**THE BURNHAM INSTITUTE** for Medical Research is located in La Jolla, California. It is a nonprofit medical research institute that focuses on cancer research. Because of the research performed at the institute, it is ranked among the top 25 such organizations in the United States. Its publication of its research findings is one of its major products. Through research, the institute's members have contributed to five approved therapies and as many diagnostic tests that are now in use. They have been credited with saving the lives of many people through earlier diagnoses. In addition, the institute has created nine innovative therapies that are now in clinical trials at dozens of medical centers around the world.

The quality of the program at the Burnham Institute is of a very high caliber. Proof is seen in the fact that the institute is the fourth largest recipient of funding grants from the U.S. National Institutes of Health. The Center for Advanced Research rates the Burnham Institute as the most efficient private research institution in America. Over 60 percent of its operating costs are covered by competitive grants awarded to its scientists.

The institute was founded by William (Bill) H. Fishman and his wife Lillian. They moved to La Jolla in the late 1970s from Boston, Massachusetts, to fulfill their goal of founding an independent research center for the study of oncodevelopment. Dr. Fishman turned down a promising career at Tufts University School of Medicine and instead moved to La Jolla to found the La Jolla Cancer Research Foundation (LJCRS). The focus of the LJCRS's medical research was on developmental biology and oncology, combined to form the study of oncodevelopment, which is an investigation into the elusive and deadly nature of cancer. The theory that Dr. Fishman held was that the abnormal development of cancer cells could be better understood if their normal development were better understood.

Dr. Fishman has served at the Burnham Institute as a trustee, president, administrator, and scientist. In 1979, his role as scientific director was given to Erkki Ruoslahti, who is from the City of Hope in Duarte, California. In the same year, the institute received a two-year planning grant from the National Cancer Institute (NCI). It soon was given five acres of land by the Whittaker Corporation on the Torrey Pines Mesa. Its nearby neighboring scientific institutes were the University of California at San Diego and the Salk Institute. From its small beginnings, the Burnham Institute has grown into an organization employing nearly 800 people. Its annual operating budget is over $100 million.

## RESEARCH

The goal of the Burnham Institute Medical Research staff is to discover the fundamental molecular mechanism of disease. With that knowledge, the power should be available to devise new therapies for curing cancer. The approach to research used by the Burnham Institute is a very collaborative one. In putting together the pieces of the puzzle that is the molecular basis of life, results are more likely to come from people working collaboratively than from those in isolation. This is because it is unlikely that any single individual will have all the knowledge and skills necessary for the task. A collaborative effort employing the partial knowledge and skills of a prize team increases the likelihood of rapidly making significant discoveries and therapeutic advances.

The research teams at the Burnham Institute are composed of very well educated and talented chemists, biologists, biophysicists, engineers, computer scientists, medical researchers, and others. Harmonious teamwork creates a scientific synergy that both inspires the researchers to greater effort and feeds their mutually shared body of knowledge. The Burnham Institute's mantra is "From Research, the Power to Cure."

The Burnham research program is three pronged. Each of the areas in which the research is organized focuses on diseases. Each area is organized into a research center, with each of these centers supported by a technology center. The three centers are the Cancer Research Center; the Del E. Webb Neuroscience, Aging, and Stem Cell Research Center; and the Infectious and Inflammatory Disease Center.

The Cancer Research Center consumes about 50 percent of the efforts of the Burnham Institute's personnel and resources. The institute joined the NCI in 1981. In that year, the NCI designed and organized cancer centers. The Burnham Institute has been placed into the "basic science" category of cancer centers. The NCI has used its grants to aid the development of the Burnham Institute into one of 13 centers that specialize in cancer drug discovery. It is also one of six centers that researches the molecular signature of cancer. The use of this knowledge can be applied to the development of powerful diagnostic tests. The institute performs this work in cooperation with other centers. In addition, the Burnham Institute is one of eight centers for cancer bionanotechnology.

The Burnham Institute's scientists have compiled a significant body of accomplishments. These include creating the enzyme-linked immunosorbent assay, which is the basis of the prostate-specific antigen test; enabling technology for the world's first biotech cancer drug, Epogen (used to promote blood cell production in cancer patients undergoing therapy); a vitamin-based cancer drug (Targretin); a DNA drug for cancer, which is in the late stages of clinical trials; and other clinical laboratory tests.

The second prong of the Burnham Institute's program is the Del E. Webb Neuroscience, Aging, and Stem Cell Research Center. This center focuses on degenerative diseases including stroke, heart disease, diabetes, Parkinson's disease, Alzheimer's, and other diseases. Because these diseases involve the loss of cells needed to function, the focus is currently on developing replacement cells through stem cell technology.

The cell replacement technologies protection strategies developed by the Burnham Institute scientists have included Memantine (Namenda), a cytoprotective drug for Alzheimer's disease or for testing in stroke victims and glaucoma patients. In addition, the institute's stem cell program was one of the first to engage in stem cell investigation in the search for regenerative medicines.

At present, the Burnham Institute has dedicated the talents of about 100 scientists to the area of stem cell research. Its program is probably the largest in the United States. Its research is supported by grants from the NIH, which has designated the institute as one of six national exploratory centers for human embryonic stem cell research. It is also one of the five centers for training scientists in human embryonic stem cell research.

For several reasons, including the protection of the stem cell line from contamination, the Burnham Institute established the Stem Cell Research Center as a safe haven for performing all types of stem cell research. The center is an exploratory center for human embryonic stem cell research and is one of six national exploratory centers. Their goal is to hasten the day when stem cell–based therapies restore the tissues in body parts to wholeness, whether the tissues were lost through disease or accident. The Stem Cell Research Center has its own state-of-the-art infrastructure. It has the capacity to derive new embryonic stem cell lines, and it can make them available to the general research community in the quest for regenerative medicines.

## EMBRYONIC STEM CELLS AND HEART TISSUE

One of the important stem cell research investigations currently underway is an examination of embryonic stem cells and heart tissue. The experiments are being conducted on mouse embryonic stem cells. The mouse embryonic stem cells that are undifferentiated are being used to grow cardiac muscle cells. If this study is successful, the future may include ways to grow human heart tissue from stem cells so that the cardiac tissue can be used to repair hearts damaged by disease or injury.

The research on mouse heart stem cells is being conducted in cooperation with the Salk Institute and with scientists at the University of California at San Diego. The close proximity of these other centers makes their cooperative efforts much easier. Some of the researchers are monitoring the presence and activity of electrically charged calcium ions inside developing mouse heart cells (cardiomyocytes). The concentration of calcium ions plays an important role in the development of electrical rhythm, and changes in calcium levels in cardiomyocytes play a vital part of cell contraction development. Further research in this area is being planned.

The Infectious and Inflammatory Disease Center investigates infectious agents and studies the way immune systems fight infections. It also has made numerous discoveries and medical contributions.

**SEE ALSO:** California; Cancer; Cells, Embryonic; University of California, San Diego.

**BIBLIOGRAPHY.** Don Monroe, "California Bets Big On Stem Cell Research," *Scientific American* (November 4, 2004); Burnham Institute for Medical Research, www.burnham.org (cited November 2007).

Andrew J. Waskey
Dalton State College

# Burns

**BURNS ARE INJURIES** to tissues caused by heat, chemicals, radiations, friction, or electricity. Burns injure the skin layers, and they may also injure other parts of the body such as muscles, nerve, lungs, and the eyes.

Depending on the severity and depth of tissue damage, burns are classified into various degrees: first-degree burns are superficial thickness burns, extending only into the epidermis (outermost layer of the skin); second-degree burns, which are partial thickness burns, involve the superficial dermis (the layer of the skin deep to the epidermis, consisting of a bed of vascular connective tissue and containing the nerves and organs of sensation, the hair roots, and sebaceous, and sweat glands) and possibly also the deep dermis; third-degree burns are full-thickness burns that include the epidermis, the entire dermis, skin appendages, and at times deeper tissue; finally, in fourth-degree burns, tissue is destroyed to the level of or below the deep fascia.

Traditionally, partial-thickness and full-thickness burns are treated by skin grafting. Skin grafting is a two-step surgical procedure in which a patch of skin is removed from one area of the body and transplanted to cover the wound. This procedure is effective but leaves the patient with a scar and may take months to heal. However, in cases of severe burns where there is not any healthy skin left to graft or the patient is not healthy enough to undergo such a surgical procedure, stem cell–based therapy provides a promising alternative.

## STEM CELL–BASED THERAPY

The basic concept of stem cell therapy in burns, and skin replacement in general, involves growing stem cells on a synthetic scaffold, and then transferring that medium on to a patient's wound or burn. The goal of this research area is to replace conventional skin grafts with a new method of healing that has better results, a faster healing rate, and no complications or rejection by the patient.

Embryonic stem cells derived by somatic cell nuclear transfer are not rejected by the recipient, who is the donor of somatic cells. In this procedure, DNA from a somatic cell (a body cell other than a sperm or egg cell) is removed, and the rest of the cell is discarded. Then this DNA is inserted into an egg cell, the DNA of which has been removed. After being inserted into the host cell, this DNA is reprogrammed by the egg. Embryonic stem cells obtained in this way can be used to develop therapies that are ideally suited for a specific person. Embryonic stem cells can be induced to differentiate into skin keratinocytes in in vitro cultures under specific conditions and can be used for generating artificial skin—an unlimited supply of graftable regenerated epithelium that is without rejection risk.

Skin has tremendous potential to regenerate after injuries. The epidermis has cells (keratinocytes) that resemble adult stem cells, which can be classified on the basis of their capacities for multiplication before they undergo differentiation. These are holoclone keratinocytes (which have tremendous potential for differentiation and can undergo 140 divisions before senescence), paraclone keratinocytes (have limited growth potential, undergo a maximum of 15 divisions), and meroclone keratinocytes (which have a proliferative potential greater than paraclones) It is holoclone keratinocytes that can be cultured in vitro in the presence of epidermal growth factors to produce a supply stratified epithelium, which retains the properties of the original epidermis. Autologous (from the patients own body) cultured keratinocytes (i.e., holoclones) can be used to treat massive full-thickness burns.

Holoclone keratinocytes grafted onto a burn site effectively proliferate and promote epidermal wound healing. However, the actual usefulness of this procedure in treating deep full-thickness burns is limited by the fact that epidermal keratinocyte sheets grown by this method contain no dermal factors. This has led to investigation into the use of some kind of dermal element or substrate to support the keratinocyte layer.

The keratinocytes are usually grown on the chosen substrates. The substrates that have been used include collagen gels (collagen is the main protein of connective tissue in animals) and cryopreserved dermis (cryopreservation is a process in which cells or whole tissues are preserved by cooling to low subzero temperatures).

Swiss doctors have also explored the potential of fetal skin cells in grafts. The therapy involves the use of skin cells grown from aborted fetuses to heal burns, sparing the need for skin grafts. Fetal cells are known to have remarkable regenerative potential. The fetal tissue promotes the growth of patients' own skin so it can be used as a biological bandage. The researchers collected skin from aborted fetuses and allowed the cells to divide in vitro. The cells were then allowed to grow on a bed of collagen (an important protein in skin). This procedure can be used to obtain several million 100 $cm^2$ patches for use in transplants from a single fetal biopsy (the removal of a sample of tissue from a living person for laboratory examination). The patches obtained in this manner were then placed on burn wounds, which took an average of 15 days to heal—considerably faster than traditional skin grafting (almost six times faster). This result gave the patients almost perfect skin. There was little hypertrophy of the new skin and no retraction. None of the fetal cells remained in the healed skin. It is not certain how exactly this happens; however, one possible explanation is that these grafts act as growth factor and cytokine secretors rather than true grafts.

Human umbilical cord blood stem cells differentiate into epithelial cells under specific in vitro conditions and therefore can also be used as a source of artificial skin for patients with deep burn injuries. Similarly, hemopoietic stem cells of the bone marrow that differentiate into blood cells can have different fates. Studies have shown that these hemopoietic stem cells, when transplanted on deep burn wounds, decreased the healing time. Thus, hemopoietic stem cells cultivated in vitro may prove to be useful in burn treatment. Growing new skin is actually possible.

## STRATATECH CORP.

In 2008, information based on clinical trials was released by Stratatech Corp., a Wisconsin biotech company. The company's approach is based on the discoveries of Lynn Allen-Hoffmann's University of Wisconsin, Madison, research lab. Lynn Allen-Hoffmann founded Stratatech Corp. in 2000. Their cell line was derived from keratinocytes, the most common and least immunogenic of the cells found in the epidermis.

The first round of clinical trials used 15 patients, with problems ranging from burns to flesh-eating bacteria at the University of Wisconsin Hospital in Madison and at the Arizona Burn Center in Phoenix. The company's tissue was used to cover the wound for one to two weeks to prepare the wound for a transplant of the patient's own skin. No problems were discovered with the company's StrataGraft patches after three months and six months examinations. In their second round of tests, the genetically altered patch will remain on the patent, instead of removing the patches and replacing them with grafts of the patient's own skin.

Stratatech Corp. is involved in developing three lines of genetically engineered material that would enhance their cell line with extra healing powers. A first version would stimulate the growth of new blood vessels. A second version would be antimicrobial, to ward off infection. A third version would neutralize substances believed to be a factor in creating skin ulcers. The company projects that their StrataGraft, human skin products, could be ready for use in hospitals by the end of 2010.

**SEE ALSO:** Cells, Embryonic; Cloning.

**BIBLIOGRAPHY.** L. Alsono and E. Fuchs, "Stem Cells of Skin Epithelium," *Proceedings of the National Academy of Sciences* (v.100, 2003); Christopher L. R. Barratt, "Cultured Keratinocytes and Keratinocyte Grafts," *BMJ* (v.299/11, 1989); R. Brychta, et al., "Cultured Skin Cells for Treatment of Burns," *Annals of the Mediterranean Burns Club* (v.71/4, 1994); Lisa Christenson, "Skin Grafting," www2.vhi.ie (cited November 2007); L.-P. Kamolza, et al., "Cultured Human Epithelium: Human Umbilical Cord Blood Stem Cells Differentiate into Keratinocytes under In Vitro Conditions," *Molecular Biology of the Cell* (v.32/1, 2006); "Keratinocytes Obtained from Embryonic Stem Cells of Mammals," U.S. Patent, March 6, 2007, www.patentstorm.us/patents (cited November 2007); R. Lovell-Badge, "Stem Cell Therapy and Research," *Mill Hill Essays* (National Institute of Medical Research, 2001); G. Pellegrini, et al. "The Control of Epidermal Stem Cells (Holoclones) in the Treatment of Massive Full-Thickness Burns with Autologous Keratinocytes Cultured on Fibrin," *Transplantation* (v.68/6, 1999); V. I. Shumakov, et al., "Mesenchymal Bone Marrow Stem Cells More Effectively Stimulate Regeneration of Deep Burn Wounds Than Embryonic Fibroblasts," *Bulletin of Experimental Biology and Medicine* (v.136/2, 2003).

Anam Imtiaz
National University of Science
and Technology

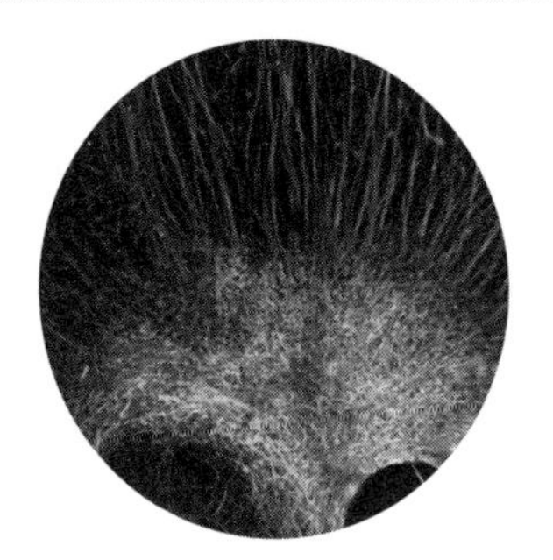

# C

## California

**HISTORICALLY AN OPEN** haven for technological innovations and scientific inquiry, with a university system that strongly supports research and a biomedical industry employing over 200,000 people, California has recently become—and is determined to remain—a leader in stem cell research. On November 2, 2004, three years after the Bush administration limited federal funding of human embryonic stem cell research to research dealing with stem cell lines already created as of August 9, 2001, the state of California passed Proposition 71, essentially electing to have the state assume a level of involvement in stem cell research that would ordinarily only be found at the federal level. In that sense, the vote is important not only to embryonic human stem cell research—it is the largest source of American funding to the field, either public or private—but to research funding in general and to the balance of power and responsibility between the state and federal governments.

Once passed (59 percent to 41 percent), Proposition 71, which was also known as the California Stem Cell Research and Cures Initiative, was codified as California Constitution Article XXXV. It established stem cell research as a state constitutional right and authorized the sale of general obligation bonds over a 10-year period to allocate $3 billion to stem cell research, with priority given to human embryonic stem cell research. Unlike Bush's August 9, 2001, executive order, it did not limit its funding to research using existing stem cell lines, but it did ban the funding of human cloning.

General obligation bonds are a secure, low-interest, tax-exempt municipal bond issued at the state, local, or county level to raise money for a government project—typically the building of a bridge or other large-scale construction project that cannot be funded gradually by tax revenue. The cost to the state over the 30 years in which the bonds will be paid off is estimated at $6 billion. To get a sense of the amount involved, Proposition 71 called for $300 million a year to be spent, favoring human embryonic stem cell research, which is 12 times what the federal government spent in the field in 2003. Universities and other institutions began exploring the creation of new dedicated laboratories, and researchers in other states sought to relocate. The University of California, San Francisco, made plans for a $109 million stem cell research facility, and its director of stem cell biology Dr. Arnold Krigstein actively recruited scientists to come work with him. Immediately, comparisons were drawn to the gold rush as well as to the dotcom boom (after all, the promise of human embryonic stem cell research remains largely potential).

## PROPOSITION 71

The Proposition 71 plan was formulated when the California legislature voted down a $1 billion stem cell research measure. The leader of the campaign was Robert N. Klein II, a Palo Alto real estate tycoon whose mother had developed Alzheimer's disease and whose young son suffered from type 1 diabetes—both conditions that stem cell research might help cure. Mr. Klein helped author the proposition, donated $3 million of the $25 million raised for the campaign, and headed the California Institute for Regenerative Medicine (CIRM) after the proposition passed.

The diverse support for Proposition 71 included actors Christopher Reeve and Michael J. Fox, both sufferers of conditions stem cell research could help alleviate, as well as other entertainment industry figures, 22 Nobel laureates, state legislators, and Governor Schwarzenegger and George Schulz, President Ronald Reagan's Secretary of State. Groups endorsing the plan included Planned Parenthood and the California chapter of the National Organization for Women; minority advocacy groups like the California National Association for the Advancement of Colored People and the National Coalition of Hispanic Organizations; dozens of patient advocacy groups for sufferers of Alzheimer's disease, sickle cell anemia, diabetes, and other diseases; and state and local hospitals and medical groups. Financial contributors included venture capitalists, the founders of eBay, Bill Gates, and Cleveland Cavaliers owner Gordon Gund.

The Republican Party as a whole opposed Proposition 71, as did the Roman Catholic Church (though various Catholic groups endorsed it), the California Pro-Life Council, and actor Mel Gibson. Opposing the plan for fiscal reasons, citing the enormous bureaucracy such a large scientific endeavor would create, were the Pro-Choice Alliance Against Proposition 71, the Green Party, and assorted smaller groups. Though opponents to the plan challenged it in court, it was upheld. In April 2006, the first grants were awarded for the training of 169 stem cell researchers; in the first quarter of the following year, CIRM began issuing its first research grants.

Two organizations were created by Proposition 71. CIRM was created to make available grants and loans for "stem cell research, for research facilities, and for other vital research opportunities to realize therapies, protocols, and/or medical procedures that will result in, as speedily as possible, the cure for, and/or substantial mitigation of, major diseases, injuries, and orphan diseases...[t]o support all stages of the process of developing cures, from laboratory research through successful clinical trials...[and t]o establish the appropriate regulatory standards and oversight bodies for research and facilities development." The Independent Citizens' Oversight Committee (ICOC), meanwhile, was created to oversee CIRM.

CIRM has up to 50 employees, in three groups: the scientific and medical research funding working group, the scientific and medical accountability standards working group, and the scientific and medical research facilities working group. The ICOC membership was established as the chancellors of the Universities of California at Davis, Irvine, Los Angeles, San Diego, and San Francisco; 12 members appointed by the governor, lieutenant governor, treasurer, and controller from other California universities, nonprofit institutions, and life science companies; Alzheimer's and spinal cord injury advocacy representatives appointed by the governor; type 2 diabetes and multiple sclerosis or amyotrophic lateral sclerosis advocates appointed by the lieutenant governor; type 1 diabetes and heart disease advocates appointed by the treasurer; cancer and Parkinson's disease advocates appointed by the controller; a mental health advocate appointed by the speaker of the assembly; an HIV/AIDS advocate appointed by the president pro tempore of the state senate; and a chairperson and vice chairperson elected by the appointees.

In establishing the state's constitutional right to pursue stem cell research, Proposition 71 clearly defined it as "research involving adult stem cells, cord blood stem cells, pluripotent stem cells, and/or progenitor cells," and then further defined those terms, leaving no room for error.

In the wake of Proposition 71, other states, including New Jersey, New York, and Washington, began to look into the possibilities of stem cell research both as a public health issue and for its potential economic benefits. Although no state committed as much money as California, the amounts were still significant, and together they dwarfed federal spending. In the long run, such state expenditures may undo a post-2001 development in academic stem cell research: Many schools had had to maintain two sets of equipment, one paid for with federal funding and another funded with state and private money, because any research done on post-2001 stem cell lines had to be done with equipment for which federal money had not been used. Sufficient state funding could make federal funding all but irrelevant for some institutions or could allow them to allocate things differently and more practically.

**SEE ALSO:** Biotechnology, History of; California Institute for Regenerative Medicine; Caltech; Cells, Embryonic; Federal Government Policies; Geron Corporation; Stem Cells, Bush Ruling; Thomson, James; University of California, Berkeley; University of California, Davis; University of California, Los Angeles; University of California, San Diego; University of California, San Francisco; University of Southern California.

**BIBLIOGRAPHY.** State of California Proposition 71, www.ss.ca.gov (cited November 2007); Don Monroe, "California Bets Big on Stem Cell Research," *Scientific American* (November 4, 2004); Keith R. Yamamoto, "Bankrolling Stem Cell Research with California Dollars," *New England Journal of Medicine* (v.351, 2004).

Bill Kte'pi
Independent Scholar

# California Institute for Regenerative Medicine

**AFTER PRESIDENT GEORGE W. BUSH** placed restrictions on stem cell funding, federal funding was restricted to adult cells and a few embryonic lines that were described by scientists as being of poor quality and unfit for research. California backers of stem cell research forced an election on proposition 71, which established a 10-year, $3 billion stem cell program. Proponents included patients, scientists, and industry. Opponents included the Roman Catholic Church, budget watchers, and conservatives.

On November 2, 2004, California voters authorized the sale of $3 billion in bonds to fund stem cell research at the state's universities and research facilities. Two months earlier, the voters were split, but late in the campaign, sentiment shifted significantly, and less than 40 percent of the voters opposed—even Governor Arnold Schwarzenegger backed Proposition 71. The proposition authorized sale of bonds and spending up to $300 million each year for a decade. Cloning for research is legal under the proposition, but cloning of babies is banned. The measure garnered seven million votes—about 59 percent of the vote.

The state-funded scientific research program is the largest ever, unmatched by any other country or state. Federal funding in all of 2004 was $25 million, and even Democratic presidential candidate John Kerry proposed to increase that amount to only $100 million. The proposition mandated establishment of a state agency to provide grants and loans to qualified research facilities. The oversight agency is the California Institute for Regenerative Medicine (CIRM). To fulfill its mandate to spend $3 billion for research into stem cell and other technologies to find therapies and cures for chronic disease and injury, the Independent Citizens Oversight Committee (ICOC) first met in December 2004.

The research focuses on therapies, diagnostics, and other life-saving medical treatments. Research involves diseases including amyotrophic lateral sclerosis, cystic fibrosis, spinal cord injury, liver disease, and multiple sclerosis. CIRM also sees applications in cancer, diabetes, arthritis, and more. It not only investigates cell replacement but also researches tissue-specific lines to test new therapies, study individual disease development, and improve immunities.

Only California institutions qualify to submit peer-reviewed proposals for the money. The process is governed by the ICOC. The ICOC membership comprises 29 professionals appointed by elected officials and university chancellors. It includes patient advocates, leaders of the state research institutions, and private sector representatives.

The ICOC approves all grants and loans, standards and policies, and regulations in open meetings. Aside from oversight and establishment of regulations, policies, and procedures, the ICOC develops annual and long-term plans, approves research standards and grants, and establishes policies regarding intellectual property rights over research results. In the first 18 months, ICOC working groups and subcommittees quickly established ethical standards as well as administrative and regulatory policies.

CIRM established working groups that included patient advocates and scientists or other experts (both Californian and outside the state) to establish ethical standards, evaluate research proposals, and develop research facilities. The first director of scientific activities was Arlene Chiu, Ph.D. CIRM also hosted a conference, "Stem Cell Research: Charting New Directions for California," and joined the International Stem Cell Forum, whose membership represents 19 countries.

ICOC members participated in the December 2004 Board on Life Sciences of the National Research Council of the National Academies meeting to set guidelines for medical and ethical practices as well as intellectual property and grant administration. Using as its model the National Academy's Guidelines for Human Embryonic Stem Cell Research, CIRM set interim standards for stem cell research, making California the first state in the United States to have such written standards.

The ICOC also established a state bureaucracy from scratch, opening in November 2004 a competition for its headquarters and selecting San Francisco from 10 competing cities after a generous tax and other benefits package made possible by a private/public partnership group. CIRM established a research fellowship program for pre- and postdoctoral and clinical fellows and to promote cross-area research collaborations.

## OPPOSITION

Opponents questioned the ability of California to repay such a large bond obligation and, more significantly, challenged the constitutionality of the California Stem Cell Research and Cures Act (Proposition 71). The lawsuit blocked the sale of state bonds until the issue was resolved. For 18 months, CIRM was effectively out of business. Blocked from selling bonds, the institute got a $150 million loan from the state general fund, a gift of $5 million from San Francisco's Dolby family, and $45 million in bond anticipation notes.

On April 6, 2006, six individuals and foundations purchased $14 million in anticipatory debt instruments despite those bonds being subject to ongoing litigation. With those funds, CIRM approved 16 grants for training 169 stem cell researchers. On April 21, 2006, Judge Bonnie Lewman Sabraw of the Alameda County Superior Court ruled Proposition 71 constitutional. Another $31 million in bonds sold in November 2006.

Sabraw deliberated for six weeks before ruling against claims that CIRM was too independent to be a government agency and thus should be blocked from spending state money. Opponents also contended that because the grant review committee included stem cell researchers, university personnel, and businesses expected to apply for grants, conflict of interest was unavoidable. Immediately after Sabraw's ruling, opponents vowed to appeal and block CIRM well into 2007. The California appeals court ruled in February 2007, just days after CIRM had awarded its first grants, that Proposition 71 was constitutional and that CIRM could proceed. Opponents appealed to the state supreme court, which declined in May to hear the appeal (it had previously—in 2004—rejected an appeal by opponents, ordering the case to a lower court).

After California took the lead, other states began providing stem cell research funding. In 2006, Connecticut, Illinois, Maryland, and New Jersey were the only other states to fund stem cell research. Total stem cell funds were $72 million for the five states and $90 million in federal funds. Then California's Governor Schwarzenegger committed $150 million in state funds, and Illinois provided $5 million. The ICOC provides comprehensive research grants up to $80 million over four years, seed grants up to $24 million over two years, and shared research laboratory grants up to $47.5 million over three years.

In February 2008, the *San Diego Union-Tribune* reported that CIRM chairman Robert Klein's plan to lend up to $750 million to stem cell firms might be overly ambitious. Industry was generally supportive because quick loans of a few million would speed clinical trials and the commercialization of their products. The Foundation for Taxpayer and Consumers Rights was not pleased, however, that qualifying standards for the loans were more relaxed than the stringent standard CIRM set for grants. One member of the CIRM oversight committee had doubts that the staff—only 26 people—could handle the volume of loans. Not surprisingly, when CIRM indicated that it anticipated a 30–40 percent failure rate, the reaction was negative.

CIRM took issue in February 2008 with President Bush for what it regarded as his distortion and mischaracterization of stem cell research in his State of the Union address. Bush lauded the November 2007 reprogramming of adult skin cells to imitate stem cells, and he called for further restrictions on cloning and commercial use of human cells. CIRM charged Bush with wanting further restrictions on human embryonic stem cell research. It noted that had Bush had his way, several lines would have failed to develop, and that federal restrictions have already cost years of productive research. CIRM said Bush's proposals would cause further years of suffering for those suffering from Parkinson's, spinal cord injury, degenerating sight, and other diseases.

**SEE ALSO:** California; Cells, Embryonic; Stem Cells, Bush Ruling.

**BIBLIOGRAPHY.** California Institute for Regenerative Medicine FAQ, www.cirm.ca.gov (cited February 2008); California Institute of Regenerative Medicine, "Annual Report, 2006," www.cirm.ca.gov (cited February 2008); California Stem Cell Report, "Biotech Loans: Industry Reaction, 30–40 Percent Failures, IP Qualms," February 3, 2008, californiastemcellreport.blogspot.com (cited February 2008); California Stem Cell Report, "CIRM to Bush: Harmful and Wrong," February 3, 2008, californiastemcellreport.blogspot.com (cited February 2008); Joyce E. Cutler, "State Supreme Court Rejects Challenge, Clearing Way for Stem Cell Bond Initiative, Bureau of National Affairs, Center for Genetics and Society," May 17, 2007, geneticsandsociety.org (cited February 2008); MSNBC Staff, "California Gives Go-Ahead to Stem-Cell Research. Proposition 71 Provides $3 billion in State Funding over Next Decade," November 3, 2004, www.msnbc.msn.com (cited February 2008); Jodi Rudoren, "Bypassing Bush, 2 States Speed Stem Cell Funding," *International Herald Tribune*, July 25, 2006, www.iht.com (cited February 2008); Stem Cell Community, "California Stem Cell Proposition 71 Upheld After Appeal," February 27, 2007, stemcellcommunity.org (cited February 2008); TheScientist.com, "California Stem Cell Program Is Legal: Judge," April 24, 2006, www.the-scientist.com (cited February 2008).

John H. Barnhill
Independent Scholar

# Caltech

**THE CALIFORNIA INSTITUTE** of Technology, located in Pasadena, California, was founded in 1891 and is known by its common nickname Caltech. Caltech is a private teaching and research institution specializing in science and technology offering undergraduate and graduate education is a variety of scientific disciplines including physical sciences, engineering and math offerings and also addressing the cross-disciplinary nature of biotechnology research. To further address the complexities of issues raised by biotechnology and stem cell research and applications, Caltech developed and offers a bioethics course focused on ethical, social and legal issues related to the biotech research.

In working with stem cells and other biomedical concepts, Caltech is dedicated to providing an interdisciplinary education and research structure. Participation in stem cell research crosses multiple departments; some of the departments involved include the divisions of biology, chemistry and chemical engineering and engineering and applied science. The Division of Biology's education and research is focused on structural, molecular, and cell biology; development and regulation and cellular and integrative neuroscience.

Offshoots of these academic programs are specifically designed to address the crossing of multiple discipline boundaries. Examples of these programs are the interdisciplinary Bioengineering and Biochemistry programs. The bioengineering program focuses on understanding biological systems using mathematical models, computation, and abstraction-based synthesis to create system models of functional life systems. The bioengineering program is intended for both teaching and research, applying engineering principles to biology and medicine for the development of biomedical products for use in clinical application. The biochemistry program incorporates biology and chemistry for understanding cell development, growth and interaction in living systems.

## TRAINING PROGRAM

In 2004 California's voters passed a proposition authorizing a $3 billion bond to fund adult and embryonic stem cell research and the founding of the California Institute of Regenerative Medicine (CIRM). In distributing these research funds, CIRM provided a $2.3 million grant to Caltech for the creation of a Stem-Cell Training Program. Designed specifically for postdoctoral scholars, the program focuses on training in stem cell fundamental concepts and technology as well as the potential use of stem cell discoveries in medical therapies and industrial applications. In addition to stem cell science, the training program will also included the various social, ethical, and legal issues related to stem cell research. Caltech is collaborating with the Keck School of Medicine at the University of Southern California and the Children's Hospital of Los Angeles and will offer courses at all three institutions. Participants in the program will also have opportunities of attending and participating in stem cell seminars and journal club programs and an annual scientific symposium.

## RESEARCH

Caltech researchers have access to resources across the disciplines including access to a mouse embryonic stem cell facility and advanced technologies. Caltech researchers working with stem cells want to improve basic scientific understanding of stem cell development, differentiation into various cell types, function and cell interaction in the living human system with a goal of moving this basic science knowledge into developing clinical and industrial applications for the treatment of chronic and debilitating human diseases. Toward this goal, researchers in the various departments have a wide range of interests including embryonic and adult stem cell plasticity, stem cells and cancer, embryonic development, tissue engineering and macromolecular fabrication and the basic science of hematopoietic, muscle, endothelial, and neural stem cells.

Caltech can claim a variety of firsts in stem cell research. In the David Anderson research laboratory, researchers were the first to isolate a peripheral nervous system stem cell with multipotency and self-renewal, identifying the signaling responsible for stem cell differentiation (along various lineages and into a glial cell) and isolating transcription factors regulating neuronal cell fate. Researchers in this group use neural stem cells, with a specific focus on the ability of the stem cell to self-renew and differentiate into all of the different neurons by using progenitor neural stem cells to determine what genetic elements regulate stem cell fate.

Researchers in the Wold Lab (Biology/Bioinformatics Lab) are studying stem cell networks in relation to cell fate during cell development and regeneration using genomic and proteomic assay to determine what regulates the mechanism from multipotent stem cell through progenitor cell and further to a fully differentiated cell using the mouse model for muscle, bone, skin and fat cells. The team is also working with researchers at Children's Hospital on how the out-of-control myogenic cells become cancerous with the hopes of improving cancer treatment and outcome. The team in collaboration with a team at the NIH has discovered that oxygen level in cell culture must be optimal for the growth of dopaminergic neurons, muscle and fat cells and how oxygen influences cell fate in culture, leading to additional focus on the identification the cell networks responsible.

Funding for stem cell research at Caltech comes from a variety of sources including public and private grants and research sponsored by companies. One of the company sponsored grants was received in 2007 from Arrowhead Research Corporation (a nanotechnology company for commercial applications of technology from the life sciences, electronics, and energy). The research will be focused on reengineering of the internal control systems of cells to drive cell differentiation and development. The agreement means Caltech receives $255,000 annually for three years and in exchange Arrowhead will retain the exclusive right to license the resultant technology.

## COLLABORATIONS

In 2006, the Caltech/MIT Enterprise Forum program focused on stem cell research and development in Southern California to discuss areas of interest to biomedical application, reasons for limited private funding, the future of stem cell research and the reality of using human stem cells for therapeutic applications. Caltech joined with other research institutions in southern California to establish the Southern California Stem Cell Scientific Collaboration in an effort to combine resources and expertise to take basic science and translate advances into clinical applications. Each participating institution will have a faculty member on the joint scientific advisory committee.

Caltech also maintains international working collaborations. Working with the researchers at the University of Rome, researchers are working on a characterizing cell lines sourced from mouse embryo dorsal aorta for gene expression. These cells have the capacity to differentiate into muscle, cardiac cells, bone or other derivatives by culturing. Researchers have identified a marker CD34 on these cells which could be used to mark stem cells. Among genes in common with stem-like cells is CD34, a putative marker of stem cells in several other contexts.

## OFFICE OF TECHNOLOGY TRANSFER

Caltech's Office of Technology Transfer was established in 1995 to assist Caltech researchers in licensing and developing the results of their research into industrial or clinical application. The service is available to faculty, students and allied researchers to protect their intellectual property and enhance medical care for patients by providing a mechanism for rapid translation of discoveries made in the laboratory into products (devices, drugs, and services) for use in the clinical setting to enhance patient quality of life. Of Caltech's more than 800 patents, those related to stem cell research include the identification, isolation, methods of differentiation and induction of stem cells including neural crest stem cells, melanoma tumor cells) and related to stem cells in living systems the stimulation of nerve growth, gene blocking, and pain signaling.

The Office of Technology Transfer provides patent portfolio management, technology license negotiation and assistance with entrepreneurial startup businesses. One business start-up success using Caltech discoveries in stem cell research is StemCells, Inc. The company was established to develop future possible clinical treatments for treating human diseases in such organ systems as the central nervous system, liver, and pancreas with non-embryonic–sourced stem cells.

**SEE ALSO:** California; California Institute for Regenerative Medicine; StemCells, Inc.

**BIBLIOGRAPHY.** California Institute of Technology, "The David Anderson Research Group," www.dja.caltech.edu (cited November 2007); California Institute of Technology, "Division of Biology," www.biology.caltech.edu (cited November 2007); Caltech Biology/Bioinformatics Lab, www.woldlab.caltech.edu (cited November 2007); Caltech Office of Technology Transfer, www.ott.caltech.edu (cited November 2007); "Caltech Receives $2.3 Million for Stem Cell Research," www.pr.caltech.edu (cited November 2007); Eileen Conrad, "Stem Cell Research Collaborations Spread," *USCB Newsletter*, January 7, 2008, www.ia.uscb.edu/93106 (cited November 2007); Engineering and Science, "The Stems of Brain Cancer," www.eands.caltech.edu (cited November 2007).

Lyn Michaud
Independent Scholar

# Cambridge University

**CAMBRIDGE UNIVERSITY, ALSO** known as the University of Cambridge, in Cambridge, England, is one of the oldest universities in the world. The first record of scholastic activity at Cambridge is from 1209, when the future city was only a trading post of the Romans. Recently, Cambridge University opened a state-of-the-art research facility for stem cell science.

Over the centuries since 1209, the university has undergone numerous renovations in mission and philosophy. The current university has developed since 1945, with the end of World War II. A major boon occurred in 1951, when Cambridge was declared an official city. The "Cambridge Phenomenon" followed, whereby many scientific industry firms were founded within Cambridge and in the outskirts. Many of these firms were established based on principles developed in Cambridge scientific laboratories. This phenomenon cemented Cambridge's position as a center of international science and industry.

In 2006, the Wellcome Trust Centre for Stem Cell Research was established within the School of the Biological Sciences at Cambridge University. The center, supported primarily by the Wellcome Trust as well as the Medical Research Council and the Wolfson Foundation, opened its doors on December 18, 2006. A symposium was held in Cambridge in celebration of the opening. It highlighted research breakthroughs in stem cell science that had taken place in this city over the past 25 years. The pioneer director of the center is Professor Austin Smith, formerly the director of the Centre for Stem Cell Research at Edinburgh University; the deputy director is Professor Fiona Watt. According to Professor Smith, the Wellcome Trust viewed the restrictions on public funding of stem cell research in the United States as an opportunity to advance research and understanding in the United Kingdom, establishing this nation as a world leader in stem cell research.

A chief focus of research at the Wellcome Centre is the mechanistic establishment of a stem cell and its derivative cells. Therefore, these genetic and biochemical pathways will be investigated, with the goal of developing therapeutics in the future. Specifically, stem cells could be transplanted and guided to differentiate into the needed tissue, or clinicians could potentially activate resident stem cells within the individual patient to restore the effete tissue.

As of the spring of 2008, the center had six founding members and was still hiring. These six members include Austin Smith and Fiona Watt, as well as Michaela Frye, Brian Hendrich, Jenny Nichols, and Juan-Jose Ventura. The Smith group studies the mechanisms regulating maintenance and differentiation of both pluripotent and tissue-restricted stem cells. The Watt group examines the mammalian epidermis, or skin, and the stem cells within that develop into a variety of lineages. In the Frye group, regulators of stem cell division and growth are studied, with an attention to the difference between stem cell division and cancer cell division, as uncontrolled stem cell proliferation becomes cancerous. The Hendrich group investigates the step that occurs in stem cells that makes them no longer pluripotent, or able to develop into any future cell type. Focusing on the embryo and where pluripotent cells are compartmentalized, the Nichols group aims to understand embryonic stem cells and a better way to maintain a line of embryonic stem cells for research and therapeutics. The Ventura group, like the Watt group, studies a particular tissue—in this case the lung. The group investigates the stem cells within the alveolar epithelium and their development and role in repair of this tissue.

Scientists at the Wellcome Centre have at their disposal numerous resources and excellent facilities for their research. To house the Wellcome Centre, the former Wellcome Trust/CR-UK Institute was revamped, complete with core facilities for imaging, bioinformatics, and flow cytometry. In the future, the center plans to offer a four-year Ph.D. program in the science of stem cells to train future stem cell researchers.

**SEE ALSO:** European Consortium for Stem Cell Research—EuroStemCell; Human Embryonic Stem Cells; Oxford University; UK National Stem Cell Network; United Kingdom; University of Edinburgh.

**BIBLIOGRAPHY.** M. Bellomo, *The Stem Cell Divide: The Facts, the Fiction, and the Fear Driving the Greatest Scientific, Political and Religious Debate of Our Time* (AMACOM/American Management Association, 2006); C. B. Cohen, *Renewing the Stuff of Life: Stem Cells, Ethics, and Public Policy* (Oxford University Press, 2007); C. Fox, *Cell of Cells: The Global Race to Capture and Control the Stem Cell* (Norton, 2007); K. R. Monroe, R. Miller, and J. Tobis, eds., *Fundamentals of the Stem Cell Debate: The Scientific, Religious, Ethical, and Political Issues* (University of California Press, 2007); M. Ruse and C. A. Pynes, eds., *The Stem Cell Controversy: Debating the Issues (Contemporary Issues)* (Prometheus Books, 2006).

Claudia Winograd
University of Illinois, Urbana-Champaign

# Canadian Stem Cell Network

**THE CANADIAN STEM CELL NETWORK** is one of Industry Canada's 21 Networks of Centres of Excellence (NCE) that bring together researchers and partners from the public, private, and nonprofit sectors to conduct research and work in areas of science to improve the well-being of Canadians. The NCEs are federally funded programs in the fields of information and communication technology, engineering and manufacturing, environmental and natural resources, and health and life sciences. The NCEs comprise academics, researchers, and industry and government professionals who work collaboratively to advance specific fields of science. The NCE programs are administered and funded by three federal Canadian agencies: the Natural Sciences and Engineering Research Council, the Canadian Institutes of Health Research, and the Social Sciences and Humanities Research Council, in partnership with Industry Canada.

The NCE has been providing these resources for the last 15 years, although it established long-term stability when the Canadian government established it as a permanent program. In 2006 the NCE's budget was increased to $82.4 million. The network has grown to support 6,000 researchers and specialized individuals in 71 Canadian universities. The network operates in collaboration with 329 provincial and federal government facilities, 525 Canadian agencies, and 430 international partners. Outside grants and in-kind giving for 2006 was almost $70 million. The Canadian Stem Cell Network was named as a Centre for Excellence in 2001, and new networks have continued to evolve, including six new networks in 2006.

The Canadian Stem Cell Network evolved out of the desire for a group of devoted researchers whose interest in stem cell research included the scientific potential of treating diseases along with consideration of the ethical and policy implications of this cutting-edge science. The group now includes over 70 highly specialized talents that include expertise in ethics, engineering, and the fields of science and medicine.

The vast interest in stem cells has exploded over the last decade, although the potential of stem cells and their ability to develop into specialized cells was identified over 25 years ago. Stem cells, with their potential to differentiate into any specialized cell within the body, can repair and regenerate damaged tissue and organs. Stem cells can be used to treat a variety of degenerative disorders, such as Alzheimer's disease, Parkinson's disease, and diabetes, along with spinal cord injuries and hematological disorders. In 2001 researchers interested in the area of stem cell research formed the Genomics Technologies and Society. The same year, this group received a four-year, $21.1 million grant from NCE to continue to study the potential of stem cell use to benefit the citizens of Canada. The network is a nonprofit organization that functions under a board of directors with guidance from an executive director from the University of Ottawa. The executive director receives scientific guidance from a scientific and deputy scientific director along with four specialized theme researchers. The theme researchers each have specialized fields of study that collaboratively meet the objectives of the Stem Cell Network.

The main goal of this NEC is to develop and implement a research program to identify what technologies allow for the advancement of stem cell use in the treatment of disease. The network develops multidisciplinary projects with goals and objectives that advance and expand the current knowledge within the organization. Because considerable financial resources are devoted to this NEC, the development of facilities that support the new technology are created and housed in core facilities across Canada so scientists can use technologies that would be impossible to replicate in multiple locations because of financial constraints. At present, the Stem Cell Network has scientists and trainees in 23 facilities. These technologies can then be translated into practice and used to guide the development of commercial products that will benefit the health and well-being of Canadians that have degenerative diseases. There are 19 industry partners that collaborate in developing products to efficiently use the advances made in the field. The Stem Cell Network partners with industry to facilitate development and advancement of specific products that aid in and advance stem cell research.

The organization has been continually seeking top-notch researchers in the field, which has grown and evolved as the science in stem cell research has advanced from its infancy. In a highly competitive environment, where scientists with expertise are in high demand, the Canadian Stem Cell Network attempts to attract new scientists by offering matching student funds. There are over 150 student trainees supported at least in part by the NEC.

Finally, the group functions to identify and address legal and ethical issues that are in constant public view. They are tasked with creating a positive public image to generate public support of the new science. Groups of scientists, social scientists, and clinicians collaborate to ensure that scientific and clinical research is planned and conducted ethically. The group has vast partnerships with government, industry leaders, health advocacy groups, and other organizations that work together to advance stem cell research, support the scientific community, and promote the science to the public at large. Along with industry partners, there are nine charitable organizations that support the organization and its goals and mission.

The Canadian Stem Cell Network has managed to make impressive gains in their six years in existence. They have a generalized goal to "cure people" and have dedicated teams that work in specific clinical areas to unlock the key to curing multiple diseases and injuries. The organization has been recognized globally by various organizations including the Juvenile Diabetes Research Foundation, Muscular Dystrophy Canada, and the Foundation Fighting Blindness in Canada. The diverse group of researchers has received various grants, awards, and government subsidies to continue to develop and evolve their research. Industry partnerships also have continued to expand, along with public support.

**SEE ALSO:** International Laws; UK National Stem Cell Network.

**BIBLIOGRAPHY.** Canadian Stem Cell Network, www.stemcellnetwork.ca (cited November 2007).

Michele R. Davidson
George Mason University

# Cancer

**THERE CURRENTLY DOES** not exist a full understanding of the underlying mechanisms of cancer. Identification of various carcinogens helped develop an understanding of how healthy cells mutate and lose normal cellular controls leading to the development of cancer. However, it remains unclear which cells in the body are associated with these accumulated mutations. Similarly, it is not clear how the tumor maintains itself, proliferates, and metastasizes.

The origins and nature of malignant cells in cancer have still not been definitively determined. Two potential models to explain the development, maintenance, and recurrence of cancer include the stochastic model and the stem cell model. Recent advances in technology related to isolation and identification of stem cells have allowed researchers to develop a strong supporting argument for the stem cell model.

Distinguishing between the stochastic and stem cell models is critical for directing the future of cancer research. A thorough understanding of the origins of cancer will generate new cancer research paradigms that can result in improved treatments. These treatments have the potential for better efficacy and less damage to patients than current methods such as radiation and chemotherapy.

## MODELS

The stochastic model, taking from the concept of stochastic probability, describes the development of cancer as a completely random process. The model proposes that cancer can arise in any cell of the body, including highly differentiated cells. This occurs by an accumulation of multiple mutations leading to a loss of normal control over the cellular life cycle. The multiple mutations result in the cell developing the phenotypes of cancer, developing into a tumor, and potentially metastasizing. The key features from this model are the concept that any cell in the body can become cancerous, and that any cell in the tumor mass has the ability to divide. As a result, any cell within the tumor mass should be able to metastasize or create tumors when experimentally transplanted into a mouse.

In contrast, the stem cell theory hypothesizes that mutations accumulate in somatic stem cells. The development of this theory considers two critical properties of stem cells. First, they have sufficiently long life spans to accumulate the necessary mutations. Second, they can asymmetrically divide providing cell populations that develop and maintain a tumor. This links with the concept that tumors consist of a mass of differentiated cells maintained by a small subpopulation of cancer stem cells. These populations of cancer stem cells possess the ability to develop new tumors by either metastasis or transplantation.

Understanding whether the stochastic or stem cell model is the predominant model of cancer development is essential to developing new effective therapies to prevent and treat cancer. Ideally, new therapies will more successfully target malignant cells while preserving healthy cells. With a thorough understanding of how cancer develops, maintains a tumor, and metastasizes, researchers can identify cellular markers useful in targeting treatments to malignant cells. Ongoing research in the field has begun to distinguish between these two models and provided initial evidence of potential molecular targets.

## EVIDENCE

The first model developed to describe cancer and the model initially subscribed to by most researchers was the stochastic model of cancer. However, during attempts to develop mouse models of human cancer, researchers began to suspect that cells within a tumor mass might have different properties than had been originally anticipated. Attempts to develop tumors in mice required the injection of a large number of malignant cells to guarantee tumor development. The idea that so many cells would be necessary to develop a tumor was not consistent with the rates of metastasis of many forms of cancer in humans.

Using the developed theories on how cancer may originate, two explanations for the low tumor formation rates arose. If the stochastic model applied, then the findings would suggest that each cell could colonize and lead to tumor development, but that the difficulties associated with starting a new tumor just meant that each individual cell had a low probability of achieving a tumor. The general view is that cancer is an aggressive and unregulated cellular process. This suggests that cells should not have such a low probability of successfully generating a tumor. The stem cell hypothesis counters that only a small subset of stem cells within the tumor mass can lead to tumor proliferation. Proving this theory required the development of recent technology capable of identifying and separating stem cells within a tumor.

In the hematopoiesis (blood formation) field, researchers began to develop the technology to identify and separate stem cells based on cell surface markers that varied between stem cells and differentiated cells. Researchers studying leukemia were able to apply this new technology and gain insight into the tumorgenic capabilities of various cell populations. Initially, it was determined that only one percent of the tumor bulk developed new tumors in methyl-cellulose assays or mouse spleen colony-forming assays. Since it was not possible to differentiate between stem cells and their terminally differentiated progeny, the stem cell hypothesis still required stronger verification.

Then, in a series of experiments examining severe combined immunodeficient (SCID) mice, utilization of flow cytometry allowed for separation of subpopulations of leukemia cells with repopulation activity. Many of the methods they used matched those used initially in identifying stem cells of the hematopoietic system. Interestingly, the tumorgenic cells from the SCID mice experiments were $CD34^{+}$ and $CD38^{-}$, a characteristic that matches the surface markers of hematopoietic stem cells.

This study convincingly showed that the tumor mass does consist of a population of differentiated cells maintained by a smaller population of stem cells. In addition, the studies showed that tumor metastasis or clone development requires tumor stem cells. The remaining question is the premalignancy nature of these stem cells. The stem cell hypothesis would suggest that the tumor stem cells come from a population of cells that have always been stem cells. However, it is possible that during the carcinogenic process a differentiated cell reobtained stem cell characteristics. The answer to this dilemma followed from some leukemia studies analyzing the effects of certain oncogenes.

Early studies examined the MLL-ENL and MOZ-TIF 2 oncogenes using a retrovirus system. The experiments submitted committed, but still not fully differentiated, progenitor cells to the oncogenes and found that the oncogenes could transform these early progenitor cells. The transformed progenitor cells developed tumor clones in mice. Cells from the initial tumors could be extracted and injected into a secondary recipient and once again develop a tumor. This ability to transform progenitor cells varies based on the oncogene. For example, the Bcr-Abl oncogene could not transform progenitor cells into tumorgenic stem cells.

The tumorgenicity and transformation studies primarily support the stem cell hypothesis as a more accurate description of the cancer development process than the stochastic model. However, the transformation studies, in particular, show that the stem cell hypothesis is not a complete description of how cancer can develop. Further analysis and characterization of the processes incurred by various oncogenes may aid in developing a complete description of the carcinogenic process.

## ADDITIONAL STUDIES

Some additional studies and observations have been brought forth to provide additional support for the stem cell hypothesis. Once such observation is that breast cancer incidence increases exponentially with age. This seems to suggest that the stem cell population serves as a critical reservoir for the accumulation of mutations. Short-lived differentiated cells have the same probability of accumulating mutations at any point in the life span and would therefore not correlate as strongly with age. Importantly, additional studies in breast cancer identified a stem cell population in breast tumors. CD44 and CD24 are key surface markers for breast tissue. The studies determined that cells that were $CD44^{+}$ and $CD24^{-}$ had 10–50-fold increased ability to develop tumors over any other CD44/CD24 combinations. The tumors that arose from the $CD44^{+}/CD24^{-}$ cells had heterogeneity that mimicked tumors taken from patients.

These studies from leukemia and breast cancer provide a solid foundation for developing further studies to examine the role of stem cells in cancer. One of the key questions is what properties change in stem cells as they develop a malignant phenotype. Equally important is to determine the intrinsic and extrinsic factors that aid in the development and maintenance of the malignant state. Further application of these results may lead to developing effective treatments that specifically target and eradicate malignant stem cells. Perhaps thorough eradication of malignant stem cells will prevent the regrowth or reoccurrence of a patient's tumors.

## DEFINING CHARACTERISTICS

A series of studies have already begun to outline some of the defining characteristics of stem cells. All stem cells have the ability to self-renew and asymmetrically divide. Malignant stem cells enhance this behavior by exhibiting an active telomerase enhancing their ability to divide indefinitely. Further characteristics associated with the malignant phenotype are the ability to migrate, to avoid apoptosis (cell death), enhance membrane transport properties, and grow independent of anchorage. Unsurprisingly, these are all characteristics typically associated with cancer. The search for key characteristics has unearthed several unique cell surface markers found on various malignant stem cell populations (Table 1). Last, three intrinsic signaling pathways, Wnt, Sonic hedgehog, and the Notch family, show increased activity in certain types of cancers (Table 2).

**Table 1** Associated Stem Cell Cellular Markers for Various Cancers

| *Cellular Marker* | *Tumor Type* |
|---|---|
| $Cd34^{+}$ / $Cd38^{+}$ | Leukemia |
| $CD138^{-}$ | Multiple Myeloma |
| $Cd44^{+}/CD24^{+}$, $Oct4^{+}$, $CX43^{-}$ | Breast Cancer |
| $CD133^{+}/nestin^{+}$ | Brain Tumor |
| $CD133^{+}$ | Colon Cancer |
| $CD44^{+}/\alpha_2\beta_1{}^{hi}/CD133^{+}$, $Scal^{+}$ | Prostate Cancer |

Of these properties, enhanced membrane transport, provides insight into why it is critical to develop treatments specific for malignant stem cells. For example, imatinib is an effective tyrosine kinase inhibitor against differentiated leukemia cells but does not have the same effect on leukemia stem cells. It is not entirely clear whether the leukemia stem cells avoid death due to their enhanced membrane transport ability or just their general resistance to apoptosis. What is clear though is that stem cells have developed unique methods to avoid death. This is important in their normal state, but problematic when it comes to malignant stem cells.

**Table 2** Dysregulated Signaling Pathways and Associated Cancers

| *Signaling Factor* | *Tumor Type* |
|---|---|
| Wnt | Colon Cancer, Chronic Myelogenous Leukemia |
| Sonic Hedgehog | Pancreatic Tumors, Basal Skin Carcinoma, Gastric Cancer, Breast Carcinoma, Prostate Tumor |
| Notch | Human T-Cell Acute Lymphoblastic Leukemia, Breast Cancer, Cervical Cancer |

The effects of enhanced membrane transport play a significant role in the development of multiple drug resistant (MDR) cancer. In these instances, the cells possess a surface transporter that binds chemotherapeutic drugs and utilizes ATP to pump the drugs out of the cell. The MDR transporter, first identified in breast cancer, prevents intracellular accumulation of drugs leading to toxicity. Roughly, 58 percent of cancer stem cells in lung, breast, ovarian, and gastric cancers test positive for the MDR transporter. These cells provide a reservoir of drug-resistant cells that are likely to be responsible for relapse and metastasis of cancer after seemingly effective treatment.

This seems to indicate that not only are new therapies necessary, but they must also target stem cell populations that have developed effective methods to avoid death. It may be easy to target these cells based on their surface markers; however, those surface markers are not always unique to malignant cells.

Often the malignant cells share these markers with their normal stem cell counterparts. Targeting and destroying these cells based on their cell surface markers may damage the normal stem cells, potentially hindering the body's ability to recover from the trauma or maintain the normal cellular recycling. Exploration into some of the other defining characteristics of cancer is providing insight into routes that may prove fruitful in defeating cancer.

## TREATMENT AND PREVENTION

Surface markers may not always be the optimal strategy for eliminating malignant stem cells. Some research has begun to focus on mechanistic differences between normal and malignant stem cells. Similar to the research done to understand how cancer develops, the first work to identify mechanistic differences examined leukemia. Their intriguing finding was that normal hematopoietic stem cells depend on the Pten suppressor gene, while leukemia stem cells in mouse models do not. Conveniently, there is also a treatment, rapamycin, with potential benefit in this situation. In leukemia, the cells produce mTOR to mediate the effects of the deleted Pten gene.

Rapamycin inhibits mTOR. In experiments that treated mice with rapamycin, the result was the elimination of leukemia and restoration of normal hematopoiesis. This is only one mechanistic difference between normal and malignant stem cells, but it provides hope that further research will reveal other therapeutic differences.

Another potential avenue for therapeutic targets is the activated signaling pathways, such as Notch and Hedgehog. These signaling pathways are associated with certain malignant stem cells. In the Notch pathway, the processing of the enzyme γ-secretase regulates many of its effects. Inhibition of this enzyme by GSI led to a decreased number of proliferating transformed human fibroblasts in both in vitro and in vivo studies. Another potential avenue for decreasing Notch signaling pathway activity is to activate the antagonistic Numb signaling pathway.

Activation of the Hedgehog signaling pathway provides another avenue for therapy. Constitutive expression of Hedgehog in the prostate is associated with the development of highly metastatic malignancy. A concern in this situation is that healthy prostate epithelium still expresses Hedgehog at regulated levels. As a result, complete inhibition of Hedgehog is not a valid therapeutic option. A potential target that differs between malignant and benign cells is the expression of Smoothened, a responsive element. Currently, there are no concrete methods for monitoring or manipulating the Hedgehog pathway for treating prostate cancer. One promising study showed that cyclopamine, a Hedgehog inhibitor, led to complete regression of human prostate tumors in athymic mice. In transgenic mouse models for medulloblastoma the molecular inhibitor HhAntag bound to Smoothened with higher affinity than cyclopamine and thus could inhibit signaling in neuroblastoma cells.

The current state of knowledge for treating the effects of stem cells in cancer is expanding. Current research shows that stem cells have a specific role in forming tumors. Researchers are using these pathways to develop very specific and effective targets for cancer therapy. Recognizing that stem cells play a central role in the development, maintenance, and metastasis of cancer provided a wealth of knowledge, which will hopefully lead to a promising treatment that combats cancer.

**SEE ALSO:** Birth Dating of Cells by Retrovirus; Bone Marrow Transplants; Cells, Adult; Clinical Trials Within U.S.: Blind Process; Clinical Trials Within U.S.: Cancer; Sloan-Kettering Institute.

**BIBLIOGRAPHY.** M. Al-Hajj, et al., "Prospective Identification of Tumoregenic Breast Cancer Cells," *Proceedings of the National Academy of Science USA* (v.100, 2003); D. Bonnet and J. E. Dick, "Human Acute Myeloid Leukemia Is Organized as a Hierarchy that Originates from a Primitive Hematopoietic Cell," *Nature Medicine* (v.3, 1997); W. R. Bruce and H. Van Der Gaag, "A Quantitative Assay for the Number of Murine Lymphoma Cells Capable of Proliferation In Vivo," *Nature* (v.199, 1963); A. Cozzio, et al., "Similar Mll-Associated Leukemias Arising from Self-Renewing Stem Cells and Short-Lived Myeloid Progenitors," *Genes & Development* (v.17, 2003); A. Giordano, et al., "Carcinogenesis and Environment: The Cancer Stem Cell Hypothesis and Implications for the Development of Novel Therapeutics and Diagnostics," *Frontiers in Bioscience* (v.12, 2007); T. Gudjonsson and M. K. Magnusson, "Stem Cell Biology and the Cellular Pathways of Carcinogenesis," *Acta Pathologica, Microbiologica et Immunologica Scandinavica* (v.113, 2005); B. J. Huntly, et al., "MOZ-TIF2, but Not Bcr-abl, Confers Properties of Leukemic Stem Cells to Committed Murine Hematopoietic Progenitors," *Cancer Cell* (v.6, 2004); S. S. Karhadkar, et al., "Hedgehog Signaling in Prostate Regeneration, Neoplasia and Metastasis," *Nature* (v.431, 2004); F. Michor, et al., "Dynamics of Chronic Myeloid Leukemia," *Nature* (v.435, 2005); C. H. Park, et al., "Mouse Myeloma Tumor Stem Cells: A Primary Cell Culture Assay," *Journal of the National Cancer Institute* (v.46, 1971); S. Pece, et al., "Loss of Negative Regulation by Numb over Notch Is Relevant to Human Breast Carcinogenesis," *Journal of Cell Biology* (v.167/2, 2004); G. Romano, "Perspectives and Controversies in the Field of Stem Cell Research," *Drug News Perspectives* (v.19, 2006); J. T. Romer, et al., "Suppression of the Shh Pathway Using a Small Molecule Inhibitor Eliminates Medulloblastoma in Ptc+/- p53-/- Mice," *Cancer Cell* (v.6, 2004); K. D. Sabbath, et al., "Heterogeneity of Clonogenic Cells in Acute Myeloblastic Leukemia," *Journal of Clinical Investigations* (v.75/2, 1985); K. D. Sabbath and J. D. Griffin, "Clonogenic Cells in Acute Myeloblastic Leukaemia" *Scandinavian Journal of Haematology* (v.35, 1985); S. Weijzen, et al., "Activation of Notch-1 Signaling Maintains the Neoplastic Phenotype in Human Ras-transformed Cells," *Nature Medicine* (v.8, 2002); W. A. Woodward, et al., "On Mammary Stem Cells," *Journal of Cell Science* (v.118, 2005); O. H. Yilmaz, et al., "Pten Dependence Distinguishes Haematopoietic Stem Cells from Leukaemia Initiating Cells," *Nature* (v.441, 2006).

Justin Glasgow
Aliasger K. Salem
University of Iowa

# Case Western Reserve University

**CASE WESTERN RESERVE UNIVERSITY,** a private research and teaching institution located in Cleveland, Ohio, was established in 1826 as Western Reserve University and was strengthened by a 1967 merger with the Case Institute of Technology, which was founded in 1880 by philanthropist Leonard Case, Jr. Case Western Reserve University has positioned itself as a leading research institution, and in addition to academic programs in the arts and sciences, engineering, law, management, dentistry, nursing, and social sciences, Case's School of Medicine is internationally recognized; research funding from the National Institutes of Health ranks it 13th largest in the United States. The School of Medicine maintains affiliations with University Hospitals of Cleveland, the Cleveland Clinic, MetroHealth Medical Center, and the Louis Stokes Cleveland Veterans Affairs Medical Center.

Case's early success in stem cell research led to the filing of patent applications in 1986 by the Department of Biology for mesenchymal stem cells and in the years from 1989 to 2000 for the clinical application of mesenchymal stem cells, including but not limited to transplantation, gene therapy, and support of hematopoietic stem cell transplantation. The first United States clinical trials using mesenchymal stem cells began in 1996.

Case received funding in 2006 from the state of Ohio to create the Ohio Cell-Based Therapy Consortium—an effort focused on coordinating clinical trials within the state of Ohio. In 2007 Case and its partners in the National Center for Regenerative Medicine (NCRM) hosted the Adult Mesenchymal Stem Cells in Regenerative Medicine Conference from August 27 to 29, 2007, in Cleveland, with international attendees representing 127 institutions from 27 countries. The conference focused on mesenchymal stem cells technology and clinical application.

The Cell Production Facility was opened in November 2005 on the Case campus. This facility complies with U.S. Food and Drug Administration regulations in providing an ultrasterile environment for the preparation and expansion of stem cells for use in human clinical trials at University Hospitals of Cleveland and the Cleveland Clinic in the Department of Stem Cell and Regenerative Medicine.

## CENTER FOR STEM CELL AND REGENERATIVE MEDICINE

The Center for Stem Cell and Regenerative Medicine (CSCRM) was established in 2003 with funding from the state of Ohio and continues its work with funding awards from a variety of sources. CSCRM is a nonprofit partnership between Case Western Reserve University and University Hospitals of Cleveland (a nationally recognized medical center known for its excellence as a pediatric hospital and receiving the nation's highest recognition as a National Cancer Institute–designated Comprehensive Cancer Center), the Cleveland Clinic (a not-for-profit medical center founded in 1921 that provides medical care as well as research and education opportunities), Athersys Inc. (a private biopharmaceutical company founded in 1995 to develop a variety of therapeutic products to treat cardiovascular disease, stroke, diabetes, blood, and immune system disorders), and the Ohio State University (a public research university founded in 1870 offering study in numerous academic areas including various medical and scientific professional programs).

CSCRM's mission is the treatment of human disease through human stem cell and tissue engineering. The center supports scientific research at the member institutions and has 62 investigators at these institutions working on six different adult stem cell types in the research areas of cancer, orthopedics, musculoskeletal, cardiovascular, neurodegenerative, and vascular disease.

CSCRM uses adult or nonembryonic stem cells derived from bone marrow, umbilical cord blood, and other adult tissues in all of its research. The center has completed or has ongoing a total of 51 clinical trials, treating 250 patients with adult stem cells and 60-plus patients with cell therapies.

Stem cell transplants (also called blood/bone marrow transplants) can cure some diseases and put others into remission. Once the unhealthy cells in the body are destroyed (often with chemotherapy) in a process called conditioning, the stem cell transplant is expected to signal the body to produce healthy replacement blood and stem cells. The transplant might be autologous, coming from the patient's own blood or bone marrow, or allogenic, coming from a human lymphocyte antigen (HLA)–compatible related or unrelated donor. The complications that may occur include rejection in graft-versus-host disease, stem cell failure, damage to organs and blood vessels, and secondary cancers or diseases.

In CSCRM's current clinical trials, researchers are investigating basic stem cell science, the collection of cells for transplant, treatments, how to limit complications, and safety and efficacy. For basic stem cell science, researchers are determining the role of DNA repair on human hematopoietic stem cell function as well as setting up a sample repository and database of allogenic unrelated hematopoietic stem cells.

Using technology to collect and increase cells for transplant, researchers at the center are inducing the mobilization of peripheral blood stem cell and peripheral blood progenitor cells, seeking cost-effective alternative sources for allogenic hematopoietic stem cells and improving the characteristics of stem cells in the treatment of some cancers.

After treatment to destroy diseased cells, blood and bone marrow transplants have become a standard method of care for treating a range of childhood and adult diseases such as amyloidosis, aplastic anemia, inherited or genetically caused cancers, and solid tumors. CSCRM's researchers are investigating how to improve current treatments and to expand treatment options in other diseases. They are researching using umbilical cord blood for high-risk malignancies and blood disorders, adjusting conditioning dosage changes, maintenance therapy, biochemical targeting, comparing drug therapies, monoclonal antibody treatment, the effectiveness of HLA-compatible peripheral blood stem cells that have been enriched for

CD34+ cells and depleted T cells, and comparing the transplant of peripheral blood stem cells versus bone marrow.

Before any treatment can be approved as a standard therapy, it is tested for safety and effectiveness. CSCRM's researchers are currently involved in clinical trials to determine the effectiveness of laboratory-expanded stem and progenitor cells and survival after protocol therapy. In an attempt to limit complications related to stem cell transplant, CSCRM's researchers are investigating the prevalence of late iron overload and oral mucositis—prophylaxis treatments to prevent graft-versus-host disease and cytomegalovirus. In addition, CSCRM is researching possible treatments for graft-versus-host disease. Research done by CSCRM has led to the formation of four biotech firms, creating new jobs and commercializing viable new therapies.

### NATIONAL CENTER FOR REGENERATIVE MEDICINE

Regenerative medicine relies on controlling cell development to regrow healthy tissue and improve the innate function of diseased or injured organs or tissues using cell-based therapy, as opposed to drugs or devices to create artificial functionality. NCRM was founded in 2004 as a partnership between Case Western Reserve University and the Cleveland Clinic Foundation and University Hospitals of Cleveland. NCRM's mission is the research, development, and clinical application of nonembryonic stem cells and tissue-engineering therapeutics for human disease including cardiovascular, cancer, genetic disorders, musculoskeletal, hematopoietic, and neurodegenerative diseases.

By combining their scientific strengths and areas of expertise, researchers from the partner institutions work under the auspices of NCRM. They use specialized research facilities, including the science laboratories at Case Western University and University Hospitals of Cleveland, as well as clinical research spaces at University Hospitals of Cleveland and the Cleveland Clinic. Their efforts are aimed toward providing optimal patient care in making advanced technology available in a timely and safe manner. Their work is accomplished through funding provided by the state of Ohio, grant awards from the National Institutes of Health and the National Institute of Aging, and from its partner institutions.

**SEE ALSO:** Blind Process Transplants; Cells, Adult.

**BIBLIOGRAPHY.** Case Western Reserve University, "The Center for Stem Cell and Regenerative Medicine," ora.ra.cwru.edu/stemcellcenter (cited November 2007); "Center for Stem Cell & Regenerative Medicine Receives $8 million from Third Frontier Program," www.eurekalert.org (cited November 2007); National Center for Regenerative Medicine, "About Us," www .ncrm.us (cited November 2007).

Lyn Michaud
Independent Scholar

# Cells, Adult

**SINCE THE DISCOVERY** of stem cells, scientists have been trying to find ways and means to isolate and use them for the treatments of many diseases. Their ability to transform into different types of cells under a suitable environment has led to growing interest in them and to rapid discoveries. The primary source of stem cells has been either embryo or adult tissue.

Although scientists were able to isolate the embryonic stem cells in animal models in 1981 and from human tissue in the late 1990s, stem cells have not been tried as a treatment for clinical diseases thus far. However, adult stem cells have been used for the treatment of various diseases for quite some time now and have yielded excellent results.

Previously, it was thought that the potential to transform into different types of cells resided only in an embryonic stem cell, but it now has been shown that adult stem cells also have the ability of doing so, provided they are nurtured in a suitable environment. These cells, however, have a lesser potential to transform into other types of cells compared to embryonic stem cells.

Because of the potential for these cells to experience aberrant growth and to transform into cancerous tissue in animal model studies, an ideal stem cell is the one that has the least chance of mutations (a sudden structural change within a gene or chromosome resulting in the creation of a new character or trait not found in the parental type). Although there have been concerns that adult stem cells may develop mutations, this may not be true unless they are forced to pass through more than 30 doublings—a practice that is not performed clinically.

One of the properties of adult stem cells is that they can be derived from and later infused or transplanted back to the same individual, so the need for immunosuppression therapy can be avoided, whereas other sources of stem cells may still need immunosuppression therapy to avoid rejection and immune intolerance as a result of a mismatch between recipient and donor tissue.

Another advantage of using adult stem cells is that they can be obtained without harming an embryo—the moral dilemma that surrounds embryonic stem cells. At present, scientists can no longer generate embryonic stem cells using federal funding. Adult stem cells, in contrast, are not engulfed by any such limitation and, therefore, can be used as an excellent alternative source of such cells.

Adult stem cells are found in a number of tissues, some of which have been used in clinical practice to treat several diseases. Scientists have been working on bone marrow stem cells since 1960s. Other tissues in which they have been identified are the kidney, brain, spinal cord, and connective tissue of many other organs.

At present, a number of clinical trials are exploring their promising roles; for example, some of the diseases that are being investigated are spinal cord injuries, Parkinson's disease, corneal repair, multiple sclerosis, leukemia, and so on. Bone marrow transplantation using bone marrow stem cells has been used for quite some time now and has shown excellent results.

Recently, scientists have also used adult stem cells for patients who had a myocardial infarction and who were not suitable for other invasive therapies such as angioplasty and coronary bypass. It has been shown that these cells grow into new vessels in the damaged area of the heart, which in turn helps improve the output function of the failing heart. Their role in regeneration of nerves has also been studied in animal models and has proved beneficial.

The future of adult stem cells seems very promising because of their unique properties and easy availability. However, additional work needs to be done to meet the challenges involved in the identification of adult stem cells and the cost effectiveness of the potential treatments so that their benefits can be seen on a larger scale. As in all emerging fields of science, there is hope that adult stem cell research will one day reveal details that are still shrouded in mystery, and the day is not far off when they will play an integral role in treating ailing humanity.

**SEE ALSO:** Cells, Embryonic; Cells, Fetal; Cells, Mouse (Embryonic).

**BIBLIOGRAPHY.** "Stem Cells," www.explorestemcells.co.uk (cited November 2007); "Stem Cells Facts," www.massgeneral.org (cited November 2007); National Institutes of Health, "Stem Cell Information," stemcells.nih.gov (cited November 2007).

Faris Khan
Wasiq Rahman
Faisal Habib Cheema
Columbia University Medical Center

# Cells, Amniotic

**AMNIOTIC CELLS ARE** those cells found within the amniotic fluid of pregnant women. Although the benefits of embryonic stem cells are widely known, knowledge regarding the potential of amniotic fluid cells is still in the infancy stage. Amniotic cells may possess the same qualities as stem cells as far as having the capability to transform into brain, muscle, and other tissues, and using this technology could have an enormous effect on tissue repair and organ regeneration.

Scientists have produced nonembryonic stem cell lines that have been termed amniotic fluid–derived stem cells (AFS). It is theorized that these cells are shed by the fetus as it develops and may be easier to harvest than embryonic stem cells. Stem cells can be harvested by amniotic cells as early as 10 weeks postconception. Amniotic fluid is currently extracted for genetic testing procedures including chorionic villus sampling and amniocentesis. Researchers also hope that future advances could include harvesting these cells from placenta tissue.

The use of embryonic stem cells has been the topic of diverse debate and political activity since 2001, when President George W. Bush severely limited funding related to stem cell research. In 2006, legislators in a Republican-controlled Congress voted to expand stem cell research. The subsequent veto issued by President Bush in response was the first in his presidency. In 2007 a Democratic-controlled Congress passed a bill to expand research, but the vote was not enough to override the June 20, 2007, presidential veto by President Bush. Congress was acting in response to the many citizens who could be potentially helped or cured by stem cell research developments. Researchers have viewed the process of cloning amniotic stem cells as a new process in studying genetic disease. This advancement would appear to be ethically neutral and nonthreatening to almost all political, special interest, and religious groups.

Amniotic cell use could greatly expand the treatment options for children born with certain birth defects because these cells would be a direct genetic match to the fetus. Worldwide, an estimated 8 million children are born with a birth defect that is genetic or with a partially genetic-related birth defect. These millions of children could potentially benefit from advances in stem cell research. Amniotic stem cells also theoretically can be used for treating diseases or serious injuries in individuals who had these cells banked during the gestational period. These cells could be collected and stored in much the same manner that cord blood is stored and banked today. Embryonic stem cells vary from adult cells that can be harvested from bone marrow in their ability to adapt and change into other types of tissue. Although adult bone marrow cells are relatively easy to obtain, their use is much more limited.

Amniotic cells have some advantages over the more studied and publicly scrutinized embryonic stem cells. They would not likely meet with the social, religious, and political controversy that has surrounded the advancement of embryonic stem cell research. When news of the potential use of AFS first broke, the Vatican's top healthcare official issued a statement offering strong support to the researchers and stated that there was no ethical problem involved in the use of AFS as long as the mother and fetus were in no danger when the cells are obtained. The report further stated that the Catholic Church does not support stem cell research because human embryos are destroyed.

From a scientific perspective, amniotic stem cells also are easier to obtain, are found in greater supply, and are easier to store for longer periods of time. Embryonic stem cells often become unstable and develop chromosomal instability after long term growth. Although amniotic fluid stem cells may have great potential, however, they do not have the same capabilities as embryonic stem cells. It is unlikely that amniotic stem cells would ever surpass or replace the use of embryonic stem cells within the scientific and research communities, although amniotic cells also have pluripotentiality—the ability to differentiate into other types of tissue.

Amniotic cells are capable of diversifying into 36 different types of tissue. The cycle repeats itself every 36 hours, and mutations and aging do not appear to occur. The cells retain the same number of chromosomes as they self-renew. Research has shown that the cells have the capability of differentiating into cell types represented in each of the three embryonic germ layers, including cells of adipogenic, osteogenic, myogenic, endothelial, neuronal, and hepatic tissue.

Worldwide, research has shown promising results. In Taiwan, researchers were able to isolate mesenchymal stem cells that were obtained from amniotic fluid samples from women who had undergone an amniocentesis. The scientists reported that under ideal circumstances, 12 percent of the samples were able to differentiate into adipocytes and osteocytes. Researchers in Greece had similar results, differentiating their cells into osteoblasts, adipocytes, and chondrocytes. Researchers in California also have yielded success with the manipulation of unmodified pluripotential cells for kidney regeneration.

Early animal studies have also yielded encouraging findings. Rodent studies that used amniotic fluid mesenchymal stem cells to regenerate the sciatic nerve after a crush injury showed increased nerve regeneration when amniotic fluid mesenchymal stem cells were used, and other studies have shown that when amniotic fluid mesenchymal stem cells are transplanted into the brains of adult rats, regeneration of brain cells occurs. Another study used amniotic fluid–derived stem cells compared to embryonic whole brain stem cells in mice who had suffered a focal cerebral ischemia-reperfusion injury. Mice who received the amniotic fluid–derived stem cells significantly reversed the focal cerebral ischemia-reperfusion–induced behavioral deficits. Mice who received these cells showed improvement in short-term memory, motor coordination, sensorimotor ability, and somatosensory functions. Other research has shown improvement in the smooth cells of the bladder in rats that have received amniotic fluid–derived stem cells.

Anthony Atala, one of the first to identify amniotic stem cells, has theorized that if 100,000 women donated their amniotic cells to collection banks, there would be enough cells for treatment for virtually every United States citizen. With the number of births in the United States exceeding 4 million annually, this donor pool would be relatively easy to obtain and sustain. Although these recent developments have emerged out of privately funded studies, the need for federal funding in this area is imperative for the continuation of research studies.

**SEE ALSO:** Cells, Adult; Cells, Embryonic.

**BIBLIOGRAPHY.** "Explore Stem Cells," www.explorestemcells.co.uk (cited November 2007); National Institutes of Health, "Stem Cell Information," stemcells.nih.gov (cited November 2007).

Michele R. Davidson
George Mason University

# Cells, Developing

**ANIMAL DEVELOPMENT IS** a process in which a single cell (a fertilized egg or zygote) is transformed into an adult organism. The animal development is a lifelong process including stages of fertilization, embryogenesis, organism development after birth, sexual maturation, adulthood development, aging, and death. Because the formation of a multicellular embryo is key to early development, many cell types must be differentiated from the fertilized egg to form organs and tissues in the body. Stem cells play important roles and are involved in every step of development, from early embryogenesis to adulthood replenishment of damaged cells and maintenance of body function. A zygote is considered to be the earliest-stage stem cell, as every cell and organ in the body stem from zygote division and differentiation.

## FERTILIZATION

The animal development event is initiated by a process called fertilization—the fusion of male and female gametes by binding of sperm to egg—and brings together the nuclei of both gametes to form a fertilized egg. The fertilization is the process of generating the zygote—the earliest-stage parental stem cell. Sperm are formed in the male testis and stored in epididymis. During mating, sperm are mixed in the seminal vesicle with prostate secretion and travels through the male reproductive tract. When sperm travels through the female reproductive tract, capacitation occurs. During this process, the receptors on the sperm surface are modified by secretions in the female reproductive tract. The capacitation increases the ability of sperm to fertilize eggs.

The female gamete is called an egg and is formed in the ovary. The ovulated egg is moved through the oviduct and meets the sperm there. The sperm head receptors bind on the egg surface's glycoprotein zona pellucida in a species-specific manner. When sperm and egg cell surface receptor bind together, the sperm empties its enzyme contents within the acrosome. These contents digest a path through the egg's surface glycoprotein layer, allowing the sperm to pass through. This process triggers a series of events leading to the activation of the egg. An activated egg modifies the egg surface receptors and prevents more than one sperm from fertilizing the egg. After a sperm enters the egg, male and female pronuclears are fused together to form a zygote. The zygote starts dividing immediately after fertilization and continues division during zygote movement from oviduct to uterus.

## EMBRYOGENESIS

Embryogenesis involves cell division, specialization of different types of cells, and the shaping and patterning of the body. Fertilization forms the diploid zygote and triggers the onset of embryonic development, which involves cell division, differentiation, and morphogenesis. During embryogenesis, the division of the zygote results in an increase in the number of cells to form organs and tissues in the body. Differentiation is a development of specialized cell types from zygote or different levels of stem cells. Both the internal clock of the specific cell type and the environmental factors affect the gene expression pattern, which in turn regulates the differentiation and organogenesis in embryos. Morphogenesis is a process by which different types of cells are organized into tissues and organs and give shape to the animal's body and organs.

At the early stage of cell division, the cell numbers increase, but the embryo does not increase in size. Therefore, the cells in the embryo become smaller and smaller with each division. Before the embryo reaches the 16-cell stage, each cell in the embryo can develop into a fully functional individual, and each cell in the embryo has the capacity to give rise to all the different cell types in the body.

After this stage, the embryonic tissue is differentiated into two groups of cells. The cells in the outer layer will develop into the fetal portion of the placenta, called the trophoblast. The trophoblast starts implanting into the uterus by secreting enzymes to digest part of the inner layer of the uterus. In the initial stages of pregnancy, the corpora lutea from the ovary produces the hormone progesterone to maintain embryo survival. In a later stage of embryogenesis, the trophoblast also secretes chorionic gonadotropin in humans, which keeps the corpus luteum secreting progesterone. The progesterone also plays a role in preventing menstruation and uterus contraction. A mass of cells within the trophoblast is called the inner cell mass; it will eventually develop into a fetus. It is from these inner cell mass cells that embryonic stem cells are derived.

The embryo continues its growth and differentiation in the uterus after fertilization. The embryo is further developed into three layers of tissue called the ectoderm, endoderm, and mesoderm. The ectoderm gives rise to the skin and nervous system. The endoderm forms the lining of the gut, liver, kidney, and other internal organs. The mesoderm becomes the muscle, skeleton, and circulatory and reproductive systems. In the third week of development of the human embryo, the nervous system begins to form, as indicated by neural tube formation. At this stage, the heart starts to form and begins to beat, and the limbs begin to appear.

Allantois develops and will form the blood vessels of the umbilical cord. In the placenta, projections of chorionic villi grow into the endometrium of the uterus that increases the surface area of contact between the mother and fetus to facilitate material exchange between these two membranes. At four weeks, eyes, ears, and respiratory systems begin to form. At about eight weeks, the entire body system is present, but most organs are not yet functionally mature. At 11 weeks, spontaneous breathing movements start. At about 25 weeks, 80 percent of all babies can survive a premature birth.

At birth, the baby acquires the basic ability to survive outside the uterus by forming functional circulation, respiration, and other systems. It continuously grows and matures from infancy to child-

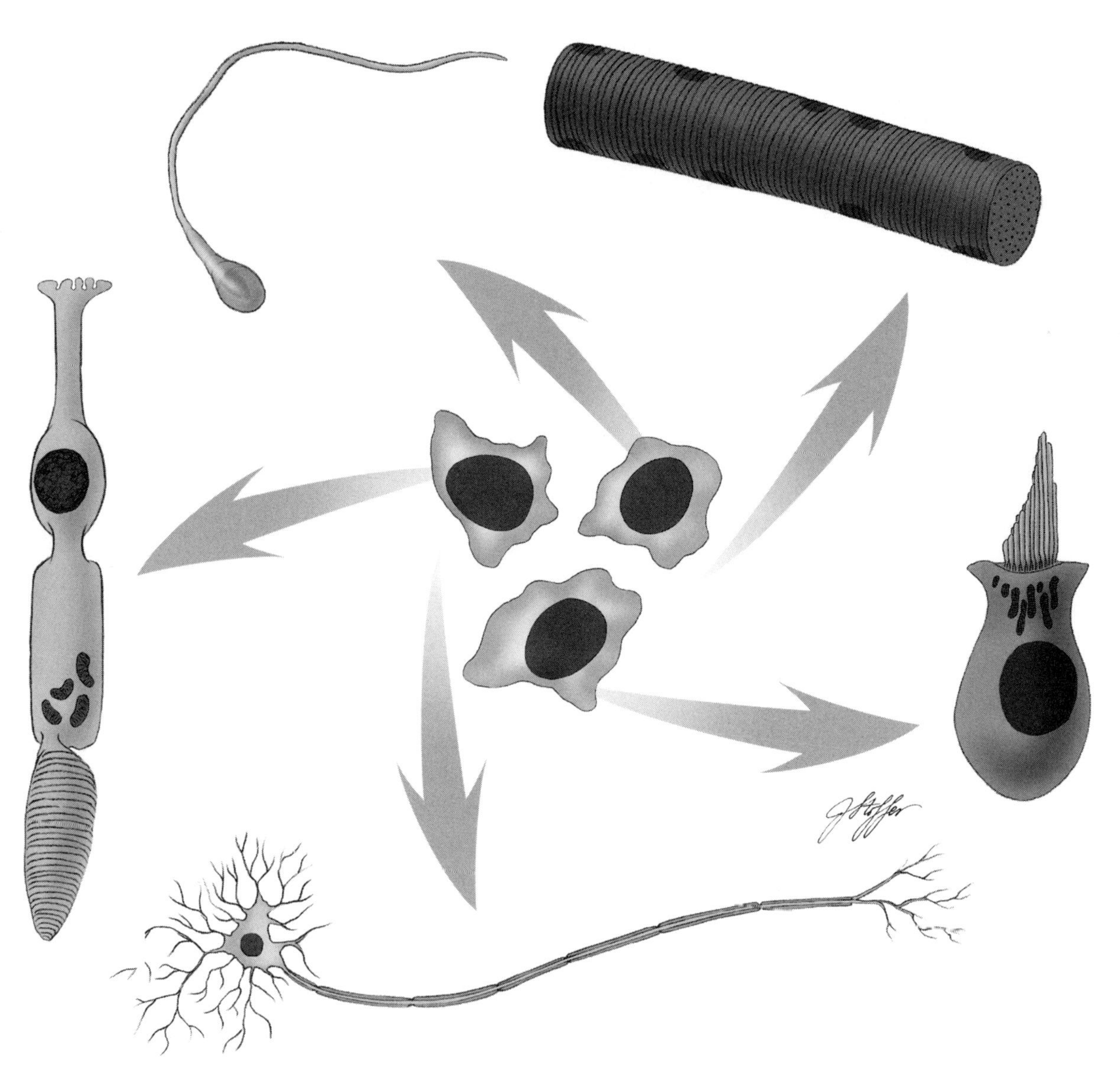

*Stem cells are involved in every step of development, from early embryogenesis to adulthood replenishment of damaged cells. The graphic depicts embryonic stem cells differentiating into different types of tissue.*

hood and during sexual maturation, until it reaches adulthood. The progressive changes in size, shape, and function of an organism after birth lead to the generation of a functioning adult system. In the early stages of life—from babyhood to childhood, childhood to adolescence, and adolescence to adulthood—enormous changes take place. Each stage of development has specific markers; however, each individual may reach various stages of development earlier or later than others. After adulthood, the development process continues, but no drastic changes in body size occur. The main developmental process is the maintenance of body function by replenishing injured or damaged cells and tissue by stem cells. This process involves adult stem cells.

Numerous organs and tissues in adult organisms contain stem cells. These tissue-specific stem cells can give rise to the defined cell types in a specific tissue. Most adult stem cells can only form a few types of cells in a specific tissue. In adulthood, stem cells continue differentiation to maintain and replenish cells injured and damaged as a result of aging and apoptosis, to maintain appropriate function of body system.

### RECENT PROGRESS IN STEM CELL RESEARCH

Developmental process continues in adulthood, and stem cells play an important role in replenishing and repairing cells and tissues damaged as a result of internal or environmental factors. Our knowledge of stem cells is continuously growing over time, and exciting new findings in adult stem cell research appear every day. Until recently, it was assumed that neurons could not be renewed when the animal reaches adulthood. However, recent studies suggest that the mammalian brain is capable of regenerating new neurons via the differentiation of neuron stem cells.

The researchers used a method to label the newly formed nerve cells and found that thousands of new nerve cells are generated each day. The deficiency in neuron stem cell self-renewal and differentiation may be related to several neurodegenerative diseases. It is commonly accepted that adult stem cells can only differentiate to the same cell types in the original tissue from which the stem cells are isolated. However, more and more researchers found that isolated adult stem cells from one tissue can differentiate to cell types specific to other tissues, such as stem cells from bone marrow differentiating to blood, neuron, and muscle cells.

Adult stem cells are also able to be integrated into early-stage embryos and express embryonic stem cell markers, and they are functionally similar to embryonic stem cells. These embryonic stem cell marker–expressing cells may represent rare embryonic stem cells present in adult tissue, or the adult stem cells can regain embryonic properties under certain conditions. This study suggests a close relationship between adult and embryonic stem cells and microenvironment that may guide stem cell function.

Some studies found that overexpressing genes unique to embryonic stem cells into somatic cells from adult mice makes these cells functional as embryonic stem cells. These studies showed a surprisingly close relationship between embryonic stem cells and differentiated adult cells—only four genes are needed to make the transition from differentiated adult cells to embryonic stem cells. Using a similar method, researchers found that adult somatic cells in humans can also be induced by these embryonic genes to function as embryonic stem cells. These cells are termed induced pluripotent stem cells, and these studies open the door for individualized medicine to regenerate patient-specific tissues and for embryonic stem cell research without destroying embryos.

**SEE ALSO:** Cells, Adult; Cells, Embryonic; Cells, Fetal; Cells, Mouse (Embryonic); Induced Pluripotent Stem Cells.

**BIBLIOGRAPHY.** Scott F. Gilbert, *Developmental Biology* (Sinauer, 2006); "Fetal Development," dir.yahoo.com/Health/Reproductive_Health/Pregnancy_and_Birth/Fetal_Development (cited November 2007); National Institutes of Health, "Stem Cell Information," stemcells.nih.gov (cited November 2007); Scientific Information Page on Adult Non-Hematopoietic Stem Cells, "Adult Stem Cells," www.adultstemcells.info (cited November 2007).

Daniel Shi
University of Wisconsin

## Cells, Embryonic

**EMBRYONIC STEM CELLS** were first identified in the 1980s in animal models, and the breakthrough of their successful isolation from human embryonic tissue came after about two decades. They are derived from embryos that are in their initial stages of development. After an ovum is fertilized by a sperm, a zygote is formed, which then transforms into a loose clump of cells, called the morula, around the fourth day of embryonic development.

The morula then forms an inner and an outer cell mass, which transform into embryonic and extra embryonic tissue (necessary for the initial development of the embryo), respectively. The inner cell mass gives rise to three germinal lay-

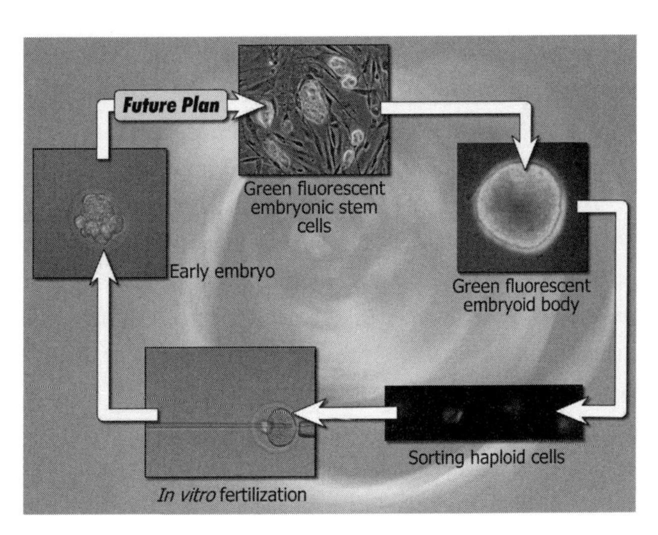


*The illustration shows the derivation of embryonic germ cells and male gametes from embryonic stem cells.*

ers—ectoderm, endoderm, and mesoderm—which go on to form different organs and tissues as the embryo matures. Embryonic stem cells are derived from the inner cell mass around day four or day five postfertilization. After isolation, the embryonic stem cells are cultured in the laboratory.

Scientists have also isolated cells with the potential of self-replication from the gonadal ridge—a part of the embryo that later produces eggs or sperm. These cells are called germ cells and are usually derived between week five and week nine of development.

Embryonic stem cells possess the property of pluripotency, which means that they can differentiate into all other cell lines except placenta and extra embryonic membranes, which are formed during embryonic development to support the embryo but are not needed after birth. Their growth is either initiated spontaneously or after the provision of appropriate environmental signals; they have been shown to have the highest potential for self-renewal and differentiation when compared with other sources such as germ, umbilical, and adult stem cells.

Because of the moral dilemmas surrounding the method of obtaining human embryonic stem cells, a policy was drafted by the U.S. federal government in August 2001 obstructing scientists from isolating stem cells by the destruction of human embryos.

However, the policy did allow them to continue to work on embryonic stem cell lines that had already been obtained or for which the derivation process had been initiated before the policy's implementation, resulting in more than 20 well-characterized human embryonic stem cell lines for widespread distribution to scientists for research purposes as of March 2007.

Most of the work using embryonic stem cells has been done on either animal models or during in vitro experiments, in which they have shown promising results for the cure of Parkinson's disease, myocardial infarction, diabetes, and spinal cord injury; however, human trials have not been conducted thus far. Scientists have shown that embryonic stem cells can be successfully made to differentiate and grow into neural, vascular, and other tissues. They are also trying to find acceptable ways of deriving new human embryonic stem cell lines without destroying living embryos. A group of scientists is focusing their efforts on retrieving them from dead embryos, and there is hope that if the tissues from some of these dead embryos can be cultured in the laboratory, they can be ultimately used to cure diseases or form various organs.

Although embryonic stem cell research is still in the budding phase, the results thus far look promising, and scientists are gradually heading toward the stage at which they may be able to use these cells as a treatment modality for many diseases.

**SEE ALSO:** Cells, Adult; Cells, Developing; Cells, Fetal; Cells, Mouse (Embryonic); Moral Status of Embryo.

**BIBLIOGRAPHY.** "Explore Stem Cells," www.explorestemcells.co.uk (cited November 2007); National Institutes of Health, "Stem Cell Information," stemcells.nih.gov (cited November 2007).

Faris Khan
Wasiq Rahman
New York Presbyterian Hospital
Nadia Farid
Khyber Medical College

# Cells, Fetal

**ON THE BASIS** of National Institutes of Health guidelines, a human fetal stem cell is defined as a cell derived from either a human embryo or a fetus harvested after abortion, whether intentional or incidental. However, this definition fails to highlight the primary difference between embryonic and fetal stem cells. This difference is a question of degree of multipotency. Where the embryonic stem cell is considered to be pluripotent—able to differentiate into any cell type in the human body—most fetal cells are believed to only be multipotent to a limited degree. To put it into layperson's terms, an embryonic stem cell is like the seed of a plant, whereas a fetal cell is a sprout. The seed could grow into any plant type, but the sprout already shows some of the properties of the full-grown plant.

In practical terms, fetal cells typically demonstrate many of the same characteristics of embryonic stem cells. Both cell types are multipotent, albeit to varying degrees; both cell types are able to renew their own populations; and both types are able to proliferate to increase cell number. Therefore, research using fetal stem cells has the potential to achieve many of the same objectives as embryonic stem cell research.

In addition, fetal cells express many of the same cell surface protein markers that can be found on embryonic stem cells, including Notch, CD133, and CD34, though at different concentrations, depending on the source of the fetal cells. Although the immune response to the surface antigens on the fetal cells or embryonic stem cells may be minimal compared to using other cells, patients receiving cell transplants may still require immunosuppression.

There are some advantages to using fetal stem cells in conducting stem cell research. Fetal cells are more robust than many strains of embryonic stem cell, making the culture of fetal cells less difficult. With regard to legal policy, there is wider access and fewer restrictions with fetal cells compared with embryonic cells. A more practical set of concerns solved by fetal cells is the potential for teratoma formation when transplanting embryonic stem cells. Using the more differentiated fetal cells could reduce the risk of teratoma formation and thereby make the usage of stem cells in transplants more practical.

Although culture of fetal cells is typically simpler than culture of embryonic stem cells, there are still several distinct aspects to fetal cell culture that is not common to culture of differentiated cells. Isolation of fetal cells typically involves isolation of the chosen tissue region, followed by culture of whole or lightly dissociated tissue. Following initial cell growth, cells are often dissociated by trypsin or similar chemicals before being replated or frozen.

In some instances, fetal cells can survive without serum; in fact, some fetal lines require culture in defined serum-free mediums for optimum growth of a highly pure population of the desired cell type. Likewise, plating conditions will vary between separate cell types, ranging from simply plating the cells to the use of a three-dimensional polymer scaffold with imbedded proteins. Much like embryonic cells, many fetal lines are able to survive multiple passages without a reduction in the cell's vitality, suggesting that the cells are stable for multiple generations.

## HISTORY

The history of fetal cell usage in medical science began in the 1930s, when fetal cells were used in culture. Particularly prominent in the 1950s was the usage of a fetal cell culture in the production of the polio vaccine and several contemporary antiviral vaccines. More recently, fetal cells have gained some prominence in transplant medicine, with a great deal of research directed toward the use of fetal cells in causing brain regeneration; early work in the area was conducted by Dr. Freed and his associates, showing initially promising responses to implantation of fetal cells.

This initial work has been highly controversial, with numerous studies either supporting or rejecting the treatment's benefits. However, research using fetal cells to treat Parkinson's disease continues; for example, work using fetal cells has been conducted by Dr. Svendsen at the University of Wisconsin, Madison, during research into Lou

Gehrig's disease. Other areas of research involving fetal cells include studies in the fields of immunology, virology, and developmental biology. Fetal stem cells are also used in place of embryonic stem cells in many studies.

## POLICY AND ETHICS

Policy shifts within the United States have had a great effect on the role of fetal cells in research. Following work using fetal cell transplants in 1988, a federal ban was placed on National Institutes of Health funding of research using fetal tissue. In 1993 the Clinton administration released the National Institutes of Health Revitalization Act. The existing ban on fetal cell research was lifted to a limited degree with this law, permitting the creation of fetal tissue for therapeutic research. The creation of a ban on embryonic research in 2000 was not accompanied by any major change in fetal cell policy.

Any discussion of fetal cells is incomplete without a brief overview of the ethical issues involved. Proponents of research involving fetal stem cells will emphasize the enormous achievements that have been conducted using these cell types, that the cells are acquired from an already dead fetus, and that a great deal of the work using fetal cells can be traced back to established lines of fetal cells. Opponents of the use of fetal cells will undoubtedly point out that fetal cells are acquired from fetuses, thereby bringing into question what we consider a human being, and the moral grounds on which we can claim access to fetal tissue. However, the focus on fetal tissue ethics is in many ways eclipsed by the debate surrounding embryonic cells.

**SEE ALSO:** Cells, Adult; Cells, Amniotic; Cells, Developing; Cells, Embryonic; Moral Status of Embryo.

**BIBLIOGRAPHY.** NIH Stem Cell Information Home Page, stemcells.nih.gov (cited November 2007); Bioethics Resources on the Web—National Institutes of Health, bioethics.od.nih.gov (cited November 2007).

John Kuo
University of Wisconsin

# Cells, Human

**THE CELL IS** the structural and functional unit of all living organisms. In the study of cells, its classification is of prime importance. Cells can be broadly classified into two types: prokaryotic (Greek: before the nucleus) cells and eukaryotic cells (Greek: new nucleus). The prokaryotic cell differs from the eukaryotic cell by the absence of a true nucleus (double membrane bound structure containing genetic information), membraned organelles (subcellular structures having a distinct function), and has a 70 S ribosome.

The eukaryotic cells again can be further classified into plant and animal cells. Both the plant and the animal cell has a true nucleus, membrane bound organelles and an 80 S ribosome. In contrast to the plant cell, the animal cell lacks a cell wall and chloroplasts (double membrane structure participating in photosynthesis) but has additional mitotic apparatus called the centrioles.

## THE HUMAN CELL

The human cell is a typical animal cell and is partitioned into two major components: protoplasm and nucleus enclosed within a cell membrane. Although different human cells have specific functional and structural characteristics, their basic structure is similar. The cell membrane is made up of lipids (phospholipids, glycolipids, and steroids) and different membrane proteins. The membrane proteins may be peripheral (attached to the peripheral parts of the cell membrane), transmembrane (communicates with the external and the internal environments) or lipid anchored (covalently bonded with the lipid molecules). Apart from giving shape to the cell the main functions of the cell membrane include: antigenic functions, containing of receptors and ion channels, participation in enzyme activity and maintaining a cell potential.

The nucleus, as described earlier, is a double membrane bound structure containing genetic information of the cell, which is encoded in the form of DNA. The protoplasm, with a gel-like consistency, harbors the different organelles of the cell: endoplasmic reticulum (ER), a system of membrane bounded channels with the main function of transportation of substances within the cell; 80 S ribosome, a subcellular entity usually associated with the ER and participates in protein synthesis; mitochondria, a double membrane bound structure carrying out respiratory functions in the cell; Golgi complex (GC), a system of vesicles that helps in transportation of different materials outside the cell; lysosome, membrane bound vesicles containing different enzymes like nucleases, phosphatases and proteases; and centrosomes and centrioles, cellular entities characteristic only for animal cells that participate in the process of cell division.

Other components of the human cell include the peroxysomes, different cytoplasmic inclusions, pigments (lipofuscin, lipochrome, etc.), microtubules and microfilaments (e.g., actin and myosin found in the human muscle cells), intermediate filaments and locomotory structures like the cilia (e.g., epithelial cell of the trachea) or flagella (e.g., spermatozoa). The principal activities common in human cells include cell division, endocytosis, exocytosis, cell locomotion, impulse conduction, and storage of different substances.

All cells of the human body are derived from stem cells (SC). SC are defined as primal cells found in multicellular organisms that have the ability to divide by mitosis and differentiate into specialized cells. SC are further classified as: embryonic stem cells derived from blastocysts, adult stem cells found in adult tissues, and cord blood stem cells found in the umbilical cord. Thus, each cell of the human body is derived from a SC and then it differentiates into specialized cells and gets organized into higher functional units.

## TYPES

There are five types of tissue in the human body: epithelial, connective, blood, muscle, and nervous tissue. Each of these tissue types consists of characteristic cellular and extracellular components. The epithelium consists of epithelial cells that form a lining of the external surface of the body and the luminal surface of body cavities. All the epithelial cells have a basic structure similar to that of a typical human cell, but they are capable of rapid mitotic division, and some of them have special apparatus like the cilia or brush borders. The cilia and brush borders are responsible for transportation of substances (e.g., mucous in the trachea) and for absorption of substances (e.g., nutrients in the gut), respectively.

The cells of the blood are of various kinds and each of them has a specific function. In general, the blood cells can be classified into red blood cells (RBC), white blood cells (WBC), and platelets (PT). All types of blood cells are derived from hemopoetic stem cells located in the bone marrow of different bones. Each type of blood cell has a unique function and hence its structure is modified to meet such demands: an RBC transports gases ($O_2$ and $CO_2$) in the body and hence to increase its surface area to carry gases it lacks a nucleus and has a biconcave shape. It also lacks mitochondrias so as not to use up the oxygen the cell is carrying.

WBCs are further divided into granulocytes (neutrophils, eosinophils, and basophils) and a-granulocytes (lymphocytes and monocytes) based on the presence and absence of granules in their protoplasm. Neutrophils are responsible for phagocytosis and eosinophils act against parasitic invasions, whereas basophils are responsible for allergic and antigen response by releasing different mediators (e.g., histamine). Among a-granulocytes, lymphocytes participate in production of antibodies against different antigens and monocytes share the phagocytic function of the neutrophils.

The platelets, like the RBCs, are anuclear and discoid in shape and participate in hemostasis (clotting of blood). The cells of the muscle tissue are called as myocytes. Myocytes have specialized contractile units called as myofibrils and usually have multiple nuclei. Myocytes organize themselves to form principally three different types of muscle tissue: skeletal, cardiac, and smooth muscle tissue. Each of these kinds is differentiated on the basis of the myofibrillar arrangement inside the myocytes and also on the basis of their innervations.

The next type of human cell of great importance is the neuron. The neuron is a very specialized cell that has a cell body that gives out principally two types of processes: an efferent axon and afferent dendrites (may be single or multiple). The cell body of the neuron is provided with a rich supply of mitochondria, a developed system of Golgi complex (GC), and neurofibrils. Conduction of impulses (with the help of different neurotransmitters located inside the GC) is the main function of neurons. Besides the former function, the neuron has another special feature: It does not undergo mitosis—but this is a topic of much debate as recent researchers in neurosciences look into the possibility of neurogenesis in certain parts of the brain. The neuron is also supported by a vast number of other non-neuronal cells like the Schwann cells, microglial (e.g., dendritic cells) and macroglial cells (e.g., astrocytes, oligodendrocytes, ependymal cells).

Finally, the cells of the connective tissue include the fibroblasts that synthesize collagen; adipocytes containing fat droplets; chondrocytes in cartilages, pigment cells with various pigments (melanin, lipochrome, etc.), and macrophages of connective tissue or histocytes. Bone, another type of connective tissue, comprises mature bone cells called osteocytes along with osteoblasts or bone producing cells, osteoclasts or bone removing cells, and osteoprogenitor cells from which the osteoblasts and osteocytes are derived.

Another important cell of the human body is the macrophage, which along with some other cells of the body forms the so-called mononuclear phagocytic system. In this system, the blood monocytes are the precursor of the tissue macrophages, which include: the Kupffer cells of the liver; microglial cells of the central nervous system; histocytes of connective tissue; dendritic cells of the epidermis; and macrophages in the pleura, peritoneum, lung alveoli, spleen, and synovial fluids. The macrophage is the body's defense against infectious agents as it actively participates in phagocytosis and also plays a key role in the immune response by T lymphocytes.

**SEE ALSO:** Cells, Adult; Cells, Developing; Cells, Sources of.

**BIBLIOGRAPHY.** Don Fawcett, *Bloom and Fawcett: A Textbook of Histology*, 12th ed. (Chapman and Hall Medical, 1994).

RAHUL PANDIT
ST. PETERSBURG STATE MEDICAL ACADEMY

# Cells, Monkey

**STEM CELLS ARE** unique cells in the body of many multicellular organisms that have the ability to develop and change into many different cells of the body. Stem cells have been studied in many animals including mice, monkeys, and humans and scientists have been able to unravel a great deal about their important properties.

Embryonic stem cells (as their name indicates) are found in embryos during very early stages of life and are responsible for the formation of different tissues of the body. Scientists have been able to manipulate the development of such cells in animals including monkeys and have made them convert into specific tissues that could potentially be used to treat different medical conditions.

Embryonic stem cells derived from monkeys have many similarities with human embryonic stem cells in terms of their growth and differentiation. This makes them suitable candidates for studying their potential in coming up with treatments for different medical conditions. Scientists have used them to study various disease models in monkeys, the results of which may have an impact on solving some of the problems that lie ahead in stem cell research. Scientists were able to transform the embryonic stem cells into special dopamine producing neurons, which when transplanted into the brains of monkeys suffering from Parkinson's disease, were able to reverse their symptoms. If cell therapies like these are successful in the future and enter mainstream medicine they would revolutionize the lives of many patients suffering from such diseases.

Embryonic stem cells in monkeys have also been made to transform into pancreatic beta cells that could produce insulin. Such cells could be used to study various therapies that can be used to treat diabetes mellitus. Mesenchymal stem cells have also been used for transformation into corneal epithelial cells in monkeys. Such techniques, if perfected, could go a long way in the treatment of patients who are in need of corneal transplants. Another group of scientists were also able to make cardiac muscle cells from stem cells in monkeys, thus opening a new arena for research in cardiovascular cell therapy.

A problem attributed to stem cell therapy is the native organism's immune response to "donor" cells and a probable solution to this is to somehow use the body's own stem cells for this purpose. In 2007 scientists overcame this problem by another novel method in which they were able to clone stem cells in monkeys by transferring the DNA from a normal body cell to an unfertilized egg, from which its own genetic material was removed. The egg developed into an embryo under the influence of the implanted DNA. Later on during the course of development scientists were able to extract stem cells from the developing embryos. The DNA in stem cells was the exact clone of the DNA present in the monkey cells initially. If these stem cells are transformed into specialized cells and implanted into the monkey whose stem cells were cloned then they would not face rejection by the immune system.

Although there has been much progress in stem cell research there are still problems to be overcome. For instance, many unfertilized eggs were used to isolate the very few monkey stem cell lines that were cloned in 2007. There is a great deal about the process of development of stem cells that scientists have yet to understand.

There are other issues in primate stem cell research as well. In the future there might be a need to study the effects of implantation of human cells into brains of monkeys in order to find treatments for disorders like Alzheimer's disease. Ethicists and scientists are pondering the moral grounds of such an undertaking. Research on monkeys can be invaluable because biologically they are very close to humans, and principles learned during this process could help us overcome some of the hurdles that lie ahead in human stem cell research.

**SEE ALSO:** Cells, Human; Cells, Mouse (Embryonic); Non-Human Primate Embryonic Stem Cells.

**BIBLIOGRAPHY.** David Cyranoski, "Cloned Monkey Stem Cells Produced," November 14, 2007, www.nature.com (cited April 2008); Yuan Jing, et al., "Induction of Corneal Epithelial Progenitors from Bone-Marrow Mesenchymal Stem Cells of Rhesus Monkeys In Vitro," *Chinese Science Bulletin* (v.52/16, 2007); L. B. Lester, et al., "Directed Differentiation of Rhesus Monkey ES Cells into Pancreatic Cell Phenotypes," *Reproductive Biology and Endocrinology* (v.2/42, 2004); Kristin Schwanke, et al., "Generation and Characterization of Functional Cardiomyocytes from Rhesus Monkey Embryonic Stem Cells," *Stem Cells* (v.24/6, 2006); Y. Takagi, et al., "Dopaminergic Neurons Generated From Monkey Embryonic Stem Cells Function in a Parkinson Primate Model," *Journal of Clinical Investigation* (v.115/1, 2005).

Wasiq Rahman
Faris Khan
Columbia University Medical Center
Nasir Malik
Punjab Medical College, Pakistan

# Cells, Mouse (Embryonic)

**STEM CELLS ARE** a special variety of cells that have been identified in some multicellular organisms. Most of the cells in the body transform into and reproduce only the parent cell type; stem cells, in contrast, have the capacity to transform into multiple cell types throughout their life spans. We also know that stem cells are of two types—adult and embryonic. As the name indicates, adult stem cells are found in adults and serve to replenish cells in certain parts of the body where they are lost because of a continuous turnover for a variety of reasons.

Examples of such tissues include skin, bone marrow, and the lining of gastrointestinal tract, and so forth. Embryonic stem cells, in contrast, are found in the body at a very early stage of its development and play an important role by forming different tissues of the body.

Since the 1960s, when the presence of stem cells was first elucidated in some cancers, these cells have been the center of attention for scientists. However, it was only in 1981 that researchers were able to isolate these cells in tissues derived from mice; since then, murine models have been a major source of our understanding regarding the functioning of these fascinating cells. Mouse stem cells have provided invaluable information regarding how stem cells proliferate and are affected by different external, as well as internal, growth factors during the process of differentiation. These growth factors, which are mainly proteins in nature, affect stem cells' behavior at different stages. Because there is a lot of similarity between the DNA of mice and that of humans, the two species make excellent candidates for research and help us appreciate the ways they might work in human beings. Furthermore, mice offer the advantage of being raised at a lower cost with relative ease and do not need any special environment when compared with other animal models. They also have a short generation time, thus enabling researchers to study successive generations with respect to a particular trait or disease without having to wait for long periods of time.

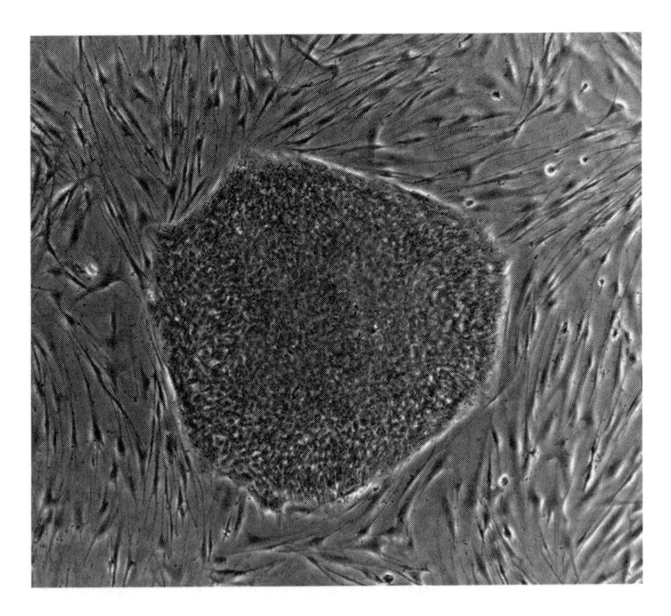

*The photo shows a human embryonic stem cell colony on a mouse embryonic fibroblast feeder layer.*

There has been a lot of debate regarding ethical issues surrounding human stem cell research, especially when it involves embryonic stem cells, because embryos need to be killed at a very early stage of their development to extract them. This approach raises the question of taking a human life and at the same time offers the prospect of providing researchers with the material that might one day be used as a treatment for many diseases. The gray area between the two doctrines has been the source of a big dilemma for the scientific world. Under the present legislation, the National Institutes of Health does not fund studies that involve human embryonic stem cell lines derived after August 2001, and that is where mouse stem cells come in.

They have played a pivotal role by being free of such controversies. Mouse stem cells have not only provided insight into some of the core principles regarding human development but have also shed light on novel ways to scrutinize the pathology of various medical disorders. They also offer hope for innovative modalities of treatment for diseases with significant morbidity and mortality despite currently available therapies.

The most exciting prospect in futuristic therapies involving stem cells is in the treatment of Parkinson's disease, a condition in which dopamine-producing neurons at a specific area of the brain degenerate. Scientists have shown from experiments in mice that stem cells could be made to differentiate into nerve cells and that these cells, when transplanted into the brains of mice lacking the dopamine-producing neurons, started producing dopamine and hence produced improvement in the severity of the disease. Other researchers have shown that stem cells improved cardiac function in mice that underwent myocardial infarction experimentally, by forming new muscle tissue and vessels.

If such techniques were perfected for humans, they would revolutionize the lives of many patients who suffer because of the lack of availability of suitable modalities of treatment. Stem cell therapy thus offers a ray of hope for such people and would have a significant effect on their lifestyle. Scientists have also been successful in transforming embryonic stem cells into corneal cells in mice, which could then be transplanted and thus used to treat corneal injuries.

In the past, it was indicated that the skin contains stem cells that could be used to regenerate new skin cells that could be used for skin grafting and to treat baldness; recently, however, scientists have gone a step farther and have transformed skin cells in mice into embryonic stem cells. This technique, if perfected for humans, would open new arenas for stem cell research because it does not involve the loss of life on the part of human embryos.

There have also been reports of successful studies using mice models in which stem cells grew into muscle cells that could be used to replace diseased skeletal muscle. Similarly, insulin-producing pancreatic cells have been regenerated that could open a new avenue into how we can treat diabetes mellitus. All these prospective treatments could eventually materialize and potentially be used in the future to treat a variety of disorders. Furthermore, advances in gene therapy and stem cell research have enabled scientists to make disease models in mice that, in turn, have greatly enhanced our ability to understand the disease process.

Mouse stem cells can also prove useful in comprehending the difficulties that we might encounter in the future. One such example would be that of immune intolerance resulting from a mismatch between the donor and the recipient genes. In addition, stem cells have also shown aberrant growth and a potential to transform into cancerous tissue. Such problems would limit their clinical applications; further research on mouse stem cells would permit us to analyze the intricate physiological processes that govern their behavior, helping us in finding solutions to these dilemmas.

Although modern science has taken big strides in stem cell research by studying mouse models, there are still hurdles in the process of identification, growth, and differentiation of stem cells that need to be overcome to achieve much-needed progress in this field. Mouse stem cells, however, have given us clues about ways to approach similar cells found in human tissue and thus have laid the basis for research that might one day change the principles and practice of medicine.

**SEE ALSO:** Cells, Adult; Cells, Embryonic; Cells, Fetal; Cells, Human.

**BIBLIOGRAPHY.** "Adult BM Stem Cells Regenerate Mouse Myocardium," *Cytotherapy* (v.4/6, 2002); "Establishment in Culture of Pluripotential Cells from Mouse Embryos," *Nature* (v.292/5819, 1981); "From Skin Cell to Stem Cell," www.nature.com/stemcells (cited November 2007); "Mouse, Human Genomes Share Similarities," www.case.edu/pubaff/univcomm/2002/june/mouse.htm (cited November 2007); "Stem Cell Information," stemcells.nih.gov (cited November 2007); Y.-T. Tai and C. N. Svendsen, "Stem Cells as a Potential Treatment of Neurological Disorders," *Current Opinion in Pharmacology* (v.4, 2004); "What Does the Mouse Genome Draft Tell Us about Evolution?" www.evolutionpages.com (cited November 2007).

Wasiq Rahman
Faris Khan
Faisal Habib Cheema
Columbia University Medical Center

# Cells, Neural

**MANY ORGANS IN** the body have stem cells. However, stem cells in the adult nervous system have only been discovered recently as the brain is traditionally thought of as containing nondividing mature cells. However, in 1960, Dr. Joseph Altman demonstrated, using radioactive thymidine, a compound that is included in DNA of dividing cells, that there are dividing cells in the dentate gyrus of the hippocampus. In the 1980s, it was shown that the dividing cells gave rise to new neurons. The term *adult neural stem cells* (NSCs) was coined for stem cells isolated from the nervous system. Interestingly, similar cells can be isolated from most regions of the brain during development, but then from only two major areas in the adult brain—the hippocampus and subventricular zone—which are discussed in detail below. These two areas of the adult brain continue to make new cells during the whole of life and can be thought of as "brain marrow." NSCs can self renew and in that way maintain the stem cell pool in these adult brain regions; they can also differentiate to all cell types of the nervous system.

Since the 1990s, it has been generally accepted that neural stem cells reside in the brain of mammals. The process whereby new neurons are generated is termed *adult neurogenesis*. In mammals, neurogenesis occurs in two defined regions of the brain: the subventricular zone, which lies next to the lateral ventricles, and the dentate gyrus, a part of the hippocampus. Cells in the subventricular zone migrate along the so-called rostral migratory stream toward the olfactory bulb, where as many as 30,000 new neurons are generated to replace the olfactory neurons. In contrast, cells from the dentate gyrus spread their axons toward the nearby regions in the hippocampus, which may be required for processes such as learning.

Once it became clear that neural stem cells remain in postnatal mammalian brains, a quest was on to isolate these cells and expand them in vitro. Dr. Samuel Weiss and Dr. Brent Reynolds were the first to isolate stem cells from the subventricular zone in 1992, and in 1995, Dr. Fred Gage and Dr. Ron McKay isolated stem cells from the dentate gyrus. Culture of fetal or adult NSCs in vitro in medium supplemented chiefly with two growth factors, namely basic fibroblast growth factor and epidermal growth factor, yields neurospheres. These neurospheres are aggregates of proliferating stem cells that float in the medium and can be dissociated and replate, where they give rise to new clusters (demonstrating the renewal ability of neural stem cells). Another method for growing the NSC is on coated culture dishes. These cells respond best to fibroblast growth factor

Transplantation of neural stem cells or their more mature progeny is considered a potentially curative therapy for patients suffering from neurodegenerative disorders, such as stroke or Parkinson's disease. Because adult neural stem cells, in contrast with fetal neural stem cells, have a more limited capacity to proliferate in vitro, fetal neural stem cells may be the most promising cells for cellular therapy of neurodegenerative disorders. However, many approaches are being considered. In addition, neural stem cells can now be isolated from human embryonic stem cells giving yet another source of tissue. Several studies in animals have transplanted fetal or adult neural stem cells in injured brain. Because the cells receive signals from the brain microenvironment, further maturation to either glial support cells or neurons can be seen. In some cases these cells integrate and contribute to physiological neural circuits. In other cases the cells make glial support cells that can also have significant effects in some animal models of disease.

While early results suggested that adult stem cells obtained from the bone marrow or other non-neural tissues may "transdifferentiate" into neurons, this has recently been shown not to be true. While some cells may look like neurons, they do not function as neurons. In some cases there was fusion between the adult cell and a mature neuron in the brain, which confused many of the studies. While a debate still continues, many believe that true neural stem cells have to be generated from neural tissues. However, it may not be necessary to always use neural stem cells for brain repair. Often improved function appears to be the result of factors released by the stem cells that improve plasticity of existing neurons, induce endogenous neurogenesis, or improve blood flow.

**SEE ALSO:** Brain; Cells, Adult; Cells, Embryonic; Cells, Fetal; Gage, Fred; Neurosphere Cultures; Stroke.

**BIBLIOGRAPHY.** Olle Lindvall and Zaal Kokaia, "Adult Stem Cells for the Treatment of Neurological Disorders," *Nature* (v.411, 2006); Philippe Taupin and Fred Gage, "Adult Neurogenesis and Neural Stem Cells of the Central Nervous System in Mammals," *Journal of Neuroscience Research* (v.69/6, 2002)

Annelies Crabbe
Katholieke Universiteit Leuven

# Cells, Sources of

**THE TURN OF** the 21st century brought about dazzling advances in biomedical research. The progress made in the field of medicine, and particularly the discovery of stem cells, opened new avenues for treating conditions that would have been incurable otherwise. Though much experimental work has been done on stem cells, the clinical translation is still in initial phases.

Stem cells were identified in the early 1980s from a mouse blastocyst; it took scientists almost two decades before successfully isolating them from human blastocysts. The striking features of stem cells are their qualities of self-renewal and pluripotency, which enable them to develop into various kinds of adult tissue if a suitable environment for nurturing is provided.

By regenerating damaged tissue using stem cells, scientists are trying to find ways to treat many diseases including, but not limited to, Parkinson's disease, myocardial infarction, diabetes, and spinal cord injury. Although it is too early to say how far the scientists will succeed in treating these conditions, the results so far have been very promising, and researchers are working enthusiastically toward finding a cure for such diseases using stem cells.

Stem cells have been derived from sources such as embryos, umbilical cords, and adults. They have the potential to proliferate multiple times and differentiate into various kinds of tissue. The differentiation of the stem cells can be either spontaneous or occur through a directed mechanism when certain stimuli or agents are present to initiate a specific process. By retaining the property of plasticity, they have the ability to transform into any kind of cell, with the exception of placenta and the extraembryonic membranes that are formed during the embryonic development. Among all the stem cells, those derived from embryonic tissue have the highest potential for self-renewal and differentiation.

## EMBRYONIC STEM CELLS

Embryonic stem cells, the original building blocks of life, are the body's founder cells. Being undifferentiated in nature and capable of self-renewal, they can differentiate into any kind of tissue. They are isolated from the developing embryo.

An ovum and a sperm fertilize to form a zygote, which serially divides to develop into a ball of loosely connected cells, called a morula, by the fourth day of development. The morula then gives rise to an inner and an outer cell mass, which transform into an embryo and extraembryonic tissue (necessary for the initial development of embryo), respectively. The inner cell mass gives rise to three germinal layers—ectoderm, endoderm, and mesoderm—which go on to form different organs and tissues as the embryo matures.

Embryonic stem cells are derived from the inner cell mass of the blastocytes around day four or five postfertilization. After isolation, the embryonic stem cells are cultured in the laboratory, and the stem cell lines are obtained with the potential to differentiate into various kinds of cells when provided with a cytokine cocktail in a suitable environment.

So far, using animal models, researchers have successfully isolated stem cells and shown them to differentiate into various types of cells in both in vitro (outside the body in an artificial environment) and in vivo (within the body) studies. Successful differentiation of embryonic stem cells into neural, vascular, and other solid organ cells was an important milestone that provided enough evidence for scientists to reproduce similar experiments, using human embryonic stem cells. Stem cells therefore were obtained from human embryos that were otherwise to be discarded following in vitro fertilization (a scientific approach to fertilization).

A stem cell policy was immediately drafted by the U.S. government in August 2001 that restrained scientists from using federal funding to obtain any further stem cells by destroying human embryos.

However, it allowed them to continue to work on the almost 60 embryonic stem cell lines that had already been obtained or for which the derivation process had been initiated before the policy's implementation. The National Institutes of Health (NIH) funded infrastructure awards for the development and distribution of the existing embryonic stem cell lines; this played a vital role in providing

21 well-characterized human embryonic stem cell lines for widespread distribution to scientists for research purposes by March 2007.

Because the federally funded studies can only use the lines registered with NIH before August 2001, passionate scientists have continued their efforts to find other ethically acceptable ways to generate human embryonic stem cells. One such group of scientists is focusing on retrieving stem cells from the dead embryos, and another is trying to come up with a proper definition of embryonic death. There is a hope that if all the scientists, ethicists, and politicians agree on a proper definition of embryonic death, then perhaps some of these dead embryos can be cultured in the laboratory with the hope of retrieving some individual revivable cells, which can be ultimately used to cure diseases or form various organs. In addition, exciting new developments in nuclear transfer techniques hold the promise of patient-specific embryonic stem cell lines.

Germ cells, just like embryonic stem cells, have also been shown to have the potential of self replication. Germ cells are usually derived between week five and nine of development from the gonadal ridge—a part of the embryo that later produces eggs or sperm. However, as compared with the embryonic stem cells, germ cells have less potential for self replication and for tumor formation (an uncontrolled, abnormal, circumscribed growth of cells in any animal tissue; neoplasm). The germ cells will, however, also make tumors if they are not carefully manipulated before implantation.

## UMBILICAL CORD STEM CELLS

Although the pluripotency of stem cells obtained from umbilical cords has been controversial in the past, there is now evidence that they are a rich source of stem cells and can be used as an alternative to blastocyst- or gonadal ridge–derived embryonic stem cells.

Containing two arteries and a vein surrounded by some connective tissue, the umbilical cord is a vital structure that connects the developing fetus to the placenta. The stem cells from cord blood are much easier to get because they can be readily obtained from the placenta at the time of delivery. The stem cells isolated from the stromal tissue around the vessels have been shown to transform into chondrogenic, osteogenic, neurogenic, adipogenic, and several other types of cells. A broader range of recipients may benefit from cord blood stem cells. They are a rich source of early stem cells, particularly hematopoietic cells (blood-forming stem cells), which are used to treat a host of blood-related diseases. Cord blood stem cells also offer some exciting possibilities for gene therapy for certain genetic diseases, especially those involving the immune system.

Because there are few ethical issues surrounding the stem cells derived from umbilical cord, they remain an excellent alternative to embryonic stem cells. Once banked, the umbilical cord stem cells can be transplanted back into the donor, to a family member, or to an unrelated recipient. The high scale of cost for storing cord stem cells makes their use limited to only a few privileged individuals, and prohibitively expensive for the general population.

## ADULT STEM CELLS

Although adult stem cells have the potential for differentiation and self-renewal, unlike embryonic and umbilical cord counterparts, they can only differentiate into a limited number of single or multiple cell lines. There is no consensus on their origin. Some think they are the remnants of embryonic stem cells, but others believe them to be a separate entity. They have been isolated from brain, bone marrow, peripheral blood, blood vessels, epithelia of the skin and digestive system, cornea, liver, and pancreas; thus, adult stem cells have been found in tissues that develop from all three embryonic germ layers, that is, ectoderm, endoderm, and mesoderm.

The most common source of adult stem cells has been the bone marrow–derived hematopoietic stem cells that have been used extensively in bone marrow transplantation for treating blood cancers like leukemia, multiple myeloma, and so on. Recently, they have also been used to repair damaged cardiac muscles by injecting them into the affected areas to induce the formation of new vessels and improve the functional capacity of the heart. A subset of CD34+ stem cells also has the

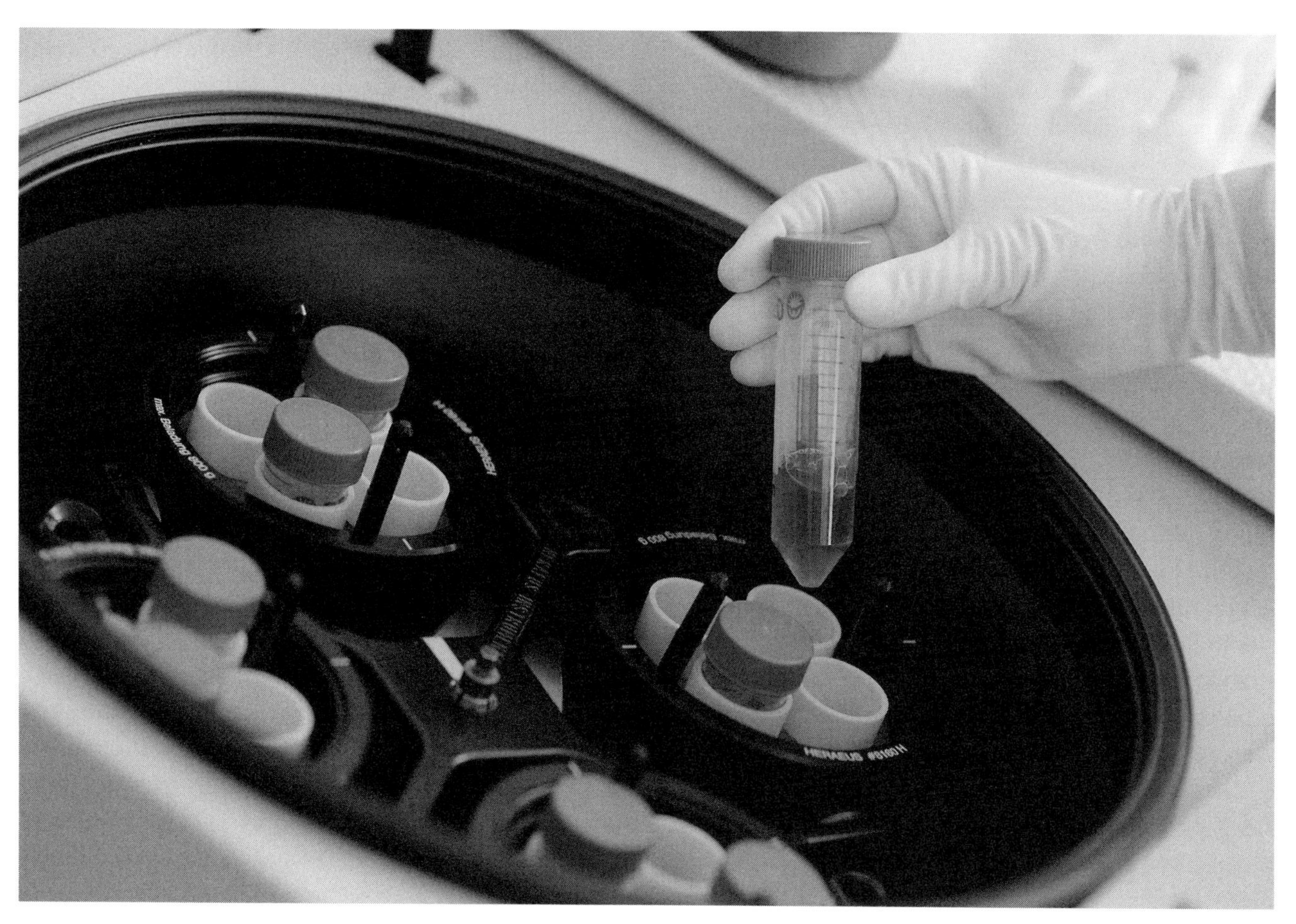

*While debate has centered around embryonic stem cells, stem cells can be derived from a number of sources, including from umbilical cords and adult patients.*

ability to home into ischemic sites, allowing potential intravenous delivery of such adult stem cells.

Researchers have also isolated adipogenic, osteogenic, and chondrogenic cell lines from bone marrow–derived cells in addition to blood cell lines. Adult stem cells in the central nervous system have been shown to develop into astrocytes, neurons, and oligodendrocytes and are usually concentrated in some specific areas of the brain. Because adult stem cells are derived from, and later are transplanted back to, the same patient, there is no risk of immune reaction, unlike with embryonic stem cells, where immunosuppression therapy may be needed to avoid cell rejection.

Some scientists have shown a concern that adult cells may have comparatively higher chances of mutation (a sudden structural change within a gene or chromosome resulting in the creation of a new character or trait not found in the parental type) and less pluripotency; however, this may not be true unless adult stem cells are made to pass through more than 30 doublings—a practice that is not done clinically, per U.S. Food and Drug Administration regulatory guidelines.

## CONCLUSIONS

Although stem cell research has progressed tremendously over the last two and a half decades, scientists are still facing many challenges that need to be addressed before stem cells can be safely and regularly used for treating various diseases. However, there is a consensus that they can have a lot of advantages and may play a pivotal role in treating various medical illnesses.

Scientists are also trying to obtain embryonic stem cells by alternative ways that will be ethically as well as scientifically acceptable. Given the successful use of mesenchymal stem cells in bone marrow transplant and the preliminary promising results of some clinical trials from Europe involving human stem cells, there is no doubt that stem cell therapy—if and when applied after having addressed all the current concerns revolving around it—will revolutionize the practice of medicine in the future.

**SEE ALSO:** Cells, Adult; Cells, Amniotic; Cells, Embryonic; Cells, Fetal; Cells, Human; Cells, Mouse (Embryonic); Cells, Umbilical.

**BIBLIOGRAPHY.** "Explore Stem Cells," www.explorestemcells.co.uk (cited November 2007); National Institutes of Health, "Stem Cell Information," stemcells.nih.gov (cited November 2007).

Faris Khan
Faisal Habib Cheema
Columbia University Medical Center
Nasir Malik
Punjab Medical

# Cells, Umbilical

**UMBILICAL CELLS ARE** a type of adult stem cells derived from umbilical cord blood. More specifically, umbilical cells refer to the hematopoietic stem cells, also known as undifferentiated blood cells, found in the umbilical cord. Because the umbilical stem cells are the precursor blood cells, they can develop into other cell types such as platelets, macrophages, and thymus cells, commonly known as T-cells. In light of this unique property, physicians use umbilical cord stem cells to treat patients who cannot generate normal blood cells as a result of genetic diseases such as leukemia.

Because these cells exhibit characteristics similar to embryonic stem cells, some researchers state that umbilical cord cells could have the potential to differentiate into liver cells, neurons, heart muscles, or even cartilage—a property known as plasticity. Because the umbilical stem cells possess a degree of plasticity similar to that of embryonic stem cells, researchers have engaged in rigorous investigation and hope to use umbilical cells in extensive stem cell therapy.

Considering the aforementioned properties, umbilical cord cells can have lifesaving therapeutic effects and may be useful in treating more diseases. In light of these beneficial characteristics, more and more parents are choosing to store umbilical blood for future use. Compared with adult stem cells derived from bone marrow, umbilical stem cells yield fewer complications during treatment and are also more responsive to drugs.

Controversy surrounds the use of embryonic stem cells because the extraction of cells results in the destruction of the embryo—an act some equate to the destruction of human life. The use of umbilical cord stem cells, in contrast, does not raise the aforementioned concern. Although the use of umbilical cord stem cells raises less debate, some disagreement still exists regarding the viability of the cells after long-term storage and the therapeutic efficacy of umbilical stem cells.

Public or private umbilical cord banks are available for those who wish to donate or store their cord blood cells. Otherwise, parents can choose to discard the umbilical cells.

Depending on the consensus reached between the physician and the chosen cord blood bank, umbilical cord blood can be obtained in one of two ways. First, the cord blood can be collected by draining the blood into a sterile bag that is sealed on completion. The second method obtains umbilical cord cells by drawing the blood into a syringe.

To ensure the quality of the umbilical cells, health professionals consider the first 15 minutes after birth to be the prime time to collect cord blood. Collecting cord blood after this window results in poor cell quality. On receiving the collected umbilical blood, scientists conduct a series of tests to eliminate bacterial contamination. Once the cord bank has conducted all the necessary tests, the sample is then processed and stored cryogenically (in liquid nitrogen). During regular intervals, umbilical cord blood banks would perform viability tests on the stored cells to determine the percentage of live cells. At present, there is no indication as to how long the umbilical cells will stay viable.

The breakthrough in stem cell research brought hope to patients suffering from cancers and rare genetic disorders. More specifically, ailments such as sickle cell anemia, non-Hodgkin's lymphoma, Kostmann syndrome, and osteoporosis can now be treated with stem cells. In the aforementioned illnesses, implanted healthy stem cells in the patients can replace blood cells either damaged or destroyed by the diseases or during chemotherapy. In addition to treating the patients suffering from cancers and various genetic disorders, umbilical cord cell therapy could also benefit those plagued by cardiovascular diseases. Japanese researchers discovered that implanting umbilical cells in the heart would not only stimulate new vessel growth but also increase blood flow. Such discovery holds promise for patients for whom heart bypass surgery and angioplasty have proven to be ineffective.

Aside from the ability to give rise to many different blood cell types and stimulating vessel growth, umbilical stem cells also demonstrate the potential to develop into other cell types such as neuron and muscle cells. In a recent experiment performed on rats with amyotrophic lateral sclerosis, a debilitating and lethal neurodegenerative disease, scientists reported that umbilical cells injected into the blood vessels slowed down the disease's progression and increased the rats' survival rate. Moreover, the umbilical cells migrated to the damaged areas such as the spinal cord and the brain.

A different study involving rats with spinal cord injuries also showed that umbilical cells could travel directly to the damaged area and restore certain functions lost as a result of the injury. These results provide hope for patients who have multiple damaged regions because stem cells implanted surgically are unable to circulate to other areas. Furthermore, once the umbilical cells' pluripotency (cells' ability to give rise to many different cell types) is fully realized, then these cells may be able to treat diseases ranging from diabetes to other neurological and autoimmune diseases such as Alzheimer's, Parkinson's, and lupus.

## ADVANTAGES AND DISADVANTAGES

Umbilical cells and embryonic cells have many differences. Although embryonic stem cells offer greater versatility, umbilical cells are less controversial. Researchers have observed that embryonic stem cells exhibit the ability to differentiate into all kinds of cells in a body. Until now, umbilical cells (a type of adult stem cells) were thought to be able to give rise to certain types of cells. However, evidence suggests that umbilical cells appear to exhibit a degree of versatility very similar to that of embryonic stem cells. Once versatility of umbilical cells is fully realized, scientists foresee a major advancement in stem cell therapy. Cells derived from embryonic cells can be rejected by the patient's immune system. However, if umbilical stem cells are given back to the patient from which they were derived, the patient is less likely to reject the cells. Furthermore, using a patient's umbilical cord stem cells also reduces the rate of disease transmission.

Moreover, extracting embryonic stem cells not only raises ethical concerns but also poses technical difficulties of obtaining embryos and isolating the cells. Often, surgeons are unable to acquire enough cells from embryos. Recent research findings claim that extracting stem cells from umbilical cord blood could overcome these obstacles because umbilical cord stem cells can be extracted and stored without encountering the ethical issues raised by embryonic stem cell research. In many parts of the world, extracting umbilical stem cells is socially and ethically acceptable.

Although extracting umbilical cells would not raise the same controversy as that of embryonic cells, umbilical cells also have disadvantages. Some argue that certain congenital disorders cannot be detected at the time of birth, and so the collected umbilical cells could be rendered useless once the disorder develops. Another disadvantage lies in the limited quantity of stem cells that are present in the umbilical cord blood; it is not possible to obtain additional umbilical cells. Although umbilical cells are hailed as an alternative to embryonic stem cells, researchers continue to examine their properties and expand their applications.

**SEE ALSO:** Cells, Adult; Cells, Embryonic; Diabetes; Stroke.

**BIBLIOGRAPHY.** BBC News, "Umbilical Cord Cells Could Create Heart Bypasses," news.bbc.co.uk (cited November 2007); BBC News, "Umbilical Cord 'Stem Cell' Hope," news.bbc.co.uk (cited November 2007); National Geographic News, "Umbilical Cord Blood: The Future of Stem Cell Research?" news.nationalgeographic.com (cited November 2007); National Institutes of Health, "Stem Cell Basics," stemcells.nih.gov (cited November 2007); Daniel A. Peterson, "Umbilical Cord Blood Cells and Brain Stroke Injury: Bringing in Fresh Blood to Address an Old Problem," *Journal of Clinical Investigation* (v.114, 2004); ScienceDaily, "Cells from Human Umbilical Cord Blood Help Rats Recover from Stroke Faster, New Study Finds," www.sciencedaily.com (cited November 2007); ScienceDaily, "Intravenous Infusions of Human Umbilical Cord Blood Stem Cells Benefit Rodents with ALS, Spinal Cord Injury," www.sciencedaily.com (cited November 2007); Society of Obstetricians and Gynecologists of Canada, "Umbilical Cord Blood," sogc.medical.org (cited November 2007); ViaCord, "What Is Cord Blood Banking?" www.viacord.com (cited November 2007); Ruth Warwick and Sue Armitage, "Cord Blood Banking," *Best Practice & Research Clinical Obstetrics & Gynaecology* (v.18, 2004).

Charlene Wu
Johns Hopkins University

# Cell Sorting

**CELL SORTING IS** a procedure that separates a group of mixed cell types into fractions of a single cell type that can then be studied in isolation; cells can be sorted on the basis of a number of operator-specified characteristics. The most commonly used type of cell sorting is fluorescence-activated cell sorting, although other methods such as magnetic cell sorting, density gradient cell sorting, and so on are also often used—the first most commonly in human therapeutics. Fluorescence-activated cell sorting finds its application in stem cell research in the separation of adult stem cells.

The first prototype cell sorter was built in 1965 at the Los Alamos National Laboratory and was developed by Mack J. Fulwyler, who combined the Wallace and Joseph Coulter volume sensing system—a system for detecting particle size—with the principle of the then-newly developed inkjet printer. The sorter's potential biological uses were recognized by Leonard Herzenberg from Stanford University, who developed the first fluorescence-activated cell sorter in 1970.

Cell sorting has a number of applications in physiological and biotechnological research. It has been used for studies regarding respiratory dysfunction in yeast and the distribution of cellular properties and has uncovered previously undetected patterns of gene expression in biological samples, which are usually complex mixtures of several cell types. Biotechnologically, cell sorting has found uses involving the study of enzymatic action and protein overproduction, screening for enzymatic activity and binding properties of certain ligands to cells, and cell engineering.

Cell sorting has also been used for the detection of the emission spectrum of marine diatoms and for the analysis of cell cycles. Most of its applications involve the detection of protein activity and production, and a review suggests that the potential of cell sorting for nonprotein products is still underutilized. Broadly, cell sorting may be divided into bulk sorting or single cell sorting.

## BULK SORTING

In this form of cell sorting, sorting and classification are accomplished in a single step, usually on the basis of a single cell characteristic. Although they are extremely rapid, and a very large number of cells can be run through them in a given time, the yield obtained lacks purity and has a lower recovery, and these methods are rarely used independently; they are most often used as enrichment methods before a single-cell sort, especially when sorting for a rare event.

The density gradient cell sorting method employs the use of a centrifuge and a medium with a density appropriate to the cells that are to be sorted. A polymer gradient column is coated with the cell suspension and then centrifuged. At the end of centrifugation, the denser cells are found at the bottom of the column and the least dense cells at the top. A new continuous cell separation method pairs centrifugation with the use of monoclonal antibodies for higher purity and recovery.

The dielectrophoretic field flow fractionation method makes use of the cell's intrinsic dielectric properties to facilitate enrichment. It is based on the equilibrium heights achieved by a cell under opposing dielectrophoretic and sedimentation forces and the velocity profile obtained when the cells are transported under these conditions within the chamber.

## SINGLE CELL SORTING

Before the process of cell sorting commences, a single-cell suspension in an appropriate sort buffer is first prepared from the sample and filtered to remove any clumps or aggregations; this suspension should be of optimal concentration—if it is too concentrated, there will be a lower recovery, and if it is too dilute, the processing time will increase. To minimize stress, the solution should be prepared as rapidly as possible, and cells should be maintained at the appropriate temperature and pH throughout the procedure.

In case of "rare event" sorts, or sorts for cells in which the desired characteristic is rare, it is usually better to enrich the suspension first to ensure a higher recovery. Enrichment can be carried out by processes such as panning, or using centrifugation for the formation of a density gradient, and so on. If a sterile environment is maintained before, during, and after the sort, the recovered cells can be cultured directly. This can be achieved by using ethanol to clean around the collection area, by running it through the sheath streams, and by using sterilized sheath fluid.

For flow sorting, the cells must be appropriately labeled with fluorescent dyes (fluorochromes) that bind to one or more cell component. These labels are used to identify positive and negative cells (i.e., cells that possess or do not possess the characteristics for which they are being sorted). Cells may carry one or more labels.

When a concentrated beam of light shines on a cell, it scatters in a distinctive pattern; it also excites the cell and causes the emission of fluorochrome molecules that fluoresce when appropriately excited. These principles of light scattering and light excitation are what flow sorting is based on. When a cell carrying a fluorochrome label passes the detectors, it releases a flash of fluorescence. These flashes are detected and documented by a photomultiplier tube that converts flashes of light to electric pulses. Apart from these flashes of fluorescence, the cell's density and size are also detectable—light from the incident laser is scattered forward and at right angles to the light beam. The light scattered forward is directly related to the diameter of the cell and can be used to determine the cell size from it; the light scattered sideways helps estimate cell density: the denser the cell (as a result of the presence of intracellular organelles and granules), the more light it reflects. Flow sorting methods help obtain a target population of very high purity and are useful in cells with a low density of surface receptors or when internal organelles are stained.

There are the two types of flow sorting methods: electrostatic and mechanical flow sorting. The first method, electrostatic flow sorting, involves the injection of cells through a nozzle into air as a focused stream. This is based on the tendency of a stream in air to break into droplets and is stabilized by use of a transducer to vibrate the nozzle and produce droplets; some of these droplets contain cells and are positively, negatively, or neutrally charged. An electrostatic field is then applied, and the charged droplets are attracted to the oppositely charged pole and collected.

In mechanical flow sorting, the cell suspension is forced into a fast-moving stream of buffer that acts as a sheath to center the particles in the flowing stream. A transducer (often a piezoelectric crystal) causes the sheath to vibrate and break into several droplets: Each cell is encased in a droplet, but not every droplet contains a cell. If a droplet fluoresces and meets the other preset criteria for a positive cell, it is detected as an event, and a charge is placed on the droplet. This permits the droplet and the cell it contains to be separated from the other cells and empty droplets as it passes an oppositely charged deflecting plate and is collected.

Electrostatic flow sorters are faster than mechanical sorters but are relatively more expensive; also, as the drops are released as an aerosol, they are potential biohazards. They can carry out two sorts simultaneously and directly sort cells onto slides, tubes, or wells. Mechanical sorters are significantly slower but are fully enclosed and can be used when working with potentially infectious materials.

Magnetic-activated cell sorting is a method used for the separation of complex cell mixtures into their constituent cells on the basis of the differences in their surface antigens. In this method, magnetic beads are coated with antibodies specific to the antigen expressed on the surface of the desired cells. When the cells are incubated with these beads, the antibodies bind with the surface antigens. The cell solution is then passed through a column to which a strong magnetic field is applied. The cells that are bound to the beads remain attached to the sides, and the other cells flow through.

The beads may bind either to the cells of interest or the cells to be eliminated, and the antibody that coats them may be varied accordingly. In case the beads bind to the cells of interest, these cells are harvested after the remaining cells have flowed past; this is called positive selection. In case the beads bind to the cells that are not of interest, the unbound cells are collected and the rest are discarded; this is called a negative sort.

Magnetic bead sorting is extremely fast and was originally used for bulk separation, but difficulties arose when more than one surface marker was used; new developments have now permitted the detection of multiple surface markers by a multistep process that includes the removal of the beads by enzymatic action and the incubation of the positively selected cells with new beads that bind to another surface antigen. The primary drawback now is the method's inapplicability to cells with intracellular markers, multiple simultaneous markers, or cells that are sorted according to size or their pattern of scattered light.

**SEE ALSO:** Cells, Adult; Fluorescence-Activated Cell Sorting.

**BIBLIOGRAPHY.** IngentaConnect, www.ingentaconnect.com (cited November 2007); Herman B. Wells Center for Pediatric Research, www.wellscenter.iupui.edu (cited November 2007); Miltenyi Biotec, www.miltenyibiotec.com (cited November 2007); Peter O'Toole, "Cell Sorting—the Basics," RMS Flow Cytometer Course 2005, University of York.

Azara Singh
Christian Medical College

# Charo, Robin Alta

**A BIOETHICIST FROM** the University of Wisconsin, Madison, Robin Alta Charo has written or collaborated on nearly 100 journal articles, book chapters, and government reports on a wide variety of topics ranging from environmental law to family planning regulations to abortion law and reproductive policy, playing an important part in the debate over medical genetics and cloning laws, as well as general science bioethical issues and dilemmas.

Robin Alta Charo was born in 1958 in Brooklyn, New York, and completed her Bachelor's in biology at Harvard-Radcliffe, graduating from Harvard University Law School in 1979 as Robin Anne Charo. She then studied for a law degree from Columbia University, and from 1982 until 1985, she served as associate director of the Legislative Drafting Research Fund of Columbia University, living in Brooklyn, New York. She then spent a year as a Fulbright Junior Lecturer in American Law at the University of Paris I, the Sorbonne, in France, from 1985 to 1986, returning to the United States in 1986 to take up an appointment as a legal analyst for the Biological Applications Program of the Congressional Office of Technology Assessment. She held this position until 1988, by which time she was also an American Association for the Advancement of Science diplomacy fellow for the Policy Development Division of the Office of Population at the U.S. Agency for International Development. In 1989 Charo was appointed to the School of Law at the University of Wisconsin, Madison, and from July 1, 2002, on, she was the associate dean for research and faculty development at the School of Law at the University of Wisconsin, Madison.

During Charo's time at the University of Wisconsin, Madison, she has been a visiting professor at a range of medical schools and law schools around the world including in Argentina, Australia, Canada, China, Cuba, France, Germany, and New Zealand. In 2006, from January until December of that year, she was a visiting professor of law at the School of Law at the University of California, Berkeley. Charo is now a member of the University of Wisconsin, Madison's Medical School's Department of Medical History and Bioethics, serves on the faculty of the University of Wisconsin, Madison's Masters in Biotechnology Studies program, and lectures in the Master's of Public Health program of the Department of Population Health Sciences. She also offers courses at the university on health law, bioethics and biotechnology law, food and drug laws, medical ethics and problems arising from them, reproductive rights, torts, and legislative drafting. A member of the university's Bioethics Advisory Committee, Charo is also a member of the university's Institutional Review Board.

Making a wide contribution to ethical problems facing medical researchers, Charo has always been cautious about new developments being applied to humans because of the possible medical complications that might arise. As a result, when she had to deal with the issue of cloning, she argued for more research into the possible risks that such advances might contribute to higher rates of birth defects, miscarriages, and other medical problems and complications. Her ideas have influenced a large number of books on bioethics, and Charo has written extensively on many subjects.

## CONTROVERSY

In 1994, she served as a member of the National Institutes of Health Human Embryo Research Panel, and from 1996 until 2001, she was also a member of the U.S. Presidential National Bioethics Advisory Commission under President Bill Clinton. In these last two roles, Charo was seen by some as controversial, with religious and evangelical groups attacking her support for stem cell research and the keeping of embryo banks.

This assault was particularly fierce after her involvement in the drafting of such reports as "Cloning Human Beings" in 1997 and "Research Involving Persons with Mental Disorders that May Affect Decision Making Capacity" in 1998; "Research Involving Human Biological Materials: Ethical Issues and Policy Guidance" and "Ethical Issues in Human Stem Cell Research" in 1999; "Ethical and Policy Issues in International Research: Clinical Trials in Developing Countries" in 2001; and "Ethical and Policy Issues in Research Involving Human Participants" in 2001. Charo, in an interview with *New Scientist* magazine in 1998, pointed out that "The average person doesn't realize they leave tissue around all the time" and that many newborn babies often have blood taken from them for routine genetic screening; this blood can then be stored for decades.

Charo is currently a member of the editorial board of the *Journal of Law, Medicine and Ethics*, as well as *Cloning: Science and Policy* and the *Monash Bioethics Review*. She is also a member of the board of the Alan Guttmacher Institute in New York City and Washington, D.C., as well as the Foundation for Genetic Medicine, and has been a member of the board for the Society for the Advancement of Women's Health Research, the American Association of Bioethics, and the

National Medical Advisory Committee of the Planned Parenthood Federation of America, as well as the program board of amfAR—the Foundation for AIDS Research.

In the past, Charo has also been a member of the steering committee established to found the International Association for Bioethics and has served as a consultant to the National Academy of Science's Institute of Medicine and the National Institute of Health Office of Protection from Research Risks. She has also been on the board of the Society for the Advancement of Women's Health and what had been the American Association for Bioethics, as well as being on the ethics advisory board of the Howard Hughes Medical Institute. In 2005 she helped draft the National Academies' Guidelines for Embryonic Stem Cell Research and was appointed to the ethics standards working group of the California Institute for Regenerative Medicine.

In 2006 Charo was appointed as a cochair of the National Academies' Human Embryonic Stem Cell Advisory Committee.

**SEE ALSO:** Cloning; Columbia University; Ethics; Harvard University.

**BIBLIOGRAPHY.** "We Ask the Answer," *New Scientist* (May 9, 1998); *Who's Who in American Law, 7th ed., 1992–1993* (Marquis Who's Who, 1991); *Who's Who in the Midwest, 27th ed., 2000–2001* (Marquis Who's Who, 2000–2001); *Who's Who in the Midwest, 28th ed., 2002* (Marquis Who's Who, 2000–2001); *Who's Who in Science and Engineering 2000–2001* (Marquis Who's Who, 1999).

Justin Corfield
Geelong Grammar School

# Children's Hospital, Boston

**CHILDREN'S HOSPITAL (CHILDREN'S)** is a pediatric hospital located in Boston, Massachusetts. It is the teaching hospital for pediatric care under Harvard Medical School. The vision of the hospital is concise: to "be the worldwide leader in improving children's health." To achieve this goal, Children's has outlined eight chief strategic objectives. One such objective is Frontiers of Knowledge, whereby interdisciplinary research is carried out in the basic and clinical sciences. Research topics aim to better understand preventions, treatments, and cures of pediatric afflictions; stem cell research falls within the Frontiers of Knowledge objective.

## STEM CELL RESEARCH

The history of science and research at Children's is rich with breakthroughs in stem cell understanding and use. The hospital first opened in 1869 in the South End neighborhood of Boston with only 20 beds. In 1985 Children's received a $17 million grant from the Howard Hughes Medical Institute to develop a molecular genetics research program. Out of that program came work from Drs. Louis Kunkel and Eric Hoffman that deduced the genetic mutation involved in Duchenne muscular dystrophy that leads to the absence of a critical protein.

At present, Dr. Kunkel is collaborating with scientists in an effort to restore this protein to patients' muscles, using healthy muscle stem cells. Dr. Evan Snyder of Children's obtained human neural stem cells from fetal tissue in 1998.

Embryonic stem cells are the only stem cells that are truly omnipotent, meaning that they can differentiate into any cell type in the human body. In 2003 Dr. George Daley, a scientist with both medical and doctoral degrees, developed germ cell lines (precursors to sperm and egg cells). An understanding of how germ cells develop could lead to the ability to re-create germ cells from further developed cells and, potentially, to create embryonic stem cells. Further research is needed to discover how to direct embryonic stem cells to become a desired cell type.

Stem cell research is not based solely on regeneration or guided differentiation; much research has been conducted in the field of cancer stem cells. Cancer stem cells are presumably the core of a cancer, reproducing and providing the impetus for the cancer to spread. One theory is that if cancer stem cells could be isolated and killed, the cancer would be killed as well. In 2006, Dr. Scott Armstrong's research team identified cancer stem cells for leukemia. By understanding the differences between leukemia stem cells and healthy blood stem cells, it may be possible to engineer drugs that specifically target cancer stem cells while leaving healthy blood stem cells intact.

That same year, Drs. Sean Wu and Stuart Orkin, together with their research teams, discovered a particular heart stem cell that is the precursor to two important cardiac cell types. Research into this stem cell is important because by harnessing the cardiac stem cell and directing its differentiation into a particular heart cell, doctors may be able to treat or cure devastating heart defects.

Also in 2006, Dr. George Daley and his team showed that a woman's unfertilized ova, or eggs, could be used to generate custom stem cells genetically tailored to the woman herself. Tissue transplantation is often difficult because of the risk of the recipient's immune system rejecting the transplant; in contrast, custom stem cells could lead to the creation of custom tissues that would not be rejected by the patient's immune system.

Dr. Stuart Orkin and his team have continued to contribute to understanding stem cell biology through their work with myeloproliferative cells. Myeloproliferative syndromes, characterized by an excessive production of blood cells in the bone marrow, cannot be treated by a transplant of healthy blood stem cells into the bone marrow, as these healthy cells frequently become sick themselves. In 2007 Dr. Orkin's work showed that these diseases may not be stem cell related but, rather, related to the environment within the bone marrow.

In addition, results came in 2007 from Dr. Leonard Zon's team, showing an increase in immune stem cell production after treatment with a prostaglandin analog. These results from studies in the zebrafish could someday help restore immune function to patients who have undergone chemotherapy, which is often toxic to immune cells, as well as other procedures. This work followed earlier work from Dr. Zon's team that discovered a crucial gene for blood stem cells. The team hopes to use this knowledge to develop a technique that would allow the growth of blood stem cells to be given to patients with severe congenital anemia or blood stem cells that were injured as an adverse effect of chemotherapy.

**SEE ALSO:** Cancer; Cells, Embryonic; Harvard University; Massachusetts; Massachusetts General Hospital; Self-Renewal, Stem Cell; Transdifferentiation.

**BIBLIOGRAPHY.** Archives Program of Children's Hospital, *Children's Hospital Boston (MA) (Images of America)* (Arcadia, 2005); R. Bertolotti and K. Ozawa, eds., *Autologous and Cancer Stem Cell Gene Therapy (Progress in Gene Therapy)* (World Scientific, 2008); K. Bridges, *Anemias and Other Red Cell Disorders* (McGraw-Hill Professional, 2007); D. W. Parsons, *Stem Cells and Cancer* (Nova Science, 2006); P. E. Petrides and H. L. Paul, eds., *Molecular Basis of Chronic Myeloproliferative Disorders* (Springer, 2004); O. D. Wiestler, B. Haendler, and D. Mumberg, eds., *Cancer Stem Cells: Novel Concepts and Prospects for Tumor Therapy (Ernst Schering Foundation Symposium Proceedings)* (Springer, 2007).

Claudia Winograd
University of Illinois, Urbana-Champaign

# Chimera Formation (Animal and Human)

**A CHIMERA IS** an organism that is made up of more than one genetically distinct type of cell. Chimeras can either form naturally or be artificially produced in the laboratory by three mechanisms: mixing stem cells from two different individuals, introducing stem cells into a fully developed tissue, or combining two fully developed tissues into one organism. Scientists study chimeras to answer fundamental questions about stem cell biology, organ transplant biology, embryonic development, human diseases, and genetics, as well as to test drug effectiveness. Although many types of chimeras are possible, the formation of human-only, animal-only, and human–animal chimeras is described here.

## HUMAN CHIMERAS

In 2002, human chimerism (the condition of being a chimera) was publicized in the popular media with the case of a 52-year-old woman who needed a kidney transplant. To find a potential kidney donor, the woman and her immediate family submitted blood samples for genetic screening. The results were surprising: The tests indicated that the woman did not have biological similarities to two of the three sons to whom she had given birth. To solve this conundrum, doctors examined samples of the woman's mucus, hair, and skin and determined that she was a tetragametic chimera; that is, a chimera formed when two of a mother's eggs are fertilized by two of the father's sperm, and the resulting two embryos fuse to form one person. Tissues (e.g., the skin, muscle, etc.) of tetragametic chimeras either can be composed of cells from both original embryos or can be made up of cells from only one of the embryos. In the case described above, the woman's blood cells were derived from only one of the fused twins, whereas her other tissues were made up of cells from both twins.

With only 30 reported cases, human chimeras appear to be relatively rare. However, because naturally occurring chimeras rarely have identifiable features, the rate of human chimerism may be higher than reported. Genetic testing of several tissue types can usually identify human chimeras, although these tests can be complicated and expensive.

Thus, testing for human chimerism usually only occurs when rare, outward physical symptoms of chimerism are observed. The physical symptoms of chimerism may include ambiguous genitalia, hermaphroditism (having both male and female sex organs), patchy colored skin, or two differently colored eyes.

Recently, in vitro fertilization has been shown to increase the rate of tetragametic chimerism in embryos. This may result from the embryos being grown in close contact before implantation into the mother's uterus or from an increased chance that an egg with two nuclei will be fertilized by two different sperm. Either way, with the increased use of in vitro fertilization, diagnosing chimerism may be increasingly relevant when considering maternity/paternity cases, blood donation, or organ donation.

In addition to tetragametic chimeras, other types of chimeras exist in the human population. These include parthenogenetic chimeras, androgenetic chimeras, microchimerism, and organ transplant patients. A parthenogenetic chimera is formed when an egg that has not undergone meiosis (a cellular process that decreases the egg's genetic material by half) is fertilized by two sperm. In this case, the two sperm provide double the typical dosage of genetic material from the father, which pairs with the doubled genetic material from the mother and results in chimera formation. Only one case of human parthenogenetic chimerism has been reported.

The reverse scenario, androgenetic chimerism, occurs when one sperm fertilizes one normal egg and another sperm fertilizes an egg that is empty of genetic material. Normally, this second fertilization event would not produce a living zygote (fertilized egg). However, in some rare cases, the genetic material from the father in the empty egg may duplicate itself, producing a zygote that contains genetic material from only the father. This father-only zygote then fuses together with the normal zygote to form a chimera. In contrast to parthenogenetic chimeras, no known androgenetic chimeras have been born alive.

Microchimerism occurs when a small amount of cells are transferred between the mother and the fetus during pregnancy. Recently, scientists have run studies showing that microchimerism might be very common in humans. In fact, up to 50 percent of mothers may carry their children's cells in their blood decades after giving birth. During pregnancy, the fetus may also absorb some of the mother's cells. After birth, children could possibly carry their mother's cells with them throughout their lives. In cases in which a mother has multiple children, the mother may absorb cells from the first child into her body and then pass these cells onto other children during her subsequent pregnancies. Thus, individuals who have older siblings may have cells in their bodies that are derived from their older brothers and sisters. Researchers think that microchimerism may help the mother's immune system tolerate the fetus during pregnancy. Some scientists also believe that the breakdown of this system of tolerance may cause some autoimmune diseases in women.

Finally, humans that have undergone organ transplants or bone marrow transplants using human donors can be considered artificially created chimeras.

## ANIMAL CHIMERAS

Animal chimera formation occurs by the same methods as in humans. Because animal models are used to help understand human disease and mammalian development, many tetragametic chimeras are artificially generated for research. Both same-species and cross-species animal chimeras have been generated in the laboratory. In the 1960s, scientists showed that same-species mouse chimeras could be created by juxtaposing stem cells from two different mice in a test tube and then transferring these cells into a female mouse.

Scientists have expanded this technology to other animal types such as rats, birds, and sheep. Cross-species chimeras have also been created by scientists. In 1984, researchers combined embryos from a sheep and a goat. The resulting "geeps" were sterile and could not produce living offspring. Despite this setback, researchers believe that the practical benefits of producing interspecies chimeras will enable the rearing of embryos from endangered species using females from other species.

## HUMAN–ANIMAL CHIMERAS

Artificially created human–animal chimeras can be formed using fully differentiated, mature adult cells or by transplanting embryonic cells into either an adult or another embryo.

In cases using fully differentiated adult cells, tissues can be grafted from an animal to a human and vice versa. In the medical clinic, these chimeras are formed by organ transplantation when a human receives an organ (e.g., a heart) from an animal donor (e.g., a pig). In the lab, scientists often create human–animal chimeras for their research. Frequently, scientists will create a human–animal chimera by transplanting diseased human cells into a mouse with no immune system. Cancer researchers use this technique to graft human cancer cells into mice and then study how cancer grows and is affected by drug treatments. In contrast, liver biologists have found that a mouse transplanted with human liver cells can grow a functional human liver. These mice are used to study how viruses affect the human liver and how the human liver responds to certain drugs.

The most ethically controversial human–animal chimeras created with fully differentiated adult cells are those generated by mixing human nerve cells with an animal's central nervous system. The ethical consideration for these studies stems from the idea that human cognizance might be transferred to animals. Nevertheless, these neural chimeras have been created by two methods: human neural stem cells are purified from fetuses and transplanted into embryos or newborn animals, or human embryonic stem cells are differentiated into neurons in the lab and then transplanted into embryos, newborns, or adult animals. Neural human–animal chimeras have been created using rats, mice, and monkeys with the aim of using them as models for studying human neural development and neurodegenerative diseases.

Finally, stem cell biologists create human–animal chimeras with embryonic stem cells by injecting human embryonic stem cells into adult or embryonic animals. To create human–animal chimeras using stem cells, human stem cells are injected into an immune-deficient adult animal to produce a special type of tumor called a teratoma. This type of tumor can grow all of the different types of cells in the body. Stem cell biologists use chimeras generated from stem cells to understand how the different cells of the body are generated from stem cells.

U.S. law does not currently prohibit the production of human–animal chimeras. In 2005, a

Human Chimera Prohibition Act was proposed in the Senate by Senator Samuel Brownback, but this act was never voted into law. However, recommended ethical standards for experiments involving human–animal chimeras were published by the International Society for Stem Cell Research in 2007.

**SEE ALSO:** Bone Marrow Transplants; Cells, Embryonic; Developmental Biology; Differentiation, In Vitro and In Vivo; Human Embryonic Stem Cells; In Vitro Fertilization.

**BIBLIOGRAPHY.** Claire Ainsworth, "The Stranger Within," *New Scientist* (v.180, 2003); Richard R. Berhinger, "Human-Animal Chimeras in Biomedical Research," *Cell Stem Cell Review* (v.1/3, 2007); GovTrack.us, "S. 1373 [109th]: Human Chimera Prohibition Act of 2005," www.govtrack.us (cited November 2007); Insoo Hyun, et al., "Ethical Standards for Human-to-Animal Chimera Experiments in Stem Cell Research," *Cell Stem Cell* (v.1/2, 2007); V. Malan and M. Vekemans, "Chimera and Other Fertilization Errors," *Clinical Genetics* (v.70, 2006); George E. Seidel, Jr., "Mammalian Oocytes and Preimplantation Embryos as Methodological Components," *Biology of Reproduction* (v.28, 1983); "It's a Geep," *Time*, February 27, 1984, www.time.com (cited November 2007); Neng Yu, et al., "Disputed Maternity Leading to Identification of Tetragametic Chimerism," *New England Journal of Medicine* (v.346, 2002).

Renee C. Ireton
University of Washington

# China

**THE PEOPLE'S REPUBLIC** of China is one of the few nations in the world to support embryonic human stem cell research with minimal restrictions. Although the opposition to such research in Europe and the Americas is often predicated on a view of life drawn from those continents' Christian heritage, such a heritage does not exist in Asia. Chinese thought instead draws from the many schools of philosophy and religious traditions of its own heritage, with the teachings of Confucius prominent among them. In his writings, Confucius no more specifies the moment at which life begins than the Bible does—and so consensus about his extrapolated position is not uniform, but traditionally in Confucianism, life (i.e., personhood, humanity, selfhood) begins at birth—not conception or during gestation. In Confucianism, and Eastern philosophy in general, personhood denotes the presence of a psyche, a mind; the Western Christian idea of a soul that resides in the unborn fetus is a foreign one. In China, the embryo does not have the special mystique that it seems to have for so many Westerners.

In 2004 a British delegation declared that China was "at, or approaching, the forefront of international stem cell research." A recurring question is whether China—with a per capita income of about 4 percent of America's ($1,284 a year in 2005)—has the funding to seriously pursue stem cell research. At present, funding is more limited than even that provided by the federal government in the United States, coming mostly from grants allocated by the Ministry of Science and Technology for both basic stem cell research and applied stem cell research. Local governments sometimes contribute additional grant money.

Though the funding may be limited, labor and supplies are cheaper in China as well, although not so cheap as to completely offset the difference. The ministry has announced its intention of ramping up funding to keep up with Chinese progress in the field, but it remains to be seen where the ceiling is and when it will be hit. Compared with in Western countries, private sources of funding are severely limited.

Notable laboratories in China include, in Beijing, the Stem-Cell Research Center at Peking University, the National Institute of Biological Sciences, and the Institute of Zoology at the Chinese Academy of Sciences; in Shanghai, Xinhua Hospital and the Shanghai Institutes for Biological Sciences of the Chinese Academy of Sciences; in Changsha, Xiangya Medical College; and in Guangdong, the

Guangzhou Institute of Biomedicine and Health of the Chinese Academy of Sciences. Those advanced students who are able to tend to go overseas for their education and training, and collaboration within China is more limited than in most countries. Findings are often presented internationally and in English-language journals before, or in lieu of, domestic presentation.

A 2006 article in the *New England Journal of Medicine* noted the lack of a social infrastructure—true scientific community—among Chinese stem cell researchers, and some have suggested that this may limit China's contributions as much as funding does. In particular, the commentators worried about the lack of informal exchange among Chinese researchers and concluded that the lack of infrastructure alone would be enough to marginalize China's role in worldwide stem cell research.

## RESTRICTIONS

Medical trial and testing protocols also are different in China than in much of the Western world; which is to say, there are fewer of them. The bulk of the burden of protocol is borne by the review boards of the institution where a given trial or study takes place, rather than being written and enforced at a distance by a federal agency as in the United States, and for various reasons, China generates much less red tape in this area.

The Ethical Guidelines for Research on Human Embryonic Stem Cells as released by the Ministry of Science and Technology and the Ministry of Health on December 24, 2003, set these rules:

- All human reproductive cloning is prohibited;
- Human embryonic stem cells used for research must only be derived from donated germ cells, blastocysts obtained by somatic cell nuclear transfer, spared gametes or blastocysts from in vitro fertilization, or fetal cells from miscarriages or voluntary abortions;
- The in vitro period of blastocysts prepared for such research must not exceed 14 days;
- Such embryos must not be implanted into any womb, human or otherwise;
- Human germ cells must not be hybridized with those of other species;
- There must not be any trade in human gametes, fertilized eggs, embryos, or fetal tissues;
- All subjects and donors must have their privacy protected, must give informed consent, and must make informed choices in the matter of their participation;
- All institutions engaging in human embryonic stem cell research must have or establish an ethical committee staffed with researchers and administrators from the fields of biology, medicine, sociology, and law to supervise and review research activities;
- All such institutions must also develop their own procedures and rules in compliance with the principles set forth by the ministries.

China's fairly lax restrictions, as compared with Western nations, and the ample supply of tissue from the millions of fetuses aborted in the country each year because of the country's population limit laws, have been expected to encourage Western biotech companies to outsource their research and development there, or to enter into other joint ventures with Chinese institutions and researchers. Intellectual property law is weaker in the East, though, and that, combined with a number of small scandals surrounding falsified results and plagiarism in other research fields, has discouraged what might otherwise be a surge of cooperative efforts.

## MEDICAL TOURISM

Asian countries have always been among the most popular destinations for medical tourists, and stem cell research has helped attract foreigners to China who are seeking treatments unavailable in their homelands. Stem Cells China Limited, a company that provides information on stem cell treatments to Westerners, lists on its Web site testimonials and blogs from patients suffering from amyotrophic lateral sclerosis, ataxia, autism, Batten disease, brain injuries, cerebral palsy, epilepsy, Friedrich's ataxia, Huntington's disease, multiple sclerosis, Parkinson's disease, spinal muscular atrophy, spinal cord injuries, and strokes.

Researchers at several universities have used stem cell injections to treat an amyotrophic lateral sclerosis-like disease in rats. In China, one doctor, Huang Hongyun, has treated mostly Americans with his amyotrophic lateral sclerosis treatment, which involves injections of stem cells into the forebrain; the treatment is not a cure and is not permanent, and Western medical authorities caution patients that there is too little information to know whether such treatments are safe, much less effective. Some patients have reported a return of leg and arm strength, but others have expressed disappointment that their posttreatment improvement is not more pronounced. Huang has claimed that medical journals have refused to publish his articles on the treatment because of his nationality, but he refuses to submit his work to randomized trials.

**SEE ALSO:** Amyotrophic Lateral Sclerosis; Batten Disease; Cells, Embryonic; China Stem Cell News; Ethics; Korea, South; Medical Tourism and Stem Cells; Moral Status of Embryo; Multiple Sclerosis; Regulations Overview; Religion, Buddhist; Singapore.

**BIBLIOGRAPHY.** *Stem Cell Mission to China, Singapore, and South Korea: Report of a DTI Global Watch Mission* (Department of Trade and Industry, September 2004); Benfu Li, "The Principles of Embryo Stem Cell Research," *Chinese Medical Ethics* (October 2001); Fiona Murray and Debora Spar, "Bit Player or Powerhouse? China and Stem Cell Research," *New England Journal of Medicine* (v.355, 2006); Renzong Qiu, "Ethical Issues of Human Embryo Stem Cell Research," Proceedings of Third International Conference of Bioethics, Institute of Philosophy, National Central University, Chungli, Taiwan, June 2002; Jie Wu, "Thinking of Stem Cells," *Beijing Science and Technology Daily* (August 6, 2001); Shusheng Xie, "What Is the Way of Stem Cell Research, Medicine, and Philosophy," *Dalian* (v.23, 2002); Geoffrey York, "Chinese Stem Cell Surgeon Stirs Passion, Shuns Trials," *Toronto Globe and Mail* (December 6, 2004).

Bill Kte'pi
Independent Scholar

# China Stem Cell News

**CHINA STEM CELL NEWS** is a means of communicating the latest information on stem cells, stem cell research, and current treatments available in China to the general public. It was established on the World Wide Web by Stem Cells China Limited, a company whose mission is to inform and educate the world via increased communication on the fast-breaking and leading-edge medical opportunities available to those in need by offering the latest facts and information about stem cells and their use in China. The Web site offers news, frequently asked questions, hospitals and laboratories conducting research, patient experiences, educational material, a newsletter, information on clinical trials and case studies, a list of treatable conditions, means of contacting the company, past and upcoming conferences, and links to other Web sites with similar content.

The team at Stem Cells China Limited continues to build their network of healthcare providers and medical professionals who serve as their source of knowledge on various groups conducting research and performing treatments in China. The company has built partnerships with several of China's leading hospitals.

The company created the China Stem Cell News Web site in order to provide a user-friendly environment for people afflicted with conditions that could possibly be treated with the most up-to-date treatments using stem cells in China.

The news page provides links to the latest news on research and treatments in China. The links are grouped alphabetically into categories including diseases, disorders, stem cells, and other sources of news. The diseases mentioned include amyotrophic lateral sclerosis (ALS), Alzheimer's, ataxia, autism, Batten disease, eye diseases, heart disease, Huntington's disease, kidney, liver, lung and peripheral vascular disease. It includes links to sources on hearing disorders, eye disorders, brain and spinal cord injury, and stroke. This page provides information on world news related to China, research from China, and China healthcare news. It also covers the different types of stem cells, such as fetal, embryonic, menstrual, and umbilical cord. This section also contains a multitude of articles regarding stem cell research and treatment in China. The frequently asked questions page provides information regarding the processing of cells, types of stem cells, including embryonic or fetal stem cells, genetics, and general information on stem cells.

The who's who page presents company backgrounds on the hospitals, laboratories, doctors, and scientists conducting stem cell research and stem cell treatments in China. The Web site makes it possible to search by groups or hospitals with treatments, by laboratories, or by people. Hospitals include Huashan Hospital, Tiantan Puhua Hospital, Huan Wu Hospital, and Xinhua Hospital. Other involved institutions include Beike Biotechnology Company Limited, the Institute of Zoology, Military Medical Sciences Academy, Peking Union Medical College, and Beijing University Stem Cell Center.

## PATIENT INFORMATION

The patient experiences page provides patient written testimonials on both positive and negative experiences with treatments. Each patient creates a profile with his or her name, age, home country, diagnosis, reason for treatment, and treatment used. Some are links to other sites and to articles, while others are the full explanations directly on the Web site. Patients have also written Web site logs narrating their trip to China, their treatments, and their experiences after treatment. Doctors have also submitted their experiences with research, treatment, and patients.

Patient experiences and Web site logs include the following diseases or disorders: ataxia, autism, ALS, brain injury, cerebral palsy, dysuria, encephalatropy, epilepsy, Guillain-Barre syndrome, Huntington's, optic nerve hypoplasia, multiple sclerosis, Parkinson's, spinal cord injuries, spinal muscular atrophy, and stroke. These patients are not solely from China, but from other countries as well, including the United States, the United Kingdom, Australia, Canada, and many more. Patients include men, women, teenagers, and children, all affected by disease that was treated with new therapy developed from research with stem cells.

The Web site also provides a discussion group with new updates on treatments and research in China, as well as the rest of the world. Ultimately, this allows those people who are interested in seeking treatments to get in touch with those who have already had treatment or those who conduct the treatment.

Prospective patients can send a general inquiry via the Web site if seeking treatment for a particular ailment. The Web site also provides a page with a list of treatable conditions. Each condition listed has a link that leads to a detailed synopsis of the condition, including a detailed definition, list of symptoms, list of tests to diagnose the condition, and current treatments available for the specific condition.

The educational material page allows prospective patients to learn more about the human brain or the vast field of alternative medicine. The information on the human brain includes an article on brain formation, as well as several pages of brain anatomy, activity, and function. The list of diseases provides direct links to detailed informative material on each condition treated by the stem cell research population in China.

The company's newsletter offers information on a specific topic related to stem cell research. The company also includes two links on clinical trials and case studies. The page on clinical trials is categorized by condition, which then shows the current clinical trials under examination. Each clinical trial includes detailed information regarding doctors and hospitals involved, the purpose of the clinical trial, as well as details about the condition. In addition to information on clinical trials associated with stem cell research in China, the China Stem Cell News Web site offers similar information on case studies in China.

The conferences page includes several articles on the many stem cell research conferences held around the world. These conferences share information on new stem cell research and resulting treatments. The China Stem Cell News Web site shares information from all over the world, as well as China. China Stem Cell News, created by the company Stem Cells China Limited, provides a multitude of information for the general public looking for the most recent research associated with stem cells and treatments developed from stem cell research.

**SEE ALSO:** China; Medical Tourism and Stem Cells.

**BIBLIOGRAPHY.** *China Stem Cell News*, www.stemcellschina.com (cited April 2008).

Jennifer Yoohanna
University of California, Los Angeles

# Christopher Reeve Foundation

**CHRISTOPHER REEVE IS** a name that most everyone immediately recognizes as synonymous with saving lives, usually as an actor on the big screen. However, in 1995, this "superman" changed roles, going from a self-sufficient man to a quadriplegic. He and his wife Dana sought out the help of the American Paralysis Foundation; later, this organization merged with the couple's efforts, adopted their names and funding, and became known as the Christopher and Dana Reeve Foundation.

This organization has since helped thousands of paralyzed individuals around the world improve their quality of life, as well as supporting hundreds of scientists in their research efforts regarding spinal cord injuries. The organization's mission reads:

> The Christopher and Dana Reeve Foundation is dedicated to curing spinal cord injury by funding innovative research, and improving the quality of life for people living with paralysis through grants, information and advocacy.

Funding is done through many avenues, one of which is the Individual Research Grants Program. The Individual Research Grants Program supports examining the most basic, molecular mechanisms of spinal cord damage and possible means of repair. Immunology and neuroscience fields are also included in grant money.

Major categories of research the foundation supports are axon guidance (regenerating axons must often grow several feet and end up joining with the correct nerves); synapse formation (connections between the nerves—synapses—must work correctly if information is to get from one part of the body to another); neurotransmission (proper chemicals—neurotransmitters—in correct amounts must be present and must have proper receptors to continue the transmission of information); cellular replacement (damaged neurons and their support cells must be coaxed to regrow); therapeutic cells (stem cells can be transplanted in and encourage the missing or damaged cells to regrow); substrates (transplanted cells can serve as scaffolding for the new cells to grow within); concomitant function (many functions controlled by the spinal cord are impaired with spinal cord injuries [SCI]; scientists are trying to address these problems); neuroprotection (after injury, the body's natural immune system responds to the trauma; decreasing this immune response could save many nerve cells that were not initially damaged); growth inhibition (inhibiting the inhibitory effects nerve support cells have on neuronal growth); and promotion of axon growth and remyelination, rehabilitation, and stem cell research (using primitive cells to restart development of the spinal cord).

The foundation also has an International Research Consortium on SCI, facilitating collaboration of many international research labs. Through these relationships, contributions have been made to treatments for Parkinson's and Alzheimer's diseases, multiple sclerosis, and amyotrophic lateral sclerosis.

Getting over the hump from bench science research and results to actual patient treatment can be tough. The Translational Research Fund helps bridge that transition. Once protocols can be applied to people, clinical trials are needed to ensure safety and efficacy. Clinical trials are also included in the foundation's work, under the umbrellas of the foundation's North American Clinical Trials Network and NeuroRecovery Network. Through this encouragement and support of scientific research on SCI, neuroscientists everywhere have come to shift their perspective from one of possibly finding a cure for SCI to one of knowing a cure is possible and that it is only a matter of time until it is found.

In addition to monies going to the labs, there is funding put aside for Quality of Life Grants. These grants serve to encourage and support programs that help improve the daily standard of living for those with spinal cord injuries, paralysis caused by any injury, and birth defects leading to paralysis. The categories these grants support are accessibility, advocacy, arts, assistive technology, children, counseling, education, employment, health promotion, independent living, practical services, sports and recreation, and therapeutic riding. The Health Promotion Grants are given in conjunction with funding from the Centers for Disease Control and Prevention and can be as large as $25,000. No grants are made to individuals, only to nonprofit agencies working with those paralyzed for any reason.

One might ask why it is important to further research in these fields. To answer that question, it is important to see what science used to know about spinal cord injuries versus what they know now. It used to be thought that if axon growth alone was encouraged, this would be enough to facilitate function return. We now understand that all the support cells (microglia, oligodendrocytes) must also be present for axons to be able to grow and function. It used to be thought that if an axon died, that was it—that function was lost. Scientists are now working on ways to use neurons, and their axons, that survived the initial trauma to take over function of the dead axons, restoring abilities that were previously thought unredeemable. After injury, scar tissue forms, and it is understood that this tissue acts as a firewall against nerve transmission.

Researchers now have ways to encourage nerves to bridge scar tissues, circumventing a previous roadblock. Scientists are also learning which stem cells are best suited to regrowing spinal cord tissues. It used to be thought that Schwann cells with olfactory ensheathing glia worked best; it is now thought that neural progenitor cells are best. Previously, natural scaffolding material was searched out, now synthetic material is being touted. Finally, advances in genetic testing such as gene mapping and chromosome visualization are helping elicit the distinct functions of each biological molecule in the spinal cord during embryonic development.

In addition to monetary support, the foundation also uses its voice to push for good legislation for those living with spinal cord injuries. In October 2007, the House of Representatives passed the Christopher and Dana Reeve Paralysis Act, H.R. 1727. (It had yet to pass the Senate.) The point of this act is to reduce redundancies in research, expand research done at the National Institutes of Health, and encourage open communication between scientists working on similar projects. There is also the inclusion of a Clinical Trials Network to examine how effective rehabilitation techniques are, as well as encouragement for sharing between those researching rehabilitation techniques.

## FUND-RAISING

All this research and support does not come free, however, and one can imagine that with this many projects in the pipeline, funding is a critical part of the foundation's successes. Over $20 million has been given to the categories discussed above since 1982. As the Christopher and Dana Reeve Foundation is a nonprofit organization, most of the money raised comes from contributions from individuals as well as corporations. Other forms of income are through planned giving (such as bequests in wills and life insurance plans), corporate-sponsored giving (joint giving of employees and their employer), and fund-raisers by groups of individuals and organizations.

Of the total money raised, 84.6 percent of it goes to program expenses, such as the many research grants mentioned earlier. Administrative costs account for 4.8 percent, and fund-raising expenses take up 10.5 percent. This translates to a fund-raising efficiency of $0.11, and an efficiency rating of 31.71, meaning that the foundation exceeds or meets industry standards and performs as well as most charities in its cause. Overall, the Christopher and Dana Reeve Foundation has a rating of 47.73, according to the Charity Navigator service.

Christopher Reeve and his wife Dana took a negative event and turned it into something positive. The development of new research projects, scientific advancements, and political action is having a far more substantial effect than the Reeve family ever initially imagined. By using his fame, Christopher Reeve has shown that there is indeed hope in the face of devastation. The power of one man's hope and desire has shaped a movement that has the potential to change scientific perception, in addition to the lives of those affected by spinal cord injuries. As Christopher Reeve said:

> What I do is based on powers we all have inside us; the ability to endure; the ability to love, to carry on, to make the best of what we have—and you don't have to be a Superman to do it.

**SEE ALSO:** Amyotrophic Lateral Sclerosis; Congress: Votes and Amendments (Cloning/Embryos); Spinal Cord Injury.

**BIBLIOGRAPHY.** Charity Navigator, www.charitynavigator.org (cited October 2007); Christopher and Dana Reeve Foundation, www.christopherreeve.org (cited October 2007); GovTrack.us, H.R. 1727: Christopher and Dana Reeve Paralysis Act, www.govtrack.us (cited October 2007).

Caroline M. Sebley
Kansas City University of Medicine and Biosciences

# Clinical Trials (Adult Cells)

**STEM CELLS ARE** specialized types of cells that differ from typical cells because of two distinct qualities. First, stem cells can renew themselves for long periods of time. Second, stem cells have the potential to differentiate into many types of cells. For example, hepatocytes or liver cells can regenerate to eventually return a liver to its original size following surgical removal of part of it. Stem cells can be divided into three main categories: embryonic, umbilical, and adult. One major difference among the three is that they are all obtained differently. For example, embryonic stem cells are collected from the very early stages of a fertilized egg, called a blastocyst—whereas umbilical stem cells are obtained from the umbilical cord of a newborn baby, adult stem cells can be derived from tissues or organs of living adults.

The advantage of using adult stem cells is that they are already somewhat differentiated, so inducement into a specific type of tissue may be easier. For example, embryonic stem cells can become differentiated into any cells in the body; hence they are called pluripotent. However, these differentiation procedures are timely and complicated. In contrast, hematopoietic stem cells, a type of adult stem cell, are called multipotent because they have the capacity to only become cells of the blood system and generally not other cell types making the differentiation relatively straightforward. Also, when recipients receive transplantation of their very own cells, these cells will usually be recognized by the recipient's immune system, and an immune response to the transplanted cells will most likely not be triggered, causing a rejection.

Although researchers are finding more and more locations from which adult stem cells can be isolated, they are still available only in select tissues and organs and are found in limited quantities. Among these locations are the bone marrow, the liver, and the brain. Another disadvantage of adult stem cells is that the harvested adult stem cells may carry genetic mutations that may be harmful to the receiving host.

Some very useful applications of adult stem cells in clinical medicine are bone marrow transplant (BMT) and peripheral bone stem cell transplant (PBSCT). BMT and PBSCT are used to facilitate patients' receiving very high dose chemotherapy or radiation therapy. Essentially, stem cells are used to restore cells that were destroyed by high-dose chemotherapy or radiation therapy. At present, BMT and PBSCT are most commonly used in the treatment of cancers such as leukemia, lymphoma, and multiple myeloma, as well as other noncancerous diseases such as sickle cell anemia and aplastic anemia.

BMT is a lifesaving advance for many people, but there are numerous complications associated with it. One serious complication is graft-versus-host disease, or GVHD. GVHD is a potentially fatal incompatibility reaction mediated by antigens or small proteins found on the surface of the cells of the receiver that are not found on the cells of the donor. These antigens are usually recognized by the transplanted white blood cells (lymphocytes). These lymphocytes start attacking the recipient's cells and can lead to death in some cases.

Clinical trials are underway to avoid serious GVHD by using PBSCT instead of BMT. PBSCT allows transplantation of the necessary stem cells and removal of the lymphocytes that are chiefly responsible for GVHD. The stem cells used in PBSCT are collected from the bloodstream rather than the bone marrow. A few days before transplantation, the donor may be given a medication to increase the number of stem cells released into the bloodstream. This medication is called a growth factor or a granulocyte colony-stimulating factor (G-CSF).

Then, in a process called apheresis or leukophoresis, blood is removed from a large vein in the arm or a central venous catheter (a tube inserted into a large vein, typically in the neck). The blood that is removed through apheresis is then fed through a machine that separates and removes the stem cells from the other cells. The blood is then returned to the donor, and the stem cells are collected and frozen until the time of transplantation.

## G-CSF IN CANCER PATIENTS

One clinical trial sponsored by the National Heart, Lung, and Blood Institute is called "Use of Granulocyte Colony Stimulating Factor (G-CSF) Mobilized Leukapheresis Collections from Normal Volunteers to Develop Improved Methods of Stem Cell and Lymphocyte Selection for Allogeneic Transplantation." The trial has been ongoing since 1996. The purpose of this clinical trial is twofold. The first purpose is to improve the method of processing of the cells that are collected by removing the lymphocytes after stimulation with G-CSF, while at the same time keeping the stem cells healthy for transplantation and blood cell building. In addition, this trial allows researchers to study whether or not G-CSF has an effect on the function of lymphocytes, which may affect the immune reaction.

G-CSF is used not only in stem cell transplant but also in cancer patients receiving chemotherapy to increase those cells that are destroyed as an adverse effect of chemotherapeutic agents. Although research is being conducted to make more target-specific chemotherapeutic agents, the most common chemotherapeutic agents currently still affect a wide variety of cells. In general, chemotherapy usually kills those cells that are dividing at the fastest rate, which is precisely why chemotherapy is effective—because cancer cells divide faster than normal cells. In addition, this is the reason why patients have symptoms such as hair loss or diarrhea—because the cells that account for these tissues usually are rapidly dividing.

Another type of cell that is also proliferating at a rapid pace is the blood cell. Therefore, myelosuppression, or a reduction of the ability of the bone marrow to make red blood cells, white blood cells, or platelets, commonly occurs in patients receiving chemotherapeutic agents. Common manifestations of this include anemia (abnormally low red blood cell count), leukopenia (abnormally low white blood cell count), and thrombocytopenia (abnormally low number of platelets). Anemia can cause fatigue, paleness, and in severe cases, even heart attacks. Leukopenia, in contrast, can put a patient at risk for severe infections because white blood cells are the primary immune cells responsible for fighting infections. Thrombocytopenia can cause patients to bleed excessively because of the platelets' vital role in helping with clotting.

One of the first clinical trials using G-CSF for the purpose of decreasing the incidence of leukopenia was completed in 1988 by the Cancer Research Unit at the Walter and Eliza Hall Institute of Medical Research of the Royal Melbourne Hospital in Australia. In this trial, 30 cancer patients were chosen to receive two cycles of G-CSF. During the first cycle, patients were treated with G-CSF for five days, followed by a three-day therapy-free period. The second cycle, which was done to investigate the effects of G-CSF during myelosuppression, was then begun. After a dose of the chemotherapeutic agent (melphalan), G-CSF was started for nine consecutive days. The results of this clinical trial were very promising. The precursor cells that form red blood and white blood cells showed an increase of up to 100-fold after four days of treatment with G-CSF and remained elevated for up to two days after cessation of therapy. In addition, the number of progenitor cells (slightly differentiated stem cells) slightly decreased in most patients.

Today, because of this and other early clinical trials, G-CSF is commonly used in patients with many types of cancers who are receiving chemotherapy to reduce the incidence of leukopenia and infections that are usually associated with it. Filgrastim is the name that has been chosen for one of the most common G-CSF agents used in clinical practice today. The use of G-CSF to increase white blood cell count is a great example of manipulating adult stem cells for clinical benefit, and it has had a profound effect on adult stem cells.

## G-CSF IN PATIENTS FOLLOWING A MYOCARDIAL INFARCTION (HEART ATTACK)

Although G-CSF has been used for many years in the treatment of chemotherapy complications, a new clinical trial has begun at the University of Ottawa under the auspices of the Canadian Institutes of Health Research, looking at whether or not G-CSF can help repair heart muscle cells after a myocardial infarction. Patients in this study will have their heart function, blood flow to the heart, and heart cell function monitored, using nuclear cardiology scans, before they are enrolled in the study to have a baseline function of the heart. Then one group will receive G-CSF for four days and the other group will receive a placebo.

The patients will then have nuclear cardiology scans done at six weeks and six months, as well as an angiogram, to assess whether any improvement is noted. The rationale behind this study is that it has been thought that when a cell is injured, stem cells are released from the bone marrow that can differentiate and transform into the injured type of cell.

## STEM CELLS FOLLOWING A TRAUMATIC BRAIN INJURY

The role of stem cells in helping patients is not limited to hematological applications but expands far into the realm of medicine. Stem cells are also being researched in helping patients after traumatic brain injury, which is the cause of 50 percent of deaths resulting from trauma; up to 25 percent of children who receive traumatic brain injury die. Bone marrow stem cells preferentially migrate to areas of brain injury and differentiate into brain cells or neurons and other supporting elements of the brain.

A clinical trial started in 2006 at the University of Texas Health Sciences Center in Houston is researching this migration in children. Children who have experienced traumatic brain injury, following appropriate consent, will have bone marrow extracted from their hip. The study is recruiting children instead of adults for various reasons. First, children have a greater neurological plasticity, or the ability of brain to reorganize after an injury. In addition, children are more likely to have isolated traumatic brain injuries that will not have associated fluid collection, as might more commonly occur in adults.

This bone marrow is then separated into two components, mesenchymal cells and hematopoietic cells. Whereas hematopoietic cells have the capacity to differentiate only into blood cells, mesenchymal cells have the ability to differentiate into many types of cells, including bone, cartilage, fat cells, and most important, neurons. A specialized center will process these particular cells, and within 48 hours of the injury, the cells will be returned back to the patient intravenously. Then the children will be monitored at one and six months after infusion to compare their progress with historical data about normal recovery after traumatic brain injury in similarly aged children.

## STEM CELLS FOLLOWING A MYOCARDIAL INFARCTION (HEART ATTACK)

One promising avenue for the use of stem cells to benefit patients is in the setting of a myocardial infarction. A large clinical trial in Vienna, Myocardial Stem Cell Administration after Acute Myocardial Infarction (MYSTAR), is currently being performed to look at whether or not stem cell transplantation could benefit patients in recovering after a heart attack. Outcomes being measured include looking at whether the damage to the blood perfusion of the heart could be decreased or the amount of blood the heart pumps be increased via bone marrow stem cell administration.

This trial will divide patients into four different groups. These groups will include patients who receive early treatment and ones who receive late treatment. In addition, these groups will be subdivided into patients who receive bone marrow in the cardiac muscle itself (intracardiac) and those who receive the marrow in the blood vessel feeding the heart (intracoronary). This is the first study of its kind looking at both methods of delivery.

## STEM CELLS FOLLOWING HEART FAILURE

Heart failure is a condition in which the heart does not pump well. Although there are numerous causes of heart failure, it is usually a complication of either a heart attack or high blood pressure. As the disease gets worse over many years, patients can even die from it. A study at the University of Pittsburgh has been looking at the safety and effectiveness of stem cells injected into the heart. Stem cells injected from the bone marrow of an eligible patient are aspirated and injected into their own heart muscle.

This clinical trial has a very novel design. These patients will not need to have any extra procedures but will simply get the stem cell injections during a ventricular assist device placement or partial artificial heart surgery. These patients all will be awaiting a heart transplant for the heart failure. While they await heart transplant, however, their heart function will be monitored. After the heart transplant is completed, the heart muscle will be examined under the microscope to look for changes at the site where the stem cells have been injected. This study will allow us to understand better exactly how stem cells are able to transform into other cells when an injury is detected.

## LIMITATIONS AND PROBLEMS

One issue with clinical trials using stem cells is how much stem cell to harvest from each patient. Stem cells in each patient are available at a finite amount; therefore, a threshold level needs to be determined through further research. With respect to the heart, another issue that has not yet fully been elucidated is when to inject the stem cells into the heart muscle—early on, or later following a myocardial infarction.

In addition, where to inject the stem cells (in the heart itself or in the blood vessels feeding the heart) is a question that has yet to be answered. Patient safety also should always be the primary goal. Stem cells injected into a patient can form other cells than the cell of interest, forming scars with potentially deleterious consequences. Further study needs to be done to make sure that these stem cell transplantations are not just effective but, more important, safe.

**SEE ALSO:** Cancer; Cells, Adult; Cells, Amniotic; Cells, Embryonic; Cells, Human; Cells, Umbilical; Heart Attack; United States.

**BIBLIOGRAPHY.** Clinical Trials: National Library of Medicine, 2007, clinicaltrials.gov/ct/show/NCT00001529 (cited October 2007); Clinical Trials: National Library of Medicine, 2007, clinicaltrials.gov/ct/show/NCT00254722 (cited October 2007); Clinical Trials: National Library of Medicine, 2007, clinicaltrials.gov/ct/show/NCT00384982 (cited October 2007); Clinical Trials: National Library of Medicine, 2007, clinicaltrials.gov/ct/show/NCT00394498 (cited October 2007); Clinical Trials: National Library of Medicine, 2007, clinicaltrials.gov/ct/show/NCT00128258 (cited October 2007); U. Dührsen, et al., "Effects of Recombinant

Human Granulocyte Colony-Stimulating Factor on Hematopoietic Progenitor Cells in Cancer Patients," *Blood* (v.72/6, 1988); M. S. Lee and R. R. Makkar, "Stem-Cell Transplantation in Myocardial Infarction: A Status Report," *Annals of Internal Medicine* (v.140/9, 2004); University of Texas Health Sciences Center at Houston: News Room, publicaffairs.uth.tmc.edu (cited October 2007).

Devin Edwin Shahverdian
Maricopa Integrated Health System

# Clinical Trials Outside U.S.: Amyotrophic Lateral Sclerosis

**AMYOTROPHIC LATERAL SCLEROSIS** (ALS), also known as Lou Gehrig's disease, is a progressive disorder of motor dysfunction that leads to paralysis and eventually death. A few published and unpublished clinical trials around the world have been begun using stem cells in humans and are in their very early stages. With all the excitement and possibilities stem cells have to offer as a therapy, it is critical that scientists and clinicians are cautious, plan rigorous studies, and most important, focus on key laboratory experiments that will provide answers to the many challenges that still face this therapeutic approach. For this therapy to be safe and have potential in the clinic, it is critical that the appropriate studies are conducted for us to learn more about the properties and complexities of the various stem cells.

## STRATEGIES

ALS is a fatal neurodegenerative disease causing the progressive loss of brain and spinal cord motor neurons. The most prominent pathology of the disease involves the death of large motor neurons in the spinal cord and brainstem. Patients eventually become paralyzed, and approximately 50 percent die within three years after onset of symptoms, usually as the result of respiratory failure.

The disease is rare before age 40, and incidence rises with advancing age, peaking at around age 70. Approximately 10 percent of cases are familial, displaying an autosomal dominant pattern of inheritance. However, familial patients cannot be distinguished clinically or pathologically from sporadic ALS patients. About 20 percent of familial ALS cases have been linked to mutations in the gene encoding the cytosolic $Cu^{2+}/Zn^{2+}$ superoxide dismutase 1, suggesting that an abnormal function of this enzyme may play a pivotal role in the pathogenesis and progression of familial ALS. The mechanism of motor neuron death in ALS remains unclear. However, the most prevalent hypothesis for motor neuron death has been that mutant SOD1 protein within motor neurons elicits oxidative stress, causing multiple cellular changes and eventually triggering cell death. Motor neuron death in ALS is complex and may involve multiple pathways including formation of protein aggregates, axonal transport defects, oxidative damage, mitochondrial defects, and alterations in calcium homeostasis, triggering cell death.

There are at least two major strategies for using stem cells to treat ALS. The first, and most obvious, is to produce new motor neurons to replace those lost in the disease. The second is to produce support cells to protect existing motor neurons from ongoing degeneration, either with or without genetic modification to express enzymes, transporters, or specific growth factors. This idea has gained much momentum recently as a result of inroads made regarding the contribution of different cellular subtypes to disease initiation and progression. In more and more studies, glial cells are being shown to modulate many neuronal functions including glutamate uptake, synaptic plasticity, trophic factor support, and even neural transmission. Astrocytes and microglia surrounding motor neurons have now also been shown to play a crucial role in motor neuron health and survival in ALS.

## STEM CELL TREATMENTS IN CHINA

Although a number of centers outside the United States advertise stem cell therapies for ALS, very few of these have been subject to serious preclinical and postoperative follow-up. A Chinese neurosurgeon, Huang Hongyun, provided stem cell treatments in Beijing, China, although there is not sufficient information about his work to indicate with scientific certainty that the treatment is safe and effective. He reported that he has treated patients with ALS with spinal cord and forebrain injections, each including 1 million olfactory ensheathing cells, which are the part of the brain involved in the sense of smell (olfaction), taken from fetuses. All treatments were performed in a Beijing hospital. Doctors inserted these olfactory ensheathing cells directly into the brains of the patients after drilling holes in their skulls under local anesthesia. Dr. Hongyun said he began his work in this area by transplanting olfactory ensheathing cells into patients with spinal cord injury. He added that he had operated on about 500 spinal cord patients and 200 others with ALS by June 2005.

Dr. Hongyun reported that within both patient groups (those with ALS and spinal cord injuries), there was rapid improvement of partial function. However, there were no data presented from the patients with spinal cord injury to demonstrate the effects—positive or negative—on any of these patients. Video clips were shown for a total of eight ALS patients before and after treatment. Two patients did not demonstrate any change in their condition after transplantation. Furthermore, there were no data or information presented about the long-term effects of the treatment. Without peer review of objective data on each patient before, immediately after, and at specific long-term points following the transplantation, the study lacks sufficient scientific evidence to demonstrate that the treatment is safe and effective.

Taken together, reports of stem cell transplantation performed in China for either ALS or spinal cord injury lack sufficient peer review and patient treatment records to fully understand if the treatments are safe and effective. A placebo response to treatment is a well-documented medical phenomenon. Without objective, long-term data collection or controls, it is very difficult to conclude with any scientific certainty that the treatment is responsible for the positive response. The work to answer key scientific questions and overcome inherent challenges to the treatment is moving forward.

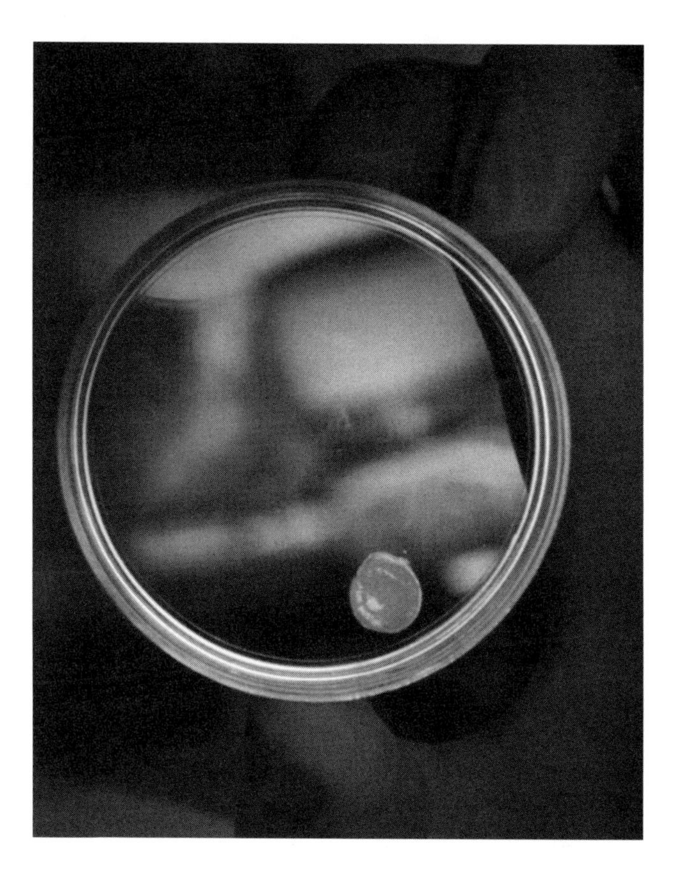

*A clinical trial of stem cell transplants for ALS in Italy reported some slowing of muscular strength decline in four patients.*

## CLINICAL TRIALS IN ITALY

In 2003 Italian researchers reported transplanting marrow cells taken from ALS patients' own pelvic bones into their spinal cords. This clinical trial was carried out by Italian researcher Letizia Mazzini (Department of Neurology, Eastern Piedmont University of Novara, Italy), with autologous mesenchymal stem cells transplanted into the thoracic region in ALS patients. Mesenchymal stem cells have been shown to possess great somatic plasticity because they are capable of differentiating into nonmesenchymal lineages. In fact, it has been demonstrated that mesenchymal stem cells are capable of differentiating into neurons and astrocytes both in vitro and in vivo. These cells have been shown to improve neurological performance in rodent models with neurological abnormalities such as brain ischemia.

The research group enrolled nine patients with ALS showing severe functional impairment of lower limbs and mild impairment of upper limbs. A bone marrow aspirate from each patient was used to prepare mesenchymal stem cell cultures that were expanded for three to four weeks. Cells were then suspended in autologous cerebrospinal fluid and directly transplanted into the surgically exposed spinal cord in the thoracic region (around the level of the shoulder blades, T7–T9).

No patients experienced severe adverse events following transplantations. Magnetic resonance imaging scans performed three and six months following transplantation did not show structural changes of the spinal cord or abnormal cell proliferation when compared with the baseline. Three months after cell implantation, a mild trend toward a slowing down of muscular strength decline was observed in the proximal muscle group of lower limbs in four patients. These preliminary results do not allow us to draw any conclusions about the efficacy of stem cell transplants for ALS treatment; nevertheless, they pave the way for further studies and trials aiming to treat neurological diseases.

Although there were no adverse effects or significant improvements in these patients, the location of the transplants was below the main cervical regions of the spinal cord controlling arm movement and breathing. The use of bone marrow–derived cells may be less than optimal for maximal integration and full differentiation into functional cells within the spinal cord. The study was designed only to test the feasibility and safety of the procedure, and it passed those tests. No benefits were seen. However, this study does provide "proof of concept" that large volumes (1 mL) of cells can be infused into the spinal cord without the formation of cysts or other pathology, as determined using magnetic resonance imaging data.

**SEE ALSO:** Amyotrophic Lateral Sclerosis; China; Italy.

**BIBLIOGRAPHY.** ALS Association, "Clinical Update, Stem Cell Treatments in China," www.alsa.org (cited October 2004); ALS Therapy Development Institute, "Clinical Trials," www.als.net (cited November 2007); Lucie Bruijn, "A Primer on Stem Cells," ALS Association Web site, www.alsa.org (cited November 2007); Letizia Mazzini, et al., "Stem Cell Treatment in Amyotrophic Lateral Sclerosis," *Journal of the Neurological Sciences* (v.265/1, 2008).

Masatoshi Suzuki
University of Wisconsin, Madison

# Clinical Trials Outside U.S.: Avascular Necrosis

**AVASCULAR NECROSIS (AVN),** or osteonecrosis, is a painful condition in which bone tissue dies as a result of ischemic injury and is unable to regenerate itself. The head of the femur is affected in 90 percent of patients and is caused most commonly by traumatic hip injury but can also result from alcoholism, excess steroid use, vasculitides or coagulopathies, Caisson disease, iatrogenic injury during hip surgery, radiation exposure, and sickle cell disease. In children, AVN of the femoral head can result from Legg-Calvé-Perthes disease, slipped capital femoral epiphysis (SCFE), and congenital hip dysplasia. Other sites of avascular necrosis include the humerus of the upper arm, femoral condyles of the knee, scaphoid and lunate bones of the wrist, calcaneus and navicular bones of the foot, and the jaw.

AVN mostly occurs in adults age 25 to 50 and in younger children, and it is more common in males than females (ratio 8:1). Up to 20,000 new patients are diagnosed with AVN each year in the United States, and thousands more go unrecognized worldwide. The femoral head eventually collapses if left untreated, leading to joint instability and arthritis that require total hip replacement. At present, there are no drugs for the definitive prevention or treatment of osteonecrosis, and current therapies have limited efficacy. The development of effective treatments has been problematic because three distinct tissues are involved in AVN: bone, bone marrow, and blood vessels.

However, researchers worldwide have recently started to explore stem cell therapy as a therapeutic approach to regenerating all of these tissue types. Histostem, a Korean company, was the first to treat AVN of the femoral head and various other disorders using umbilical cord stem cells, and this group has branched out to India and other nations for further research. Orthopaedic researchers in Taiwan have recently used mesenchymal stem cells in bone marrow to restore damaged blood vessels in AVN. Aastrom, an American company, has also started a clinical trial in Spain to determine whether its patented bone tissue repair cells can treat AVN.

The trials presented here are a testament to the potential for stem cell therapy to treat previously incurable diseases such as avascular necrosis. New directions in the treatment of AVN will continue to evolve; however, it is important to continually evaluate and retain proper ethical standards for stem cell research.

## RESEARCH

The Korean biotechnology company Histostem is pioneering human stem cell–based therapies in the treatment of presently incurable diseases such as liver cirrhosis, spinal cord injury, multiple sclerosis, type 1 and 2 diabetes, Buerger disease, and femoral head avascular necrosis. This Seoul-based research group patented a technique for isolating and culturing stem cells from umbilical cord blood in 2000 and rapidly became the world's largest cord blood bank as of 2004. Researchers were able to differentiate the stem cells into osteoblast (bone) and chondrocyte (cartilage) lines, and these cells can be used for transplantation into adult patients to attempt to treat various musculoskeletal pathologies. Researchers have also collaborated with Peking University in China to study stem cell therapy in blood vessel disorders. In 2005 the Korean researchers succeeded in treating several patients with AVN and other blood vessel diseases, using stem cell therapy. In this 74-patient trial, which examined AVN, nonunion bone fracture, Buerger disease, and cerebral infarction, seven of 11 patients (64 percent) with femoral head AVN showed significant improvement without any adverse effects. Success rates also ranged from 60 to 94 percent for the other disorders.

Histostem has recently announced plans to establish four umbilical cord blood banks in India and also branched out to Indian research institutions in Chandigarh in 2007 to pursue stem cell research and future trials for AVN and other disorders. A national stem cell bank hub and cell therapy center will likely be launched within the next five years in Mumbai, pending ethical considerations by the Ministry of Health and private contributions from Reliance Life Science and Histostem.

Researchers in Taiwan at the Taipei Veterans General Hospital Department of Orthopaedics also reported promising results for stem cell therapy for AVN in September 2007. They used mesenchymal stem cells from bone marrow, which have been shown to restore damaged blood vessels and potentially treat stroke, myocardial infarction, and avascular necrosis. Mesenchymal stem cells can overcome oxygen deprivation by producing factors that prevent apoptotic cell death and promote new blood vessel formation. Therefore, the researchers proposed that endothelial cell regeneration would occur; they confirmed this in an animal model. This research was completed in collaboration with Tulane University in Louisiana and published in *Stem Cells* journal in late 2007.

Aastrom Biosciences, a Michigan-based company studying the use of autologous stem cells for cellular regeneration, recently began a clinical trial for femoral head osteonecrosis at the Centro Medico Teknon in Barcelona, Spain. In January 2007, the first two patients in a cohort of 10 subjects were treated with Aastrom's patented Tissue/Bone Repair Cells (BRCs). BRCs are unique mixtures of stem cells and progenitor cells derived from the patient's own bone marrow that have been shown to regenerate all three tissue types involved in AVN: bone, bone marrow, and blood vessels. BRCs have shown promising initial results in the treatment of atrophic nonunion fractures in long bones, spinal fusion, and vascular regeneration. Therefore, a trial for the treatment of avascular necrosis is also underway. The therapeutic approach will involve necrotic tissue removal from the femoral head, followed by BRC implantation into the area. The goal of this treatment is to delay or eliminate AVN progression and the need for total hip replacement in patients. Although the results from this 24-month clinical trial are currently pending, successful outcomes may eventually influence stem cell research decisions made by government authorities internationally.

A variety of approaches to treating avascular necrosis using stem cell therapies are currently being evaluated and are beginning to show promising results. As there are currently no definitive pharmaceutical treatments for AVN, stem cells could begin to provide a novel therapeutic modality for this previously incurable disease. It is important to note that the aforementioned clinical trials have been established only recently. Therefore, any forward-looking statements may or may not be confirmed by the results of these studies, and readers must be careful about preemptively making broad conclusions from the paucity of current data regarding AVN stem cell research. It is equally important to constantly assess and uphold appropriate ethical standards while stem cell research and medical knowledge progresses during the 21st century.

**SEE ALSO:** Aastrom Biosciences, Inc.; Bone Diseases.

**BIBLIOGRAPHY.** Aastrom Biosciences, www.aastrom.com (cited November 2007); "National Institute of Arthritis and Musculoskeletal and Skin Diseases: Osteonecrosis," www.niams.nih.gov (cited November 2007).

Anjan P. Kaushik
University of Virginia School of Medicine

# Clinical Trials Outside U.S.: Severe Coronary Artery Disease

**SEVERAL CLINICAL TRIALS** targeting heart disease have shown that adult stem cell therapy is safe and effective. Adult stem cell therapy for heart disease is commercially available on at least five continents at last count. The most well known of these companies is TheraVitae, a private company based in Bangkok, Thailand, with locations in Kiryat Weizmann, Israel; Toronto, Canada; Singapore; Taipei, Taiwan; and Hong Kong. TheraVitae is a private, multinational company focused on using stem cells from the patient's own blood in order to treat a variety of disorders, especially cardiovascular diseases. Research, development, and manufacturing are performed at the company's state-of-the-art cell therapy facility located in Kiryat Weizmann. TheraVitae's plans treatments for optical and neurological diseases in the future.

The company has already developed a proprietary stem cell technology, VesCell, that is currently being used by hospitals in Thailand to treat patients with heart disease. VesCell uses a special process that differentiates the stem cells so that they can build additional blood flow to and from the heart by creating new blood vessels and new heart muscle. While VesCell stem cell treatment may not cure heart disease, it can substantially improve the flow of blood, thus reducing chest pains and sharply increasing physical capacity More than 250 heart patients have traveled to Thailand to receive TheraVitae's adult stem cell therapy. TheraVitae reports that 75 percent of their heart patients have an improved quality of life after receiving adult stem cell treatment. The worldwide results (over 2,000 treated) are similar despite many different types of adult stem cells being implanted into very sick heart patients by doctors in over two dozen countries.

TheraVitae is conducting a clinical trial to study the safety and efficacy of the administration of endothelial progenitor cells to patients with severe angina pectoris. The study, conducted at Siriraj Hospital, the largest hospital in Bangkok, Thailand, will assess the treatment in 24 patients with severe chronic angina who meet certain inclusion and exclusion criteria. Associate Professor Damras Tresukosol of the Cardiac Center at the Siriraj Hospital is the principal investigator in the study. This trial will determine the efficacy and safety of a new heart treatment option for Thais who have severe anginal symptoms despite undergoing another revascularization therapy.

Endothelial progenitor cells, EPCs, are stem cells harvested from the patient's own blood that have the capability to form new blood vessels, or angiogenesis. EPCs are found in the bloodstream, but in a very low concentration. TheraVitae has developed proprietary technologies to harvest, expand and differentiate EPCs to an amount sufficient to induce angiogenesis in the heart. The cells are processed outside the body and then injected into the patient during standard angiography to regions of the heart suffering from reduced blood supply. Injection of EPCs in cardiac patients has proven to increase blood supply to the heart muscle and reduce symptoms of angina in several trials in the United States and Europe.

The potential success of these trials would mean that heart patients would now have another treatment option other than coronary bypass surgery. Furthermore, treating these patients with cell therapy is potentially safer, for the procedure is similar to a cardiac catheterization that is routinely performed to examine a patient's heart function and blood supply. Moreover, employing autologous EPCs (cells taken from the patient himself/herself) eliminates concerns of tissue rejection.

Using the patient's own bone marrow–derived stem cells, Dr. Amit Patel at the University of Pittsburgh's McGowan Institute of Regenerative Medicine has shown a dramatic increase in ejection fraction for patients with congestive heart failure. He has worked with many other countries such as Argentina, Uruguay, Ecuador, Greece, Japan, and Thailand, where he has taught minimally invasive techniques to companies like TheraVitae for the treatment of nonischemic (idiopathic) and ischemic heart failure. A Brazilian stem cell bank has also performed sample manipulation in more than 30 cell therapy procedures in cardiac patients.

**SEE ALSO:** Cells, Adult; Heart; Heart Attack.

**BIBLIOGRAPHY.** Clinicaltrials.gov, clinicaltrials.gov (cited April 2008); Stem Cell News, www.stemnews.com (cited April 2008); Vescell, www.vescell.com (cited April 2008).

Fernando Herrera
University of California, San Diego

# Clinical Trials Outside U.S.: Spinal Cord Injury

**THE CENTRAL NERVOUS** system, which includes the spinal cord, is abundant with factors that inhibit outgrowth and therefore regeneration of nerves. Thus, spinal cord injury has limited therapeutic options. Numerous clinical trials around the globe are carried out to find the way to induce nerve regeneration after spinal cord injury and therefore at least partially restore sensory and / or motor function to the injury patient. As of current knowledge, there is not a way of stimulating regeneration in the spinal cord and thus restoring sensory and motor function in people with spinal cord injuries, but researchers are working to gain a better understanding of the impeding factors and thus a way around them.

Recently, an international society was established to improve the prognosis for spinal cord injury (SCI) patients by discovering effective treatment measures in a safe but quick manner. This society is the International Campaign for Cures of spinal cord injury paralysis (ICCP). At a meeting in the year 2004 held in Vancouver, Canada, the ICCP established standards for clinical trials in terms of factors such as trial prerequisites, protocol design, and patient management.

Setting standards for protocol design ensures that the proper controls are always considered. In order to do a thorough clinical trial that truly carries out the intended investigation, the clinicians must carefully select participants such that these participants do not bring in outside, confounding factors. Additionally, control trials must parallel the clinical trial, in order to show a baseline against which to compare the trial results. These concepts seem simple but they become compli-

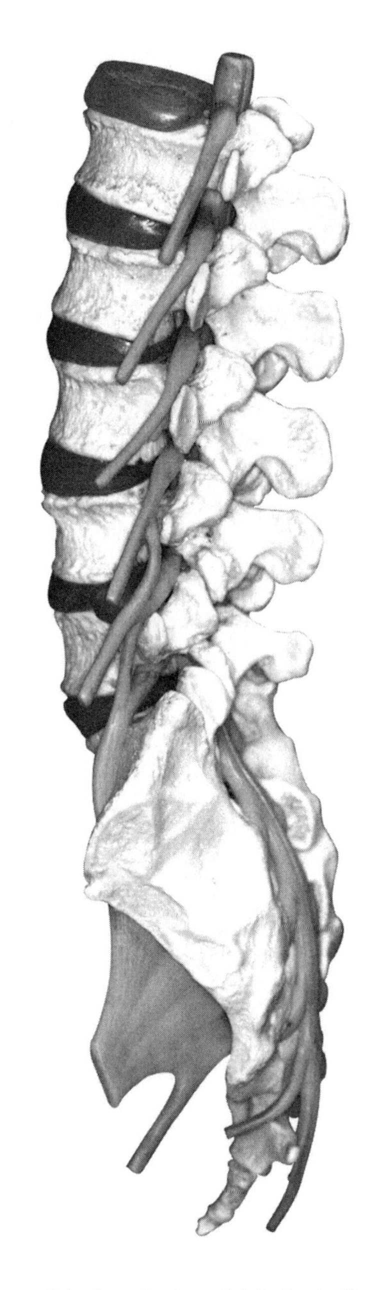

*An anatomy model of a spinal cord. Injuries to the spinal cord have limited therapeutic options.*

cated in intricate trials. Having standard rules for designing controls and proper protocols is facilitative to researchers looking to design clinical trials for SCI recovery, as well as to the clinicians and patients who need to understand the results.

Importantly, there must be an agreed upon threshold for improvement that is accepted by clinicians as proving a method for therapeutics. This threshold is equally important as one below which improvement is not seen and the techniques under trial are not considered effective. For example, a study carried out in Brazil attempted to transplant the sural nerve (a peripheral nerve from the lower leg) into SCI patients to serve as a neural bridge across a region of the spinal cord that had been severed by a gunshot injury. The technique was found to be ineffective. Although it is important to find a technique that improves the status of a SCI patient, it is also important to know what does not work, in order to gain a more thorough understanding of the physiology of a SCI.

Another study carried out in China showed that transplanting olfactory bulb cells into SCI sites showed moderate improvement in their condition. The olfactory bulb is a site in the brain with neurogenesis throughout life. In this case, the neurons were taken from fetuses and expanded in culture. The problem with this study is that there were no controls. Therefore, the "improvement" reported is not truly compared to anything except pre-trial condition, and it cannot be known what actually caused the improvement. However unlikely, it may have been merely a placebo effect. This study was carried out before the ICCP meeting. An additional concern in international clinical trials is regulation. When laboratories from multiple countries collaborate, government regulation of the studies becomes complicated for trial participants.

**SEE ALSO:** Brazil; China; Christopher Reeve Foundation; Regulations Overview; Spinal Cord Injury.

**BIBLIOGRAPHY.** D. Brunier and G. Nahler, *International Clinical Trials* (Informa Healthcare, 1999); L. M. Friedman, C. D. Furberg, and D. L. DeMets, *Fundamentals of Clinical Trials* (Springer, 1999); S. A. Sisto, E. Druin, and M. M. Sliwinski, *Spinal Cord Injuries* (Mosby, 2008); J. Steeves, J. Fawcett, and M. Tuszynski, "Report of International Clinical Trials Workshop on Spinal Cord Injury February 20–21, 2004, Vancouver, Canada," *Spinal Cord* (August 2004).

Claudia Winograd
University of Illinois, Urbana-Champaign

# Clinical Trials Within U.S.: Batten Disease

**BATTEN DISEASE IS** an inherited disorder of the nervous system that begins in childhood. Children with Batten disease suffer seizures and progressive loss of motor skills, sight, and mental capacity, eventually becoming blind, bedridden, and unable to communicate. Batten disease is often fatal by the late teens or 20s. As yet, no specific treatment is known that can halt or reverse the symptoms of Batten disease. However, seizures can sometimes be reduced or controlled with anticonvulsant drugs, and other medical problems can be treated appropriately as they arise. Physical therapy and occupational therapy also may help patients retain functioning as long as possible.

Recently, a company (StemCells, Inc. of Palo Alto, California) has initiated a phase 1 clinical trial to investigate the safety and preliminary efficacy of fetal stem cell transplantation into patients with Batten disease. It is believed to be the first-ever transplant of fetal stem cells into a human brain.

## BATTEN DISEASE

Batten disease is named after the British pediatrician Frederick Batten, who first described the condition in 1903. This disease is the most common form of a group of disorders called neuronal ceroid lipofuscinosis, which are lysosomal storage disorders brought on by inherited genetic mutations in genes that provide cells with normally secreted housekeeping lysosomal enzymes. Lack of these enzymes causes a buildup of lipofuscin (aggregates of lipids and proteins) that leads to neuronal cell loss, primarily in the brain. Some physicians use the term Batten disease to describe all forms of neuronal ceroid lipofuscinosis, initially classified by age of onset (infantile, late infantile, and juvenile) and now more precisely classified in terms of the specific enzyme deficiencies causing the disease.

The disease is inherited in an autosomal recessive manner. Six genes have now been identified that cause different types of Batten disease in children or adults; more have yet to be identified. Two genes are related to two subtypes of neuronal ceroid lipofuscinosis: infantile and late infantile. These genes are CLN1, which codes for the enzyme palmityl-protein thioesterase 1 (PPT1), and CLN2, which codes for the enzyme tripeptidyl peptidase I (TPP-I). The consequence of these gene mutations is either a defective or missing enzyme that leads to accumulation of lipofuscin-like fluorescent inclusions in various cell types. The diagnosis of Batten disease is based on the presence of these deposits in skin samples as well as other criteria.

Early symptoms of this disorder usually appear at age 4–10 years, with gradual onset of vision problems, including eye discoloration causing a milky fog gloss over the eyes, or seizures. Because vision loss is often an early sign of the condition, Batten disease may be first suspected during an eye exam. Often, an eye specialist or other physician may refer the child to a neurologist. Diagnostic tests for Batten disease include blood or urine tests, skin or tissue sampling, an electroencephalogram, electrical studies of the eyes, and brain scans.

Early signs may be subtle personality and behavior changes, slow learning or regression, repetitive speech or echolalia, clumsiness, or stumbling. There may be slowing head growth in the infantile form, poor circulation in lower extremities (legs and feet), decreased body fat and muscle mass, curvature of the spine, hyperventilation or breath-holding spells, teeth grinding, and constipation. Over time, affected children suffer mental impairment, worsening seizures, and progressive loss of sight, speech, and motor skills. Eventually, children with Batten disease become blind, bedridden, and demented. Batten disease is often fatal by age 8–15 years.

Symptoms of Batten disease are linked to a buildup of lipofuscin in the body's tissues. Therefore, replacement of defective enzymes or genes is the objective of research into treatments for Batten disease and other lysosomal storage disorders. In June 2004, a phase 1 clinical trial was launched at Weill Medical College of Cornell University,

New York City, to study a gene therapy method for treatment of the signs and symptoms of late infantile neuronal ceroid lipofuscinosis.

## FIRST CLINICAL TRIAL OF HUMAN CENTRAL NERVOUS SYSTEM STEM CELLS

An alternative means of treating the disease is to provide the brain with a replacement source of a functional enzyme that can be taken up by the enzyme-deficient cells. In October 2005, the U.S. Food and Drug Administration approved a phase 1 clinical trial by StemCells, Inc. to transplant fetal neuronal cells into the brains of children suffering from the infantile and late-infantile versions of Batten disease.

The company's human neural stem cells (HuCNS-SC) are a cell therapy product consisting of neural cells prepared under controlled conditions. These cells are isolated from the human fetal brain and are immature and in an early stage of development. They are derived from aborted and miscarried fetuses, purified, expanded, and then stored and frozen in cell banks until they are transplanted. Preclinical data have shown that their neural stem cells survive transplantation, migrate to different regions of the brain, and become the specialized cells normally found in that region.

These human neural stem cells have also been shown to produce both the PPT1 and TPP-I enzymes. In preclinical models of PPT1 deficiency, the corresponding enzyme activity increases with time after transplantation. Thus, placement of human neural stem cells in appropriate places in the brain has the prospect of replacing missing enzymes. To avoid rejection of these foreign cells, the immune system of the patients has to be suppressed.

In November 2006, StemCells, Inc. initiated a phase 1 trial to investigate the safety and preliminary efficacy of their neural stem cells as a treatment of infantile and late-infantile Batten disease. The trial is an open-label study of two dose levels of the cells. The primary objective of the trial was to measure the safety of the company's stem cells. The trial has also evaluated HuCNS-SC's ability to affect the progression of the disease.

It is important to note that this was a safety trial with no blinded conditions, and results are not designed to show efficacy. In similar studies, the Tiantan Puhua Hospital Stem Cell Center in China announced that stem cells were successfully used in January 2008, with the hope of improving and potentially prolonging the life of a 6-year-old California boy. The child has shown improvements in motor skills and has become more active and alert. In another clinical trial, a 9-year-old girl died a year after receiving a brain transplant of neural stem cells. It was determined that her death was likely due to her disease.

The company began a clinical study with surgeons at Doernbecher Children's Hospital at Oregon Health & Science University, Portland, Oregon, in which purified neural stem cells were injected into the brain of a 6-year-old child suffering from Batten disease, who had lost the ability to walk and talk. The patient is expected to be the first of six individuals to receive an injection of a stem cell product from StemCells, Inc. This was believed to be the first-ever transplant of fetal stem cells into a human brain. By early December, the child had recovered well enough to return home, and it was reported that there were some signs of speech returning. The primary evaluation was at one year post–cell transplantation; patients have been asked to permit monitoring to be continued for at least a five-year period after transplantation.

This phase 1 clinical trial is being led by Robert D. Steiner, M.D., vice chairman of pediatric research and head of the Division of Metabolism at Doernbecher Children's Hospital, and professor of Pediatrics and Molecular and Medical Genetics at Oregon Health & Science University School of Medicine; Nathan Selden, M.D., Ph.D., Campagna Associate Professor of Pediatric Neurological Surgery and head of the Division of Pediatric Neurological Surgery, Doernbecher and Oregon Health & Science University School of Medicine; and Thomas K. Koch, M.D., director of pediatric neurology and professor of pediatrics and neurology at Doernbecher and Oregon Health & Science University School of Medicine.

**SEE ALSO:** Batten Disease; Oregon Health & Science University; StemCells, Inc.; Weill-Cornell Medical College.

**BIBLIOGRAPHY.** Kaspar Mossman, "The World's First Neural Stem Cell Transplant," *Scientific American* (December 2006); National Institution of Neurological Disorders and Stroke, "Batten Disease Information Page," www.ninds.nih.gov/disorders/batten/batten.htm (cited November 2007); National Institution of Neurological Disorders and Stroke, "Batten Disease Fact Sheet," www.ninds.nih.gov/disorders/batten/detail_batten.htm (cited November 2007); StemCells, Inc., www.stemcellsinc.com/index.htm (cited November 2007); Wikipedia, "Batten Disease," en.wikipedia.org/wiki/Batten_disease (cited November 2007).

Masatoshi Suzuki
University of Wisconsin, Madison

# Clinical Trials Within U.S.: Blind Process

**CLINICAL TRIALS ARE** scientific experiments designed to determine whether new procedures, drugs, or agents are beneficial to those human patients involved. Customarily, a blind process is used in which the new drug (or other treatment) is tested against a placebo, which is a harmless substitute of the same basic size and shape that will not provide any medical benefit. Patients selected to participate in the trial will be divided randomly into groups taking either the new treatment or the placebo. Only when the group not taking that placebo shows statistically significantly higher levels of outcome (however this is measured in medical terms) than the placebo-taking group can the trial be determined a success. This blind process is necessary because there is a clear incentive and a propensity for patients to report an improvement in their condition, or for carers to do so if the patient is unable to provide such a report.

Clinical trials customarily take place a considerable period of time after the initial creation and development of a new treatment, which will then proceed, depending on local legal conditions, to animal testing. This procedure is lengthy and is customarily processed with due regard to safety and scientific rigor. One important implication of this procedure is that pharmaceutical companies seeking to bring new drugs to market have generally had to sponsor many years, and even decades, of expensive research scientists and medical laboratories before new drugs can pass relevant legislative controls and be brought to the market. This makes new drugs expensive, as the costs are used not just for profits but also to cover the extensive period of testing and research that preceded entry to the market. In some countries, where undemocratic regimes are able to suppress public opinion, free speech, and the accountability of pharmaceutical companies to be responsible for the ill effects of their products, the cost of drugs and the speed with which they can be brought to market can be considerably reduced, albeit at a human cost that can be very high. In the United States, the prominence of the legal profession ensures that this form of behavior is prosecuted, if not prohibited.

The extent of national and international cooperation in medical research provides numerous opportunities for more rapid and broader-based solutions to be identified. Myeloma, for example, which is a blood cancer that occurs within the bone marrow, has been found to have promising new treatments resulting from clinical trials. Stem cell research has also provided material for clinical trials. A stream of research from the University of Texas Medical School at Houston, for example, has examined the possibility that children with brain injuries may find some relief from secondary effects by using stem cells from their own bone marrow tissue. This research has also provided some positive results.

The National Library of Medicine lists a large number of university schools and other institutions pursuing stem cell–involved clinical trials. Prospective patients may search for opportunities to participate in such trials online, and other online resources also provide advice and support for patients and their families and carers. Private-sector brokers also exist, aiming to connect would-be patients with suitable trial providers. As ever, care should be taken when determining whether such a service would be helpful in individual cases.

**SEE ALSO:** Bone Marrow Transplants; Cancer; Clinical Trials (Adult Cells); University of Texas Health Science Center at Houston.

**BIBLIOGRAPHY.** Roger Bertolotti, Keiya Ozawa, and Kirk H. Hammond, eds., *Progress in Gene Therapy: Pioneering Stem Cell/Gene Therapy Trials* (Brill Academic, 2004); Clinical Data Interchange Standards Consortium, www.cdisc.org (cited November 2007); Clinical Trials Registry, clinicaltrials.gov (cited November 2007); EurekAlert, "Clinical Trial to Test Stem Cell Approach for Children with Brain Injury," www.eurekalert.org (cited December 2005); National Library of Medicine, nlm.nih.gov (cited November 2007); Kim Waterman, "Clinical Trials Provide Hope for Bone Marrow Cancer Patients," *Medical News Today*, www.medicalnewstoday.com (cited November 2007).

John Walsh
Shinawatra International University

# Clinical Trials Within U.S.: Cancer

**STEM CELL RESEARCH** is playing an increasingly relevant role both in clinical and experimental oncology at the present time. On the one hand, the identification of cancer stem cells in different neoplasms noticeably modified general comprehension about cancer biology; on the other, the delivery of such growing knowledge from bench to bedside is starting to affect therapeutic choices in cancer treatment.

Bone marrow transplants (BMTs) were the first application of stem cells in cancer therapy. Available since 1956, and subsequently improved, this treatment is now considered a current therapeutic option for many hematological neoplasms, and much interest has been generated about the possibility of extending such procedures to solid tumors. BMT is more commonly performed as a hematopoietic stem cell transplant (HSCT), in which the infusion of HSCs previously harvested through a conditioning therapy (high-dose chemoradiotherapy) can entirely rebuild the marrow in 10–20 days. Although the traditional HSCT needs a complete myeloablation, which means that the host's marrow is completely destroyed before the infusion of the donor's HSCs, nonmyeloablative or reduced-intensity transplants require less intense conditioning regimens, which are employed just to suppress the patient's immune response so that the donor's HSC can efficiently engraft. A large amount of clinical data prove HSCT to be an effective treatment in leukemia and other hematological malignancies: With more than 200,000 transplants performed worldwide, HSCT is an advisable treatment in patients with acute myeloid leukemia who achieved a first complete remission, in patients with acute lymphoblastic leukemia obtaining a poor response to chemotherapy, and also in patients suffering from chronic lymphocytic leukemia, some high-risk lymphomas, and myelodysplastic syndromes.

Initially employed for solid tumor therapy as autografts or allografts with rescue purposes, and aiming to overcome myelotoxicity caused by the high-dose antineoplastic treatment, HSCT was demonstrated afterward to be directly responsible for an observed antitumor effect in the allograft setting. Allogeneic HSCT has in fact been proven to be a resourceful sort of immunotherapy both in myeloablative and in nonmyeloablative transplants: an antitumor immune response mediated by the graft, defined as graft versus leukemia or graft versus tumor (GVT), has been respectively demonstrated in a hematological and a solid cancer context.

The relatively high transplant-related mortality and a more complicated patient management compared with the standard treatments contributed to the scarce diffusion of such therapeutic options in the past, but the recent introduction of nonmyeloablative protocols increased interest in this treatment, as it demonstrated many fewer risks. In the recent past, many clinical trials in and outside the United States tested allogeneic HSCT as immunotherapy for solid tumors; renal cell carcinoma, breast cancer, ovarian cancer, and testicular germ cell tumors have been the most investigated.

Regarding renal cell carcinoma, in 2000, Childs and colleagues first observed a tumor regression in 10 of 19 patients treated with nonmyeloablative HSCT (53 percent)—a result that was confirmed by a 2002 update, with a 48 percent response rate. In 2005 Artz and colleagues from the University of Chicago published a review including 14 studies and 163 patients, reporting an overall response rate of 24 percent. Many phase 1–2 clinical trials are currently ongoing within the United States; some are testing the feasibility, the safety, and the efficacy of the procedure, and in many others, HSCT is combined with other forms of adoptive immunotherapy such as donor lymphocyte infusion to evaluate whether such additional treatments have an effect on HSCT efficacy.

At this time, nonmyeloablative HSCT is mainly practiced in metastatic cytokine refractory or recurrent kidney cancers. Some cases of interferon or interleukin 2 sensitization in previously refractory cancers have been described after HSCT. Randomized phase 3 trials are needed to compare HSCT with standard therapies; the European ITAC group is currently testing this hypothesis.

## BREAST CANCER

A GVT effect has also been demonstrated for breast cancer. Ueno and colleagues from the M. D. Anderson Cancer Center performed two clinical trials in the 1990s. In the first one, 16 patients suffering from metastatic breast cancer were treated with standard myeloablative HSCT, with one complete response, five partial responses, and eight stable diseases; in the second study, three of eight metastatic breast cancer patients achieved a response after receiving a reduced-intensity HSCT. A patient series published in 2003 by Bishop from the National Cancer Institute identified five partial and three minor responses from 16 metastatic breast cancer patients who had been treated with reduced-intensity allograft and donor T-lymphocyte infusion.

Because metastatic breast cancer is not considered a curable disease, a reasonable encouragement in involving HSCT in the clinical arena induced researchers to evaluate this treatment, together with other options such as trastuzumab, angiogenesis inhibitors, lymphocyte infusions, and vaccines. A wide range of phase 1–2 trials are now recruiting patients all over the United States; in 2004, Bishop started a new trial evaluating a new HSCT protocol, including a T-cell depleted SCT followed by donor lymphocyte infusion, with the aim of reducing transplant-related toxicity, mainly connected to graft-versus-host disease, and increasing treatment efficacy.

To compare HSCT efficacy with standard treatment, a phase 3 randomized clinical trial issued by Bensinger is currently ongoing at Fred Hutchinson Cancer Center. Begun in 1998, this study is comparing chemotherapy alone (busulphan, melphalan, and thiotepa) with chemotherapy plus myeloablative HSCT. A clear, evidence-based evaluation of HSCT role in metastatic breast cancer will be achieved only with further, carefully designed clinical trials. To date, HSCT for breast cancer should be recommended only in pilot studies, performed in highly specialized centers.

## OTHER TUMORS

Good results have been obtained in advanced germ cell tumors, where—notwithstanding the high cure rates provided by platinum-based chemotherapy—10–20 percent of the patients do not achieve a durable complete response, which necessitates a second-line treatment. Myeloablative HSCT is being employed with progressively declining side effects, taking advantage of the high-dose chemotherapy over a greatly chemosensitive tumor. Other tumors have been evaluated as possible candidates for HSCT. In some cases, responses were anecdotal, as in prostate, ovarian, colorectal, pancreatic, and lung cancer, that were mainly documented by single case reports or small series of patients. Given this background, the future role of HSCT depends on the results obtained by the ongoing clinical trials as well as by a better knowledge of tumor immunology. On the one hand, an improved control of toxicity and mortality should be achieved to make the risk/benefit ratio more acceptable for the patient. On the other hand, GVT-effect enhancement studies have proven that tumor cell eradication can be modulated in various ways, such as interleukin or lymphocyte infusion, with promisingly helpful reflections for allo-SCT in cancer therapy.

In addition to the previously reported employment of allo-HSCT, the possibility of genetically modifying HSCs to use them as vehicles of gene transfer is stirring up new interest in HSCT. HSCs can, in fact, be modified with a drug resistance gene to protect grafted marrow from the toxic effects of chemotherapy, therefore allowing clinicians to increase antineoplastic drug doses. Different clinical studies performed on humans demonstrated an efficient retrovirus-mediated transfer of the MDR-1 gene, codifying for p-glycoprotein—an efflux pump that prevents drugs from accumulating within the cells. Hanania, from the M. D. Anderson Cancer Center and Abonour, from the Indiana University School of Medicine, documented in two independent studies an efficient transfer among different groups of patients (breast, ovarian, testicular cancer).

Although confirming the feasibility of this approach, these data contemporaneously figure out many important issues, which actually thwart a direct clinical application of such a procedure. In fact, only 10–50 percent of the grafted cell successfully expressed MDR-1 gene at one month, showing that much still needs to be solved to prevent a transient or incomplete gene transfer. Another possible application of gene-modified HSCT is the transduction of chimeric receptor genes obtained by elaborating and combining variable sequences from the T-cell receptor and immunoglobulin receptors. These surface molecules, whose genes are transferred to the HSCs, can recognize selected antigens just like their ordinary counterparts, which are expressed by the immune system cells. In this way, HSCs can proliferate after the transplant procedure, forming a stable progeny of myeloid and lymphoid cells, which can efficiently identify and kill cancer cells in a non–major histocompatibility complex–restricted way.

## MESENCHYMAL STEM CELLS AND CANCER GENE THERAPY

Mesenchymal stem cells (MSCs) are multipotent cells that can be easily isolated from a bone marrow aspirate and expanded in vitro. Given the MSCs' property of fostering tumor stroma, migrating directly to the tumor site, and differentiating into vascular and other support cells, several investigators successfully exploited this mechanism to target delivery of agents to cancer cells.

Even though this approach is still limited to preclinical data, some encouraging results come from different U.S. studies, such as the work published by Studeny and colleagues from the M. D. Anderson Cancer Center. Genetically engineered MSCs, bearing the interferon-beta gene, were efficiently integrated within the tumor mass, determining an interferon-mediated anticancer effect in mice. Many other studies have been published with a similar rationale, but to date, none of these has been proposed for a clinical assessment yet.

## CANCER STEM CELL TARGETING

Over the last 20 years, a great paradox emerged in clinical oncology: Improving therapies do not necessarily reflect an enhanced patient survival. The identification of cancer stem cells (CSCs), a rare population of undifferentiated cells that are supposed to sustain tumor growth and recurrence, provided the explanation of such phenomena and forced the researchers to globally rethink cancer therapy. CSCs have been identified in the majority of tumors, and great efforts have been addressed to characterizing these cells from a molecular point of view to have knowledge of their metabolism and their surface markers and to exploit such knowledge for diagnostic and therapeutic purposes.

Different strategies have been hypothesized to target anticancer therapy specifically to the stem cell compartment: Stem cells can undergo elimination or differentiation. CSC elimination may be obtained in many ways: suppression of stem cell–specific signaling pathways and sensitization toward chemotherapy, but also a GVT effect induction, as described before. A stem cell–targeted therapy could be a promising approach.

Despite the fact that many aspects of CSC biology are still unknown, different key points in the cancer stem cell cycle have been identified. Molecules such as PTEN, Wnt, Notch, and Hedgehog play a relevant role in self renewal and could represent potential candidates for a selective stem cell elimination therapy. The importance of these mediators has been proven in different preclinical studies; for example, cyclopamine, a vegetal alkaloid, behaved as an efficient hedgehog inhibitor, demonstrating a valuable antineoplastic effect in mice.

Even though anti-CSC drug development is in its infancy, some compounds succeeded to cross through the preclinical phase and are currently being studied in humans. SL-401, for instance, is a recombinant protein, designed by Stemline Therapeutics, that binds to the interleukin 3 receptor—a surface protein that is overexpressed in various cancers, and especially in leukemic stem cells. Once SL-401 binds to the receptor, an attached toxin penetrates into the cell, killing it. Its antitumor properties have been tested during a phase 1 trial on 30 patients with acute myelogenous leukemia; the lack of evident toxicity and the achievement of one complete and many partial responses encouraged further investigation.

Another way of targeting CSCs could be GRN163L, a telomerase inhibitor developed by Geron that is currently undergoing a multicenter phase 1 trial within the United States. Because the CSCs' relevance in cancer therapy relies on their sustained replicative potential, which continuously supplies the tumor burden, promoting CSC differentiation would induce a reduction of tumor load. On this basis, a differentiating role has been claimed for histone deacetylase inhibitors, a novel group of drugs that interfere with the transcriptional activity of their target cells. More than 50 registered studies are testing suberoylanilide hydroxamic acid for various cancers within the United States. Independent from the strategy involved, CSC-oriented therapy is hopefully expected to modify the natural history of cancer—preventing tumor relapse and enhancing survival will be its main landmarks.

**SEE ALSO:** Cancer; Clinical Trials Within U.S.: Blind Process.

**BIBLIOGRAPHY.** C. Massard, E. Deutsch, and J. C. Soria "Tumor Stem Cell-Targeted Treatment: Elimination or Differentiation," *Annals of Oncology* (v.17, 2006); Olle Ringdén and Katarina Le Blanc, "Allogeneic Hematopoietic Stem Cell Transplantation: State of the Art and New Perspectives," *Acta Pathologica, Microbiologica et Immunologica Scandinavica* (v.113, 2005); Carol Tang, et al., "Cancer Stem Cell: Target for Anti-Cancer Therapy," *FASEB Journal* (v.21, 2007).

David James Pinato
Eastern Piedmont University
School of Medicine

## Clinical Trials Within U.S.: Heart Disease

**CARDIOVASCULAR DISEASE IS** the number one cause of death in the United States. Cell therapy is being investigated at a rapid pace worldwide and may revolutionize contemporary cardiovascular disease treatment. Progress in this field is fueled by promising results in animal studies and a societal push for effective and potentially curative therapy. Stem cells can differentiate into nearly any mature cell phenotype and can self-renew indefinitely. Adult-derived "progenitor" cells have limited differentiation capability and cannot self-renew; however, these cells are more readily accessible and are not subject to moral/ethical debate. Bone marrow and peripheral blood circulating progenitor cells have been the focus of current human trials. Future trials will explore the therapeutic potential of other adult progenitor cell sources.

Initial emphasis on cell transfer to replace myocardium has recently shifted to paracrine modulation of myocardial remodeling, mechanical strengthening of scar tissue, and promotion of tissue survival. Human trials have demonstrated feasibility of a variety of cell-based approaches with modest short-term benefits. Cells from autologous (one's own self) and allogeneic (from donors) sources have been transplanted in patients with heart disease, using a variety of delivery approaches. Safety has been confirmed in nearly all cardiovascular cell therapy trials; however, important questions such as optimal cell type, dose, delivery method, and patient type remain.

Three clinical syndromes are principal targets for cell therapy approaches: myocardial infarction (MI), chronic myocardial ischemia, and cardiomyopathy. Considerable overlap exists in the clinical presentation and pathophysiology of these syndromes; however, categorizing in this way is useful to demonstrate the rationale and study design of clinical trials. Cell therapy attempts to prevent heart enlargement following MI, develop new blood vessels and increase blood flow for chronic myocardial ischemia, and regenerate contractile heart muscle for cardiomyopathy causing heart failure.

Mechanisms underlying the benefits of progenitor cells observed in animal studies remain poorly understood. Transplanted cells may encourage the release of factors that locally activate adjacent native cells with beneficial effects. A few investigators suggest that cells "fuse" with native cells and thereby alter their behavior in some beneficial way. Others suggest that transplanted progenitor cells transdifferentiate and that the daughter cells become the cells of the target organ, such as heart muscle cells or blood vessels. Fusion and differentiation events are perhaps too rare to have meaningful treatment effect.

Several adult progenitor cell types have been studied, and many are identified by cell surface antigens measured by flow cytometry. CD34+ cells and CD133+ cells identify endothelial progenitors and may be isolated from bone marrow, adipose tissue, peripheral blood, and umbilical cord. These cells may promote new blood vessel growth in areas of ischemia. Mesenchymal stromal cells (MSCs) may induce a therapeutic effect via paracrine mechanisms. Skeletal myoblasts represent an abundant autologous source of cells that show a contractile phenotype when transplanted into the myocardium. In addition, resident cardiac stem cells have been discovered to reside in protected niches in the heart. Early-phase clinical trials using skeletal myoblast and resident cardiac stem cell transfer following ex vivo expansion are ongoing.

## MYOCARDIAL INFARCTION

MI occurs in nearly 1 million patients annually in the United States, with a mortality of approximately 25 percent over three years. A proportion of these patients will develop adverse remodeling, leading to congestive heart failure and sudden death. Cellular therapy offers the potential to improve these outcomes.

Strauer et al. first reported therapeutic cell transfer of unfractionated bone marrow mononuclear cells in 10 patients. The method used was to perform a large-volume bone marrow aspirate and then reinfuse the cells directly into the infarct-related coronary artery, using the catheters that are familiar to interventional cardiologists. Bone marrow mononuclear cells were aspirated five to nine days following emergent coronary stenting for acute MI. After overnight storage, cells were infused into the open infarct-related artery via a coronary balloon catheter. The balloon was inflated during infusion to prevent backflow of cells. At three months, infarct size decreased, wall movement increased, and cardiac perfusion was improved compared with a parallel control group. Fernandez-Aviles et al. reported improved six-month regional and global left ventricular function with cardiac magnetic resonance imaging at six months in 20 patients, using a similar cell source and delivery approach.

Following these initial results, several major trials in cellular therapy for recent MI patients have been performed. The Transplantation of Progenitor Cells and Regeneration Enhancement in Acute MI trial compared intracoronary infusion of circulating peripheral blood mononuclear cells (29 patients) compared with blood mononuclear cells (BMNCs; 30 patients). Similar functional and viability improvements were in seen in both groups, and both showed improvements over control patients. The Bone Marrow Transfer to Enhance ST-Elevation Infarct Regeneration was the first randomized control trial to compare intracoronary infusion of BMNCs (30 patients) against placebo (30 patients). At six months, cardiac ejection fraction improved in the BM-treated patients; however, this benefit was not sustained at one year. Janssens et al. reported results from a double-blind, randomized controlled trial of intracoronary infusion BMNCs. At four months, the infarct size was reduced; however, there was no significant improvement of ejection fraction, myocardial flow, or metabolism in infarcted segments, determined using highly sensitive imaging techniques such as magnetic resonance imaging.

The Autologous Stem Cell Transplantation in Acute MI trial was a double-blind, randomized trial of intracoronary BMNC infusion with 50 patients in treated and control groups. No improvement in infarct area, size, or function with intracoronary BM cell therapy was observed at six months. The Reinfusion of Enriched Progenitor Cells and Infarct Remodeling in Acute MI trial was also a double-blind, randomized trial of nearly 100 patients per group of BMNC injected via the intracoronary route versus the control group. The BMNC-treated group had a significant 2.5 percent increase in left ventricular ejection fraction at four months, assessed by cine ventriculography. Furthermore, the treatment group had a reduction in major cardiovascular adverse events at one year. The Myocardial Regeneration and Angiogenesis in MI with GCSF (granulocyte colony-stimulating factor) and Intracoronary Stem Cell Infusion study randomly assigned 27 patients to GCSF mobilized peripheral blood mononuclear cell infusion compared with GCSF alone compared with placebo following emergency stenting for MI. The treated group showed improved myocardial function and perfusion.

Cytokine therapy with GCSF is effective for mobilization of BM-derived progenitors into the peripheral circulation. Early clinical studies suggested that GCSF therapy after MI reduces ventricular remodeling and improves ejection fraction. However, recent larger and randomized controlled trials failed to demonstrate benefit with GCSF administered to post-MI patients. A similar neutral effect was observed in patients with chronic ischemia and refractory angina. With the evidence available, it appears that cytokine mobilization alone is not effective treatment for cardiovascular disease.

Investigators are now focusing on transplanting bone marrow cell subpopulations, in part because of the modest performance of unfractionated cell products. Notable among these products are endothelial progenitor cells, MSCs, and cardiac stem cells. For example, Bartunek et al. administered bone marrow–derived CD133+ endothelial progenitor cells via an intracoronary route post MI. At four months, there was a significant increase in ejection fraction and fractional shortening with ventriculography. There was a significant decrease in perfusion abnormalities. Chen et al. randomly assigned 69 patients having postprimary angioplasty for MI to undergo intracoronary MSC compared to saline at 18 days post-MI. Significant improvements in infarct size, ventricular volumes, and ejection fraction at six months were reported.

## CHRONIC MYOCARDIAL ISCHEMIA

Clinical cell therapy information for chronic myocardial ischemia stems from small-scale, nonrandomized, uncontrolled trials. A few trials have tested direct injection of endothelial progenitor cells during concomitant surgical revascularization. Catheter-based endomyocardial delivery of bone marrow–derived cells has also been tested. Overall, these small-scale studies have demonstrated reduced angina frequency, improved functional capacity, and reduced ischemic burden with cell therapy.

Losordo et al. demonstrated the feasibility, safety, and bioactivity of autologous CD34+ endothelial progenitor cell transplantation in a phase 1/2a clinical trial. Twenty-four patients were enrolled into this randomized, double-blind, placebo-controlled dose-escalating study with refractory, severe angina; these patients also were no longer candidates for mechanical revascularization. Cells were harvested by apheresis following cytokine mobilization. Unfractionated mononuclear cells were enriched for CD34+. Cells were readministered into the cardiac muscle via a catheter-needle device guided by an electro-anatomic mapping system. Ischemic areas determined by single-photon emission computed tomography (SPECT) were targets for cell delivery. There were no serious adverse events apart from one episode of ventricular tachycardia in the placebo group, which was successfully cardioverted. Angina frequency was similar at baseline between cell-treated and placebo groups. There was a significant reduction in angina frequency at three months; 27.0 ± 23.8 angina episodes in the placebo group compared with 9.6 ± 13.3 in the cell treated group. This effect was still present at six months; 16.0 ± 19.3 angina episodes in the placebo group compared with 8.6 ± 10.3 angina episodes in the cell-treated group. Of note, angina frequency declined in both groups at six months. This observation may reflect the so-called "placebo" effect resulting from better education and improved antiangina medication compliance as a result of clinical trial participation. Favorable trends were seen for nitroglycerin use, exercise tolerance, angina classification, SPECT ischemia scores, and quality-of-life measures.

Stamm et al. directly injected autologous, CD 133+–enriched bone marrow–derived progenitor cells during coronary artery bypass surgery in patients with chronic myocardial ischemia. Modest improvements in global ventricular function and regional perfusion were observed. Again, the sample size was small, and therefore, observations may be skewed by heterogeneous treatment benefit from concomitant surgical revascularization. The Prospective Randomized Trial of Direct Endomyocardial Implantation of Bone Marrow Cells for Therapeutic Angiogenesis in Coronary Artery Diseases trial randomly assigned 28 chronic ischemia patients to catheter-directed intramyocardial BMNC transplant or to control groups. Significant improvements in exercise time, cardiac function, and perfusion were observed.

Additional clinical trials are currently underway in Europe and Asia, investigating the safety and potential benefit of a variety of cell types for chronic ischemia. Notably, the ACT34-CMI (Adult Autologous CD34+ Stem Cells for Chronic Myocardial Ischemia) trial is a phase 2b, multicenter, randomized controlled, double-blind clinical trial in the United States. The aim of this trial is to test whether percutaneous endomyocardial injection of autologous CD34+ cells enriched from GCSF mobilized peripheral apheresis product can reduce angina symptoms in subjects with refractory symptomatic chronic myocardial ischemia.

## CONGESTIVE HEART FAILURE

Congestive heart failure (CHF) is a clinical syndrome resulting from myocardial injury that impairs the heart's ability to circulate blood sufficiently to meet the metabolic needs of the body. CHF is common and can lead to frequent hospitalization and sudden death. Initially, the principal goal of cell therapy for CHF was myocyte replacement; however, this paradigm is being reevaluated. Newer concepts such as paracrine factor–induced reverse geometric remodeling and neoangiogenesis are being proposed as potential beneficial mechanisms for therapy.

Autologous bone marrow mononuclear cells and skeletal myoblasts have been delivered in a small series of CHF patients with reduced ejection fractions by catheter-directed transendocardial injections, intracoronary infusion, and direct epicardial injections during concomitant coronary artery bypass surgery. Intramyocardial deposits of skeletal myoblasts lead to apparent ventricular arrhythmia, perhaps as a result of poor electrical integration within the myocardium. Nevertheless, short-term improvements in cardiac function combined with modest symptom relief was observed, forming the basis for future, larger-scale clinical trials.

Cell therapy has the potential to revolutionize the management of cardiovascular disease. Initial human studies testing adult progenitor cells have demonstrated safety with the approaches used combined with promising short-term benefits. Challenges that remain include defining the optimal cell type, dose, delivery mode, and patient population. Future, larger-scale trials are underway to demonstrate the efficacy of cell therapy in patients with MI, chronic myocardial ischemia, and cardiomyopathy.

**SEE ALSO:** Clinical Trials Outside U.S.: Severe Coronary Artery Disease; Heart; Heart Attack.

**BIBLIOGRAPHY.** B. Assmus, et al., "Transplantation of Progenitor Cells and Regeneration Enhancement in Acute Myocardial Infarction (TOPCARE-AMI)," *Circulation* (v.106/24, 2002); B. Assmus, et al., "Transcoronary Transplantation of Progenitor Cells after Myocardial Infarction," *New England Journal of Medicine* (v.355/12, 2006); L. B. Balsam, et al., "Haematopoietic Stem Cells Adopt Mature Hematopoietic Fates in Ischemic Myocardium," *Nature* (v.428/6983, 2004); J. Bartunek, et al., "Intracoronary Injection of CD133-Positive Enriched Bone Marrow Progenitor Cells Promotes Cardiac Recovery after Recent Myocardial Infarction: Feasibility and Safety," *Circulation* (v.112/9, 2005); "Chartbook on Cardiovascular Lung and Blood Diseases," *Morbidity and Mortality Weekly Report* (2004); S. L. Chen, et al., "Improvement of Cardiac Function after Transplantation of Autologous Bone Marrow Mesenchymal Stem Cells in Patients with Acute Myocardial Infarction," *Chinese Medical Journal* (v.117/10, 2004); S. Dimmeler, A. M. Zeiher, and M. D. Schneider, "Unchain My Heart: The Scientific Foundations of Cardiac Repair," *Journal of Clinical Investigation* (v.115/3, 2005); F. Fernandez-Aviles, et al., "Experimental and Clinical Regenerative Capability of Human Bone Marrow Cells after Myocardial Infarction," *Circulation Research*, (v.95/7, 2004); J. M. Hill, et al., "Outcomes and Risks of Granulocyte Colony-Stimulating Factor in Patients with Coronary Artery Disease," *Journal of the American College of Cardiology* (v.46/9, 2005); H. Ince, et al., "Prevention of Left Ventricular Remodeling with Granulocyte Colony-Stimulating Factor after Acute Myocardial Infarction: Final 1-Year Results of the Front-Integrated Revascularization and Stem Cell Liberation in Evolving Acute Myocardial Infarction by Granulocyte Colony-Stimulating Factor (FIRSTLINE-AMI) Trial," *Circulation* (v.112/9, 2005; K. A. Jackson, et al., "Regeneration of Ischemic Cardiac Muscle and Vascular Endothelium by Adult Stem Cells," *Journal of Clinical Investigation* (v.107/11, 2001); S. Janssens, et al., "Autologous Bone Marrow-Derived Stem-Cell Transfer in Patients with ST-Segment Elevation Myocardial Infarction: Double-Blind, Randomised Controlled Trial," *Lancet* (v.367/9505, 2006); H. J. Kang, et al., "Effects of Intracoronary Infusion of Peripheral Blood Stem-Cells Mobilised with Granulocyte-Colony Stimulating Factor on Left Ventricular Systolic Function and Restenosis after Coronary Stenting in Myocardial Infarction: The MAGIC Cell Randomised Clinical Trial," *Lancet* (v.363/9411, 2004); T. Kinnaird, et al., "Local Delivery of Marrow-Derived Stromal Cells Augments Collateral Perfusion through Paracrine Mechanisms," *Circulation* (v.109/12, 2004); D. W. Losordo, et al., "Intramyocardial Transplantation of Autologous CD34+ Stem Cells for Intractable Angina: A Phase I/IIa Double-Blind, Randomized Controlled Trial," *Circulation* (v.115/25, 2007); K. Lunde, et al., "Intracoronary Injection of Mononuclear Bone Marrow Cells in Acute Myocardial Infarction," *New England Journal of Medicine* (v.355/12, 2006); P. Menasche, et al., "Autologous Skeletal Myoblast Transplantation for Severe Postinfarction Left Ventricular Dysfunction," *Journal of the American College of Cardiology* (v.41/7, 2003); C. E. Murry, et al., "Haematopoietic Stem Cells Do Not Transdifferentiate into Cardiac Myocytes in Myocardial Infarcts," *Nature* (v.428/6983, 2004); J. M. Nygren, et al., "Bone Marrow-Derived Hematopoietic Cells Generate Cardiomyocytes at a Low Frequency through Cell Fusion, but Not Transdifferentiation," *Nature Medicine* (v.10/5, 2004); A. N. Patel, et al., "Surgical Treatment for Congestive Heart Failure with Autologous Adult Stem Cell Transplantation: A Prospective Randomized Study," *Journal of Thoracic and Cardiovascular Surgery* (v.130/6, 2005); E. C. Perin, et al., "Transendocardial, Autologous Bone Marrow Cell Transplantation for Severe, Chronic Ischemic Heart Failure," *Circulation* (v.107/18, 2003); R. S. Ripa, et al., "Stem Cell Mobilization Induced by Subcutaneous Granulocyte-Colony Stimulating Factor to Improve Cardiac Regeneration after Acute ST-Elevation Myocardial Infarction: Result of the Double-Blind, Randomized, Placebo-Controlled Stem Cells in Myocardial Infarction (STEMMI) Trial," *Circulation* (v.113/16, 2006); V. Schachinger, et al., "Intracoronary Bone Marrow-Derived Progenitor Cells in Acute Myocardial Infarction," *New England Journal of Medicine* (v.355/12, 2006); C. Stamm, et al., "Autologous Bone-Marrow Stem-Cell Transplantation for Myocardial Regeneration," *Lancet* (v.361/9351, 2003); B. E. Strauer, et al., "Repair of Infarcted Myocardium by Autologous Intracoronary Mononuclear

Bone Marrow Cell Transplantation in Humans," *Circulation* (v.106/15, 2002); H. F. Tse, et al., "Prospective Randomized Trial of Direct Endomyocardial Implantation of Bone Marrow Cells for Treatment of Severe Coronary Artery Diseases (PROTECT-CAD trial)," *European Heart Journal* (v.28/24, 2007); K. C. Wollert, et al., "Intracoronary Autologous Bone-Marrow Cell Transfer after Myocardial Infarction: The BOOST Randomised Controlled Clinical Trial," *Lancet* (v.364/9429, 2004); D. Zohlnhofer, et al., "Stem Cell Mobilization by Granulocyte Colony-Stimulating Factor in Patients with Acute Myocardial Infarction: A Randomized Controlled Trial," *Journal of the American Medical Association* (v.295/9, 2006).

Amish N. Raval
University of Wisconsin

# Clinical Trials Within U.S.: Peripheral Vascular Disease

**LOWER-EXTREMITY PERIPHERAL ARTERY** disease (PAD) is a common, debilitating, and potentially life-threatening illness affecting nearly 10 million people in the United States and fully 10 percent of those older than 60 years. PAD unfortunately remains an underrecognized disease, however, and can be difficult to treat. Obstructive PAD is most commonly caused by atherosclerosis and can initially manifest as intermittent claudication, defined as leg muscle pain with walking that is relieved with rest. PAD may progress to critical limb ischemia (CLI), defined by pain at rest, skin ulcers, and gangrene. In the latter condition, limb amputation is threatened unless blood flow can be restored.

Risk factor modification, exercise therapy, and antiplatelet, antihypertensive, and antilipid therapy are mainstay therapy for PAD. Unfortunately, a significant number of patients fail medical therapy. Mechanical revascularization includes invasive surgical bypass and minimally invasive catheter-based approaches. Surgical bypass to restore blood flow may be limited by arteries that are too small and diseased to successfully graft into. Patient comorbidities also make surgical options risky. Use of percutaneous revascularization such as angioplasty and stenting is limited by small, distal, diseased arteries; technical difficulty accessing the target artery; and high restenosis rates. Incomplete revascularization may result in poor distal arterial runoff and inadequate tissue perfusion. Amputation may be the only treatment option for nonhealing ulcers or gangrene in many patients. Afflicted patients may have significant physical and emotional disabilities. Psychological testing of patients with CLI shows quality-of-life indices similar to those of patients with terminal malignancy. The magnitude of the clinical problem, the effect of the disease on quality of life, and limitations of conventional treatment make this patient subset ideally suited for clinical investigation of novel regenerative cell-based therapies.

Stem cells can differentiate into nearly any cell type and can self-renew indefinitely. Adult progenitor cells differ from stem cells in that they have reduced differentiation capacity and lack the ability to self-renew. However, adult progenitors are more easily accessible, have significant proliferative capability, and can generate large numbers of mature cells. Hypoxia results in the enhanced ability of certain "endothelial" progenitor cells (EPCs) to ameliorate ischemia. EPCs are typically defined by their expression of certain surface markers such as CD34+, CD133+, and Flk-1. As EPCs differentiate, they acquire mature endothelial lineage markers such as vascular endothelium cadherin, CD31+, and von Willebrand factor. Adult-derived bone marrow and circulating progenitor cells have been the focus of current human trials to treat severe, obstructive PAD.

## RATIONALE FOR CLINICAL TRIALS IN PAD

The chief goal behind cell therapy for PAD is to restore blood flow to the lower extremities. Locally administered unfractionated bone marrow–derived mononuclear cells (BMNCs) or select EPCs have shown improved perfusion in animal models of ischemia. For example, mice with surgically induced hind limb ischemia demonstrated improved vasculogenic response when CD34+ endothelial progenitors were administered directly into the lower extremity muscle. In another study, when peripheral blood human CD34+ progenitor cells were injected into the tail veins of immunocompromised mice with hind limb ischemia, increased capillary growth in the affected limb was observed. Improved collaterals, capillary density, and tissue perfusion were similarly observed when BMNCs were administered intramuscularly in a rat hind limb ischemia model. Yoshida et al. administered unselected BMNCs by both intraarterial infusion and direct intramuscular injection into rats with hind limb ischemia. The rats then demonstrated improved collateralization by angiography and increased capillary density by histology with both routes of administration compared with controls. These initial promising early benefits have paved the way toward initial human trials.

## CLINICAL CELL THERAPY TRIALS AND PAD

Small human trials exploring cell therapy for patients with PAD have focused on safety and exploratory efficacy. Study designs have typically been small prospective cohort studies with baseline comparisons. In general, these investigational therapies are being tested in medically refractory CLI patients for whom mechanical revascularization is not ideal. At present, adult progenitor cells are harvested by direct bone marrow aspiration or cytokine mobilization followed by peripheral blood leukophoresis. Safety of cell implantation and delivery is of paramount importance and has been the focus of early trials.

Several clinical studies of autologous bone marrow and peripheral blood–derived progenitor cell transplantation for cardiac disease have emerged; however, there still remain little published data of cell-based therapy in PAD patients. A phase 1 clinical study from Japan compared peripheral blood mononuclear cell (PMNC) preparation with unselected BMNCs directly injected into the gastrocnemius muscles of patients with bilateral leg ischemia, defined by an ankle brachial index (ABI) of less than 0.6.10 This group demonstrated improved lower extremity blood flow, transcutaneous tissue oxygen pressure, and pain-free walking time in the lower extremities receiving BMNC compared with the lower extremities receiving PMNC.

A small pilot study evaluated direct intramuscular administration of granulocyte colony-stimulating factor (GCSF) mobilized, unselected PMNCs into the lower extremities of patients with nonhealing ulcers or gangrene. This group observed improved ABIs, wound healing, limb perfusion by laser Doppler, and neocollateralization. There were no major adverse events resulting from the administration of GCSF. Improved endothelium-dependent vasodilatation was also observed in CLI patients who received autologous BMNCs. Improved ABI, pain-free walking time, and transcutaneous oxygen pressure (TcPO2) were also observed in this small cohort. Intramuscular injection of CD34+ cells derived from GCSF-mobilized blood leukophoresis product was considered safe and resulted in improvements in angiographically visible collaterals and transcutaneous tissue oxygen pressure in no-revascularization-option CLI patients.

In a small, eight-patient cohort, Saigawa et al. demonstrated that unselected BMNC lower extremity transplant resulted in significant symptoms, ABI improvement, wound healing, and collateral scores. An interesting observation was that the individuals who improved the most with the cell therapy had a greater relative number of CD34+ cells in the administered cell fraction. These data suggest that the dose of EPCs may directly affect potential therapeutic effects; however, these results have not been replicated in other clinical cell therapy trials.

Recently, a Spanish group reported the very first results of CD133+ implantation in CLI patients. Specifically, this group reported results on three patients who underwent GCSF mobilization for 4 days, followed by leukophoresis and cell sorting, using a magnetic separation system to isolate CD133+ cells. Between 2.1 and 3.0 × $10^6$ CD 133+ cells/kg were obtained, and half of the product (1.05–1.5 × $10^6$ CD 133+ cells/kg) was divided into 10 doses and injected into 10 sites in the gastrocnemius muscle. The safety of this approach, the prevention of amputation, and improved pain-free walking all were demonstrated in this small cohort.

Durdu et al. recently reported the results of intramuscular administration of unselected BMNCs in patients with a condition called thromboangiitis obliterans (also known as Buerger's disease). The cause of this condition remains unknown, and treatment modalities have been unsatisfactory in this type of nonatherosclerotic, segmental, inflammatory vasculitis. In the 28 patients who underwent cell transplant, there was a significant improvement at six months in rest pain scores, peak walking time, ABI, ulcer healing, and quality of life compared with baseline.

The goals of therapy for PAD include improving symptoms, objective measures of improved lower-extremity circulation, and limb salvage rates. Clinical trials exploring cell therapy for PAD have demonstrated safety and feasibility with the approaches and methods tested. Exploratory efficacy signals have shown some short-term benefits, but this needs to be confirmed in larger studies. Current trial sample sizes are too small to conclude evidence of efficacy, although trends toward benefits are being seen, and safety with the cell transplant method and delivery modes are being confirmed. Future challenges include the need to optimize cell type, dose, delivery method, and patient population likely to benefit from this potential revolutionary therapy.

**SEE ALSO:** Cells, Adult; Cells, Human.

**BIBLIOGRAPHY.** M. Albers, A. C. Fratezi, and N. De Luccia, "Assessment of Quality of Life of Patients with Severe Ischemia as a Result of Infrainguinal Arterial Occlusive Disease," *Journal of Vascular Surgery* (v.16/1, 1992); T. Asahara, et al., "Isolation of Putative Progenitor Endothelial Cells for Angiogenesis," *Science* (v.275/5302, 1997); M. H. Criqui, "Peripheral Arterial Disease—Epidemiological Aspects," Vascular Medicine (v.6/3, 2001); U. M. Gehling, et al., "In Vitro Differentiation of Endothelial Cells from AC133-Positive Progenitor Cells," *Blood* (v.95/10, 2000); K. Hamano, et al., "Therapeutic Angiogenesis Induced by Local Autologous Bone Marrow Cell Implantation," *Annals of Thoracic Surgery* (v.73/4, 2002); Y. Higashi, et al., "Autologous Bone-Marrow Mononuclear Cell Implantation Improves Endothelium-Dependent Vasodilation in Patients with Limb Ischemia," *Circulation* (v.109/10, 2004); P. P. Huang, et al., "Autologous Transplantation of Peripheral Blood Stem Cells as an Effective Therapeutic Approach for Severe Arteriosclerosis Obliterans of Lower Extremities," *Journal of Thrombosis and Haemostasis* (v.91/3, 2004); S. Ikenaga, et al., "Autologous Bone Marrow Implantation Induced Angiogenesis and Improved Deteriorated Exercise Capacity in a Rat Ischemic Hindlimb Model," *Journal of Surgery Research* (v.96/2, 2001); F. A. Kudo, et al., Autologous Transplantation of Peripheral Blood Endothelial Progenitor Cells (CD34+) for Therapeutic Angiogenesis in Patients with Critical Limb Ischemia," *International Journal of Angiology* (v.22/4, 2003); M. Peichev, et al., "Expression of VEGFR-2 and AC133 by Circulating Human CD34(+) Cells Identifies a Population of Functional Endothelial Precursors," *Blood* (v.95/3, 2000); M. Pesce, et al., "Myoendothelial Differentiation of Human Umbilical Cord Blood-Derived Stem Cells in Ischemic Limb Tissues," *Circulation Research* (v.93/5, 2003); F. M. Sanchez-Guijo, et al., "Peripheral Endothelial Projenitor Cells (CD133+) for Therapeutic Vasculogenesis in Critical Limb Ischemia of the Lower Extremities (Abstract)" (European Group for Blood and Marrow Transplantation, 2006); E. Tateishi-Yuyama, et al., "Therapeutic Angiogenesis for Patients with Limb Ischaemia by Autologous Transplantation of Bone-Marrow Cells: A Pilot Study and a Randomised Controlled Trial," *Lancet* (v.360/9331, 2002).

Amish N. Raval
University of Wisconsin

# Clinical Trials Within U.S.: Skin Transplants (Burns)

**THE SKIN IS** a vital organ for maintaining body homeostasis, and is a major immunologic defense against infection. When the integrity of the skin is compromised, such as in severe burn injuries, the person is at risk for complications such as dehydration as well as infection. Therefore, a skin transplant is often performed by splitting skin from a less damaged region of the body to another, more damaged region. The process of skin transplantation, particularly after a burn, is still undergoing improvement, and the way to test novel techniques is via a clinical trial.

A clinical trial is a critical method for determined the safety, efficacy, and benefit of a potential new clinical technique. This technique may be for treatment, therapy, diagnostic purposes, prevention, or improvement of the patient's quality of life. Although based on promising laboratory research, clinical trials are not guaranteed to work and must be understood as trials. For example, the volunteers for clinical trials of a novel therapy are not guaranteed an improvement in their condition and in fact are taking a significant risk. Nevertheless, while these volunteers may not see improvement themselves, they are doing a great service to others with the disease, as clinicians will learn about therapeutics and the potential benefits or harms of a particular technique.

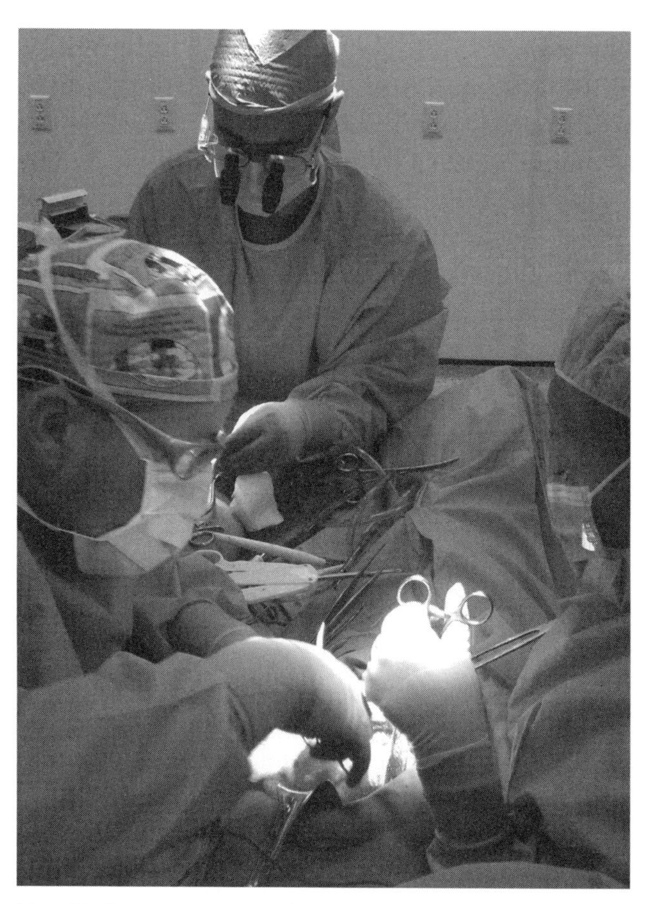

*U.S. Air Force surgeons perform a procedure involving skin grafting at Bagram medical facilities in Afghanistan.*

According to the U.S. National Institutes of Health, there are two major classes of clinical trials. These classes are interventional, which measure a treatment type, and observational, where the clinicians monitor a particular patient group. A clinical trial involving a skin transplant, particularly in the treatment of a burn, would be an interventional clinical trial.

Clinical trials that have been completed in the United States include trials examining the optimal method of affixing the transplant to the new location. Options included skin staples, stitches, or medical adhesive such as cyanoacrylate glue. Severely damaged skin especially after a burn injury, is fragile and can be difficult to work with using tools such as sutures or staples, and some studies showed a benefit to using a medical adhesive.

Other trials investigate the use of certain topical healing agents such as anti-inflammatory creams or ointments, or anti-scarring treatments. One study examined the use of cultured skin substitute over using split skin from a less-affected body area. Cultured skin substitute (CSS) is a biopolymer generated in the laboratory that contains an artificial matrix onto which human cells are encouraged to grow using growth factors to induce the differentiation of skin cells. Another type of cultured skin transplant is a cultured epidermal autograft (CEA), which is a cultured skin from the patient's own cells. CEAs do no necessarily have a matrix.

Given the nature of the skin excision and graft process, bleeding can be a devastating issue. In order to prevent severe bleeding during and after the procedure, clinical trials have investigated the utility of anti-bleeding factors when used in the adhesives for the graft. A recent study presented at the 2008 American Burn Association meeting showed that a novel product called Recothrom, a recombinant form of Thrombin, made by the company ZymoGenetics, can be used effectively to seal the borders of a skin transplant on a burn patient. This product is a spray and therefore easy to administer. The study was carried out at the University of California, Davis Medical Center and led by Dr. David G. Greenhalgh. Thrombin is physiologically considered a coagulation factor, involved in the cessation of blood flow. An earlier study, in which Greenhalgh also participated, showed that fibrin, a blood clotting factor, was also effective as a spray-on treatment to prevent bleeding.

**SEE ALSO:** Clinical Trials Worldwide; National Institutes of Health (NIH); University of California, Davis.

**BIBLIOGRAPHY.** J. W. Fluhr, P. Elsner, E. Berardesca, et al., *Bioengineering of the Skin: Water and the Stratum Corneum*, 2nd Edition (Dematology: Clinical & Basic Science) (Informa Healthcare, 2004); L. M. Friedman, C. D. Furberg, and D. L. DeMets, *Fundamentals of Clinical Trials* (Springer, 1999).

Claudia Winograd
University of Illinois, Urbana-Champaign

# Clinical Trials Within U.S.: Spinal Cord Injury

**WITHIN THE UNITED** States, no clinical trials using stem cells for the treatment of spinal cord injury have been approved. This is not altogether surprising, as the field of stem cell research is still in its youth. With that said, there are several promising projects that are preparing to enter the clinical study phase.

Physiologically speaking, spinal cord trauma differs from other types of central nervous system injuries. Instead of cell bodies (as in the brain), the spine is predominantly composed of long axon tracts. As such, spinal cord damage results in loss of sensory, motor, or autonomic function. More specifically, damage to the spinal cord prevents transmission of sensory information to the brain, as well as transmission of motor and autonomic commands from the brain to the body. Effectively, areas below the level of injury lose sensation and control, which manifests as numbness and paralysis. Full loss of sensation and control is considered a "complete" spinal cord injury, whereas partial loss of function is "incomplete." Characteristic of the central nervous system, neurons of the spinal cord have limited regenerative abilities, rendering most injuries permanent.

The advantage of damaging an axon is that it does not necessarily imply the death of its corresponding neuron. Rather, via a process known as Wallerian degeneration, only the severed portion of an axon is lost; the remaining, nucleus-containing segment remains viable, with the potential for regrowth. However, a cocktail of inhibitory biochemical signals produced by the microenvironment of the spine seems to be partially responsible for its limited regenerative properties. An associated process of Wallerian degeneration is the demyelination of damaged axons. This important component of neurons normally surrounds the axon tract to effectively serve as an electrical insulator. Through this mechanism, speeds of signal propagation through the axon can increase up to 70-fold. Without myelination, axons in the spine transmit information too slowly to support a functional human being.

Lest one believe that the full extent of spinal cord injuries arises only from the primary event, it should be noted that a secondary insult comes about from physiologic causes. Local invasion of inflammatory components and changes in vascular integrity results in fluid and cellular accumulation, which exacerbates cord compression. This added impingement on healthy tissue induces further destruction and demyelination. Following acute inflammation, a scar is formed at the lesion site, which creates yet another barrier against future growth. The incredible complexity of this process means that there are numerous points of possible intervention. From restoring myelin of injured neurons to creating a growth-facilitating microenvironment to stimulating neuronal regrowth, the sheer scope of the issue has required over a decade for studies to finally advance to the clinical trial phase.

## CLINICAL TRIALS: ALMOST THERE

Although numerous countries (Australia, Brazil, China, France, India, Portugal, Russia, and South Korea, to say the least) have started clinical studies using stem cell transplantations to treat spinal cord injuries, the United States has yet to approve one. Known for its tight restriction on human experiments, the Food and Drug Administration insists on the replication of published preclinical studies that supposedly demonstrate safety and proof-of-principle results. Perhaps this is for the best, as it is not uncommon for promising outcomes from one laboratory to deviate when attempted by another. However, because of the expanse of the field, there has been little desire to devote precious man hours and funding toward replicating experiments. As a result, this lack of confirmatory studies has led to a delay in the development of clinical trials.

To address this delay, the National Institutes of Health has established three centers within the nation to contend with important, but often overlooked, research-related issues. Each Branded Facility of Research in Spinal Cord Injury (FOR-SCI) is funded to study a unique subset of spinal cord issues. Of the three, the Miami Project of the University of Miami and the Reeve-Irvine Research Center have each been contracted to focus on replication studies that have been deemed crucial to the development of treatments.

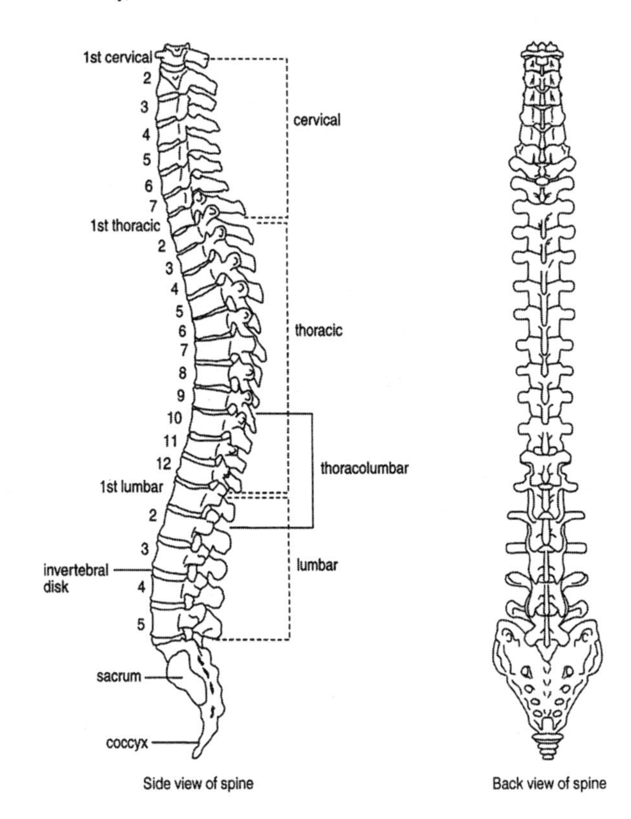


*Despite the hype, even repeated spinal injections of 50 million embryonic stem cells have failed to achieve full recovery.*

## TRIALS OF THE NEAR FUTURE: OLFACTORY ENSHEATHING CELLS

One of the FOR-SCI priorities was a 2002 study conducted by Jike Lu and colleagues. The experiment asserted the ability of olfactory ensheathing cells (OECs) to promote recovery of motor functions. Furthermore, the protocol was said to be effective even after a month-long delay between injury and transplant. The success of the project was said to stem from the use of OECs. Functionally, olfactory neurons are unusual in that they have regenerative abilities because of their constant exposure to the external environment (much like how skin is continually renewed). As a supporting cell, OECs surround the growing axons of olfactory neurons and stimulate them toward their target—a function that Lu hoped to use to his advantage in the spinal cord. In the experiment, biopsies of rat and human nasal cavity linings (olfactory lamina propria) were taken and transplanted into damaged rat spines. The experiment used the lamina propria to function doubly as a reservoir for OECs and as a neuron-guiding cellular scaffold within the damaged region. Within two to three weeks of the procedure, motor abilities of the test subjects had already surpassed those of their untreated control counterparts. This progressive improvement of the test rats continued for the remainder of the study, while the control group remained at the same deficient level.

Aside from its obvious benefits of facilitating functional improvement, this study also provided solutions to many questions plaguing stem cell researchers across the board. First and foremost, nasal cavity lamina propria was show to be not only a reliable source of OECs but also to exist in relatively high quantities and is easy to obtain. Thus, the often controversial issue of fetal tissue is easily bypassed, and a clinically practical source of therapeutic cells has been identified. Second, the use of differentiated supporting cells and not embryonic stem cells eliminates the possibility of uncontrolled differentiation, and the possible proliferation, of implanted cells. Third, because tissues are patient derived, there is no fear of immunologic rejection. Subsequently, the patient does not have to undergo dangerous, lifelong immunosuppression. Fourth, the experiment appears to have been unaffected despite a month-long delay between injury and treatment. Physicians prefer to wait at least a week after spinal trauma before beginning any interventions, to allow the inflammatory process to resolve. The success of this study holds strong implications for the development of a clinically viable protocol.

Fortunately for all, researchers at the Reeve-Irvine Research Center have confirmed the success of Lu's work. In fact, physicians in Portugal, China, and Russia, where the regulations are more lax, have already reported using OEC transplantation as a therapy.

## TRIALS OF THE NEAR FUTURE: OLIGODENDROCYTE PROGENITOR CELLS

Another study that is soon to reach clinical trial in the United States is the use of oligodendrocyte progenitors. Derived from human embryonic stem cells, these oligodendrocyte precursors are functionally comparable to OECs. Both cell types support neurons, myelinate axons, and secrete a host of growth factors.

Led by Dr. Hans Keirstead of the Reeve-Irvine Research Center, this project was effectively a duplicate of the previously discussed study with a few tweaks. The most striking difference was choice of implant material. For this study, human embryonic stem cells were in the spotlight. These cells were induced by a series of signaling chemicals to differentiate into oligodendrocyte progenitors and then subsequently encouraged to proliferate en masse. The result of this procedure created high-purity samples of progenitor cells, and in practical quantities. From there, researchers hypothesized that if the appropriate stimuli were administered simultaneously with the tissue transplant, progenitors would further differentiate into mature oligodendrocytes, where they could then remyelinate damaged axons. From here, the transplant procedure was the same, with a minor difference in the time delay before initiation of therapy. Instead of waiting four weeks between insult and treatment, transplantation was timed to occur at either seven days or 10 months following an injury. Results of the study showed that day seven implantations demonstrated functional improvements and increased remyelination of damaged axons. Progenitors implanted in month 10, in contrast, though able to demonstrate differentiation and survival, failed to remyelinate axons. Accordingly, there was no significant recovery of function. This implies that there is a limited window of time in which this particular treatment course may be effective.

Perhaps the most significant finding of this series of experiments is the fact that the oligodendrocyte progenitors seem to have no deleterious effects on normal tissue. Part of the study included using different-sized lesions, in which the smaller ones exhibited little or no demyelination. When comparing results between injuries, it appeared that there were no unfavorable changes in the morphologic makeup of cells in the smaller lesion (i.e., no excessive myelination or increases in cell density). Because the incidence of uncontrolled proliferation is always a looming question, this demonstrable lack of adverse growth or dysfunction is very promising for clinical trials.

In using differentiated cells, Keirstead's strategy decreases the possibility of tumor formation but carries two potential problems. For one, differentiated cells are more prone to triggering an immune response by the host. This has the ramification of destroying the foreign implant or exacerbating the original lesion. (Keirstead did, however, prove in later studies that the immunologic privilege accorded to embryonic stem cells could be extended to the oligodendrocyte progenitors.) The other, and more obvious, problem with this sample protocol is that use of embryonic cells opens the floodgates to controversy regarding the procurement of these cells, which has yet to be resolved.

In spite of this, a phase 1 trial funded by the Geron Corporation in California is supposedly slated to begin sometime in 2008. Also conducted by Keirstead, the use of these oligodendrocyte progenitors (branded as GRNOPC1, for GeRoN Oligodendrocyte Progenitor Cells) will be in keeping with his work on the aforementioned studies. It should be noted, however, that the Geron Corporation is frequently criticized for touting its initiation of clinical trials "next year"—which it has been saying since 2004.

### CONTINUED SEARCH FOR A CURE

In the grand scope of spinal cord injuries, partial recovery of function is easy, relatively speaking, to bring about. After all, reestablishment of as little as 10 percent of the destroyed axon tracts is enough to induce a disproportionately increased enhancement of functional skills attributable to the plastic, or adaptive, quality of neurons.

Subsequently, with all the hype surrounding stem cell research, it is important to keep in mind that none of these studies, preclinical or clinical, have demonstrated a full recovery. Even a radical attempt at forcing a cure by repeated injections of 50 million embryonic stem cells directly into the spinal cord (as performed by researchers in India) has failed to restore subjects to their preinjury state. Nonetheless, these attempts have made some significant improvements in the lives of patients. In an extreme case, an informal report claimed to have restored a patient's ability to walk (i.e., using a walker for 10 steps), but the average case gets nowhere near this level.

Still, it is amazing how much stem cell research has achieved. Yet its potential has barely been tapped. The sheer expanse of the field means that much work remains to be accomplished. Future studies will undoubtedly reveal more incredible qualities of these cells and how they can be used to develop a clinically viable cure for patients with spinal cord injuries.

**SEE ALSO:** Cells, Embryonic; Geron Corporation; Reeve-Irvine Research Center; Spinal Cord Injury.

**BIBLIOGRAPHY.** Geron Corporation, "Press Release: Geron Presents New Data that Documents Progress in Development of Therapeutic Products from Human Embryonic Stem Cell," www.geron.com (cited July 2006); Laurance Johnston, "Embryonic Stem-Cell Therapy," www.healingtherapies.info (cited August 2007); Hans Keirstead, et al., "Human Embryonic Stem Cell-Derived Oligodendrocyte Progenitor Cell Transplants Remyelinate and Restore Locomotion after Spinal Cord Injury," *Journal of Neuroscience* (v.25/19, 2005); Jike Lu, et al., "Olfactory Ensheathing Cells Promote Locomotor Recovery after Delayed Transplantation into Transected Spinal Cord," *Brain* (v.125/1, 2002).

Priscilla Pang
Case Western Reserve University

# Clinical Trials Within U.S.: Traumatic Brain Injury

**TRAUMATIC BRAIN INJURY** refers to brain damage caused by an external mechanical force. It is a relatively common event, with 1.5 million people in the United States incurring some sort of head trauma annually. Fortunately, 75 percent of the cases turn out to be mild, with little or no consequences. However, survivors in the remaining 25 percent suffer from moderate to severe functional deficits, which greatly decrease quality of life as well as life expectancy. Although there has been much work dedicated to helping patients with this condition, the complexity of the brain has rendered it extremely difficult to develop a successful regenerative or restorative treatment. Despite over a decade of stem cell research, it is only just recently that the first clinical trial in the United States was approved by the U.S. Food and Drug Administration for using stem cells to treat brain injuries.

The full extent of damage from a traumatic brain injury arises from the combination of multiple processes. Obviously, destruction would be incurred by direct external force. "Contrecoup" injuries, in which a moving brain is slammed into the skull opposing the impact side (e.g., in a car accident), are also direct causes of cerebral wounding. However, following that, the injured organ and surrounding tissues undergo subsequent waves of damage caused by secondary structural, biochemical, and inflammatory mechanisms. Pressure within the brain increases (generally as a result of fluid accumulation, be it blood or invasion of inflammatory components), neurotransmitters are inappropriately released in toxic quantities, or integrity of vasculature is lost. The end result is the death of other neurons not initially involved with the original injury.

Because of how the brain is organized, injuries to the organ can give rise to drastically different clinical manifestations, based on location and severity of the lesion. For survivors, injuries are classified according to the Glasgow Coma Scale as "mild," "moderate," or "severe," based on eye, verbal, and motor abilities. Although 75 percent of cases are mild, approximately 50,000 people die per year (about half of all traumatic deaths) because of severe head trauma.

In terms of treatment for individuals with head injuries, acute care is limited to minimizing the secondary wave of damage. The most important part of this care is reducing intracranial pressure and maintaining adequate blood perfusion through the use of pharmacologic or surgical interventions. Poststabilization, supportive management of symptoms, physical therapy, and cognitive therapy make up the basis of chronic care because no restorative treatments exist as of yet.

## ENTERING THE CLINICAL TRIAL PHASE

The intricacy of the brain has proven to be a difficult obstacle to creating an effective treatment. Along with replacing neurons (or inducing regeneration of damaged neurons), supporting cells such as astrocytes, oligodendrocytes, and glial cells must also be restored, and in the appropriate proportions. The microenvironment of the brain must contain all the correct biochemical signals and growth factors to direct reformation of neural connections. Renewal of neural coherency must occur not only on a local cell-to-cell scale but also in the anatomical scope of rebuilding functional neural tracts. In consideration of all this, it seems amazing that after only a decade of work, clinical trials with stem cells have finally been approved. This onset of human experiments comes only after extensive studies have demonstrated "proof-of-principle" results using animal and cell models.

In April 2006 Dr. Charles S. Cox Jr. and Dr. James E. Baumgartner of the University of Texas Health Science Center at Houston began a phase 1 trial to determine the safety of stem cell treatment for traumatic brain injury in children. Their study aims to use autologous (harvested from the individuals themselves) bone marrow precursor cells because of their many advantages: autologous transplants eliminate the need for lifelong immunosuppression, and bone marrow precursor cells contain both mesenchymal and hematopoietic stem cells. Hematopoietic stem cells are valuable for their reported ability to stimulate blood vessel formation, and mesenchymal stem cells are particularly promising because of their ability to differentiate into multiple tissue types, their capacity for almost limitless proliferation, and the quantity and ease with which they can be harvested and cultured. In addition, these cells exhibit a preference for migration to the damaged area and differentiation into neural components.

The rationale for using children is that their immature brains carry a greater capacity for remodeling based on experiences and circumstances. This state of neuroplasticity lends itself to creating a growth-supportive environment for transplanted cells. Moreover, as plasticity responds to the experiences of the person, growth will—ideally—be regulated in an individualized manner to repair the injured brain.

Although the primary goal of their study is to evaluate the safety of such harvesting and transplantation procedures within a clinical setting, the researchers will concurrently assess whether this protocol facilitates functional improvements. Using subjects aged 5–14 years, harvesting and transplantation will occur within 24 to 36 hours of trauma. During the procedures, intracranial pressure will be monitored and controlled to stay below 40 mmHg, as there is a chance that additional volume could increase intracranial pressure to unacceptable levels. Safety will be evaluated during the postprocedural hospital stay ("acute injury phase") through the observation of neurologic and systemic manifestations. For six months following the transplant, subjects will undergo tests to measure functional capacity and will be compared against known control patients (those treated in the conventional manner).

Even though the study only intends to use 10 subjects, the rigidity of the criteria lends itself to exclusion of many potential candidates. Each child must be enrolled within 24 hours of trauma that has been graded as "severe." The harvesting and transplantation must occur 24–36 hours after the injury, which effectively limits participants to the local Houston area. Subjects must have no known history of previous brain injury, developmental delay, neurologic impairment, renal or hepatic disorders, cancer, or a state of immunosuppression. Other conditions include that the trauma must be limited solely to the head, that the patient undergoes no extended periods (>30 minutes) of hypoxia, and that the patient must be willing to return for six months of follow-up visits. As of November 2007 the study is still open for enrolling, proving the difficulty in recruiting suitable patients.

Granted, as one of the first trials of its kind in the United States, this study cannot cover every aspect of stem cell therapy. In the best possible scenario, this experiment will prove to be fully effective, with complete restoration of functional abilities. However, even then, there are still hurdles to be overcome. The idea that childhood neuroplasticity regulates the differentiation and growth of progenitor cells implies that older individuals carry a decreased potential for regeneration. Other studies have shown that as the current study only caters to new traumas, it neglects the hundreds of thousands of people who have been living for years with their deficits. It also overlooks those who cannot access medical centers that have the ability to perform such a technique within the narrow time frame. For these individuals, there is hope to be found in preclinical studies that report the ability of stem cells to provide some reestablishment of function long after the acute injury phase.

## CHALLENGES

One potential and significant problem with this investigation—as well as other stem cell research—is that the mechanisms for how bone marrow progenitor cells actually achieve this restorative response remain unknown. It could be that these cells simply take the place of the damaged cells, restoring the brain to its original state. It may also turn out that these progenitor cells do not actually replace the damaged neurons but, rather, possess some unknown property that facilitates functional connections. (This is actually supported by the fact that improvements in functional deficits are seen within days or weeks of implantation, which is not enough time for differentiation and replacement of the damaged neurons.) Armed with only a basic understanding of the complex signals governing a damaged brain, it is unlikely that enough is known about these cells to predict the complete effects of implantation. Subsequently, it would not be improbable for progenitor cells to deviate from the intended path, resulting in no improvements, neural dysfunction, or worse yet, tumor formation. Until these mechanisms can be elucidated, clinical trials should proceed with caution.

It should be noted that in 2005, Russian researchers, headed by Victor Seledtsov, published their results on the ability of fetal stem cells to reanimate patients with severe head injuries. Although the patients did not experience a full recovery of function, this experiment provides proof that stem cells carry the potential to be a cure for traumatic brain injury. Hopefully, with the help of international collaborations, a safe and clinically viable treatment can one day be developed.

**SEE ALSO:** Brain; Spinal Cord Injury.

**BIBLIOGRAPHY.** Charles S. Cox Jr. and Mary-Clare Day, "Safety of Autologous Stem Cell Treatment for Traumatic Brian Injury in Children," www.clinicaltrials.gov/show/NCT00254722 (cited April 2006); Luca Longhi, et al., "Stem Cell Transplantation as a Therapeutic Strategy for Traumatic Brain Injury," *Transplant Immunology* (v.15/2, 2005); David A. Olson, "Head Injury," www.emedicine.com (cited October 2006); Victor I. Seledtsov, et al., "Cell Transplantation Therapy in Reanimating Severely Head-Injured Patients," *Biomedicine and Pharmacotherapy* (v.59/7, 2005).

Priscilla Pang
Case Western Reserve University

# Clinical Trials Worldwide

**FOUR PIONEERING STUDIES** in neurological disorders include a phase 1 study at the University of Texas Health Science Center at Houston that is evaluating the safety of autologous (using the patient's own cells) bone marrow treatments in 10 children aged 5–14 years with traumatic brain injury; a phase 1/2 study at the University of Cambridge to determine the safety and effectiveness of bone marrow–derived autologous mesenchymal stem cells in multiple sclerosis; a phase 1 safety study on the use of autologous bone marrow stem cells for acute stroke, sponsored by the Federal University of Rio de Janeiro in Brazil; and a recently completed phase 1 evaluation at Inha University in Incheon, Korea, where autologous bone marrow stem cells were used to treat acute and chronic spinal cord injuries. Thirty-five patients were treated in this study, and there were no serious adverse effects.

Azienda Unità Sanitaria Locale di Piacenza, in Italy, has been evaluating the safety of autologous bone marrow mononuclear cells for acute heart attack. Similar studies are under way at Nantes University Hospital in France, at Odense University Hospital in Denmark, at the University of Oulu in Finland, at the Minnesota Heart Institute in Minneapolis, and in a multicenter phase 3 national program in Brazil. Emory University in Atlanta, Georgia, is using autologous bone marrow CD34+ stem cells for acute heart attack. Rigshopitalet, in Denmark, is using autologous bone marrow–derived mesenchymal cells for treating severe chronic myocardial ischemia. Chronic damage from a heart attack is also being treated by BioCardia, Inc., in Buenos Aires, Argentina, and a similar study is in progress in Leiden University, Netherlands, and in a multicenter national program in Brazil.

The Texas Heart Institute is using autologous bone marrow mononuclear cell injections to help increase blood vessel development in patients with endstage ischemic cardiomyopathy, and the University of Pittsburgh in Pennsylvania is using autologous bone marrow progenitor cells for congestive heart failure.

Heinrich-Heine University in Duesseldorf, Germany, and Aastrom Biosciences, Inc., are using autologous bone marrow stem cells for peripheral artery disease, and CHU de Reims in Nantes, France, and the University of Naples in Italy are evaluating mononuclear cells for peripheral artery disease. The Franziskus Hospital in Berlin, Germany, is evaluating the use of autologous bone marrow treatments for critical, limb-threatening ischemia in a phase 2/3 study in patients with atherosclerosis or diabetes.

Researchers at the Federal University of Rio de Janiero, Brazil, are evaluating the safety of bone marrow–derived mononuclear cells in patients with liver cirrhosis. Shaheed Beheshti Medical University in Iran is sponsoring a phase 1/2 study of autologous bone marrow mesenchymal stem cells being differentiated into liver progenitor cells for end-stage liver disease.

Type 1 and type 2 diabetic patients are being treated at Shandong University in China with autologous bone marrow mononuclear cells infused directly into the pancreas. In wound healing, the University of Heidelberg in Germany is sponsoring a clinical trial using autologous bone marrow cells to treat diabetic ulcers and diabetic nonhealing wounds.

At Nagoya University in Japan, mesenchymal cells and mesenchymal-derived bone cells have been surgically implanted in 10 patients with periodontitis in a phase 1/2 clinical study. Osiris Therapeutics, Inc., in the United States is sponsoring a multicenter phase 2 study of its trademarked version of bone marrow–derived mesenchymal cells for intravenous infusion into patients with Crohn's disease.

## TYPES OF STEM CELLS IN USE

The Institute of Biomedical Research and Innovation in Kobe, Hyogo, Japan, has started a phase 1/2 safety and effectiveness evaluation of using autologous peripheral blood CD34+ stem cells to treat chronic critical limb ischemia.

Duchenne muscular dystrophy is a genetic disorder that causes progressive muscle weakness and premature death as a result of the absence of the gene that produces dystrophin. The CD133+ progenitor cell, found in peripheral blood, muscle, and umbilical cord blood, has been found to increase the production of dystrophin. The University of Milan, Italy, recently completed a phase 1 safety evaluation of muscle-derived CD133+ cells that were taken from the legs of eight boys with the disorder and then infused back to each person. The boys showed an increase in muscle fibers, and no adverse effects were observed.

Paul R. Sanberg, Professor and Director of the Center of Excellence for Aging and Brain Repair, Department of Neurosurgery at the University of South Florida College of Medicine, reported in October 2007 that South Korean scientists have shown that mesenchymal stem cells (MSCs) from human umbilical cord blood can promote recovery of motor function in rodent models of stroke and spinal cord injury following direct injections into the damaged area. The Korean Food and Drug Administration (FDA) has approved the injection of these cells directly into the brains of 13 chronic stroke patients.

A 20-year-old U.S. male patient sought stem cell treatment after facing amputation of his legs and arms due to tissue decay from meningitis. He was able to receive the experimental treatment at the Metropolitan Hospital of Santiago in the Dominican Republic, as the FDA has not approved the treatment in the United States. At two weeks after treatment, his circulation had improved, he was able to move one foot, and the therapy may save his extremities.

Umbilical cord blood–derived stem cells are the best kept secret for treatments that extend beyond blood or immune system–related diseases. In 2006 Dr. McGuckin and his associates isolated embryonic-like pluripotent stem cells from umbilical cord blood that has potential use in neurological disorders. The University of Florida has begun a phase 1/2 study of autologous umbilical cord blood transfusions to reverse hyperglycemia in 23 children with type 1 diabetes whose parents have stored their cord blood. Also in the United States, cord blood is being collected and stored for the treatment of sickle cell disease. Case studies of successes with cerebral palsy are accumulating in Mexico with the use of umbilical cord blood–derived stem cell injections. For donor treatments, umbilical cord blood–derived multipotent and pluripotent stem cells have a significant contribution to make to regenerative medicine.

The Rajavithi Hospital in Thailand is beginning a phase 1 safety evaluation of the use of oligodendrocyte progenitor cells for the possible treatment of demyelinating diseases such as multiple sclerosis.

StemCells, Inc., in conjunction with Oregon Health & Science University in Portland, have started a phase 1 safety evaluation of the surgical implantation of central nervous system (CNS) stem cells into children with infantile or late infantile neuronal ceroid lipofuscinosis, also using immune suppressants. This disorder causes the body to lack two enzymes that CNS stem cells are able to produce, so treatment may prevent further death of the person's neurons.

Ciliary neurotrophic factor (CNTF) is a growth factor that has been shown to protect the black and white rod photoreceptors that are responsible for seeing in the dark. CNTF also helps the survival of retinal ganglion cells and the regeneration of axons that relay visual information through the optic nerve to the brain. Neurotech Pharmaceuticals has sponsored a phase 2/3 multicenter clinical trial in the use of CNTF-producing human retinal pigment epithelium cells in an implant for retinitis pigmentosa and choroideremia and macular degeneration. The CNTF growth factor is gradually released through a capsule membrane into the surrounding fluid to help protect the cell of the retina.

Olfactory ensheathing cells have the ability to protect and help regenerate axons that extend from neurons. They secrete several types of growth factors for brain cells, which allow neurons to move across a glial scar. This is an important factor in treating brain and spinal cord injuries. One of the first researchers to explore the use of these cells for spinal cord injuries is Dr. Huang at Beijing Hongtianji Neuroscience Academy in Bejing, China.

## GENE THERAPY

X-linked severe combined immunodeficiency is a genetic disease that lacks a common gamma chain protein. Patients with this disorder are not able to produce T lymphocytes, and their B lymphocytes are not able to produce antibodies. A phase 1 safety study on the use of peripheral blood–derived and expanded CD34+ stem cells that contain the gene for the gamma chain protein is ongoing.

X-linked chronic granulomatous disease is caused by the lack of a protein called gp91 phox. This protein is needed to produce hydrogen peroxide in immune cells called neutrophils. Without this protein, a person is vulnerable to life-threatening infections. In addition, the neutrophils aggregate into a granuloma, an abnormal collection of cells that can then cause a blockage in organs. The patient's peripheral blood is taken, and CD34+ cells with the gene for the gp91 phox are expanded and given back to the patient.

## EMBRYONIC CLINICAL TRIALS

The Hadassah Medical Organization in Israel is beginning a clinical study of collecting human embryonic stem cells. The purpose is to establish a new stem cell line according to U.S. FDA guidelines that will be suitable for clinical trials, including those for infertility. The cell line will not be contaminated by animal feeder cells, and the donor eligibility will be based on current health and medical history.

There are a number of factors that have slowed the progress of clinical trials from embryonic and embryonic-derived cell research. These factors include the risk of tumor development and immune complications. It has been stated by experts in this field that "no rational medical research would consider using undifferentiated embryonic stem cells in a human therapeutic strategy." What can be exciting is their use in pharmaceutical and nutritional research to determine what products can be toxic to stem cells and what products can promote normal stem cell growth, mobilization, and differentiation. An entire new line of regenerative products is now being developed that will help promote the repair of damaged and diseased tissue by mobilizing our own stem cells.

**SEE ALSO:** Bone Marrow Transplants; Brazil; Cells, Embryonic; Japan; University of Texas Health Science Center at Houston.

**BIBLIOGRAPHY.** L. P. Cen, et al., "Chemotactic Effect of Ciliary Neurotrophic Factor on Macrophages in Retinal Ganglion Cell Survival and Axonal Regeneration," *Investigative Ophthalmology and Visual Science* (v.48/9, 2007); G. G. Cezar, "Can Human Embryonic Stem Cells Contribute to the Discovery of Safer and More Effective Drugs?" *Current Opinion in Chemical Biology* (v.11, 2007); H. Y. Huang, et al., "Influence of Patients Age on Functional Recovery after Transplantation of Olfactory Ensheathing Cells into Injured Spinal Cord," *Chinese Medical Journal* (v.116, 2003); H. Y. Huang, et al., "Influential Factors for Functional Improvement after Olfactory Ensheathing Cell Transplantation for Chronic Spinal Cord Injury," *Chinese Journal of Reparative and Reconstructive Surgery* (Zhongguo Xiu Fu Chong Jian Waike Za Zhi) (v.20/4, 2006); C. McGuckin, et al., "Embryonic-Like Stem Cells from Umbilical Cord Blood and Potential for Neural Modeling," *Acta Neurobiologiae Experimentalis* (v.66, 2006); G. Raisman and Y. Li,

"Repair of Neural Pathway by Olfactory Ensheathing Cells," *Nature Reviews Neuroscience* (v.8/4, 2007); F. Ramirez, D. A. Steenblock, A. G. Payne, and L. Darnall, "Umbilical Cord Stem Cell Therapy for Cerebral Palsy," *Medical Hypotheses Research* (v.3, 2006); K. D. Rhee, et al., "Molecular and Cellular Alterations Induced by Sustained Expression of Ciliary Neurotrophic Factor in a Mouse Model of Retinitis Pigmentosa," *Investigative Ophthalmology and Visual Science* (v.48/3, 2007); D. A. Steenblock and A. G. Payne, *Umbilical Cord Stem Cell Therapy, the Gift of Healing from Healthy Newborns* (Basic Health Publications, 2006); Y. Torrente, et al., "Autologous Transplantation of Muscle-Derived CD133+ Stem Cells in Duchenne Muscle Patients," *Cell Transplantation* (v.16/6, 2007); S. H. Yoon, et al., "Complete Spinal Cord Injury Treatment Using Autologous Bone Marrow Cell Transplantation and Bone Marrow Stimulation with Granulocyte Macrophage-Colony Stimulating Factor: Phase I/II Clinical Trial," *Stem Cells* (v.25, 2007).

David A. Steenblock
Personalized Regenerative Medicine

# Cloning

**CLONING IS A** process by which identical copies, or clones, of something are made. In biological sciences, it is concerned with making identical copies of biological material such as DNA fragments (molecular cloning), cells (cell cloning), or organisms. It is an asexual (involving only one parent) method of reproduction.

Stem cell research is often confused with cloning as both involve the use of embryonic stem cells. While reproductive and therapeutic cloning only involve the use of embryos, stem cell research involves the use of adult stems cells, stem cells from fetuses, umbilical cord blood cells, and amniotic fluid, along with embryonic stem cells, to find cures for a variety of degenerative diseases.

There are three main types of cloning: recombinant DNA technology or DNA cloning, reproductive cloning, and therapeutic cloning. Recombinant DNA technology or DNA cloning technology has been in use since 1970s and involves isolating a defined DNA sequence and then obtaining its multiple copies in vivo (within a cell). The DNA sequence of interest is transferred from one organism to a self-replicating genetic element, for example, a bacterial plasmid (self-replicating extra chromosomal circular DNA molecules).

There are four steps involved in DNA cloning, namely, fragmentation, ligation, transfection and screening/selection. In fragmentation, restrictive enzymes are used to isolate the required DNA sequence from chromosomal DNA. In the second step, ligation, the plasmid that serves as a vector and is originally circular is first linearized using restrictive enzymes and then the DNA fragment of interest is inserted into it by incubating them with an enzyme called ligase. In the next step the vector containing the DNA of interest is transfected into the host cells. Mostly bacteria, yeast cells or mammal cells are used as hosts. The transfected cells are then grown in culture. In the process of selection, only cells transfected are allowed to grow; this is done by antibiotic resistance marker or color selection markers on permissive media.

Reproductive cloning involves unicellular as well as multicellular cloning. In unicellular cloning a population of cells is derived from a single cell. In organism cloning a genetically identical copy of an organism is produced. This type of cloning involves a process called somatic cell nuclear transfer (SCNT) in which the nucleus containing the genetic material of the donor's somatic cell (e.g., skin cell) is removed and placed in an egg whose nucleus has already been removed. The reconstructed egg is first given some time for the nucleus and the cytoplasm to adapt to each other, and then it is stimulated, either chemically or electrically, for division. The developing embryo is then implanted into the uterus of a host female where it completes development until birth. This type of cloning has a very low success rate.

## ANIMAL CLONING

The first organism ever to be cloned was a tadpole in 1952, but many scientists questioned if the cloning had actually occurred and experiments conducted by other labs were not able to give satisfactory results. The first mammal ever reproduced by this method was Dolly the sheep in 1996 (Dolly was one success out of 276 tries). Most Finn Dorset sheep live 11–12 years, but Dolly was put down by lethal injection in February 2003 as she was suffering from lung cancer and arthritis. During her short life Dolly gave birth to six lambs.

After the first success, many animals have been cloned to this date, including sheep, cattle, mice, and goats. On the other hand, cloning of animals such as horses and chickens present certain complications and has not succeeded. This proves that certain species are more resistant to somatic nuclear transfer than others and the techniques used for cloning still need to be refined for greater success rates. Scientists at Oregon National Primate Research Center recently showed that macaque monkey embryos could be cloned to generate embryonic stem cells suggesting that generating human cells using the procedure may one day be possible. However, no cloned monkey embryos survived implantation.

Reproductive cloning has many disadvantages and is expensive and inefficient. The success rate is less than 10 percent. Cloned animals tend to have a suppressed immune system and so are prone to infections, tumor growth, and other disorders. Defects in the genetic imprints of DNA from a single donor cell may lead to abnormalities in the developing embryo. Even if they are born healthy, cloned animals tend to die at an early age.

## REPRODUCTIVE VS. THERAPEUTIC CLONING

Therapeutic cloning involves the production of human embryos for the purpose of research. The cloned human embryo is used to extract embryonic stem cells, which in turn are used for potential therapies for a wide variety of diseases. The removal of stem cells destroys the embryo, and for this purpose cloned embryos are used. Cloning in stem cell research, i.e., therapeutic cloning has yet to succeed. As yet no embryonic stem cells derived from a cloned embryo have been successful.

The first human embryo ever to be cloned was in November 2001 by scientists of Advanced Cell Technology (ATC), a biotechnology company in Massachusetts. The somatic nucleus from a skin cell was transferred into an enucleated egg. The egg containing the new genetic material was chemically stimulated by using ionomycin. Out of eight eggs used in the experiment only three began division, and only one reached a six-cell stage before division ceased completely.

The cloning procedure for reproductive and therapeutic cloning is similar. The only differentiating point between them is the application of the cloning. In reproductive cloning the new embryo, which is created by SCNT, is implanted into the uterus of a female in order to bring it to term while in therapeutic cloning the new embryo, which is also created by SCNT, is used to isolate stem cells for therapeutic purposes.

Recombinant DNA technology is important in understanding other major medical technologies including gene therapy, genetic engineering, and sequencing genomes. In 2005, South Korean scientist Hwang Woo-suk and his coauthors claimed that by cloning human embryos, they had created 11 stem cell lines that genetically matched certain patients. The paper was later found to have a large amount of fabricated data, and Hwang was indicted on embezzlement and bioethics law violations. Investigators did find that Hwang's claim of creating Snuppy, the "world's first" cloned dog, was genuine. In their efforts to clone the dog, the team obtained only three pregnancies from more than 1,000 embryo transfers into 123 recipients.

Reproductive cloning can be used for medical research purposes for production of a population of genetically identical animals, such as mice for the study of human disease. A series of laboratory mice can be cloned to produce genetically identical mice. In doing so, the mice could be used to test gene therapy or medicines to see the effects of them on living beings, and it could be confirmed that the effect that has taken place is due to the therapy, and not genetic differences of the mouse.

Reproductive cloning can also be used to revive endangered or extinct species. The first endangered animal ever to be cloned was a gaur (a wild ox) in 2001. A cow was used as a host to bring the baby gaur to term. The baby gaur, named Noah, died two days after birth from a common bacterial infection. In the same year, scientists in Italy successfully cloned a mouflon (an endangered wild sheep). The cloned mouflon is currently living in a wildlife center in Sardinia. The cloning of extinct animals presents a problem because of the lack of appropriately preserved DNA.

### CLONING STEM CELLS FOR RESEARCH

Stem cell lines created by therapeutic cloning are genetically identical to that of the adult cell donor. In the future, embryonic stem cells, which can form all types of functional adult cells, may potentially be used to produce cells or tissues to grow entire hearts, livers, and even kidneys, thus solving the problem of the shortfall of organ donors. This may be a feasible approach to growing an exact tissue match for a patient in need—if the donor nucleus came from the patient, the resulting embryonic stem cell line will be a perfect match. This would avoid problems such as tissue rejection and use of strong immunosuppressives during implantation. Still, many complications need to be overcome before this can become a reality.

In February 2002 the researchers at Advanced Cell Technology reported that they had successfully transplanted kidney-like organs in cows. A cloned cow embryo was produced using the skin cell from a donor's ear to extract the somatic nucleus.

The cloned embryo was then allowed to grow and develop into fetuses. Fetal tissue was then harvested from the clones and transplanted into the donor cow. The cow was under constant observation for three months after the transplant and it showed no sign of immune rejection.

Possible diseases that can be treated using cloned cells, tissues, and organs include all degenerative diseases, including conditions and disabilities such as Parkinson's and Alzheimer's diseases, spinal cord injury, stroke, burns, heart disease, type 1 diabetes, osteoarthritis, rheumatoid arthritis, muscular dystrophies and liver diseases.

Even though cloning has vast potential for applications in the future, it gives rise to a number of moral issues as it involves the use of an embryo, which may be considered a human being in early stages of life. As already mentioned, the embryo used is destroyed in the process. Some believe that research using cloned human embryos should not be permitted as they find it morally questionable, while others insist that this research is morally necessary because it offers the only hope of finding a cure to serious diseases such as Parkinson's, Alzheimer's, and multiple sclerosis.

**SEE ALSO:** Cells, Embryonic; Cells, Fetal; Cells, Sources of; Congress: Votes and Amendments (Cloning/Embryos); Differentiation, In Vitro and In Vivo; Egg Donation; Ethics; Nuclear Reprogramming; Nuclear Transfer, Altered; Nuclear Transfer, Somatic.

**BIBLIOGRAPHY.** American Medical Association, "Report 5 of the Council of Scientific Affairs (A-03)," www.ama-assn.org (cited November 2007); International Society for Stem Cell Research, "Stem Cell Science," www.isscr.org (cited November 2007); K. Takahashi and S. Yamanaka, "Induction of Pluripotent Stem Cells from Mouse Embryonic and Adult Fibroblast Cultures by Defined Factors," *Cell* (v.126/4, 2006); J. Thomson, et al., "Induced Pluripotent Stem Cell Lines Derived from Human Somatic Cells," *Science* (v.318, 2007); Jeffrey M. Perkel, "Life Science Technologies—Beyond Somatic Cell Nuclear Transfer," *Science*, April 20, 2007, www.sciencemag.org (cited November 2007); I. Wilmut, et al., "Somatic Cell Nuclear Transfer," *Nature* (v.419, 2002).

Sameen Arshad
National University of Science and Technology

## Coalition for the Advancement of Medical Research

**THE COALITION FOR** the Advancement of Medical Research, based in Washington, D.C., was founded in 2001 as an advocacy group to support research involving both adult and embryonic stem cells and somatic cell nuclear transfer. The coalition reaches out to state and federal legislators as well as to media outlets to educate them on the sciences of stem cell research and to present the position of the public scientific community and medical professionals regarding the need for this research as a means of developing treatment for human illness.

Memberships and opportunities for involvement are open to anyone, and the coalition has over 20,000 members from a broad spectrum of people throughout the United States, including patients and families who would benefit from the advances in treatment resulting from the research, as well as academic and medical professionals, foundations, scientific societies, and allied industry stakeholders.

## COALITION GOALS

Member groups are invited to meetings on Capitol Hill to discuss embryonic stem cell research, group link on the coalition's Web site, participate in advocacy activities as a network for media interviews, and receive e-mail updates of news relating to the field of stem cell research. These benefits are currently used by recognized organizations as members.

The activities of the coalition are focused on several goals: promoting fundamental scientific research and the translation to medical treatment by advocating for federal and state legislation, educating policy makers and the general public about the advances toward regenerative medicine, and expanding research using embryonic stem cells and somatic nuclear transfer, also known as therapeutic cloning.

By working toward these goals, the coalition seeks to protect current funding and to expand embryonic stem cell research because of the potential for these cells to develop into a new cell in the body. This research is possible with the use of excess embryos created for assisted reproduction through in vitro fertilization. More fertilized embryos are created than will be used, to increase the chance of a viable pregnancy. The coalition supports legislation to inform couples of the possibility of donating these excess embryos to researchers.

The coalition provided information to congressional lawmakers regarding the federal Stem Cell Enchancement Acts to provide federal funding as well as regulation and oversight that have passed the House Representatives in 2005 and 2007 and passed in the Senate in 2006 and 2007. Both bills were vetoed by President George W. Bush in 2006 and 2007, respectively.

Because neither bill was approved, the United States remains a leader in the field of research but without regulation or consistent funding. To fill the gap, each state is left to determine both funding and what types of stem cell research to support. The coalition has prepared position papers, sent letters on the coalition position to state legislators in states considering stem cell legislation, and prepared information for the media, as well as having the information available on the Web site.

The coalition supports increased federal funding because private funding does not ensure that research meets socioethical guidelines, nor does it give the public a voice in oversight or in how the research is carried out. Funding also gives additional opportunities to expand research to underfunded research universities and medical institutes.

In lieu of federal policy on stem cell research, the coalition supports appropriate legislation at the state level, through this creates a patchwork of states that support stem cell research and attract experts in biomedical research, as well as states that create broad legislation or bans that in effect discourage and stop stem cell research or therapeutic cloning.

In presenting public opinion, the coalition gathers information from a variety of opinion surveys, such as Gallup polls, the Pew Research Center, *USAToday*, and others, as well as performs its own opinion polls.

The coalition relies on member support and involvement by individuals to contact legislators and become involved in gaining support for stem cell research and somatic cell nuclear transfer. Their Web site (www.stemcellfunding.org) contains useful information not only on stem cell research but also on legislative initiatives and on support needed. The Web site details the coalition's activities at federal and state levels, provides a listing of organization members with links to their Web sites for additional information, and provides samples of letters to legislators and the media.

**SEE ALSO:** Cells, Embryonic; Nuclear Transfer, Somatic; Stem Cells, Bush Ruling.

**BIBLIOGRAPHY.** Coalition for the Advancement of Medical Research, www.stemcellfunding.org (cited November 2007).

LYN MICHAUD
INDEPENDENT SCHOLAR

# Colorado

**COLORADO HAS NO** specific legislation either permitting or prohibiting human embryonic stem cell research. Representative Diana DeGette, a Democrat from Colorado, has introduced and sponsored bills for Federal Stem Cell Research funding and enhancement that have later been vetoed by the president. Colorado State Legislative action from 2006 included a $2 million appropriation for the specific purpose of promoting growth in bioscience research in Colorado through the Bioscience Discovery Evaluation Grant Program. This money is earmarked for private and university research in a wide range of disciplines including diagnosing and treating human disease and improving agriculture.

To provide facilities for improving Colorado's biotechnology research, a $4.3 billion redevelopment project at the former Fitzsimons Army Medical Center created the 160-acre Colorado Bioscience Park Aurora and 217-acre campus of University of Colorado Health Sciences Center.

The first human fetal cell transplant for the treatment of Parkinson's disease in the United States was performed at the University of Colorado Hospital in November, 1988 by Drs. Curt Freed and Robert Breeze. Studies by Freed and others show that fetal tissue can be safely transplanted into the human brain and provide patients with improvements in motor function.

The Charles C. Gates Regenerative Medicine and Stem Cell Biology Program began with a $6 million grant to University of Colorado Medical School from the Charles C. and June S. Gates Family Fund in August 2006. The research center is headed by Dr. Dennis Roop, a noted stem cell researcher, who brought additional U.S. National Institutes of Health funding for the study of Parkinson's disease, cancer, and genetic skin disorders using both adult and embryonic stem cells.

The University of Colorado Health Sciences Center, founded in 1883, is a public institution in Denver, Colorado. The university confers bachelor's, master's, doctoral, and professional degrees in health sciences. A Ph.D. graduate program in Cell and Developmental Biology includes stem cell biology in addition to cell biology, developmental biology, neuroscience, and molecular biology and molecular structure.

In addition to classroom instruction, interdisciplinary research opportunities in stem cell research related to human disease include pancreatic stem cell development and molecular biology/transcriptional regulation of embryonic pancreatic development using mouse gene knockout techniques, mouse embryonic and extra-embryonic stem cells/transcriptional regulation of mouse embryonic development and the role of transcription factors in mammary gland development and breast cancer.

**SEE ALSO:** Cells, Adult; Cells, Embryonic; Regulations Overview; United States.

**BIBLIOGRAPHY.** "Biotechnology and Life Sciences," *Colorado Data Book* (August 2006); Rocky Mountain Blood and Bone Marrow Transplant Program, www.rockymountainbmt.com (cited November 2007); University of Colorado Health Sciences Center, "Stem Cell Biology Research," www.uchsc.edu (cited November 2007).

LYN MICHAUD
INDEPENDENT SCHOLAR

# Columbia University

**COLUMBIA UNIVERSITY IS** located in New York City. Its roots date back to 1754, when the King of England established the school by royal charter; it was originally known as King's College. Columbia is New York's oldest university and opened the first medical school—the College of Physicians and Surgeons—granting an M.D. degree in the United States in 1770. When the medical school formed an alliance with Presbyterian Hospital in 1922, it became the first academic medical center in the United States. Columbia offers undergraduate, graduate, and professional programs in a variety of academic disciplines with research opportunities.

The Columbia University Health Sciences campus combines medical care, education, and scientific research (both fundamental research with the ultimate goal of translation into clinical applications and clinical trials). Columbia has long been a leader in stem cell research, experiencing such successes as the first successful transfer of genes from one cell to another, the discovery that embryos and teratomas are made up of rapidly dividing stem cells, making the determination that stem cells have controls at certain points to stop them from dividing outside the uterus, and coating mouse embryonic epithelial cells and inducing them to become motor neurons in cell culture.

Columbia University Medical Center provides patient clinical services, is home to Columbia's medical school, and performs scientific research (both basic research and clinical trials). Stem cell researchers are working on the heart, eye, blood, skin, and immune system. The center's past successes include the discovery that antidepressants stimulate stem cells to form new brain cells; that embryonic stem cells can be turned into light-sensing neurons; that hair follicle epithelial cells can be used as a source of adult stem cells to regenerate skin; that neural and musculoskeletal stem cells can be differentiated into motor neurons; that activated stem and immune cells may be useful for leukemia, lymphoma, and solid tumors; and of gene and cell therapy to help pace the heart adult stem cells.

## RESEARCH CENTERS AND PROGRAMS

Audubon Biotechnology and Research Park was developed by the university, the state, and the city of New York in an area adjacent to Columbia University Medical Center. The park houses the Mary Woodard Lasker Biomedical Research building, which opened in October 1995 and is home to the Audubon Business Technology Center; the Russ Berrie Medical Science Pavilion, with specialties in diabetes, genetics, and pediatrics; and the Irving Cancer Research Center, which opened in May 2005. The Audubon Business and Technology Center is an incubator for business start-ups for private research and development in biotechnology with laboratories and regulatory and commerce assistance.

The Naomi Berrie Diabetes Center was established in 1997 and moved into the Russ Berrie Medical Science Pavilion in 1998. The center focuses on combining patient- and family-centered care and education with diabetes research. Researchers are working to create insulin-producing islet cells from stem cells because cell therapies using islet cells transplant are in short supply, and cells and stem cells that are differentiated into islet cells may be a new source.

The Herbert Irving Comprehensive Cancer Center builds on Columbia's long history for cancer research. The center provides patient care and conducts basic and clinical research, including research using stem cells. The center's eight research programs are organized into basic research, disease-specific research, and population-based research. Program activities focus on different aspects of cancer, from its molecular and cellular mechanisms through its unique behavior in different tissues to statistical aspects of its occurrence and treatment in large populations. Researchers are working with cord blood stem cells and cancer therapies to expand a rich source of stem and immune cell transplants for childhood leukemia and solid tumors. Another research project includes the genetic mechanisms that control cell division and gene expression in cancer cells and studies how cancer disrupts DNA repair mechanisms and encourages instability.

The Stem Cell Consortium brings together a variety of academic disciplines for collaboration, education, and research to use innovation in basic science and to translate that information into clinical applications for treating human disease. Researchers are working on adult and embryonic stem cells to study cell development, cell and tissue repair, and the use of stem cells as a tool for studying disease mechanisms in developing new therapies. Columbia's researchers work with embryonic and adult stem cells—both human and animal—to study cell development and the possibility of repairing or replacing cells, tissues, and whole organs.

Researchers in the Neural Stem Cell Program investigate the biology of neural stem cells derived from human embryonic stem cells or adult nervous system and the possibility of using stem cells to treat neurological disorders. Stem cells can be used to generate any cell in the central nervous system and have the potential to repair injured or diseased tissue. Research being done under the Neural Stem Cell Program includes examinations of neural development including adult neurogenesis, interactions in brain development, and signaling pathways; developmental studies of the nervous system, neural crest, and specificity to the diseases of Parkinson's and other neurodegenerative disorders to find the molecular basis of neurodegeneration; and the activity of proteins in the migration of neurons with the hope of finding a therapeutic strategy for treatment. Additional research by the various researchers includes studies of Alzheimer's disease by examining the mechanisms of stem cell activity in relation to memory.

## COLLABORATIONS

In addition to collaborative research among the departments at Columbia University and international collaboration, as with the Karolinska Institute in Sweden, Columbia University was the first to transplant retinal tissue to correct age-related vision loss in the photo receptors. The hope is that using stem cells may eliminate tissue rejection. The researchers also were able to isolate sheets of embryonic color-sensitive photoreceptors.

Research collaboration with the Whitehead Institute and MIT is focused on developing new cell treatment. The contribution by Columbia University to the program includes investigating how motor neurons in the spinal cord develop to innervate specific muscles. Researchers work to identify molecular mechanisms involved in normal development and in degeneration.

In collaboration with Stony Brook University, researchers are using mesenchymal cells from bone marrow and modifying them to express the ion channel for pacing the heart; they then connect these cells to cardiac cells in both culture medium and in animal models. This finding follows on the discovery that the genes to regulate the heart rate and rhythm were found in mesenchymal stem cells. The possibility of delivering these cells to specific regions of the heart meant that they could be made to function as pacemakers. The hope in regenerative medicine is to eliminate the complications associated with using viruses for gene therapy and in the ability of mesenchymal stem cells to carry small molecules and genetic signals.

Finally, Columbia offers the Brunie Prize in Neural Stem Cell Research, which recognizes graduate student research. To be eligible for the $2,000 award, the graduate student must have passed their qualifying exam and be enrolled in the Columbia University Graduate School of Arts and Sciences.

**SEE ALSO:** Cells, Embryonic; Lasker Foundation; Massachusetts Institute of Technology; New York; Sweden.

**BIBLIOGRAPHY.** Audubon Center, "Mission," www.auduboncenter.org (cited November 2007); Stem Cell Initiative, www.cumc.columbia.edu (cited November 2007); Naomi Berrie Diabetes Center, www.nbdiabetes.org (cited November 2007).

Lyn Michaud
Independent Scholar

# Congress: Votes and Amendments (Cloning/ Embryos)

**OVER THE LAST** decade, the federal government has taken an active role in the public debate over human cloning and stem cell research. Despite repeated attempts by the U.S. Congress to ban human cloning, all such efforts have failed, leaving cloning still legal in the United States. As far as embryonic stem cell research is concerned, the issue is not whether to permit such research (there are currently no prohibitions on private organizations from engaging in cloning research) but, rather, whether or not to allocate federal taxpayer dollars for these purposes.

Congress first placed restrictions on federal funding in 1995, and then in 2001, President Bush announced that he would permit federal funding of research on cell lines that were available before his announcement, but prohibit funding of research on cell lines obtained afterward. Since then, Congress has made two major attempts to override President Bush's policy; both attempts have resulted in insuperable presidential vetoes.

## CLONING

Shortly following the February 1997 announcement that researchers in Scotland had successfully cloned Dolly the sheep, President Clinton issued an executive order, which remains in force, banning the use of federal funds for purposes of human cloning. This order, however, did not prohibit research on cloning done by private institutions.

There are currently no federal laws in the United States that prohibit human cloning, either for research or for reproductive purposes. Research cloning refers to when scientists attempt to create a clone of an embryo only, which would then be used for scientific research. Such an embryo would not be permitted to continue to grow and develop. Reproductive cloning, in contrast, refers to creating an organism that grows to maturity. This organism would be genetically identical to the original. Thus far, scientists have been unable to successfully create a human clone for either purpose.

Nevertheless, there have been three major attempts by Congress to prohibit or regulate human cloning. The first attempt took place in February 1998, when Democratic Senators Dianne Feinstein of California and Edward Kennedy of Massachusetts formally introduced S. 1602, which sought to ban human reproductive cloning for 10 years while allowing for limited research cloning. The bill would have required scientists to eventually destroy cloned embryos rather than allowing them to grow to maturity. In response, Republican Senators Kit Bond of Missouri, Bill Frist of Tennessee, and Trent Lott of Mississippi introduced S. 1601, which was intended to prohibit human cloning for either reproductive or research purposes. S. 1601 was quickly blocked by a procedural tactic, and the Senate declined to consider a vote on the Feinstein–Kennedy version of the bill.

The second attempt came in April 2001, when independent scientists announced their intentions to clone a human being. The House considered two separate bills similar to those considered by the Senate in 1998. H.R. 2172, the Cloning Prohibition Act of 2001, introduced by Representative James Greenwood, a Republican from Pennsylvania, would have banned reproductive human cloning for 10 years and required private researchers to inform the government if human embryos were cloned for research purposes. H.R. 2525, The Human Cloning Prohibition Action of 2001, was also introduced by Representative David Weldon, a Democrat from Florida, and called for a ban on both reproductive and research cloning. The House passed H.R. 2525 in July by a vote of 265–162, with most House Republicans supporting the bill, along with several conservative Democrats. The bill failed to become law, however, because of the failure of the Senate to vote on the bill's counterpart, S. 790, proposed by Senator Sam Brownback, a Republican from Kansas.

The third attempt took place in February 2003 when Weldon again introduced a similar bill, H.R. 534, the Human Cloning Prohibition

Act of 2003, which passed the House 241–155; again, however, the Senate declined to schedule a vote on the bill. Research into human cloning by private organizations in the United States thus remains legal.

## STEM CELL RESEARCH

Embryonic stem cell research and its surrounding political controversies have received a large amount of attention over the past several years, with vocal and passionate opinions expressed by both sides of the debate. The controversy centers around whether or not one considers embryos to be, in fact, human beings entitled to protection from the government. Embryonic stem cell research involves the destruction of a human embryo in its very early stages of development. Opponents claim that the destruction of a fertilized embryo is morally wrong because the embryo, although small, is human life and must be treated as such.

Supporters, in contrast, argue that an embryo fertilized outside of the uterus with no intention to be implanted and allowed to develop normally has not achieved human status. Furthermore, supporters point out that fertilized embryos routinely are created through in vitro fertility procedures and are not then implanted back in the mother's uterus. The majority of these embryos are simply discarded, and supporters argue that they might as well be used for research that could potentially be used to save other lives by assisting in finding cures for diseases.

As stated previously, the controversial issue for Congress is not whether or not to prohibit stem cell research outright (it is still legal for private medical organizations) but, rather, whether or not taxpayer dollars should be used by the federal government to fund such research.

The first significant legislation related to stem cell research was a small section of a 1995 appropriations bill for the National Institutes of Health (NIH). Section 509 of H.R. 3010 contained a ban on federal funding to the NIH for the purpose of human embryo research. In the meantime, however, the NIH released draft guidelines in December 1999 that outlined how the organization would theoretically handle stem cell research if permitted to do so by the federal government. President Clinton delayed making a decision on the issue, deferring instead to his successor.

President Bush made a nationally televised announcement on August 9, 2001, in which he revealed his administration's official policy regarding stem cell research. The president permitted federal funding of stem cell research on cell lines already in existence at the time of the announcement. However, the national government would not support or fund research on stem cells collected after the fact because it would, as the president explained, encourage the further destruction of human embryos.

A number of minor congressional bills were introduced over the next several years seeking to ease the funding restrictions that President Bush had put into place in 2001, but none successfully made it out of committee. The first victory for supporters came in February 2005 with the passage of H.R. 810, the Stem Cell Research Enhancement Act, sponsored by representatives Mike Castle, a Republican from Delaware, and Diana DeGette, a Democrat form Colorado. Largely because of the attention that stem cell research had received during the 2004 presidential campaign, the issue gained sufficient support to pass the House with a vote of 238–194.

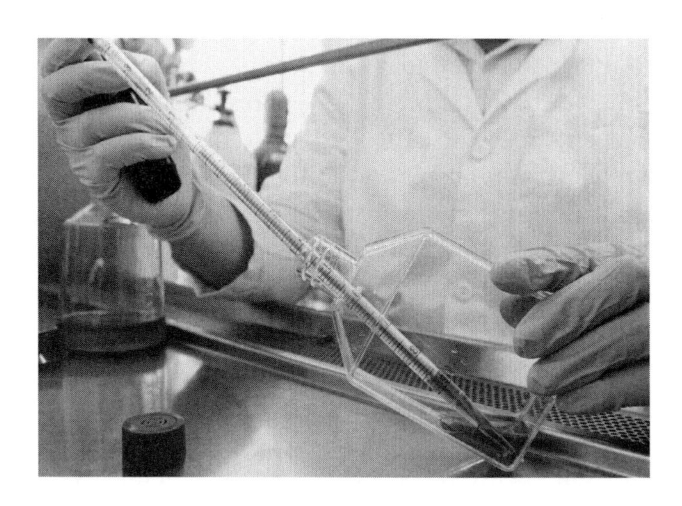

*The successful Democratic congressional campaign of 2006 included a commitment to funding for stem cell research.*

The bill still faced an uphill battle in the Senate, however. It took more than a year for Senate leaders, including majority leader and practicing physician Bill Frist, a Republican from Tennessee, to best decide how to submit the matter to a vote. In June 2006, it was determined that the Senate would vote on three separate bills. To avoid a Senate parliamentary procedure known as a filibuster, in which any senator can prevent voting on a bill by refusing to yield to the floor, each bill would require a supermajority of 60 votes. The three bills included the original H.R. 810, which would expand federal funding for stem cell research by the NIH. The second was S. 3504, the Fetus Farming Prohibition Act, sponsored by Senator Rick Santorum, a Republican from Pennsylvania, which prohibited the creation of "fetal farms," where embryos would be grown specifically for research purposes. The third bill was S. 2754, the Alternative Pluripotent Stem Cell Therapies Enhancement Act, also sponsored by Santorum, which would encourage research into investigating alternative sources from which to derive stem cells that do not involve actual destruction of human embryos (pluripotent stem cells).

Each bill passed the Senate on July 18, 2006. The two bills sponsored by Santorum received unanimous support, whereas the key H.R. 810 bill passed 63–37. The Senate bills then had to be passed by the House. The fetus farming bill passed the House unanimously, but the "alternative sources bill failed, lacking key Democratic support. It was later argued that House Democrats did not want to give President Bush the option of vetoing H.R. 810 while signing S. 2754, which would have allowed him to "save face" by indicating his support for researching alternative sources of stem cells but not specifically expanding research funding.

President Bush signed the fetal farm bill into law and vetoed H.R. 810, which would have eased restrictions for federal funding of stem cell research—the first veto of his tenure as president. In a statement, the president explained that providing federal funding for stem cell research "crosses a moral boundary that our decent society needs to respect." The House was unable to override the presidential veto.

Democrats took control of both the Senate and the House in the 2006 midterm congressional elections. A major feature of their national campaign included a commitment to pass legislation extending federal funding for stem cell research. Within days after taking office in January 2007, the new Democratic House passed the Stem Cell Research Enhancement Act by a vote of 253–174. The Senate followed in April by passing S. 5 by a vote of 63–34. Again, a bill to ease restrictions on federal funding for stem cell research went to the president, who vetoed it on June 20, 2007. There have been no additional attempts by Congress since.

## CONGRESSIONAL BILLS, 107TH–110TH CONGRESS

In the 107th Congress, H.R. 2059 and S. 723, the Stem Cell Research Act of 2001, would have amended the Public Health Service Act to provide for stem cell research. H.R. 2096 and S. 1349, the Responsible Stem Cell Research Act of 2001, would have required the federal government to create a stem cell donor bank. H. Con. Res. 17, Support for Pluripotent Stem Cell Research, was introduced to express the sense of the House on alternative sources of stem cells. H.R. 2747, the Stem Cell Research for Patient Benefit Act of 2001, sought to create specific guidelines directing research using stem cells. H.R. 2838, the New Century Health Advantage Act, would have required the federal government to conduct stem cell research and repeal the Human Embryo Research Ban. H.R. 2863, the Cell Development Research Act of 2001, would have created a federal advisory committee charged with making recommending on stem cell and cloning research. H.R. 4011, the Science of Stem Cell Research Act, would have established a Stem Cell Research Board to investigate the consequences of President Bush's stem cell policy announced in August 2001.

In the 108th Congress H.R. 534, the Human Cloning Prohibition Act of 2003, which sought to ban both reproductive and therapeutic cloning, was passed by the House 241–155. H.R. 801, to amend the Federal Food, Drug, and Cosmetic Act, would have banned reproductive cloning but allowed for therapeutic cloning. H.R. 916, the Human Cloning Research Prohibition Act, would have prohibited human cloning research funded by federal dollars. H.R. 938, the Human Cloning Prevention Act of 2003, would have prevented the federal government from contracting with any organization that "engaged in human cloning." S. 245, the Human Cloning Prohibition Act of 2003, would have prohibited both reproductive and therapeutic cloning. S. 303, the Human Cloning Ban and Stem Cell Research Protection Act of 2003, sought to ban reproductive cloning but allow therapeutic cloning.

In the 109th Congress, H.R. 162, the Stem Cell Replenishment Act of 2005, would have allowed for federal funding of stem cell research on stem cells derived after President Bush's ban took effect. H.R. 222, the Human Cloning Research Prohibition Act, intended to prohibit federal research of human cloning. H.R. 810, the Stem Cell Research Enhancement Act of 2005, would have required the federal government to support stem cell research, passed the House 238–194, passed the Senate 63–37, and was vetoed by the president on July 19, 2006, House failed to override veto 235–193. H.R. 1357, the Human Cloning Prohibition Act of 2005, sought to prohibit human cloning. S. 471, the Stem Cell Research Enhancement Act of 2005, sought to expand federal funding of stem cell research. S. 658, the Human Cloning Prohibition Act of 2005, sought to prohibit human cloning. S. 659, the Human Chimera Prohibition Act of 2005, intended to "prohibit human chimeras" (i.e., human/animal hybrids). S. 876, the Human Cloning Ban and Stem Cell Research Protection Act of 2005, intended to ban human cloning and "protect" stem cell research.

In the 110th Congress, H.R. 3, an amendment to Public Health Service Act to expand stem cell research, passed the House 253–174. H.R. 322, the Alternative Pluripotent Stem Cell Therapies Enhancement Act of 2007, would have required the federal government to research sources of stem cells other than embryos (e.g., umbilical cords). H.R. 457, the Cures Can Be Found Act of 2007, would have provided a tax credit for individuals who donate umbilical cord blood or stem cells to organizations that do not engage in embryonic stem cell research. H.R. 2807 would have intensified stem cell research "showing evidence of substantial clinical benefit." S. 5, the Stem Cell Research Enhancement Act of 2007, would have expanded federal funding of stem cell research, passed the Senate 63–34, passed by the House 247–176, and was vetoed by President Bush June 20, 2007. S. 30, the HOPE (Hope Offered through Principled and Ethical) Stem Cell Research Act, would have intensified research to derive stem cell lines, passed the Senate 70–28. S. 51, the Pluripotent Stem Cell Therapy Enhancement Act of 2007, would have required the federal government to research alternative sources of stem cells other than embryos. S. 362, the Stem Cell Research Expansion Act, would have authorized the government to fund stem cell research that did not involve the destruction of an embryo. S. 363, the Hope Offered through Principled, Ethically-Sound Stem Cell Research Act, would have prohibited federal research on embryonic stem cell and also prohibited individuals from receiving medical treatments involving the destruction of embryos. S. 812, the Human Cloning Ban and Stem Cell Research Protection Act of 2007, would have prohibited human cloning and "protected" stem cell research.

**SEE ALSO:** Cloning; Federal Government Policies; Moral Status of Embryo; National Institutes of Health; Presidential Campaigns; Regulations Overview; *Roe v. Wade*; Stem Cells, Bush Ruling.

**BIBLIOGRAPHY.** "AAAS Policy Brief: Stem Cell Research," www.aaas.org (cited March 2008); Center for Genetics and Society, "Failure to Pass Federal Cloning Legislation, 1997-2003," geneticsandsociety .org (cited March 2008); Maria Godoy, Joe Palca, and Beth Novey, "Key Moments in the Stem-Cell Debate," www.npr.org (cited March 2008); National Institutes of Health, "107th Congress Stem Cell Research," stemcells.nih.gov/policy/legislation/archive107.htm (cited March 2008); National Institutes of Health, "108th

Congress Stem Cell Research," stemcells.nih.gov/policy/legislation/archive108.htm (cited March 2008); National Institutes of Health, "109th Congress Stem Cell Research," stemcells.nih.gov/policy/legislation/archive109.htm (cited March 2008); National Institutes of Health, "110th Congress Stem Cell Research," stemcells.nih.gov/policy/legislation (cited March 2008); National Institutes of Health, "Federal Policy," stemcells.nih.gov/policy (cited March 2008).

Benjamin Knoll
University of Iowa

# Connecticut

**THE CONNECTICUT DEPARTMENT** of Health aims to make the state of Connecticut an "international center of excellence for stem cell research." On June 15, 2005, the Connecticut General Assembly approved Public Act 05-149 entitled "An Act Permitting Stem Cell Research and Banning the Cloning of Human Beings."

The act was signed by Governor M. Jodi Rell and incorporated into Connecticut law. This act made Connecticut the third U.S. state to publicly support stem cell research, budgeting $20 million for embryonic or human adult stem cell research for the fiscal year of 2007–2008. It earned Connecticut the nickname Stem Cell Central, given by the *New York Times* in a major article reporting on the act.

The first call for research proposals received 70 applications from Connecticut researchers and resulted in nearly all $20 million being allocated to researchers at Yale University in New Haven, Wesleyan University in Middletown, and the University of Connecticut, the main campus of which is at Storrs.

For the remaining fiscal years until the one ending in June 2015, an additional $10 million was to be set aside for this research. The funding for the research would come from the State of Connecticut's Tobacco Settlement Fund. As of 2007, Connecticut receives just over $375 million annually from its tobacco settlement payments, as well as from a tobacco tax.

The Connecticut Stem Cell Research Fund has supported projects of all sizes. Dr. Michael P. Snyder of Yale University received $3,815,477 to study an integrated approach to neural differentiation of human embryonic stem cells, and embryonic stem cell core facilities at three universities (one at Yale and one joint facility at the University of Connecticut and Wesleyan University) received $2.5 million each. Dr. Joseph LoTurco at the University of Connecticut received approximately $500,000 to study the migration and integration of embryonic stem cell derived neurons into cerebral cortex.

Many more researchers were granted approximately $200,000 for smaller, shorter studies that also targeted the molecular biology of stem cells, including a grant to Dr. Yingqun Joan Huang of Yale University, who studies the function of the fragile X mental retardation protein in early human neural development, and one to Dr. Gang Xu of the University of Connecticut for the study of the generation of insulin-producing cells from human embryonic stem cells.

To oversee the Stem Cell Research Fund, the State of Connecticut has a Stem Cell Research Advisory Committee, with a Subcommittee on Law and Ethics, as well as a Stem Cell Research Peer Review Committee. The Peer Review Committee reviews submitted proposals for funding by the Connecticut Stem Cell Research Fund, following guidelines established by the U.S. National Institutes of Health.

To oversee the use and research of stem cells at the University of Connecticut, this institution has organized an Embryonic Stem Cells Research Oversight Committee (UC-ESCRO). UC-ESCRO functions to guide researchers at the University of Connecticut, as well as those scientists affiliated with the university, through their research to ensure ethical compliance and proper handling of sensitive topics. If the oversight committee determines a particular project to be unethical, regardless of the funding source, this project will not be allowed at the university. Wesleyan University and Yale University have similar committees.

The Connecticut Department of Public Health, the Connecticut Stem Cell Coalition, and Connecticut United for Research Excellence sponsor the annual conference StemCONN. This conference is an international symposium for stem cell research. One result from the conference is a publicly available panel discussion on stem cells, which is targeted toward people who are not necessarily scientists. In particular, the panel aims to stimulate discussion and thereby education and awareness among youth in high schools and colleges across the state.

**SEE ALSO:** *Individual U.S. State Articles*; Biotechnology, History of; Clinical Trials Within U.S.: Batten Disease; Clinical Trials Within U.S.: Blind Process; Clinical Trials Within U.S.: Cancer; Clinical Trials Within U.S.: Heart Disease; Clinical Trials Within U.S.: Peripheral Vascular Disease; Clinical Trials Within U.S.: Skin Transplants (Burns); Clinical Trials Within U.S.: Spinal Cord Injury; Clinical Trials Within U.S.: Traumatic Brain Injury; Ethics; Federal Government Policies; Moral Status of Embryo; Special Interest/Lobby Groups; United States.

**BIBLIOGRAPHY.** C. B. Cohen, *Renewing the Stuff of Life: Stem Cells, Ethics, and Public Policy* (Oxford University Press, 2007); C. Fox, *Cell of Cells: The Global Race to Capture and Control the Stem Cell* (Norton, 2007); T. Kaplan, "Suddenly, Connecticut Is Stem Cell Central," *New York Times* (November 25, 2007); K. R. Monroe, R. Miller, and J. Tobis, eds., *Fundamentals of the Stem Cell Debate: The Scientific, Religious, Ethical, and Political Issues* (University of California Press, 2007).

Claudia Winograd
University of Illinois, Urbana-Champaign

# Coriell Institute

**THE CORIELL INSTITUTE** for Medical Research, located on the University of Medicine and Dentistry of New Jersey campus in Camden, New Jersey, is a not-for-profit research institution founded in 1953 by Dr. Lewis Coriell. Dr. Coriell designed breakthrough cell line storage and processing technologies in the early 1950s. This technology allowed other scientists to create vaccines (including the polio vaccine by Dr. Salk and Dr. Sabin) and treatments.

In 1956 laboratory space was provided to researchers by the South Jersey Medical Research Foundation. The name was changed to the Institute for Medical Research in 1966 and finally to the Coriell Institute for Medical Research to honor Dr. Coriell when he retired in 1985.

The Coriell Institute remains at the forefront of cell technology, with scientists working on cell cultures, cell characterization, and cryopreservation and electronic catalogs. The Coriell Institute focuses on research, cell banking, and public education.

## RESEARCH

Research at Coriell from the very beginning has been both basic (fundamental processes and principles) and clinical (applied research toward therapeutic use). Research topics at the institute have ranged from cancer, environmental mutagens, human cytogenetics, medical and laboratory clean rooms, and infectious diseases, to methods to improve cell culture techniques.

The Coriell Institute has developed expertise in human cell culturing techniques that has become standard in research laboratories, including the techniques for freezing and thawing cells, sterile handling of cultures, and specialized containment hoods. Dr. Coriell initiated the first studies using liquid nitrogen for very low temperature freezing and storage of skin and blood cell cultures.

Under the leadership of Dr. Michael Christman, the Coriell Institute has established the Delaware Valley Personalized Medicine Project (genetic profiling and correlation with health/disease risks and treatment response). The research will require the cooperation of area hospitals including Cooper Hospital (adjacent to Coriell Institute) to enroll patient volunteers in this genetic study correlating disease, treatment, and prognosis to the individual genetic profile. Coriell Institute researchers will attempt to discover presently unknown genes correlated with increased risk for diseases, to understand differing patient responses to treatments, and to determine confidentiality and use of the resulting information for medical applications by patients and their treating physicians and healthcare team. A current clinical research program in stem cell biology involves a partnership between Coriell Institute and the Cooper Heart Institute at Cooper University Hospital. The research focuses on repairing damaged heart cells using stem cells from cord blood.

## CELL BANKING

Coriell Institute maintains the largest, most extensive cell line and tissue repositories spanning six familial cancer classifications and 26 major diseases (their full repository profile can be accessed on the Web at www.coriell.org). In 1964 the National Cancer Institute funded the first standard characterized cell repository at the Coriell Institute. Coriell expanded its cell banking capabilities to include the Human Genetic Mutant Cell Repository in 1972 and the national Aging Cell Repository in 1974. A partnership with BioRep in Milan, Italy, has created the largest cryogenic cell line repository in the world.

In 2007 Coriell established a multimillion dollar Genotyping and Microarray Center—a facility that processes up to 2000 DNA or RNA samples per month. This high-capacity facility consists of state-of-the-art equipment and receives samples from laboratories around the world requesting genotyping and microarray analysis.

Cell cultures and DNA can be established from blood or skin for genetic disease research. Lymphocytes (white blood cells) can be immortalized with a virus and then replicated indefinitely in culture medium. Fibroblasts (cells from a skin biopsy) can be used to establish a cell line, though their growth in culture medium is time limited. These cells can then be frozen and stored at Coriell Institute. The cells are stored in 750,000 vials in 62 giant tanks full of liquid nitrogen, held at –316 degrees F.

Scientists from around the world have access to more than 120,000 cell lines for their research. Coriell reports it has distributed more than 160,000 cell lines in addition to over 50,000 DNA samples a year to researchers in 62 nations. Its cell lines have been used by the Human Genome Project (global program for mapping the human genome) and by the International HapMap Project (to identify genes causing disease).

## NEW JERSEY STEM CELL RESOURCE

In December 2005 New Jersey became the first state to finance research using human embryonic stem cells, including cell lines prohibited from use in research by federal funding restrictions. The Ellie Katz Umbilical Cord Blood Program and the Coriell Institute for Medical Research received $350,000 each in December 2005 to create the nation's first public cord and placental blood bank for stem cell research.

The New Jersey Stem Cell Resource (NJSCR), located at the Coriell Institute, was created by an executive order of the governor enacted on October 18, 2005. The Coriell Institute (also home to the New Jersey Cord Blood Bank) established a research bank to provide umbilical cord blood and placenta stem cell samples for New Jersey scientists and for researchers around the world. NJSCR also stocks cord blood mononuclear cells, CD34+ stem cells, CD34 depleted mononuclear cells, cord blood, mesenchymal stromal cells, and placental mesenchymal stromal cells. The center also accepts custom orders for fresh cord blood, fresh umbilical cords and placentas, and custom cell selection.

**SEE ALSO:** Cells, Embryonic; New Jersey.

**BIBLIOGRAPHY.** BioRep, "The Coriell Partnership," www.biorep.it (cited November 2007); Coriell Institute, "About Coriell," www.coriell.org (cited November 2007); Coriell Institute, "Coriell and Cooper to Pioneer Stem Cell Heart Research," *Discover Quarterly Newsletter* (2006); New Jersey Commission on Science and Technology, "Stem Cell Research in New Jersey," www.state.nj.us/scitech/stemcell (cited November 2007).

Lyn Michaud
Independent Scholar

# Cytogenetic Instability of Stem Cells

**DIVIDING CELLS ARE** subject to errors during cell division that can result in abnormal chromosome patterns. Cytogenetics, which involves the study of abnormal chromosomes, has shown that human and mouse embryonic stem (ES) cells from laboratories throughout the world tend to show the same chromosome aberrations. The most frequent change in human ES cells involves gain of chromosomes 12 or 17, both of which are associated with cancer, whereas mouse embryonic stem cells tend to acquire extra copies of chromosomes 8 or 11. There is no way to distinguish embryonic stem cells with abnormal chromosomes from normal stem cells without genetic testing, as both express the same proteins and typical stem cell markers, and the presence of chromosome changes does not affect the ability of these cells to give rise to different cell lineages.

Although accidents in division leading to extra or missing chromosomes occur in dividing cells of all tissues and species, most of these lead to cell death. However, when a specific chromosome change results in the affected cells having a growth advantage, cells with this change tend to increase and completely replace the normal cells in about 10 passages. Therefore, it is not surprising that the most common chromosome changes seen in human and mouse ES cells involve acquisition of those extra chromosomes that are associated with cancer when they occur in the body. For example, the presence of extra copies of chromosome 12, and often of chromosome 17, is characteristic of spontaneously developing germ cell tumors of the testis in human males.

In both cultured ES cells as well as germ cell tumors, the presence of extra chromosomes 12 and 17 tends to increase proliferation and mitotic instability, leading to acquisition of other chromosome changes. Because the most common secondary changes involve acquisition of extra copies of chromosome 20 and the X, these must also confer some growth advantage, as is shown by the fact that in rare cases human ES cell cultures have acquired an extra X or chromosome 20 as the sole abnormality. In mouse ES cells, loss of Y is a recurrent change, though not so frequent as acquisition of an extra chromosome 8.

Mouse ES cells tend to be more unstable than their human counterparts, often acquiring chromosome aberrations at early passages. The advantage of research using mouse ES cells is that these cells can undergo targeted mutations and, when injected into mouse embryos, can create chimeric offspring with specific genetic constitutions useful for research. However, if the ES cell has an extra chromosome 8, such cells are unlikely to enter the germ line. In fact, in mouse ES cells, there appears to be an inverse correlation between the efficiency of targeted mutations entering the germline and the growth rate of the ES cells in culture, perhaps because cells from the more rapidly proliferating cultures are likely to have an extra chromosome 8.

Although some researchers claim normal chromosomes in human ES cells after extended time in culture (more than 100 passages), others have reported recurrent aberrations involving chromosomes 12 and 17 occurring between passages 25 and 45. Despite optimal culture techniques, guaranteeing the genetic integrity of ES cells is difficult because of the stresses of tissue culture and the selective pressures exerted on the cells after cultures have been frozen and thawed. Because cultures of cryopreserved ES cells tend to grow poorly after thawing, a few cells with a growth advantage resulting from an extra chromosome 12 or 17 can increase in number and eventually overgrow the normal cells.

## ADULT STEM CELLS

Unlike ES cells, which can give rise to any lineage, adult stem cells can only generate cells of a specific lineage. Adult stem cells are present in specialized tissues throughout the body, such as bone marrow or skin, and are capable of unlimited production of differentiated cells. For adult stem cells to be able to divide continuously, they must have an active telomerase gene, which is characteristic of all ES cells and is needed for duplication of chromosome ends (called telomeres). The presence of the telomerase gene enables stem cells to maintain the integrity of the chromosomes throughout many cell divisions, whereas differentiated cells of the body do not have this gene and therefore can undergo only a limited number of divisions. Because several mutations are required for a normal cell to become a cancer cell, including the ability to make telomerase, it is generally believed that cancer cells derive from mutated adult stem cells because differentiated cells have a limited life-span and therefore cannot accumulate the necessary mutations for malignant transformation.

Most mutations in adult stem cells that give rise to cancer or leukemia tend to be lineage specific because certain changes will promote growth in one tissue but not another. For example, chronic myeloid leukemia is caused by specific chromosome changes in a bone marrow stem cell. Because the normal stem cells in the bone marrow divide only when more blood cells are needed, they become quiescent as a result of continuous blood cell production by the mutated stem cells. This enables the abnormal stem cells populating the bone marrow to divide continuously, thereby producing the elevated blood cell count characteristic of this leukemia. The mutation in chronic myeloid leukemia involves a specific exchange between chromosomes 9 and 22, but this chromosome aberration has no effect in any other tissue because chromosome changes associated with cancer are lineage specific.

Although there are few reports of chromosome studies of cultured adult stem cells, it has been shown that cultured human mesenchymal stem cells have spontaneously acquired an extra chromosome 8, which is a common finding in cancers of mesenchymal origin. The fact that cultured adult stem cells can undergo tissue-specific chromosome changes associated with malignant diseases emphasizes the need to ensure that any adult stem cells used therapeutically, including reprogrammed cells, be monitored for genetic changes.

**SEE ALSO:** Self-Renewal, Stem Cell.

**BIBLIOGRAPHY.** Duncan Baker, et al., "Adaptation to Culture of Human Embryonic Stem Cells and Oncogenesis In Vivo," *Nature Biotechnology* (v.25/2, 2007); M. Mitalipova, et al., "Preserving the Genetic Integrity of Human Embryonic Stem Cells," *Nature Biotechnology* (v.23/1, 2005).

Lorraine F. Meisner
University of Wisconsin

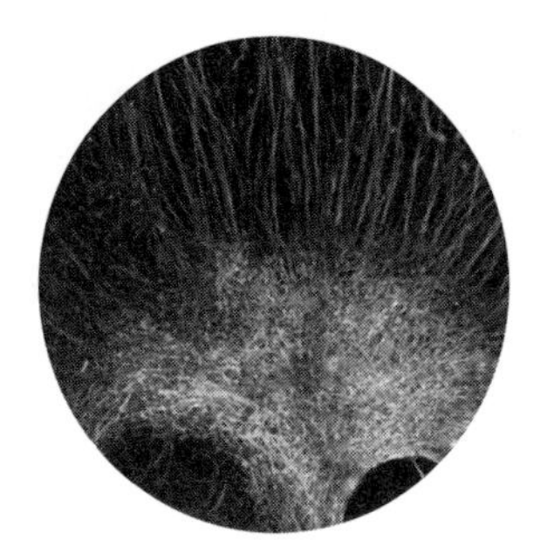

# D

## Delaware

**WITH THE FOUNDING** of the Delaware Biotechnology Institute in 1999, the state and its academic and industrial leaders made the development of biotechnology, including stem cell research, within the state a priority. Delaware has no legislation in place to regulate or fund stem cell research, though the Delaware BioTechnology Institute at the University of Delaware is a statewide collaborative network to encourage research in biotechnology including stem cell research.

At present, no federal legislation in the United States is in place to regulate stem cell research (except by executive order to not allow federal funding for generation of new embryonic stem cell research and limiting research to specific embryonic stem cell lines); this leaves each state responsible for determining its own policy and funding for stem cell research.

Although passed by the Delaware Senate in March, in June 2007 the legislators in the Delaware House of Representatives defeated a bill (State Bill 5) regarding oversight and regulation of research for regenerative medicine and human cloning and establishing regulation of stem cell research on adult, embryonic, and umbilical cord blood cells. The defeat of this bill left Delaware with no laws governing stem cell research; therefore, research being done could continue.

The University of Delaware, located in Newark, was founded in 1743. The university offers a variety of academic programs in science and medicine, as well as other academic majors. One of the research groups in the chemical engineering department is focused on stem cell differentiation and understanding the cellular processes of regulation. Current research includes cancer biology and genetically linked illness. In cancer, biology researchers are studying embryonic development and cancer tumor growth processes in both mouse and human models; the role of bone matrix in the progression of cancer following metastasis from primary sites, with the possibility of molecular drug development for prevention or control of metastasis; the study of cell adhesion molecule role in metastasis; finding fast-growing versus slow-growing cell types for drug development for cancer inhibition; tissue engineering with polymeric and organic–inorganic hybrid materials; and synthesis of model peptides for the activation of pharmaceuticals at the target organ.

The university also participates in research with industry partners through the Delaware Biotechnology Institute to work on gene editing and repair that may lead to a cure for a number of devastating hereditary diseases.

There is also clinical collaboration with Christiana Care Health Services, through a National Institutes of Health National Center for Research Resources IDeA Network of Biomedical Research Excellence grant to Delaware. The core of the program is focused on innovative research in biomedical imaging and in infrastructure to support expanded cancer research in Delaware. The network brings together state, academic, and industrial stakeholders to perform research and improve educational opportunities as a means of enhancing the biotechnology industry and promote jobs within the state.

The Delaware Biotechnology Institute was established at the University of Delaware in 1999 as a center of excellence in biotechnology and life sciences. The institute was created through funding from the state of Delaware, the National Institutes of Health, the National Science Foundation, and other government and private sources. The institute's research facility occupies land adjacent to the Delaware Technology Park, with laboratory space dedicated to plants, animals, human health, biomaterials, and bioinformatics, as well as office space and instrumentation. Though the institute is an academic division of the University of Delaware, it brings together professionals from other institutions statewide, including Delaware State University, Delaware Technical and Community College, Wesley College, Christiana Care Health System, Helen F. Graham Cancer Center, Alfred I. DuPont Hospital for Children, and Nemours Biomedical Research for collaboration.

The institute brings together all the academic disciplines for the development of new technology. The field of biomaterials is an emerging technology area creating clinical therapies, medications, and bioelectronic devices through the networking of scientists in physical sciences and those in materials science and engineering. The institute's current research includes biosurface modifications to promote or prevent protein absorption, rapid separation and sensing of proteins, and cell and tissue engineering. An example of the type of integrated research occurring is the creation of nanofibers by controlling polymer shaping by the university's department of Materials Science and Engineering and then the biology department's investigation of cell response, growth, and proliferation within the polymers.

The Delaware Technology Park, located in Newark, Delaware, is built on 40 acres adjacent to the University of Delaware and is dedicated to the creation of jobs and the growth of biotechnology and other high-tech industries in an environment with proximity (within 35 miles) to 30 educational institutions, as well as providing networking opportunities with other businesses in the park.

**SEE ALSO:** *Individual U.S. State Articles*; Biotechnology, History of; Clinical Trials Within U.S.: Batten Disease; Clinical Trials Within U.S.: Blind Process; Clinical Trials Within U.S.: Cancer; Clinical Trials Within U.S.: Heart Disease; Clinical Trials Within U.S.: Peripheral Vascular Disease; Clinical Trials Within U.S.: Skin Transplants (Burns); Clinical Trials Within U.S.: Spinal Cord Injury; Clinical Trials Within U.S.: Traumatic Brain Injury; Ethics; Federal Government Policies; Moral Status of Embryo; Special Interest/Lobby Groups; United States.

**BIBLIOGRAPHY.** Delaware BioTechnology Institute, www.dbi.udel.edu (cited November 2007); Delaware Technology Park, "About," www.deltechpark.org (cited November 2007); State of Delaware Legislature, "144th General Assembly Senate Bill # 5 w/SA 4 + HA 1, HA 2, HA 3," legis.delaware.gov (cited November 2007).

Lyn Michaud
Independent Scholar

# Denmark

**STEM CELL RESEARCH** in Denmark is able to progress as a result of government support with appropriate legislation and funding, a strong scientific research foundation, and international cooperative relationships and partnerships. Stem cell researchers benefit from networking relationships within the country, with the Danish Stem Cell Research Center, regional relationships through the ScanBalt organization to enhance biotechnology within the Nordic and Baltic sea region, and international affiliations.

Human embryonic stem cell research is permitted in Denmark, including with stem cell lines derived from leftover embryos created for in vitro fertilization. However, Danish law prohibits the creation of embryos specifically for research or procurement of human embryonic stem cells, and it also prohibits reproductive and therapeutic cloning.

## STEM CELL RESEARCHERS

The University of Southern Denmark was founded in 1966 as the Odense University, and through the years, the university has expanded and incorporated additional schools, including the National Institute of Public Health in 2007, which will remain in Copenhagen and retain its national status. The university is made up of six campuses (Odense, Kolding, Esbjerg, Sønderborg, Slagelse, and Copenhagen), offering education and research opportunities. Research being done at the university includes work by the Department of Anatomy and Neurobiology with neural stem cells for transplantation to repair tissues and by the Department of Immunology and Microbiology on differentiation markers.

Copenhagen University is the largest teaching and research institution in Denmark. The university contains numerous institutes, departments, laboratories, centers, and museums, including the Department of Life Sciences and the Department of Medical Biochemistry and Genetics. Research being done under the auspices of the Danish Stem Cell Research Center includes liver stem cells for liver regeneration and endocrine and pancreatic stem cells in the development of the pancreas and for treating diabetes.

Aalborg University was established in 1974, incorporating the existing educational institutions either entirely or partly under one organization. With an emphasis on education, along with basic and applied research, the university is at the forefront of health science technology. The Laboratory for Stem Cell Research is working with cord blood stem cells and stem cell differentiation.

Odense University Hospital is a public hospital offering medical education, research, and medical services for the region and as an area of expertise for certain rare diseases, or for specialized treatment for the entire country. The hospital also maintains a patient information center established in 1992. Research is being done by researchers in the laboratory for Molecular Endocrinology Treatment, using mesenchymal stem cells, and by the Institute of Pathology on using stem cells for muscle regeneration.

NsGene A/S was established in 1999 in Ballerup as a research company to develop cell transplantation to treat neurological diseases, with a focus on Alzheimer's disease, Parkinson's disease, epilepsy, and neuropathic pain. Methods and technology discovered by NsGene are being used by biopharmaceutical companies, and researchers continue to work with neural stem cells and creating delivery systems to ensure that the cellular therapy reaches the target tissue/organ.

The Hagedorn Research Institute is an independent basic research component of Novo Nordisk A/S and is devoted to finding a cure for diabetes and its complications. The Hagedorn Research Institute has a commitment to interdisciplinary basic research, to the education of Master's and doctoral students. Research efforts are focused on therapy to cure diabetes, and one of the areas of research is the use of stem cell research and developmental biology of the pancreas to study the cellular and molecular mechanisms involved in pancreatic beta-cell neoformation, replication, regeneration, differentiation, function, and cell death, with the aim of curing diabetes by reconstituting/preserving an adequate functional beta-cell mass. Research under the auspices of the Danish Stem Cell Research Center relates to islet cell development and replacement.

Denmark maintains international collaborations and networks in the area of stem cell research including the International Stem Cell Forum and the EuroStemCell Project. In addition, ScanBalt, an organization based in Copenhagen, Denmark, mediates and coordinates education, research, and development in biotech and life sciences within the Scandinavian Baltic Sea Region, to overcome the limitations based on small country size to be competitive in stem cell research on a global level. In addition to providing information to the public, ScanBalt maintains a members-only virtual campus via the Internet to provide up-to-date listings of courses, lectures, job openings, ongoing research projects, and requests for proposals from funding agencies.

## DANISH STEM CELL RESEARCH CENTER

The Danish Center for Stem Cell Research (DASC) was established April 1, 2002, on a five-year grant from the Danish Research Agency through the Medical Research Council. DASC consists of nine research groups located at the universities of Aalborg, Southern Denmark (Odense), and Copenhagen; Odense University Hospital; NsGene A/S; and Hagedorn Research Institute. DASC is devoted to study of adult stem cells, which are derived from already formed adult tissue, developing fetal tissue, and umbilical blood.

Research is focused on the following five areas: insulin-producing cells; brain cells, in particular dopaminergic nerves; liver cells; cartilage, bone, and connective tissue cells; and skeletal muscle cells. The objectives of the center are to provide a solid scientific basis for stem cell research in the areas of research for diabetes, Parkinson's disease, liver failure and dysfunction, and skeletal muscle disorders and malfunction; to promote research training in stem cell biology and stem cell therapy; and to communicate factual knowledge about stem cells and the potential use of stem cell therapy to the public.

Research groups include the University of Southern Denmark (neural stem cells, neuroplasticity, repair [transplantation] and anatomy and neurobiology, Jens Zimmer [Rasmussen Professor], Morten Meyer [associate professor], and Nedime Serakinci [assistant professor]; and cross-development differentiation markers [FA-1, gp340/DMBT1] and immunology and microbiology, Charlotte Harken Jensen [research fellow] and Uffe L. Holmskov [professor]), Copenhagen University (endocrine and pancreatic stem cells), Department of Medical Biochemistry and Genetics [IMBG], Jens Høiriis Nielsen [associate professor], Hans Kofod, and Mette Grønborg, Panum Institute; liver stem cells and liver regeneration, Department of Medical Biochemistry and Genetics [IMBG], Hanne Cathrine Bisgaard [associate professor] and Lene Juel Rasmussen), Aalborg University (stem cells from cord blood, stem cell differentiation, Laboratory for Stem Cell Research, Vladimir Zachar [associate professor] and Trine Fink [associate professor]), Odense University Hospital (mesenchymal stem cells, Laboratory for Molecular Endocrinology, Moustapha Kassem [professor] and Henning Beck-Nielsen [professor, consultant]; and muscle regeneration and stem cells, Institute of Pathology, Henrik D. Schrøder [professor, consultant]), NsGene A/S, Ballerup (neural stem cells [cell replacement, cell factory], Department of Developmental Biology, Lars Wahlberg [vice president, chief operating officer] and Bengt Juliusson), and the Hagedorn Research Institute, Gentofte (islet cell development and replacement strategies, Department of Developmental Biology, Palle Serup [principal scientist], Ole D. Madsen [director of research], Richard Scott Heller, Jacob Hecksher-Sørensen, and Claus Rescan).

The Danish Stem Cell Research Doctoral School (DASCDOC) is a national doctoral program in Stem Cell Research and Related Technologies. DASCDOC was established January 1, 2003, by a five-year grant from the National Research Agency after application to the Danish Research Training Council. This is an interdisciplinary school, consisting of 23 research groups from Danish universities, hospitals, veterinary research institutions, sector research institutions, and members of the biotechnology industry. The aim of the doctoral school is to train people with doctoral degrees in the field of stem cell research and related technologies, including developmental biology and cell replacement therapies in regenerative medicine.

The specialized areas of study are early embryonic development; transgene technologies; stem cell isolation and differentiation in relation to stem cell–based therapies including brain, liver, pancreas, intestines, mesenchymal tissues (skeletal muscle, cartilage, bone, heart); and the blood and the immune system.

Stem cell sources are tissue-derived, adult or fetal stem cells from the corresponding tissues and organs and umbilical cord blood, as well as embryonic stem cells derived from the early embryo of rodents, domestic animals, and human embryonic stem cells.

The purpose of the program is to gather Danish doctoral students, supervisors, and other basic science and clinical researchers in the field of stem cell research in a joint, nationwide doctoral research training program, including advanced doctoral courses, summer schools, and joint meetings on tissue-derived stem cells, embryonic stem cells, the necessary technologies, and ethical aspects. The faculty of DASCDOC is composed of active researchers in the stem cell field and related technologies, as well as those with special insight into the legal and ethical aspects of stem cell research. Faculty members are engaged in the planning, organization, and running of the doctoral courses, summer schools, and other activities.

**SEE ALSO:** Cells, Embryonic; European Consortium for Stem Cell Research—EuroStemCell.

**BIBLIOGRAPHY.** Danish Stem Cell Research Center, www.dasc.dk (cited November 2007); DASDOC, www.dascdoc.dk (cited November 2007); Hagedorn Research Institute, "History and Mission," www.hagedorn.dk (cited November 2007); International Stem Cell Forum, www.stemcellforum.org (cited November 2007); ScanBalt, "Organization," www.scanbalt.org (cited November 2007); University of Southern Denmark, "History," www.sdu.dk (cited November 2007).

LYN MICHAUD
INDEPENDENT SCHOLAR
FERNANDO HERRERA
UNIVERSITY OF CALIFORNIA, SAN DIEGO

# Developmental Biology

**DEVELOPMENTAL BIOLOGY IS** the science that studies the mechanisms of development of animals. Some would also include the development of plants within its scope, but as mechanisms differ very substantially between animals and plants, in practice the term *developmental biology* is usually used to refer only to animal developmental biology.

The subject represents a fusion between three traditions of 20th-century biological science. Experimental embryology emerged in the early 20th century, being initially based mostly on microsurgical experiments using amphibian and sea urchin embryos. Developmental genetics grew up mid-century, based mostly on the genetics of the fruit fly *Drosophila* and the laboratory mouse. Molecular biology arose from the discovery of the structure of DNA in 1953, and by the 1980s a group of new techniques enabled the isolation of individual genes by molecular cloning, the determination of their nucleotide sequences, and the study of gene expression in cells and embryos. Modern developmental biology took shape in the 1980s by combining the concepts and techniques of these three areas.

Development of animals takes place mostly during embryonic life, so developmental biology is mostly concerned with embryology. However, there are other developmental processes; for example, those associated with postnatal development, tissue renewal, regeneration, wound healing, and in some types of animal, metamorphosis.

Much use is made of "model organisms" in developmental biology research. These are particular species that have some technical advantages for one or more types of experimental work, and with which a large community of scientists agrees to work. Concentration of effort on a few model organisms has brought rapid progress because it enables the elucidation of whole genome sequences and the sharing of clones for specific genes or antibodies for specific gene products and generally speeds the development of techniques for working with the organism. The main model organisms used in developmental biology research are the nematode *Caenorhabditis elegans*, the fruit fly

*Drosophila*, the zebrafish, the frog *Xenopus*, the chick embryo, and the mouse. Each has its own strengths and weaknesses for experimental work. In general, *C. elegans*, *Drosophila*, and the mouse are good for genetic experiments, and *Xenopus* and the chick are good for microsurgical methods; the zebrafish occupies an intermediate position.

The specific problem areas addressed by developmental biology have been regional specification, morphogenesis, and cell differentiation and growth. Regional specification refers to the mechanism by which a uniform ball or sheet of cells becomes programmed such that different cell types arise at different positions. The earliest such event usually depends on the localization of a regulatory substance, or determinant, in a particular position in the cytoplasm of the fertilized egg. Following cleavage of the egg to form a cell mass, certain cells will inherit the determinant, and it then causes activation of specific genes in those cells.

Subsequent events of regional specification normally involve extracellular inducing factors, which are secreted from one group of cells (an organizing or signaling center) and diffuse away, forming a concentration gradient. The surrounding cells are competent to respond by activating or repressing specific regulatory genes in response to particular concentrations of the inducing factor. Several cycles of this process bring about subdivision of a simple cell mass into a highly complex body pattern. The inducing factors belong to a few classes: chiefly, the fibroblast growth factor, Wnt, hedgehog, and bone morphogenetic protein families.

Morphogenesis is the name given to the processes of cell and tissue movement and adhesion, as these cooperate with events of regional specification to generate a three-dimensional embryo with shape as well as pattern.

Cell differentiation involves the activation of batteries of genes encoding functional gene products for the cell type in question (e.g., a muscle, nerve, fat, or epithelial cell). Its regulation often involves a process of lateral inhibition, mediated by the Delta-Notch signaling system, whereby one cell developing to a particular phenotype will inhibit the surrounding cells from following the same pathway. Growth control at the whole-organism level is still poorly understood in terms of control of final size and of proportions between different body parts. However, the intrinsic cellular events of cell division and its regulation by extracellular growth factors have been well studied.

One of the most remarkable discoveries of modern developmental biology is that the basic mechanisms of regional specification in the different model organisms are quite similar. The same gene families tend to perform the same tasks despite the considerable difference in morphology of both embryos and adults. So, for example, it is well established that the anteroposterior (head-to-tail) pattern of animal embryos is specified by a set of genes called the Hox genes, which encode a specific subset of homeodomain transcription factors. Typically, the Hox genes form a cluster within the genome, and their expression is as a nested set such that all the genes are on at the posterior end of the body, and each gene in the set has a different anterior threshold of expression. Often the order of anterior expression limits is the same as the order of location of these genes on the chromosome. The high level of conservation of molecular and genetic mechanisms between different types of animal give good confidence that studies on the model organisms will be relevant to understanding developmental mechanisms in humans.

Developmental biology provides valuable underpinning for stem cell biology by providing information about the normal mechanisms of development and the inducing factors and regulatory genes that are required to be activated to produce a particular cell phenotype.

**SEE ALSO:** Cells, Developing; Differentiation, In Vitro and In Vivo.

**BIBLIOGRAPHY.** S. F. Gilbert, *Developmental Biology* (Sinauer, 2006); J. M. W. Slack, *Essential Developmental Biology* (Blackwell Science, 2005); L. Wolpert, *Principles of Development* (Oxford University Press, 2006).

Jonathan Slack
University of Minnesota

# Diabetes

**DIABETES IS A** disease in which there are high levels of glucose found in the blood of the patient. It is also known as non–insulin-dependent diabetes or adult onset diabetes. In this disease, the body is unable to produce an adequate amount of insulin, which is what helps sugars to change into energy and plays a major role in the metabolism of the body. In this article, we discuss the physiology behind insulin production and its role in the body; diabetes onset, signs and symptoms, and treatment; and the role of stem cells in diabetes.

The islets of Langerhans form the endocrine tissue of the pancreas. The islets are microscopic structures scattered throughout the pancreas. They comprise alpha cells, beta cells, delta cells, and pancreatic polypeptide cells. Insulin is only produced by the beta cells of the islets of Langerhans. Insulin performs a number of roles in the body's metabolism, particularly related to carbohydrates, lipids, and proteins. In carbohydrate metabolism, insulin increases glucose transport to muscles and adipose tissues, performs glycogenesis and glycolysis, and decreases gluconeogenesis. In lipid metabolism, insulin increases fatty acid synthesis and triglyceride synthesis and decreases lipolysis, ketogenesis, and fatty acid oxidation. In protein metabolism, it increases amino acid transportation and protein synthesis and decreases protein degradation.

There are two types of diabetes: primary diabetes mellitus and secondary diabetes mellitus. Primary diabetes mellitus is divided into insulin-dependent diabetes mellitus (IDDM, or type 1 diabetes) and non–insulin-dependent diabetes mellitus (NIDDM, or type 2 diabetes). Secondary diabetes mellitus is caused by number of factors including pancreatic diseases such as pancreatitis and hemochromatosis; drugs such as corticosteroids and thiazide diuretics; endocrine diseases such as Cushing's syndrome, acromegaly, and thyrotoxicosis; and diabetes of pregnancy.

## TYPE 1 DIABETES

Type 1 diabetes is common in children and young adults. The body is unable to produce insulin, so insulin is injected on daily basis. This condition is caused by autoimmune destruction of the pancreatic islets beta cells. There are number of factors that can play a role in type 1 diabetes, such as environment, inheritance, genetic susceptibility, viral infections (e.g., Coxsakie's virus), and autoimmune factors.

Symptoms that may be found in a patient with type 1 diabetes include increased urination as a result of osmotic diuresis, which is caused by blood glucose levels exceeding the renal threshold, causing a sustained hyperglycemia; increased thirst as a result of osmotic diuresis and a hyperosmolar state, which causes the loss of fluid and electrolytes; blurring of vision, when hyperosmolar fluids cause destruction to the lens and retina; weight loss; postural hypotension; paresthesias, in which peripheral sensory nerves are affected; and ketoacidosis in acute conditions.

## TYPE 2 DIABETES

In type 2 diabetes, there is inadequate production of insulin, which therefore cannot meet the body's daily requirements. In type 2 diabetes, there is a increased resistance found in the body against the insulin, and there are also defects in insulin production. Although the exact cause of the disease is unknown, scientists do believe that following factors may play role in developing type 2 diabetes: a sedentary lifestyle; overeating and obesity; being identical twins of a patient with NIDDM; having a decreased response by body cells to insulin, or in other words, tissue resistance to body insulin; decreased insulin production; and delayed production of insulin in response to the food we eat. The patients with type 2 diabetes mellitus develop symptoms such as visual blurring, increased susceptibility to infections, and delayed wound healing.

There are a number of investigations that are helpful in the diagnosis of diabetes, such as, if fasting blood sugar is more than 126 mg/dL on more than one occasion, if random blood sugar tests at more than 200 mg/dL, a glucose tolerance test, checking the level of glycosylated hemoglobin, checking serum fructosamine, performing a urine analysis to find glucose in the urine, looking for

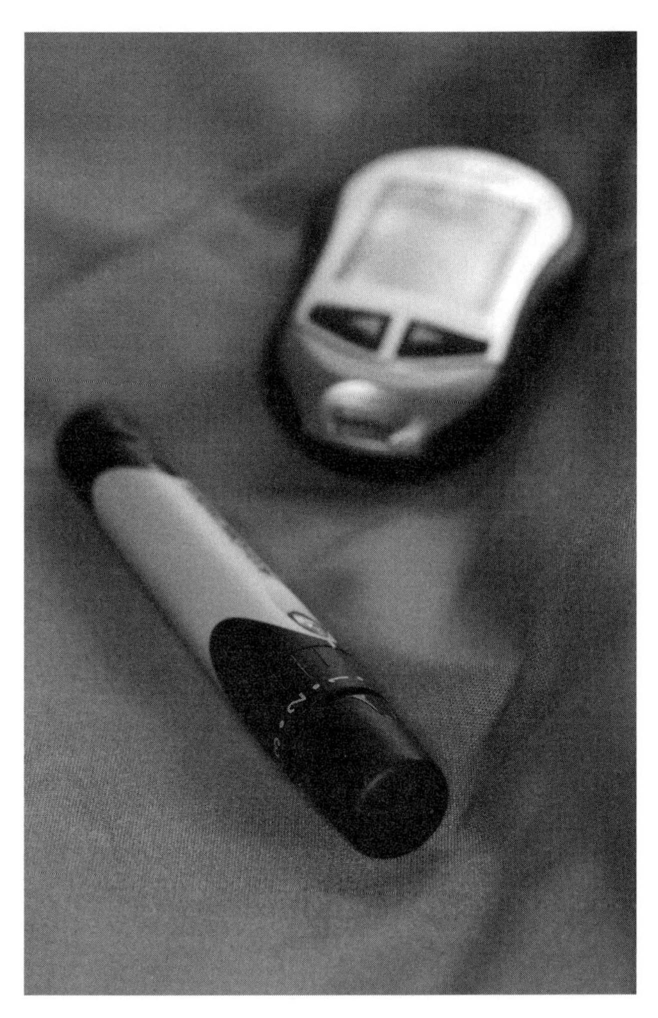

*Treatments derived from stem cells have the potential to free diabetes patients from blood sugar monitors and injections.*

proteinuria, doing a complete blood count, and measuring urea, creatinine, and electrolytes.

At present, there is no cure for diabetes. Once the patient develops type 1 diabetes, he or she must take insulin throughout his or her lifetime and check his or her blood glucose levels three to four times a day. To minimize the complications of diabetes, such as retinopathy and heart disease, the patient must keep his or her blood glucose level close to normal values. In type 2 diabetes, the patient can control his or her glucose levels by proper diet, oral medications, and daily exercise. The education of the patient is an important issue in the treatment of the disease. The patient must know how to check blood sugar with a glucometer, how to measure an accurate dose of insulin, how to check ketone bodies on urinalysis, how to identify hypoglycemic symptoms and their management, and how to maintain good hygiene, especially of the feet. One of the treatments for diabetes is a transplanted pancreas. To prevent the body from rejecting the transplanted pancreas, however, for the rest of his or her life, the patient is kept on drugs that suppress the immune system.

These patients are susceptible to infections, and the steroid immunosuppressant therapy also increases the metabolic needs of transplanted cells and, ultimately, their capacity to produce insulin decreases with the passage of time. Researchers are trying to find a substitute for insulin-producing cells in the pancreas, which are destroyed by the immune systems of patients with this disease.

The goal of curing diabetes can be achieved by injecting pancreatic islets cells in the patient. These islets cells are obtained from cadavers; the procedure needs at least two cadavers. There are certain criteria for the transplantation, such as, the tissues must be obtained within eight hours of the donor's death and should be immunologically identical to the patient. Islets cell transplantation is preferred over the transplantation of the entire pancreatic organ because once immunogenicity of islets cells is decreased by immunosuppressive drugs, the cells are ready to be transplanted; instead of general anesthesia, islets cells can be isolated and placed in the patient by means of portal vein percutaneous catheterization; and to protect them from the patient's own immune system, the islet cells can be encapsulated, allowing the insulin to exit while protecting the islet cells. Scientists are facing some problems with islet cells transplantation, however, as they are unable to get a sufficient amount of islet cells to transplant. In addition, the need for immunosuppressive therapy leads to increased insulin resistance in the body and a decline in insulin production.

## STEM CELLS

Stem cells are a special type of cells that are capable of transforming into different types of cells in the human body. Stems cells are necessary for the development, growth, and maintenance of skin, blood, brain, nerves, muscles, and other organs of the body. Stem cells are very important as therapeutic agents. Scientists are finding out under which conditions stem cells can replicate themselves for long periods of time and how stem cells can be processed to differentiate into a specialized type of cells under different conditions. There are two main types of stem cells, embryonic stem cells and adult stem cells. Embryonic stem cells are capable of differentiating into various types of cells and can be found in embryos. Adult stem cells modify themselves according to the tissues of the body and have the ability to form different varieties of a specific cell type. Stem cells are available from various sources including peripheral blood, at the time of birth from the umbilical cord, and from bone marrow.

Peripheral blood contains a small number of stem cells. Our bone marrow naturally releases blood-forming stem cells in our circulation, which can be collected by a special procedure called apheresis. These stem cells are collected by inserting a needle into the vein of donor.

Cord blood is taken from the placenta or umbilical cord at the time of birth of a baby. After the cord blood is collected, it is stored and frozen for future use.

Adult stem cells are found to be more demanding to maintain in culture medium compared with the embryonic stem cells. However, in a given tissue, it is difficult to recognize and isolate different varieties of adult stem cells. These stem cells may be found between ductal cells during the fetal developmental period. The difference between the ductal cells and the endocrine cells is based on their gene expression (also called cell markers) and their particular structure. Scientists are using different approaches toward the isolation and cultivation of stem cells from adult pancreatic tissues or fetal tissues. Ductal epithelium contains pancreatic stem cells, which have been used to generate human or mouse islet-like cells and have shown good results in insulin-dependent diabetes. However, this process cannot be applied on a large scale, as these stem cells have a low proliferation rate. Embryonic stem cells are easily available and can be managed adequately compared with adult stem cells, but at the same time, embryonic stem cells are much more difficult to handle and may form benign tumors called teratomas when they are placed in organisms.

## EMBRYOGENESIS

During embryogenesis, islet cells start to proliferate within the pancreas. They are likely to develop from undifferentiated precursor cells, which are associated with the ductal epithelium of the pancreas. Scientists are working on how to isolate the stem cells, which are responsible for the formation of the endocrine system of the pancreas. Specifically, Islets of Langerhans then appear to emerge from the stem cells, which are capable of differentiating into alpha cells (glycogen producing), beta cells (insulin producing), gamma cells (somatostatin producing), and delta cells (pancreatic-polypeptide producing).

Once the stem cells proliferate to produce the specific islet cells, these cells start to move into the surrounding exocrine tissue. The exocrine tissues begin developing vessels as a result of angiogenesis, and neurogenesis occurs, which induces nerve formation in islet cells with parasympathetic, sympathetic, and peptidergic neurons. Finally, islet cells mature and start giving a response to the changes in levels of blood glucose.

## STEM CELLS IN LABS

As discussed previously, in type 1 diabetes, the islet cells are attacked and destroyed by the immune system of the body, making the disease difficult to cure. Stem cells could play a vital role if islet cells could be cultured in vitro. This could provide a good solution to islet cell transplantation problems. Because of the increased availability of islet cells in a culture medium, a greater amount of these cells could be given to diabetic patients.

Theoretically, some researchers believe that stem cells can be engineered in such a way that they can express a specific type of genes that could not be detected by the immune cells of the patient. In experimental models, the islet progenitor cells can be induced to proliferate from the ductal epithelial cells, which form monolayers of cells. The islet progenitor cells grow and form islet-like structures that are well organized and are capable of producing endocrine hormones, insulin, glucagon, somatostatin, and hepatocyte growth factor. However, there are many factors responsible for the failure of stem cells to become fully mature. Experimental studies on mice showed that if undifferentiated stem cells are induced to grow in a culture medium, they start to express specific genes and begin producing mouse insulin 1 and 2, islets and amyloid, and the glucose transporter GLUT-2. Pancreatic alpha cells start producing somatostatin. In vitro, islet cell clusters are encircled by nerve cells, similar to the arrangement in vivo, which shows positive stains for neuron-specific tubulin.

In adult tissue, different progenitor cells have been identified, and some of them are capable of being cultured for multiple generations. However, embryonic stem cell results show that these cells will hopefully soon produce good results in self replication and will be able to overcome the body's own immune system.

**SEE ALSO:** Cells, Embryonic; Cells, Mouse (Embryonic); Mouse ES Cell Isolation.

**BIBLIOGRAPHY.** "Diabetics Cured in Stem-Cell Treatment Advance," www.timesonline.co.uk (cited November 2007); "The Promise of Stem Cells: Diabetes," www.stemcell.umn.edu (cited November 2007); "Stem Cell Discovery Could Aid in Diabetes Treatments," www.sciencedaily.com August 27, 2004 (cited November 2007); "Stem Cells Key to Diabetes Cure," www.wired.com, September 20, 2002 (cited November 2007).

G. Ishaq Khan
Dow University of Health Sciences

# Dickey Amendment

**THE DICKEY AMENDMENT** was enacted by the U.S. Congress and signed by former President William J. Clinton in January 1996 as a rider to an appropriations bill for the Department of Labor and Health and Human Services. The amendment to the appropriations bill prohibits federal funding for the creation of human embryos for research that would cause embryos to be destroyed, discarded, or knowingly subjected to risk of injury or death greater than that allowed for research on fetuses in utero. Consequently, this amendment also banned the use of federal funds for in vitro fertilization research. However, the Dickey Amendment only affected federally funded research and did not affect the private research sector.

Although this amendment blocked federal funding for research that created or destroyed an embryo, federal funds could still be used for research on established embryonic stem cell lines after President George W. Bush's announcement on August 9, 2001. Congress has included the Dickey Amendment in the Department of Labor and Health and Human Services Appropriations Bill every year since its enactment in 1996.

Human embryo research had been discussed and assessed in the years before the Dickey Amendment. In 1993, President Clinton authorized through his executive power the use of tissues from aborted fetuses for research on a number of diseases. In 1994 the National Institutes of Health (NIH) Revitalization Act had given the NIH direct authority to fund human embryo research for the first time in history. In 1994 the NIH created the Human Embryo Research Panel with 19 members including three embryologists, six physicians, three biomedical ethicists, two lawyers, a sociologist, two political scientists, and two representatives of constituents affected by infertility and sickle cell anemia. Four of the physicians were in reproductive medicine, one was in public health, and the last was in medical ethics. Two of the three ethicists were Roman Catholics. This panel would work together to assess the standards of human embryo research.

The Gingrich-era Congress questioned the ethical concerns of human embryonic stem cell research. Then, in 1996, the Dickey Amendment was drafted as a rider to an appropriations bill for the Department of Health and Human Services. The amendment is also commonly known as the Dickey-Wicker Amendment, after Jay Dickey and Roger Wicker, the two U.S. Representatives who drafted it. Jay Dickey was a Republican Congressional Representative from Arkansas who served from 1993 until 2000, when he lost his reelection campaign to Democratic candidate Mike Ross. Congressman Dickey served on multiple committees, including the U.S. House Committee on Appropriations; subcommittees on agriculture, national security, energy and water, transportation and labor, health and human services, and education. Roger Wicker was then and is currently a Republican Congressional Representative from Mississippi. Congressman Roger Wicker has held his position in Mississippi's First Congressional District since 1995.

The full text of the Dickey-Wicker Amendment can be found repeated annually in the Labor/Health and Human Services Appropriations Bill. The law clearly states that none of the funds made available in this act may be used for the creation of a human embryo or embryos for research purposes or for research in which a human embryo or embryos is destroyed, discarded, or knowingly subjected to risk of injury or death greater than that allowed for research on fetuses in utero under 45 CFR 46.204 and 46.207, and subsection 498 (b) of the Public Health Service Act (42 U.S.C. 289g(b)).

For the purposes of the amendment, the term *human embryo or embryos* included any organism not protected as a human subject under 45 CFR 46 as of the date of the enactment of the governing appropriations act that is derived by fertilization, parthenogenesis, cloning, or any other means from one or more human gametes or human diploid cells.

The creation of the Dickey-Wicker Amendment affects all research involving human embryos from 1996 onward. Although the Dickey-Wicker Amendment ceased federal funding for human embryonic research, it did not affect the private sector, and therefore, privately funded research on human embryos still occurred. Biotechnological companies such as Geron conducted human embryonic stem cell research in the private sector. They even organized their own Ethics Advisory Board and created their own guidelines regarding the ethical concerns of human embryonic stem cell research.

In the summer of 1996, Dolly, the famous cloned sheep, was born. President Clinton reacted to Dolly's birth with an executive moratorium on any federal research that could possibly lead to human cloning, and in October 1996, he issued a presidential directive prohibiting the use of federal funds to clone humans.

The Dickey-Wicker Amendment raised important ethical concerns on the topic of human embryonic stem cells. If stem cell research on human embryonic stem cells raises ethical concerns, it also questions whether or not the nation should federally fund the research. When Jamie Thompson of the University of Wisconsin created the first human embryonic stem cell line in 1998, questions were raised asking whether or not stem cell lines are considered human embryos by definition. As a result, the NIH was allowed to allocate federal funding to any experiment on the cells themselves.

## NIH GUIDELINES

The White House then formed a committee appointed by the president called the National Bioethics Advisory Committee. In August 2000, the NIH published its Guidelines for Research Using Human Pluripotent Stem Cells in the Federal Register, stating that federal money could be used only for research on stem cell lines derived from embryos or fetal tissue, not for the creation of human embryos for stem cell research. President Clinton signed these guidelines into effect that same month.

One year later, however, newly elected President Bush stopped federal funding altogether on August 9, 2001. He stated that any embryonic stem cell lines created before August 9, 2001, could remain federally funded, but no new lines could be created or studied using federal funds. Therefore, only 22 embryonic stem cell lines in existence are federally funded in their research. All research on embryonic stem cell lines created after this date must have private funding.

The Dickey-Wicker Amendment began a series of ethical concerns regarding human embryonic stem cell research. It questioned the idea and perhaps the repercussions of human cloning. It questioned the true definition of a human embryonic stem cell and whether or not human embryonic stem cell lines fit into that particular category of human embryos. It was a valued rider to the Health and Human Services Appropriations Bill in 1996. From 1996 on, the language of the Dickey-Wicker Amendment has been included in the Health and Human Services Appropriations Bill, and the scientific world continues to analyze the ethics of human embryonic stem cell research.

**SEE ALSO:** Cells, Embryonic; Cells, Human; Funding for IVF; Human Embryonic Stem Cells; Stem Cells, Bush Ruling.

**BIBLIOGRAPHY.** The White House, "Current Federal Law and Policy on Stem Cell Research," www.whitehouse.gov (cited November 2007); NOVA Science Now, "The Politics of Stem Cells," www.pbs.org (cited November 2007); National Institutes of Health, "Research Ethics and Stem Cells," stemcells.nih.gov (cited November 2007).

Jennifer Yoohanna
University of California, Los Angeles

# Differentiation, In Vitro and In Vivo

**CELL DIFFERENTIATION,** or cellular differentiation, is the process by which the cells of a multicellular organism develop the specialized abilities required by each of the organism's several structures. In the context of stem cell biology, it should be noted that the two defining characteristics of stem cells are the ability to pass through several mitotic cycles without differentiating—a property known as self-renewal—and the ability to differentiate into any mature cell type. This property is known as totipotency. There are some cells that can differentiate into many, but not all, mature cell types. Although these cells are not totipotent, they are occasionally considered to be stem cells and are called multipotent.

Cell differentiation occurs via the differential expression of cellular genes, so that the cellular proteins formed vary from cell type to cell type. It may take place in vivo, or in the body of the living organism, or be induced in vitro, in the laboratory. Differentiation is an essential stage in the development of an organism and is necessary for maintaining its particular form and identity.

Cell differentiation is closely regulated by cellular signaling substances called cytokines and by the extracellular matrix that surrounds the cell. It affects some disease states—some genes that were known to inhibit the growth of tumors have been found to act by promoting the differentiation of tumor cells, inhibiting their spread. In others, it is affected itself; for example, infection by the HIV virus has been found to induce differentiation in some cells. Certain factors, such as the products of oncogenes, have been found to reverse differentiation—in this way, a differentiated adult cell may be reverted to pluripotency. However, because this reversal of differentiation involves the use of oncogenes, which can transform normal cells into malignant tumor cells, its application is likely to be restricted.

Cell differentiation requires the cell to turn through the cell cycle several times, as the promotion of the expression of certain genes and the simultaneous suppression of others is a molecularly complex process. Certain cells remain undifferentiated into adulthood and are called adult stem cells. Reservoirs of these cells exist in the bone marrow, and the cells are present in smaller quantities in the brain, muscle, and heart.

## CELL DIFFERENTIATION IN VIVO

Differentiation is the third phase of embryonic development, the first two being growth and morphogenesis. It results in the formation of tissues and organ systems that are capable of performing certain specialized functions. In the context of embryogenesis, most major differentiation processes begin at the stage of gastrulation; this is the process in which cells migrate to the interior of the blastula and subsequently give rise to two or three germ layers from which the body's various organs develop; the embryo at this stage is known as a gastrula.

The embryo's organs and tissues differentiate rapidly in the fourth to eighth weeks and are at risk for congenital anomalies if exposed to teratogens during this period (teratogens are agents—chemical, physical, or biological—that can increase the incidence of such anomalies. Notorious examples are X-ray radiation, thalidomide, and the rubella virus).

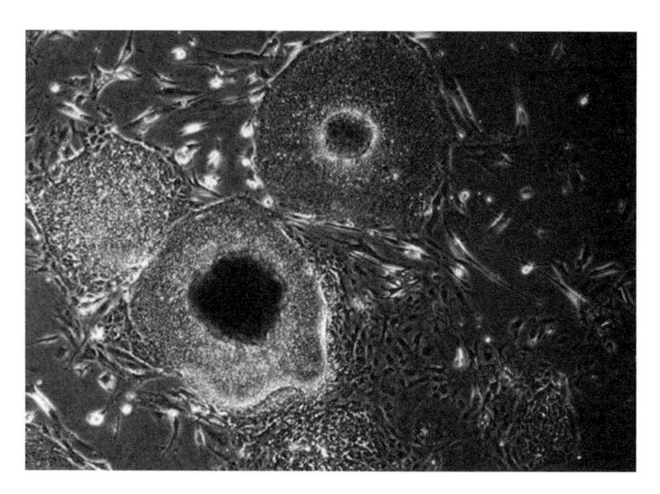

*During cell differentiation, as shown above, cells develop specialized abilities to serve the body's different structures.*

## FACTORS AFFECTING CELL DIFFERENTIATION IN VIVO

The process of cell differentiation is one that is made possible by the simultaneous up-regulation and down-regulation of several genes, and any factors that affect gene expression are likely to affect cell differentiation and other cellular processes.

Enzyme-linked receptors are cellular receptors for growth factors and hormones that span the cellular membrane (transmembrane proteins) and possess intrinsic catalytic abilities by virtue of being associated with various enzymes. Their chief function is to regulate "long-term" cellular processes like apoptosis, differentiation, or division; they do this by facilitating or inhibiting intracellular cascades that signal the activation or inhibition of the expression of a particular gene, and anything that affects these receptors or the signaling pathways they trigger will affect these cellular processes.

Another category of substances that control cell differentiation is the cytokines, which are polypeptides (chains of amino acids) that serve to regulate growth and development. Cytokines also act via their receptors; although these are structurally different from the enzyme-linked receptors mentioned above, they are similar in that they also trigger signaling cascades that ultimately result in alterations in gene expression and long-term cellular effects—the intracellular substances they use to effect these changes are, however, different. Certain cytokines are known to control hematopoietic (blood-forming) cell growth and differentiation.

The extracellular matrix that surrounds cells has been found to contain several growth factors and other proteins that profoundly affect cellular differentiation; this matrix not only promotes cell differentiation but influences its direction as well. A study on nonprimate embryonic stem cells showed that "efficient cell-cell aggregation, together with less efficient cell attachment and spreading" (to an extracellular matrix) "results in more efficient cell differentiation."

## CELL DIFFERENTIATION AND DISEASE PROCESSES

Tumor cells are classified into benign (noncancerous) and malignant (cancerous) types. One of the identifying features of malignant tumors is their lack of similarity to the tissue of their origin; in other words, these tumors are poorly differentiated or undifferentiated, as opposed to benign tumors, which are well differentiated. As a general rule, less-differentiated tumors tend to exhibit a higher growth rate than well-differentiated ones.

Teratomas are benign germ cell tumors that may occur independently or in association with a malignant condition. The contents of a teratoma testify grotesquely to the pluripotent capabilities of a germ cell: they can contain differentiated elements from all three germ cell layers, and it is not uncommon to find hair, teeth, and other tissue when a teratoma is cut open. When these tumors occur as cystic (fluid-containing) swellings over the sutures of the skull (the immobile joints that hold together the bones of the skull), they are known as dermoid cysts.

A study at the University of Pennsylvania showed that when a certain type of human tumor cells that can be weakly infected by HIV were brought in contact with the virus, the virus promoted the differentiation of the infected cells into polygonal cells of a distinctive phenotype. It is speculated that disruption of these differentiation mechanisms may provide a means of controlling the HIV virus in vivo, and also that such an effect on the host's stem cells could cause severe harm.

## CELL DIFFERENTIATION IN VITRO

Cell differentiation in vitro, or in the laboratory, provides the opportunity for "directed differentiation," in which a stem cell can be manipulated to give rise to a specialized cell type. Such directed differentiation finds several applications in stem cell therapy; it may also provide an alternative to animal testing of pharmaceutical products, which is useful but limited in terms of predicting its effects in human cells.

Stem cell therapy may be pivotal in the treatment of several degenerative and traumatic conditions, but techniques of direct differentiation must be perfected before their clinical use is possible. Cellular differentiation depends on cytokines, growth factors, cellular interactions with the surrounding matrix, and intercellular association; altering the conditions in which cells are growing will affect differentiation, and each of these factors can be manipulated accordingly. This is currently the most practical method used to direct differentiation.

Another method involves the insertion of active foreign genes into the cell to trigger differentiation and guide it in the direction desired. This method is precise but requires accuracy in determining the active gene at a particular stage of differentiation, activation of this gene at the precise moment, and insertion of the gene into the right location. Another theoretically possible method is to "reprogram" these cells by injecting them into oocytes.

The directed differentiation of human embryonic stem cells has immense therapeutic potential and the methods used for directing their differentiation are similar to those used for mouse stem cells.

Cell differentiation in vitro has several applications in the treatment of diseases caused by degeneration of or damage to tissues. Some diseases that may potentially be treated by stem cell therapy are Duchenne's muscular dystrophy, osteogenesis imperfecta, Parkinson's disease, diabetes, damage to the spinal cord caused by trauma, heart failure, liver failure, and other degenerative conditions or injuries.

**SEE ALSO:** Cells, Embryonic; Clinical Trials Outside U.S.: Amyotrophic Lateral Sclerosis; Clinical Trials Outside U.S.: Avascular Necrosis; Clinical Trials Within U.S.: Batten Disease; Clinical Trials Within U.S.: Blind Process; Clinical Trials Within U.S.: Cancer; Clinical Trials Within U.S.: Heart Disease; Clinical Trials Within U.S.: Peripheral Vascular Disease; Clinical Trials Within U.S.: Spinal Cord Injury; Clinical Trials Within U.S.: Traumatic Brain Injury; Clinical Trials Worldwide; Methods of Growing Cells; Nuclear Transfer, Altered; Nuclear Transfer, Somatic.

**BIBLIOGRAPHY.** Department of Health and Human Services, *Stem Cells: Scientific Progress and Future Research Directions*, June 2001, stemcells.nih.gov/info/scireport/2001report (cited November 2007); Stephen J. McPhee, Vishwanath R. Lingappa, and William F. Ganong, *The Pathophysiology of Disease*, 4th ed. (Lange, 2002); Thomas M. Devlin, ed., *Textbook of Biochemistry with Clinical Correlations*, 6th ed. (Wiley-Liss, 2005); S. Chen, et al., "Cell-Cell and Cell-Extracellular Matrix Interactions Regulate Embryonic Stem Cell Differentiation," *Stem Cells* (v.25/3, 2007); Wikipedia, www.wikipedia.org (cited November 2007); Jonathan Phillips, Paul Murray, and Paul Kirk, eds., *The Biology of Disease*, 2nd ed. (Blackwell Science, 2001).

Azara Singh
Christian Medical College

# Division Types (Symmetrical and Asymmetrical)

**TWO DISTINCT TYPES** of cell division have been observed during the development of both invertebrates and vertebrates: symmetrical and asymmetrical cell divisions. An asymmetric cell division produces two daughter cells with different properties. This is in contrast to symmetric cell divisions, which give rise to equivalent daughter cells. Notably, stem cells divide asymmetrically to give rise to two distinct daughter cells: one copy of themselves and one cell programmed to differentiate into another cell type.

## ASYMMETRIC

Animals are made up of a vast number of distinct cell types. During development, these cell types are generated from a single cell, the zygote. Asymmetric divisions contribute to this expansion in cell type diversity by making two types of cells from one. For example, it is thought that many of the cells in the central nervous system derive from asymmetric divisions. Cells may divide asymmetrically to produce two novel cells at the expense of the mother cell. For example, in plants, an asymmetric division of an unspecialized epidermal cell can produce a guard cell mother cell that divides again to produce two guard cells—the cells that control the closing and opening of stomata.

In principle, there are two mechanisms by which distinct properties may be conferred on the daughters of a dividing cell. In one, the daughter cells are initially equivalent, but a difference is induced by signaling between the cells. In another, the prospective daughter cells are made different at the time of division of the mother cell. Because this latter mechanism does not depend on the interactions of the cells with their environment, it must rely on intrinsic asymmetry. The term *asymmetric cell division* usually refers to such intrinsic asymmetric divisions. Intrinsic asymmetric divisions rely on the following mechanism: At mitosis, certain proteins are localized asymmetrically to one half of the cell. Next, the cell is cleaved to separate the two halves. Thus, the asymmetrically localized proteins are inherited to only one of the daughter cells, causing that cell to be different from its sibling. Because these proteins determine what becomes of a cell, they are called cell fate determinants. This mechanism has two requirements: first, the mother cell must be polarized, and second, the mitotic spindle must be aligned with the axis of polarity. The cell biology of these events has been most successfully studied in three animal models: the mouse, the nematode *Caenorhabditis elegans*, and the fruit fly *Drosophila melanogaster*.

Most mechanistic insights into asymmetric cell division come from invertebrate experiments. However, discoveries in work on mammalian stem cells have revealed enormous flexibility among the progeny of individual cells. Many different cell fates can be induced by changing growth factors in the culture medium, suggesting that lineage restrictions and intrinsic asymmetries have only minor functions. However, time-lapse video microscopy shows that cortical progenitor cells divide in stereotyped lineages—even in culture, where directional extrinsic signals can be largely excluded. Although there is no clear genetic evidence for intrinsically asymmetric cell divisions in vertebrates, the observation of putative stem cells in intact tissues has revealed several examples for asymmetrically segregating proteins such as Numb and the Notch receptor.

Stem cells constitute a population of cells that continues to divide in organisms and produces cells for tissue generation. Stem cells can self-renew (they produce both differentiating daughters and daughters that maintain stem cell identity) and are pluripotent (they can give rise to all cell types in a given organ). One strategy by which stem cells can accomplish this is asymmetric cell division, whereby each stem cell divides to generate one daughter with a stem cell fate (self-renewal) and one daughter that differentiates. However, asymmetric divisions often give rise to only one novel cell type in addition to a new copy of the mother cell. Self-renewal is a hallmark of stem cells, and there is growing evidence that stem cells self-renew through asymmetric division. In this way, the production of new cell types (differentiation) is precisely balanced by the renewal of the stem cell population. Thus, an asymmetric division is a particularly attractive strategy because it manages both tasks (i.e., self-renewal and differentiation) with a single division. However, a disadvantage of this strategy is that it leaves stem cells unable to expand in number. This lack of flexibility is a problem, given that stem cell numbers can increase markedly, both when stem cell pools are first established during development and when they are regenerated after injury. Therefore, asymmetric cell divisions cannot be the complete story. Stem cells must have additional self-renewal strategies that permit dynamic control of their numbers.

## SYMMETRIC

Stem cells can also use symmetric divisions to self-renew and to generate differentiated progeny. Symmetric stem cell divisions have been observed during the development of both invertebrates and vertebrates. Symmetric stem cell divisions are also common during wound healing and regeneration. A hallmark of all three processes is an increase in the number of stem cells. This increase cannot be explained by a strategy restricted to asymmetric cell division, in which only one daughter cell maintains stem cell identity.

Although the idea that stem cells can divide symmetrically may seem counterintuitive, stem cells are defined by their potential to generate more stem cells and differentiated daughters, rather than by their production of a stem cell and a differentiated daughter at each division. When viewed as a population, a pool of stem cells with equivalent developmental potential may produce only stem cell daughters in some divisions and only differentiated daughters in others. The evidence for symmetric stem cell divisions is strong, both in model organisms such as *C. elegans* and *Drosophila* and in vertebrates.

## SWITCHING

In principle, stem cells can rely either completely on symmetric divisions or on a combination of symmetric and asymmetric divisions. Some mammalian stem cells seem to switch between symmetric and asymmetric cell divisions. For example, neural stem cells change from primarily symmetric divisions that expand stem cell pools during embryonic development to primarily asymmetric divisions that expand differentiated cell numbers in mid- to late gestation. In the developing mammalian cortex, cell divisions are confined to the so-called ventricular zone. Neural precursors divide in the ventricular zone, and daughter cells either stay in this zone and continue to divide or move away from it to differentiate. As layers of differentiated cells arise in the forebrain, neural progenitors increasingly undergo asymmetric division: one cell remains in the ventricular zone ("niche" of stem cells), and the other cell migrates into overlying layers of differentiated neurons. For these cells, divisions are classified as symmetric or asymmetric, depending on whether one or both daughter cells retain the position and morphology associated with stem cells. A caveat, however, is that mammalian stem cells cannot be distinguished from other progenitors on the basis of only morphology and position, so it remains possible that the frequency of asymmetric and symmetric divisions of stem cells differs from that observed in the overall pool of undifferentiated cells.

Switching between symmetric and asymmetric divisions has also been observed in adult mammals. Some adult stem cells seem to divide asymmetrically under steady-state conditions. However, they retain the capacity to divide symmetrically to restore stem cell pools depleted by injury or disease, as has been observed in the nervous and hematopoietic systems. In the subventricular zone of the adult forebrain, for example, asymmetric divisions predominate under steady-state conditions, although some apparently symmetric divisions can be observed. Forebrain loss after stroke increases the rate of division among subventricular zone progenitors, including a rise in symmetric cell divisions that, in turn, leads to increase in neurogenesis. A similar event has been found in the mammalian hematopoietic system. When the hematopoietic system is decimated by chemotherapy, hematopoietic stem cells begin dividing and expand about 10-fold to regenerate pools of both stem cells and differentiated cells. These data suggest that stem cells can facultatively use both symmetric and asymmetric divisions.

The prolonged symmetric divisions of mammalian stem cells during early embryonic development generate large pools of stem cells and tissues. The ability to switch back and forth between symmetric and asymmetric modes of division depends on developmental and environmental cues. A key issue for the future is how stem cells are regulated to switch between asymmetric and symmetric divisions.

**SEE ALSO:** Differentiation, In Vitro and In Vivo; Self-Renewal, Stem Cell.

**BIBLIOGRAPHY.** Gord Fishell and Arnold R. Kriegstein, "Neurons from Radial Glia: The Consequences of Asymmetric Inheritance," *Current Opinion in Neuroscience* (v.12, 2003); Juergen A. Knoblich, "Asymmetric Cell Division during Animal Development," *Nature Reviews in Molecular Cell Biology* (v.2, 2001); Sean J. Morrison and Judith Kimble, "Asymmetric and Symmetric Stem-Cell Divisions in Development and Cancer," *Nature* (v.441/29, 2006); Wikipedia, "Asymmetric Cell Division," en.wikipedia.org (cited November 2007).

Masatoshi Suzuki
University of Wisconsin, Madison

# DNA Fingerprinting of Stem Cells

**DNA FINGERPRINTING,** or genotyping, is a common name that has been given to several DNA-based methodologies for determining the DNA signature or genetic identity of an individual that differentiates him or her from another individual of the same species. Use of DNA fingerprinting is important for research involving cultured stem cells (SCs) because of the need to guarantee the genetic identity of the SC line being studied and the fact that many studies of cultured human SCs have demonstrated a significant level of intraspecies and interspecies cross-contamination. Historically, cross-contamination of cultured cells has been a major problem, with long-reaching repercussions, emphasizing the need to use DNA fingerprinting to prevent the use of accidentally cross-contaminated cultured human SCs.

## CASES OF MISTAKEN IDENTITY

The need for precise methods for cell line identification first became apparent in the 1970s, when it was found that many cancer researchers who thought they were growing different types of cancer but getting similar results to other researchers were, in fact, growing cell lines derived from HeLa, a very aggressive cervical cancer culture. It was later discovered that even small numbers of HeLa cells were capable of overgrowing the cells in other cultures to the extent that the majority of cancer researchers, unbeknownst to themselves, were basing their conclusions on HeLa rather than on the specific cancers with which they started.

Accidental cell contamination has been shown to have devastating effects, both professionally and economically. For example, HeLa-contaminated cases are estimated to have cost over $10 million, and this problem is not limited to the past. Similar results have been reported as late as 2000, with the observation that up to 18 percent of cancer cell lines were contaminated by another cell line. Similar results continue to be reported in other types of cultured cell lines and are not limited to cancer cells. In the past year, similar occurrences of mistaken identities in cultures of human SCs have been observed, which is not surprising because SC research branched out of tissue culture technology, which has a history of repeated examples of mistaken identity. Moreover, cultured SCs tend to look alike. So, if the code on a tube or flask is read incorrectly, or the culture is not labeled correctly, then the experiments can be continued on cell lines containing the wrong genome.

In addition to intraspecies cross-contamination, interspecies cross-contamination has been seen. Many human SCs are currently cultured on inactivated mouse SCs. In some cases, the latter have shown to possess growth advantages that allow them to overtake human SC cultures.

## METHODS OF IDENTIFICATION

DNA fingerprinting was invented by Sir Alec Jeffreys as a method for analyzing DNA regions containing repetitive nucleotide sequences (called minisatellites). This method provided a mechanism for determining an individual's DNA signature on the basis of their unique combination of identifiable sequences from each parent, which was successful in settling paternity, immigration, and forensic disputes.

Restriction fragment-length polymorphism (RFLP) was initially used as a method for DNA fingerprinting, involving isolating DNA from the rest of the cellular material and cutting it into different sizes with restriction enzymes (proteins that cut the DNA in specific sites). The fragments are then separated on a gel and visualized with radioactive probes, producing a specific pattern, or fingerprint. Limitations of this technology include the requirement for large amounts of DNA and the fact that it is a lengthy, time-consuming process.

An improvement to the RFLP method involved addition of polymerase chain reaction (PCR) to amplify specific DNA sequences containing variable numbers of tandem repeat regions. However this methodology still uses a gel to separate the fragments, and a high number of repeats may cluster together, thus compromising the results.

The most reliable and quickest method in current use is analysis of PCR-amplified short tandem repeats (STRs). STRs are regions of DNA containing short repeated sequences. The most commonly used STRs involve repeats of four bases. The number of repeats at each site or locus varies from individual to individual, which allows specific discrimination of an individual's DNA fingerprint. These polymorphisms have a common distribution based on population of origin. The power of discrimination based on analysis of STRs increases when comparing several sites or loci. The U.S. Federal Bureau of Investigation selected 13 loci as a basic combination of STRs that enables unique identification of each individual. This selection is known as the Combined DNA Index System, or CODIS.

Each STR locus can be amplified millions of times with PCR, and the fragments can then be separated and detected by electrophoresis. Separation is performed using a ladder or marker of known DNA size that determines, by comparison, the sample's DNA size or allele. In turn, the allele indicates the number of repeats for each locus. Capillary electrophoresis and gel electrophoresis are used to separate and visualize these PCR fragments. The former is the current gold standard because it provides the ability to determine the size of each PCR product rapidly and accurately.

Use of DNA STR profiling has enabled precise designation (authentication) of human cell lines as well as the identification of mix-ups and cross-contamination that could have disastrous effects for therapeutic uses. In light of the many new discoveries and advancements in SC biology, it is essential to know the identity of the cell lines that are used for research and therapeutic applications.

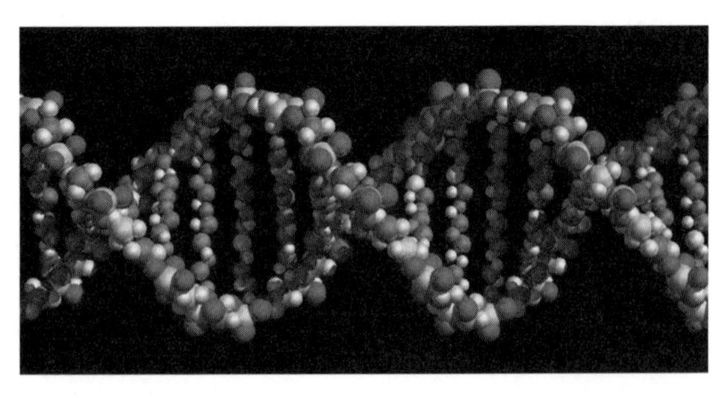

*Like the nearly 18 percent of cultured cancer cell lines found contaminated in 2000, stem cell lines also need DNA testing.*

**SEE ALSO:** Cells, Human; Cells, Mouse (Embryonic).

**BIBLIOGRAPHY.** P. Hughes, et al., "The Costs of Using Unauthenticated, over Passaged Cell Lines: How Much More Data Do We Need?" *Biotechniques* (v.43, 2007); Roland M. Nardone, "Eradication of Cross-Contaminated Cell Lines: A Call for Action," *Cell Biology and Toxicology* (v.23/6, 2007); S. Obrien, "Cell Culture Forensics," *Proceedings of the National Academy of Sciences* (v.98, 2001).

Mario Salguero
University of Wisconsin, Madison

# Do No Harm: The Coalition of Americans for Research Ethics

**DO NO HARM** is a coalition of Americans who have banded together to promote ethical stem cell research. The members are conservative Christians who see themselves as engaged in faithful and responsible ethical actions to promote both ethically responsible stem cell research and morally acceptable public policies that support stem cell research or that ban federal funding of unethical stem cell research.

The coalition's headquarters is in Washington, D.C. The founding members of Do No Harm were Kevin FitzGerald, David Lauler, Ralph Miech, Frank E. Young, Christopher Hook, David A. Prentice, and Joseph Zanga. Kevin FitzGerald is an associate professor of oncology at Georgetown University in Washington, D.C. He is also a member of the Society of Jesus (Jesuits). Christopher Hook is a physician specializing in hematology and medical oncology at the Mayo Clinic in Minnesota. He is also the chairman of the Mayo Clinical Ethics Council, Mayo Reproductive Medicine Advisory Board, and DNA Research Committee.

Ralph Miech holds doctorates in medicine and pharmacology. He is now retired but is associate professor emeritus of pharmacology at Brown University School of Medicine in Providence, Rhode Island. Not too far way and also in New England is Dr. Robert D. Orr, a physician and director of ethics at the University of Vermont's College of Medicine in Burlington, Vermont. Dr. David A. Prentice is a senior fellow for life sciences at the Family Research Council (FRC). The FRC is an organization that promotes a Judeo-Christian worldview. It seeks to promote public policies that are pro-life. Dr. Frank E. Young is a physician who has served as commissioner of the U.S. Food and Drug Administration and is also dean emeritus, University of Rochester School of Medicine and Dentistry. He is currently the director of the Reformed Theological Seminary in Washington, D.C. Joseph Zanga is director of the Office of Generalist Programs with the National Health Service Corporation. He is also Ambassador Professor of Pediatrics at the Brody School of Medicine at East Carolina University in Greenville, North Carolina.

Since the founding of Do No Harm, many other physicians, research scientists, ethicists, and supporters of a Christian ethic of stem cell research have joined the Do No Harm Coalition and subscribe to its objectives. The objectives are to advance the development of medical treatments and therapies that do not require the destruction of human life, including the human embryo; to educate and inform public policy makers and the general public regarding these ethically acceptable and medically promising areas of research and treatment; and to support continuation of federal laws prohibiting the federal funding of research that requires the destruction of human life, including the human embryo.

In its founding statement, the Do No Harm coalition went on record as opposing the decision of the Department of Health and Human Services and the National Institutes of Health to fund stem cell research that is dependent on the destruction of human embryos. It also opposed the decision of the National Bioethics Advisory Commission calling for lifting the ban against federally funded human embryo research to harvest stem cells after embryos were destroyed.

The coalition, from the beginning, has been motivated by the conclusion that human stem cell research is objectionable on legal, ethical, and scientific grounds if it requires the destruction of human embryos. This is because the members of the Coalition believe that the destruction of human embryonic life is unnecessary for medical progress, as alternative methods of obtaining human stem cells and of repairing and regenerating human tissue exist and continue to be developed.

One of the grave concerns that the Do No Harm coalition has is that the utilitarian argument that medical research that is done for the greater good is not always morally justified. Although the members of the coalition believe that it is beyond dispute that stem cells have the means for the treatment of illnesses, and the relief of suffering and treatment is a great good, the coalition does not believe that any and all means are justified to achieve this end. For example, coalition members, like most other ethicists, would not condone the murder of random individuals just to have an opportunity to harvest their organs, no matter how great the benefit might be—even if the beneficiary were a famous and prominent person who could still make great contributions to humanity. For the coalition, some methods are morally or legally unjustified no matter how great the claim that a greater good is the end result. It believes that if it were morally permissible to do harm to achieve a greater good, then the patient and the moral imperative to first do not harm could be ignored in the quest for some greater good.

The particular forms of medical research that the coalition opposes are embryonic stem cell research and human cloning, especially if they are funded by the federal government. What the coalition members believe is an example of Christian humanism, rather than secular humanism. Both forms of humanism believe that people are important. For secular humanists, however, hard things can be done to individuals that are morally justified if humanity as a whole benefits. However, in Christian humanism, individuals are important because they are worth the death of Christ on the Cross.

The coalition's members believe that the values enshrined in American law are reflective of this view that individuals are valuable. Moreover, they believe that this is a part of the tradition that affirms the dignity of every human being—a tradition of human rights belonging to every individual and even to unborn embryos. They believe that this right to life is echoed in the laws against murder found in every one of the 50 states, and in the federal law as well.

In November 2007, two scientific papers were published showing that pluripotent stem cells can be made without the use of human cloning or the destruction of embryos. The Do No Harm coalition greeted the news with cautious optimism. This is an appropriate response because scientific announcements have also been known to show graver limitations than press reports at first indicate. Still, Do No Harm's response was one that celebrated the news as a vindication of the morality of their stance and as a strong indication of future avenues of research. The best part of the news is that it means that patient-specific stem cells theoretically can be generated that will not have the likelihood of rejection.

**SEE ALSO:** Cells, Adult; Cells, Fetal; Ethics; Moral Status of Embryo; Religion, Christian.

**BIBLIOGRAPHY.** Do No Harm: The Coalition of Americans for Research Ethics, www.stemcellresearch.org (cited November 2007).

Andrew J. Waskey
Dalton State College

# Down Syndrome

**DOWN SYNDROME** (also called trisomy 21) is a genetic disorder caused by the abnormal presence of the entire or a part of an extra chromosome 21. The disease is named after John Langdon Down, a British doctor who described it in 1866. Down pointed out the striking similarity of facial features among children with the disease when they were compared with those of Blumenbach's Mongolian race. Hence, the disease is sometimes referred to as "mongolism" and "mongolian idiocy." The disorder was identified as a chromosome 21 trisomy by Jérôme Lejeune in 1959.

The typical patient suffering from Down syndrome has a total of 47 chromosomes in all the somatic cells of his body. Such an abnormality accounts for the impaired growth and development of the child. Down syndrome is the leading genetic cause of mental retardation. Latest statistics report the incidence of Down syndrome to be 1 per 800 live births, making it one of the most frequently inherited chromosomal abnormalities of modern medicine. These statistics are profoundly influenced by the age of the mother at the time of birth.

Patients with Down syndrome have certain common physical features, which may include a single transverse palmer crease (a single instead of a double crease across one or both palms), almond-shaped eyes, epicanthic folds of the eyelids, up-slanting palpebral fissures, shorter limbs, a larger-than-normal space between the big and second toes, poor muscle tone, and a protruding tongue. Individuals with Down syndrome are at a greater risk for congenital heart defects, gastroesophageal reflux disease, recurrent ear infections, obstructive sleep apnea, thyroid dysfunction, and rarely, leukemia and Alzheimer's disease.

## STEM CELL RESEARCH

The neurological signs and symptoms of Down syndrome are recognized during the prenatal and early postnatal period in humans. Stem cell research offers the generation of human neural tissue in culture—a novel model system to study alterations in developmental disorders such as Down syndrome. An article published in the *Lancet* in 2002 described an intriguing model used to study Down syndrome, devised at the University of Cambridge by Bahn and Emson.

Every fetus begins as one cell, which then divides repeatedly. These cells are pluripotent, that is, they have the capability to differentiate into multiple lineages of cells, virtually giving rise to all the cells in the body. Embryonic stem cells are often collected at a developmental stage when they are just about to differentiate into a particular cell lineage.

Bahn and Emson used stem cells from the developing human brain that are precursors to neural tissue and grew them as spherical aggregates called neurospheres. They used neurospheres from postmortem fetuses (with and without Down syndrome) that were biochemically induced to form neurons. The RNA proteins were extracted from the neurospheres and compared with the RNA proteins from normal neurospheres. Through vigorous experimental procedures, it was found that one specific protein was absent from the neurospheres of Down syndrome patients. The *SCG10* gene was relatively or absolutely functionally deficient. Further investigation discovered that certain other genes were also underexpressed; namely, *L1*, *Synapsin*, and *ß4-tubulin*. The neurons from the defective stem cells were shorter, had misshapen axons, and fewer dendrites projected from the main body of the neuron when compared with the control.

Down syndrome is a condition of extra genes, or gene overexpression. Hence, the underexpression of these four genes seemed puzzling. As it turned out, however, the transcriptional regulation for all of them was regulated by the repressor element silencing transcription factor, or the REST factor. This factor serves to repress expression of certain genes, regulating transcription and translation. Thus, it is likely that an overexpression of the REST factor causes an oversuppression of the *SCG10*, *L1*, *Synapsin*, and *ß4-tubulin* genes. This issue is subject to a lot of scrutiny.

Nevertheless, stem cell research discovered a substantial derangement in the genetics of the development of neurons that begins in the earliest stages of formation of the embryo with Down syndrome, resulting form a disruption of expression of certain genes of the neurons.

Early research performed on Down syndrome includes mimicking Down syndrome in mice. The researchers were able to plant about 90 percent of human chromosome 21, which contained over 250 genes, into the embryonic stem cells of mice. This was done by extracting all chromosomes from a human cell and transferring them into mouse embryonic stem cells, each of which absorbed one chromosome at random.

The fusion of the human chromosomes with the mouse embryonic stem cells followed. Mouse stem cells that took up chromosome 21 successfully were then isolated and injected into mouse embryos. These embryos were then implanted in the mother, whose offspring were shown to have the extra copy of chromosome 21. The offspring had problems with memory, abnormal brain function, and congenital cardiac defects similar to those that occur in humans with Down syndrome.

The genetically engineered mice had the craniofacial hallmarks of Down syndrome, resulting directly from having extra copies of a chromosome virtually identical to the one in humans. The mice looked mostly normal but had shorter noses and flattened skulls. The experimental animal has an abnormally small cerebellum, the part of the brain controlling movement, which defect is also found in people with Down syndrome. The mouse model predicted an abnormally low density of cerebellar brain cells. The researchers matched the Down syndrome mouse data with well-established characteristics of skulls of Down syndrome patients and found an absolute correspondence.

Continuing research efforts aspire to examine the role of individual genes developing Down syndrome and to determine why those individuals with this condition are particularly susceptible to diseases like leukemia and autoimmune disorders. Stem cell research in Down syndrome offers hope in unraveling the picture of individual genes responsible for complex conditions, such as diabetes, and to create artificial chromosomes for gene therapy. Researchers believe that this research would help them in the study of other aneuploidies (disorders in which patients have an abnormal number of chromosomes), such as Edward's syndrome.

There is not a specific cure for Down syndrome at present, but researchers have every reason to believe that gene therapy in the future will enhance therapeutic options for such people. Sequential functional essays of the genes present on chromosomes allow us to design specific drugs that can turn certain genes on and off. Hence, a patient with Down could benefit from drugs that could help regulate proper gene expression.

The Down Syndrome Association appreciates the research endeavors and their results. Stem cell research on Down syndrome as a whole (using either human or mouse cell) is yielding substantial results, not only for patients with Down syndrome but also indirectly for patients suffering from Alzheimer's, heart disease, and leukemia. Nevertheless, it must be recognized that this research is at the primary level of finding the basic pathology of Down syndrome, and discovering a cure or treatment through stem cell research will take a while. At the pace of present research, however, the future looks very hopeful.

**SEE ALSO:** Cells, Embryonic; Cells, Mouse (Embryonic); Cells, Neural.

**BIBLIOGRAPHY.** S. Bahn, et al., "Neuronal Target Genes of the Neuron-Restrictive Silencer Factor in Neurospheres Derived from Fetuses with Down Syndrome: A Gene Expression Study," *Lancet* (v.359/9303, 2002).

Quratulain Khan
National University of Science and Technology

# Duke University

**DUKE UNIVERSITY IS** a private coeducational research university located in Durham, North Carolina. Founded by Methodists and Quakers in the present-day town of Trinity in 1838, the school moved to Durham in 1892. In 1924 tobacco industrialist James B. Duke established the Duke Endowment, prompting the institution to change its name in honor of his father Washington Duke.

The university is organized into two undergraduate and eight graduate schools. The undergraduate student body, which includes 40 percent ethnic minorities, comes from all 50 U.S. states and 117 countries. In its 2008 edition, *U.S. News & World Report* ranked the undergraduate division eighth in the nation, while ranking the medical, law, and business schools each among the top 11 in the country. Duke's research expenditures are among the largest 20 in the United States, and its athletic program is one of the nation's best. Competing in the Atlantic Coast Conference, the athletic teams have captured nine national championships, including three by the men's basketball team.

In addition to academics, research, and athletics, Duke is also well known for its sizable campus and Gothic architecture, especially Duke Chapel. The forests surrounding parts of the campus belie the university's proximity to downtown Durham. Duke's 8,610 acres (35 km$^2$) of property contain three main campuses in Durham as well as a marine lab in Beaufort. Construction projects have updated both the freshmen-populated Georgian-style East Campus and the main Gothic-style West Campus, as well as the adjacent Duke University Medical Center (DUMC), over the past five years.

## STEM CELL RESEARCH PROGRAM

Since stem cell treatments first became a possibility in medicine during the 1960s, DUMC researchers and physicians have played a major role in advancing their increasingly complex uses. In recent years, DUMC has worked to create a number of unique methods to apply stem cells to the treatment of cancer and rare diseases. The mission of the Duke Stem Cell Research Program is to advance the understanding of stem cells and to promote their application in the clinical realm to help save lives and reduce suffering. At the basic science level, both embryonic and adult stem cell research and a variety of model organisms, including mice, flies, and fish, are being studied.

Over the past several years, Duke scientists have demonstrated the ability to reprogram adipose-derived adult stromal cells into fat, cartilage, and bone cells. All of these cells arise from mesenchymal, or connective tissue, parentage. However, the latest experiments have demonstrated that researchers can transform these cells from fat into a totally different lineage. Earlier this year, Duke researchers demonstrated that these adipose-derived cells are truly adult stem cells. As a source of cells for treatment, adipose tissue is not only limitless but does not carry the potentially charged ethical or political concerns other stem cell sources do.

Recent experiments at DUMC have demonstrated that newly transformed adipose cells expressed many similar cellular proteins as normal nerve and glial cells. Furthermore, they showed that the functions of these cells were similar to nerves. These newly formed cells were exposed to N-methyl-D-aspartate (NMDA), an agent that blocks the activity of the neurotransmitter glutamate and is toxic to nerve cells. In response to NMDA, the newly induced cells died—a response similar to that of normal nerve cells under the same conditions. The goal is to understand the rules that govern how stem cells grow and multiply and how they differentiate into many different specialized cell types. Over the past five years, Duke researchers under the direction of Farshid Guilak, Ph.D., have been investigating novel approaches to treating cartilage damage. In their experimental system, the researchers expose human adipose-derived stem cells to different cocktails of nutrients, vitamins, and growth factors. This chemical reprogramming forces these cells to progress along different paths, whether to bone, cartilage, or nerves.

In their latest experiments, the researchers added BMP-6 to the cocktail in which hADAS cells were grown in tiny spheres of a complex carbohydrate known as alginate. The three-dimensional scaffold provided by the alginate spheres promotes differentiation of treated hADAS cells into cartilage tissue. Interestingly, the Duke team also found that hADAS cells comprise a distinct lineage of stem cells. Although the treatment of mesenchymal stem cells with BMP-6 tends to stimulate a transformation into bone cells, the treatment of hADAS cells with BMP-6 stimulates cartilage cell growth, as well as the blockage of bone cell growth. On the basis of current research, it appears that hADAS cells demonstrate the potential to serve as a readily available source for creating new cells and tissues to treat cartilage damage.

The mission of the Duke Stem Cell Research Program is to advance the understanding of the basic science of stem cells and to promote their clinical application to help save lives and reduce suffering. At the basic science level they are using both embryonic and adult stem cells and a variety of animal models to further research. The goal is to understand the rules that govern how stem cells grow and multiply and how they differentiate into many different specialized cell types. The environment in which stem cells reside in adult organs and tissues, and how signals from the body normally control stem cell behavior, are also actively being studied. At the clinical level, new techniques are being explored on how both adult and embryonic stem cells can be used therapeutically and how they can be integrated into damaged or diseased tissues to promote regeneration and repair. Every effort to increase the understanding of cancer cells and the therapeutic use of stem cells in new anticancer therapies is being explored.

**SEE ALSO:** Cells, Adult; Cells, Embryonic; North Carolina; United States.

**BIBLIOGRAPHY.** Duke University, www.duke.edu (cited November 2007); DukeMedNews, www.dukemednews.duke.edu (cited November 2007); *Duke Magazine*, www.dukemagazine.duke.edu (cited November 2007).

Fernando Herrera
University of California, San Diego

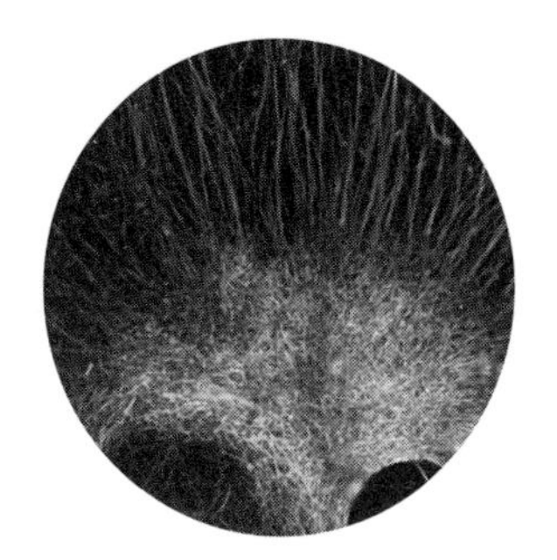

# E

## East of England Stem Cell Network

**THE EAST OF ENGLAND** Stem Cell Network was established in 2004 to facilitate and encourage collaboration and interaction between those from the academic, clinical, and commercial sectors with an interest in stem cell science in this region. The East of England network is an acknowledged center of excellence in all aspects of stem cell research. As well as being the location of the Cambridge Stem Cell Institute and the U.K. Stem Cell Bank, it hires people with expertise across the fields of developmental biology, epigenetics, clinical translation of research into practice, and the ethics and regulation of stem cell technology. The network is a collaborative effort among Cambridge University, Addenbrooke's Hospital, and a host of business and research groups.

The East of England network is host to an extensive range and depth of research activity in the field of stem cell science. It has been estimated that there are over 150 individuals and 45 research, infrastructure, and commercial organizations with independent projects in the stem cell sector that are ongoing in the region. Research in this area spans the basic sciences of developmental genetics, cellular biology, genomic imprinting, and cell signaling to the clinical application of stem cells for neuronal repair and pancreatic islet transplantation. In addition to this activity, the eastern region of the country is also home to a number of organizations with interests in the fields of scientific knowledge dissemination and education, legal and regulatory affairs, and the commercial applications of stem cell research.

The major new contributor to the East of England network's stem cell research activities is the Cambridge Stem Cell Initiative, an interdisciplinary coalition of faculty members from across the University of Cambridge that comprises investigators in both the School of Biological Sciences and the School of Clinical Medicine. The initiative is led by Professor Roger Pedersen and supports three major research programs in the areas of stem cell genetics, biology, and medicine. Its mission is to generate insights into the biology of stem cells through basic research, and thus to provide the foundation needed for novel therapies from regenerative medicine. The initiative also aims to train the next generation of stem cell researchers and to attract the best in the field to Cambridge. At present, the main hub of the initiative is the Cambridge Institute for Stem Cell Biology. The institute's chair is Professor Austin Smith, a leading figure in the human and mouse embryonic stem cell research arena. The institute has recently recruited a number of new principal investigators, and its next phase is the development of facilities dedicated to clinical stem cell research, which will be based on the campus of one of the region's leading teaching hospitals, Addenbrooke's, which is part of the Cambridge University Hospitals National Health Service Foundation Trust. Both the research conducted within the newly formed institute and the wider initiative build on existing work that is taking place within Cambridge University.

Cambridge University's School of Clinical Medicine also hosts a number of eminent researchers with major interests in the therapeutic potential of stem cells. Roger Pedersen, professor of regenerative medicine at the Department of Surgery there, is conducting research into the differentiation of human embryonic stem (hES) cells by creating stable, transgenic cell lines that express green fluorescent protein without affecting cell pluripotency. These lines therefore provide an ideal tool for the investigation of the role of specific genes involved in hES differentiation. Additional activity with a number of collaborators has centered on the study of the mechanisms involved in the maintenance of hES pluripotency and the development of stem cells for pancreatic islet transplantation for the treatment of type 1 diabetes. Professor Pedersen is also the director of the program in stem cell medicine at the Cambridge Stem Cell Initiative.

The interests of Professor Tony Green, head of the Department of Hematology, are focused on the transcriptional regulation of hematopoietic stem cells and the disorders that arise from the transformation of these cells, such as chronic myeloid leukemia. The researchers in this department have identified a number of transcriptional gene enhancers involved in hematopoiesis and endothelial development, using experimental models combined with genomics and bioinformatics. They have also characterized chromosomal abnormalities associated with chronic myeloid leukemia and other myeloproliferative disorders, and how these relate to disease prognosis.

Professor James Fawcett, head of the Cambridge Centre for Brain Repair, has concentrated his research on the capacity of the central nervous system (CNS) to recover from neurological damage. His group is involved in the study of neural plasticity, the therapeutic potential of oligodendrocyte precursors following a CNS injury, and the stimulation of axon regeneration to aid recovery from spinal cord injuries. Several other groups at the Centre for Brain Repair work on a number of different aspects of human embryonic, fetal, and adult stem cells, with regard to their therapeutic potential for the treatment of neurodegenerative conditions such as multiple sclerosis and Parkinson's disease.

Other departments within the clinical school who also have significant interest in stem cells and their application to a number of diseases including diabetes, heart disease, atherosclerosis, cancer, and stroke include the departments of Medical Genetics, Medicine, Obstetrics and Gynecology, Oncology, and the Cambridge Institute for Medical Research. Clinical research carried out in this field is also strongly supported by Addenbrooke's Hospital and Papworth Hospital National Health Service Trusts.

## OTHER INSTITUTIONS

In addition to the university, numerous institutions in the Cambridge area also have strong interests in various aspects of stem cell biology. These include the Welcome Trust Sanger Institute, where director Professor Allan Bradley's research group has used mouse embryonic stem (ES) cells to study gene function in both normal physiological development and diseases such as cancer. Other groups are involved in the production of large numbers of characterized mouse ES cell lines created by gene trap mutagenesis to identify new genetic pathways essential for mammalian development, as well as many other areas of mouse and zebra fish embryonic development. The U.K. Stem Cell Bank is also located in the East of England, within the National Institute for Biological Standards and Control. The bank provides a repository for stem cell lines of all types and will be developed to supply cell lines both for basic research and for the development of clinical applications.

**SEE ALSO:** Cells, Embryonic; Human Embryonic Stem Cells; United Kingdom.

**BIBLIOGRAPHY.** Cambridge Stem Cell Initiative, www.stemcells.cam.ac.uk (cited November 2007); East of England Development Agency, www.eeda.org.uk (cited November 2007); East of England Stem Cell Network, www.eescn.org.uk (cited November 2007).

Fernando A. Herrera
University of California, San Diego

# Eaves, Connie

**CONNIE J. EAVES** is stem cell biology researcher at the Terry Fox Laboratory in the British Columbia Cancer Research Centre. She is also the director of the Terry Fox Laboratory and professor of medical genetics at the University of British Columbia in Vancouver, Canada. In addition, she is an associate member of medicine and associate member of pathology and laboratory medicine at the University of British Columbia.

Dr. Eaves is a world-class researcher in the field of hematopoietic stem cell biology. She has made a number of discoveries that have aided the development of stem cell assays, and her research has shown that molecular regulation of stem cell fate decisions is significant in the development of breast cancer. She has also contributed to the study of leukemogenesis. Her most important recent discovery has been that breast cells include breast stem cells, which has been a breakthrough in the medical field of breast cancer research.

Eaves earned a bachelor of arts in biology and chemistry from Queen's University in 1964 and a master's of science in biology, specializing in genetics, in 1966. She studied at Paterson Laboratories and the Holt Radium Institute. She received her doctorate from the University of Manchester, England, in 1969.

In 1970 Eaves returned to Canada after completing a postdoctoral year in England to do more postdoctoral work at the Ontario Cancer Institute in Toronto. From 1970 to 1973, she worked with Dr. James Till and Dr. Ernest McCulloch. In 1973 Eaves joined the British Columbia Cancer Institute (British Columbia Cancer Agency) as a National Cancer Institute of Canada Scholar. Her research was on preclinical pius-meson radiobiology. She divided her time there with her position as an assistant professor in medical genetics at the University of British Columbia. In 1980 Eaves played an important role in the founding of the Terry Fox Laboratory at the British Columbia Cancer Agency, and in 1986 she was appointed to the post of deputy director.

Eaves' doctoral research program generated the first known evidence that there are two cell populations that contribute to the generation of antibody responses. The B and T lymphocytes are the two types of cell that are found in the blood, and thus are both scientifically and medically important. This important finding was published in *Nature* in 1967.

Other important insights gained from Eaves's work developed the concept of a hierarchy of progenitor classes with different lineages in the human body's manufacturing of blood. This led to stem cells eventually being recognized. From this early beginning in hematology, Eaves has become a world-class authority on stem cells in human blood. Her specific research focus now is chronic myeloid leukemia. An important outcome of her work in the 1990s was the contribution she made to understanding the behavior of stem cells in normal and malignant cells in the human breast.

The research that Eaves has followed has currently led her to study the unique properties of stem cells in tissues that are normal, as well as those that are cancerous. The studies have shown that cells have unique properties that can lead to the development of cancer and also to the development of anticancer treatments.

In addition to her research work, Eaves has been a teacher. Because of the quality of her research, she has attracted many undergraduate, graduate, and postgraduate students. In the case of the latter, she attracts those with clinical training, which is used to engage both research and medicine. She has been able to supervise the postgraduate training of over 50 postdoctoral students. With the establishment of the Fox Laboratory, Eaves has been able to provide postgraduate students a place to work on research projects. Many of her graduates have gone on to become nationally and internationally recognized stem cell specialists in their own rights. A dynamic group of young researchers continues to do research at the Fox Laboratory. Their collective publication record is now very impressive, with over 340 peer-reviewed articles, conference proceedings, and book chapters.

In addition to research and publication, Eaves has been successful in developing national and international collaborative research programs. She was active with the human genome project and is also a member of the Stem Cell Network, which has provided a grant to fund work in gene therapy.

Eaves served as councillor of the American Society of Hematology from 1996 to 1999. From 2000 to 2003 she served as vice president and president of the International Society of Experimental Hematology. She also has served on grant review panels for the National Institutes of Health and, as a peer reviewer, examined papers submitted on stem cell research to a variety of journals publishing in the area of hematology and stem cell research. She is a member of several editorial boards including those of *Blood* and *Biology of Blood and Marrow Transplantation*. She also has served as the editor of the new journal *Stem Cell*.

Eaves has been an active member of many scientific societies including the American Society of Hematology and the International Society for Experimental Hematology. She has also been cochair of the Canadian Breast Cancer Research Initiative and president of the National Cancer Institute of Canada. Dr. Eaves has been widely recognized for the importance of her work. In 1993, she was elected a fellow of the Royal Society of Canada, and in 2003, she was awarded the Robert L. Nobel prize for Excellence in Cancer Research. The prize is awarded by the National Cancer Institute of Canada.

**SEE ALSO:** Cancer; Cells, Adult; Cells, Human.

**BIBLIOGRAPHY.** M. B. Bowie et al., "Identification of a New Intrinsically Timed Developmental Checkpoint that Reprograms Key Hematopoietic Stem Cell Properties," *Proceedings of the National Academy of Sciences* (v.104/14, 2007); O. Christ et al., "Improved Purification of Hematopoietic Stem Cells Based on Their Elevated Aldehyde Dehydrogenase Activity," *Haematologica* (v.92/9, 2007); X. Jiang, K. M. Saw, A. Eaves, and C. Eaves, "Instability of BCR-ABL Gene in Primary and Cultured Chronic Myeloid Leukemia Stem Cells," *Journal of the National Cancer Institute* (v.99/9, 2007); X. Jiang, C. Smith, A. Eaves, and C. Eaves, "The Challenges of Targeting Chronic Myeloid Leukemia Stem Cells," *Clinical Lymphoma Myeloma* (v.7, 2007); Y. Zhao et al., "A Modified Polymerase Chain Reaction-Long Serial Analysis of Gene Expression Protocol Identifies Novel Transcripts in Human CD34+ Bone Marrow Cells," *Stem Cells* (v.25/7, 2007).

Andrew J. Waskey
Dalton State College

# EC Cell Isolation

**TERATOMAS ARE BENIGN** tumors that are formed in the ovaries or testicles, and also in other sites of an infant. Teratomas derive from oocytes that activate parthenogenetically, begin development, and grow into a disorganized mass of tissue. Similar tumors are found in the testicles and are often more malignant. One type of testicular tumor is known as germ cell tumor (GCT); this type of tumor accounts for almost all kinds of testicular cancers. GCTs are commonly found in embryos or young men who just completed puberty.

Embryonal carcinoma (EC) cells are derived from GCT. EC cells are a small population of GCT, found among the disorganized array of somatic and extraembryonic cells in a tumor. Isolated EC cells give rise to teratocarcinomas upon reinjection into mouse models, indicating their pluripotent properties.

During the 1970s, EC cells were found to be very similar to the inner cell mass and primitive ectoderm of a blastocyst. Following this observation, a hypothesis was raised that EC cells were just malignant counterparts of embryonic cells. Several experiments were carried out to increase understanding of EC cells. EC cells express similar properties as embryonic stem cells: They are able to self-renew and differentiate into a variety of cell types. However, abnormalities are often observed in chromosome structure and a number of these EC cells. EC cells are found to be more restrictive in their ability to differentiate. Some EC cell lines have even lost this innate ability of stem cells and remain undifferentiated. Despite prominent differences in properties of EC cells and embryonic stem cells, EC cells have been pivotal in the understanding of stem cells and formulation of isolation techniques of stem cells.

## PROPERTIES

GCT and teratocarcinomas were experimentally derived from mouse models in the 1970s and made possible further understanding of GCT. The discovery of undifferentiated stem cells in GCT led scientists to postulate that such cells, known as EC cells, are just malignant versions of embryonic stem cells. The understanding of EC cell properties and culture techniques led to the later success of isolation of embryonic stem cells in 1981. The similarity in properties of EC and embryonic stem cells make EC cells good models to study the differentiation of stem cells and characterize culture medium that was used to culture early embryonic stem cell lines from mouse models.

Through in-depth studies of characteristics of EC cells, scientists have devised several criteria that are widely used to identify EC cells. These studies have also led to further understanding of the similarities and differences of EC and embryonic stem cells. Variations in these criteria have also been observed between the animal models.

The first identification criteria are a set of cell-surface antigens. Alkaline phosphatase is found to be well-expressed in human and mouse models, both in EC cells and embryonic stem cells. Elevated expression of alkaline phosphatase is a common characteristic of undifferentiated pluripotent cells.

The next group of cell-surface markers is glycolipid antigens; this group of markers shown variation in expression in human and mouse models. Glycolipid antigens are found to be associated with early embryo glycolipid synthesis. Human EC and embryonic stem cells express high levels of SSEA-3 (stage specific embryonic antigen-3) and SSEA-4 but not SSEA-1 while mouse EC and embryonic stem cells express heightened levels of SSEA-1 only. These SSEA molecules are recognized by monoclonal antibodies MC631 and MC813-70. In human models, SSEA-3 has been determined as a more accurate indicator of EC cells as SSEA-4 has been expressed in other somatic cells.

The third group of identification markers is high molecular weight glycoproteins. These epitopes are defined by monoclonal antibodies including TRA-1-60, TRA-1-81, K4 and K21 and GCTM2. These antigens are not detected in the mouse model and are generally used to define human EC and embryonic stem cells. Lastly, the transcription factor Oct-4 is found to be highly expressed in both mouse and human EC and embryonic stem cells. The level of Oct-4 expression is greatly diminished once differentiation occurs.

Other than genetic and cell surface markers, the EC cells have been morphologically characterized. EC cells are observed to be about 15μm in diameter and each has a large nucleus. EC cells are also found to have very little cytoplasm. The ability to define EC cells made it possible to ensure the integrity of the derived EC cell lines. Recent techniques have also capitalized on these unique properties of EC cells to refine the isolation procedures.

## ISOLATION

In the early 20th century, researchers postulated that the development of teratomas was related to embryogenesis and that EC cells were just stem cells that went out of control. In 1967 Dr. Stevens proved this hypothesis by demonstrating that spontaneous teratomas occurred in the 129 mouse strain. Dr. Skreb and colleagues made further studies of EC cells possible by showing that teratomas

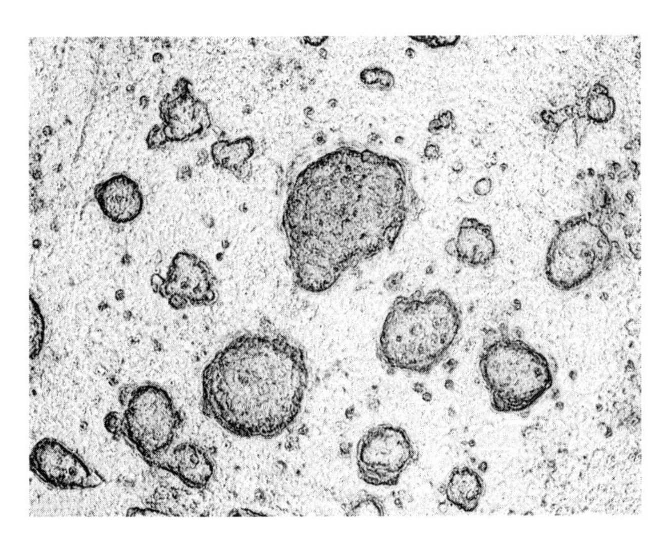

*EC cells have been pivotal in the understanding of stem cells and the formulation of isolation techniques for stem cells.*

and teracarcinomas were formed upon ectopic transplantation of embryos. The first human EC cells were obtained by Dr. Pierce in 1957 and this experiment proved EC cells to be progenitors of differentiated teracarcinomas.

With a better understanding of teratocarcinomas and teratomas, Dr. M. J. Evans reported the isolation of clonal tissue culture strain from teratoma cells in the mouse model in 1972. According to Dr. Evans's methodology, tumors also known as GCT were first obtained by implanting an embryo into an adult testis. These GCT were maintained by subcutaneous transplantation for several mouse generations and those with slower growth were chose for isolation purposes.

The selected tumors were chemically treated to remove most of the tissue components, leaving only cells. The array of cells was then disaggregated into single cell suspension before incubation with chick fibroblasts. Upon incubation, the cells grow into colonies that are then picked individually and transferred to irradiated feeder layers. Feeder layer growth was terminated once cell growth exceeded a million cells.

The successful isolation of EC cells made possible the characterization of EC cell properties and later on, the derivation of embryonic stem cells. With further understanding of EC cells and breakthroughs in technology, Dr. Stefan Przyboski further advanced the techniques for EC cell isolation. In 2001 Dr. Przyboski made use of immunomagnetic sorting technology to recognize the unique SSEA-3 expression and isolate human EC cells from explanted tumors. According to Dr. Przyboski's immunomagnetic sorting technique, confluent EC cells were first trypsinized into a single-cell suspension. The suspension was then diluted and incubated with a SSEA-3 antibody for 45 minutes. The EC cells were then isolation by direct positive magnetic separation. The magnetic particles used to select EC cells will detach themselves upon subsequent culturing in 48 hours.

These isolated EC cells were resuspended and washed several times. Single cells were selected and confirmed with microscopy techniques before being transferred into individual tissue culture plates. Following isolation, these single EC cells will be amplified into colonies and EC cell lines.

The isolation of EC cells has led to many applications and helped researchers understand mechanisms of cell differentiation and techniques of stem cell isolation. The many human and mouse EC lines available offer an alternative for scientists who are interested in studying embryo development of various animal models. Coupled with research on embryonic stem cells and other types of adult stem cells, the isolation of EC cells has brought the research community closer to realizing the goal of regenerative medicine.

**SEE ALSO:** Cells, Embryonic; Cells, Mouse (Embryonic); Embryonic Stem Cells.

**BIBLIOGRAPHY.** P. W. Andrews, "Teratocarcinomas and Human Embryology: Pluripotent Human EC Cell Lines," *Acta Pathologica, Microbiologica et Immunologica Scandinavica* (v.106, 1998); P. W. Andrews, "From Teratocarcinomas to Embryonic Stem Cells," *Philosophical Transactions of the Royal Society B* (v.357, 2002); P. W. Andrews et al., "Embryonic Stem (ES) Cell and Embryonal Carcinoma (EC) Cells: Opposite Sides of the Same Coin," *Biochemical Society Transactions* (v.33/6, 2005); M. J. Evans, "The Isolation Properties of a Clonal Tissue Culture Strain of Pluripotent Mouse

Teratoma Cells," *Journal of Embryology and Experimental Morphology* (v.28, 1972); G. R. Martins and M. J. Evans, "Differentiation of Clonal Lines of Teratocarcinoma Cells: Formation of Embryoid Bodies In Vitro," *Proceedings of the National Academies of Science of the USA* (v.72/4, 1975).

Ka Yi Ling
University of Wisconsin

# Eggan, Kevin

**KEVIN EGGAN IS** an assistant professor of molecular and cellular biology at Harvard University. He is also an assistant investigator for the Stowers Medical Institute and principal investigator of the Harvard Stem Cell Institute. His office is in Cambridge, Massachusetts.

In 1996, Eggan received a bachelor's of science degree in microbiology from the University of Illinois at Urbana-Champaign. His doctoral degree in biology was awarded by the Massachusetts Institute of Technology (MIT) in 2003. The birth of Dolly the sheep, the first cloned animal, occurred while Kevin was doing his doctoral work at MIT. Inspired, he devoted his time to mastering the techniques involved in cloning. It was a delicate technique that took a year's concentrated work to master. After graduating from MIT, Eggan became a postdoctoral fellow at the Whitehead Institute for Biomedical Research and later a junior fellow in the Harvard Society of Fellows. He joined Harvard University's Department of Molecular and Cellular Biology in 2005.

Still in his early 30s, Eggan is a pursuing a career in developmental biology. His research goal, similar to that of other developmental biologists, is to address fundamental questions about cellular differentiation and plasticity. The questions addressed to cellular development are basic research questions, rather than applied research questions, and the goal is pure knowledge. If there are applications that emerge, they will be for another day's work. Although this separation between knowledge and application is the classic ideal, in reality, the great hope of the basic research in developmental biology is to ask questions of stem cells that can provide answers for adult cells. The therapeutic goal is to develop therapeutic stem cell lines from adult cell nuclei.

The research that Eggan is conducting is an exploration of the mechanisms by which somatic cell nuclear transfers occur. The transfers are forms of cloning in which a differentiation of a cell can be reversed. The result of the reversal of the differential produces a condition in which a cell can reprogram its nucleus into a totipotent state. Totipotency is the power that a single cell has to divide and to produce all of the differentiated cells in an organism, whether mammalian or some other life form. Totipotent cells are formed during both sexual (zygotes) and asexual (spores) reproduction.

Somatic cells are the type of cells that form the body of an organism. They are the cells forming body parts such as organs, blood, bones, and connective tissue skin. They are different from germline cells. The "gametes" or germline cells are cells such as spermatozoa or ova, which create a zygote in mammals when fertilization occurs. Virtually all of the cells of a mammal, including humans, are somatic cells, with only the spermatozoa and ova cells forming gametocytes and undifferentiated stem cells.

The somatic cell nuclear transfer (SCNT) research that Eggan is conducting uses a laboratory technique to create an "ovum" in the donor nucleus. The technique is often used in embryonic stem cell research to conduct the development of therapeutic cloning and reproductive cloning. When conducting SCNT research, the DNA of a somatic cell is removed, and the remainder is discarded. The nucleus of a sperm or a ova (egg cell) is removed, and the DNA from the nucleus of the somatic cell is implanted in the enucleated egg cell. Then the egg cell is reprogrammed by the host cell. Stimulated by a shock, it begins to divide to form a blastocyst (early staged embryo) with around 100 cells. These cells all have the DNA of the original somatic cell.

The accomplishments of Eggan in this area of research have placed him at the cutting edge of this new frontier of research. Understanding the mechanism for the development of a single cell into a complex organism is very important to the advancement of developmental biology and stem cell research.

Eggan has used mouse embryos to study the X chromosome. His research has sought to understand X chromosome activation and deactivation. He has demonstrated that the nuclear transfer procedure does, in fact, lead to epigenetic reprogramming of the donor genome. The epigenetic changes that occur serve as an informational program that makes it possible to interpret the genetic code. The modifications are inheritable and give stable instructions so that specific chromatin activity to organize and structure can occur. In other recent research, Eggan has demonstrated that the nuclei of adult cells that are very specialized can also exhibit pluripotential possibilities. This means that specialized cells such as the olfactory cells of the nose, which have odorant receptors, can be used for stem cell research.

In June 2006 Eggan was granted permission to pursue embryonic stem cell lines that were taken from patients who were suffering from terminal diseases or from debilitating diseases such as Parkinson's disease. His project had been given clearance after a careful review by independent human subjects and ethics panels. The goal was to create stem cell lines from skin cells from terminal patients and to redirect the stem cells from an adult or differentiated cell so that therapeutic applications for diseases could be developed. The research also provides an experimental platform for investigating the genetic and environmental factors that contribute to disease.

The change in the focus of his research from mice embryonic stem cell research to human stem cell research also forced many changes in Eggan's lifestyle. The politically charged issue of human embryonic stem cell research means that research funds for human embryonic research have to come from private donors, and they have to be kept completely separate from federal funds, which cannot be used for human embryonic stem cell research in many cases. Eggan is a member of the Stowers Medical Institute, which privately funds embryonic stem cell research. The politics of embryonic stem cell research are such that researchers enter a political storm when they engage in human stem cell research. However, Eggan's desire to find cures for diseases such as Alzheimer's disease and diabetes through embryonic research has driven him into the fray. He is aware that although there is as yet no moral consensus on stem cell research, there is a nearly universal moral consensus to help the sick.

Eggan has been a collaborator in numerous scientific articles on stem cell research. In some he was the lead author. He is also a contributor to a new book on stem cell research.

**SEE ALSO:** Cells, Embryonic; Cells, Mouse (Embryonic); Harvard University.

**BIBLIOGRAPHY.** Stephen Sullivan, Chad Cowan, and Kevin Eggan, eds., *Human Embryonic Stem Cells: The Practical Handbook* (John Wiley and Sons, 2007).

ANDREW J. WASKEY
DALTON STATE COLLEGE

# Egg Donation

**EGG DONATION IS** not a new area of research. It has been one of the methods to address infertility for many years. Donors of both eggs and sperm have been compensated when the donations were used for the purpose of infertility, but despite this payment, there has been a lack of major discussion on the payment policy.

In the United States, the subject of reproduction has been self-regulated, mostly through the American Society for Reproductive Medicine. The society has agreed that the payment for egg donation should range between $3000 and $5000. This is in contrast to some countries, including Canada, where payment for egg donation is prohibited.

The world is facing a new era, in which there is a need for large numbers of eggs for the derivation of new embryonic stem cell lines (ESCs) and for nuclear reprogramming to generate ESCs.

Egg donation is the process by which a female is provided with hormones to stimulate the maturation of multiple eggs within the ovarian follicles, and the mature eggs are then harvested for donation. The process by which egg maturation is induced and harvested is as follows: The hormones are delivered under the skin via subcutaneous injection, and then the eggs are retrieved by an invasive procedure. The female is subjected briefly to anesthesia, and the eggs are retrieved by ultrasound with a needle being passed through the vagina to the ovary.

## GUIDELINES

The selected guides have an effect on long-term policies. It is interesting to examine a state that supports the derivation of new human ESC lines and to determine whether egg donation policies might conflict with the state's mission. California leads the emphasis of ESC research through the commitment of state funds. The state, however, prohibits payment to egg donors, except for direct expenses. This type of law, although it appears contradictory, suggests that despite the support of ESC research and the derivation of new lines, the states, such as California, are mindful of ensuring that ethical boundaries are not crossed. Although California should be applauded, the issue is confusing because its law allows for the payment to gamete donors for the purpose of conception by infertility donors, to surrogate women, and also to research subjects.

The issue of research also needs to be elaborated because its mention brings up another topic: The donation of eggs for the purpose of deriving an ESC line, or for nuclear transfer. It is open for discussion whether this type of donation falls under the umbrella of research. If one argues that the derived cells, in this case, ESCs, are intended for research, then the donors would be required to sign informed consents without undue coercion or inducement. The donors also will be required to get information on the potential risk to themselves. At present, it is difficult to determine what the risks should include, as this type of information is unclear and mostly anecdotal. The limited data suggest that there is no risk to the donor, with six percent of donors showing signs of hyperovulation. The process of preparing the donor results in an increase in the cycling of eggs toward maturation. Increased cycling of any cell could predispose them to mutations, and such changes can occur in the harvested eggs as well as in those left in the woman. Because there is no definitive scientific data that argue for safety, what would be documented in the consent form? Today's society challenges anecdotal information, leaving the subject in a grey zone of uncertainty.

In 2005 a body of scientists and ethicists, under the umbrella of the National Academy of Science (NAS), released a document titled "Guidelines for Human Embryonic Stem Cell Research." The document, however, states that the issue of payment is open to further review. The NAS document was widely accepted as a general guide, but it cannot be legally enforced. The state of California similarly adapted the NAS guidelines on payment for egg donation by allowing reimbursement only for incurred expenses. The egg donors are subjected to an invasive procedure and can be psychologically harmed, among other effects, but the reimbursable expenses incurred do not account for this form of trauma. Perhaps an exhaustive legal argument might be able to justify these types of trauma as authentic expenses. To date, such argument, if it has been made, has not been widely circulated to the public.

At the international level, a significant guide was developed by a professional stem cell society, the International Society for Stem Cell Research (ISSCR). The documentation on ethical guidelines by the ISSCR, as it extends to countries outside of the United States, could be considered a guide that embodies the input of an international community. In this regard, this document is perhaps a relatively more cohesive guide for the scientific community. The society indicates that each country should develop its own rules rather than having a global guide. This is a more liberal guide compared with the 2005 document developed by the National Academy of Science.

Although the ISSCR guide provides for the future incorporation of culture, religion, and other country-specific issues, this could be a problem for scientists around the globe who are engaged in collaborative research on stem cells. The intercountry collaboration will require common institutional agreements. Although science has been performed with collaboration among countries, the issue of egg donation might not have an easy solution. Several unfortunate incidents in ESC research between different countries have formed the impetus for countries to step back and develop their own guidelines on egg donation. The method by which these problems will be addressed is unclear, and the development of guides for intercountry collaborations might occur after several years of discussions.

As these discussions are developed, scientists and educators have the responsibility to teach the next generation of stem cell biologists that rules are necessary and science cannot be conducted at the expense of ethics. As the discussions among stem cell biologists and bioethicists continue, it is imperative to remember that different countries have their unique cultures and beliefs. Whether these fundamental beliefs are based on religion, they nonetheless need to be heeded and respected. In the end, the guidelines should be able to justify how much an egg donor is compensated.

## DONORS

Humans have been known to donate eggs for altruistic reasons, such as assisting women who are infertile. However, for the most part, egg donors are enticed by the payment. This leads to further discussion about the population that is most likely to act as egg donors. A population of women who are in dire need of money may consider egg donation a good opportunity, regardless of the knowledge that the harvesting procedure is invasive. These women could be part of the skewed cohorts of egg donors.

The following case presentation includes three groups of individuals. Women in group 1 are from a lower socioeconomic background, women in group 2 are from middle-class families, and women in group 3 are affluent. The three groups are asked to donate their eggs; the payment is set at $5000. There is no coercion, and additionally, the information on potential donor risk is transparent. What are the likely outcomes? The prediction is that a larger pool of donors would be derived from group 1. Depending on the country involved, this group also might be of a particular ethnicity. This would result in the derived ESCs being skewed towards a particular ethnic group, which would lack diversity. If group 1 made up the larger percentages of donors, they might also make up the most unhealthy population, which might lead to mutated or defective ESCs and predispose the individuals to risks.

If altruism is incorporated into the character of the individuals who are likely to donate, then the number of potential donors could be equal among the three groups. At times, altruism would be a result of knowing the final outcome of the eggs. Full knowledge could, for instance, relate to the future use of the ESCs to generate blood cells for immediate delivery and eliminate the need for a blood donation. In addition, knowledge of the eggs' final destination might involve knowing the method by which nuclear transfer might be used to treat diseases. Individuals within the lower socioeconomic group might be the least educated, as higher education in most countries could be costly. Therefore, revisiting the characteristics of the individuals who in this scenario are likely to donate for altruistic reasons, we might argue that group 3 would have the greatest participation, which could also lead to skewed ethnicity and lack of diversity.

The question, then, is why should diversity be a concern? The major point to be addressed here is the fear of rejection when ESCs are taken to patients. As with bone marrow transplantation, the probability of finding a close match is high when the ethnicity of the donor and the recipient are similar. This rule also applies to ESCs.

The final question is whether the egg donors should be paid or not. Opinion on this issue is split among individuals and even among large committees. This is not a simple question and would require years for a compromise to occur. In the case of fertility, altruistic donations from relatives cannot be encouraged because the eggs and sperm might express common genes, with a high probability of expressing carrier health defects. However, in the case of the development of ESCs for health problems, altruistic egg donation from relatives can be encouraged because the probability of rejection could decrease. In the meantime, the development of ESCs needs to use egg donations that are obtained ethically.

**SEE ALSO:** Cells, Embryonic; Embryonic Stem Cells; Ethics; International Society for Stem Cell Research; Nuclear Transfer, Altered; Nuclear Transfer, Somatic; Regulations Overview.

**BIBLIOGRAPHY.** G. Q. Daley et al., "Ethics. The ISSCR Guidelines for Human Embryonic Stem Cell Research," *Science* (v.315, 2007); E. Gerber and S. Schalman-Bergen, "California Limits Egg Donor Compensation in Privately-Funded Research," *Journal of Law, Medicine, and Ethics* (v.35, 2007); C. Holden and G. Vogel, "National Academies: Panel Would Entrust Stem Cell Research to Local Oversight," *Science* (v.308, 2005); P. Pearson, "Special Report: Health Effects of Egg Donation May Take Decades to Emerge," *Nature* (v.442, 2006); J. A. Robertson, "Compensation and Egg Donation for Research, *Fertility and Sterility* (v.86, 2006).

Pranela Rameshwar
UMDNJ–New Jersey Medical School

# Ethics

**SIMPLY PUT, ETHICS** is the study of the principles of right and wrong. Ethicists seek to know and to advise how to do good. However, this definition puts the subject into a deep quandary because, as the simple child's prayer says, "God is good, God is great…" and then goodness is an attribute of God and hence difficult to know. The difficulty of knowing what is good is at the core of the many types of ethics and many of the disputes over what is ethical and what is not. The sources of ethical principles have been nature or religion. Those who seek to develop naturalistic ethical systems use reason to identify principles that are consistent with human nature. For example, Benedict de Spinoza developed an ethic based upon reasonings about humans. Religions have long developed ethics that are in agreement with the discerned nature of the divine or with the revealed will of God.

Seeking to do well and to avoid evil has been a universal human activity. It is the quest for the moral life that has separated saints and sinners, good citizens from rogues, or those who seek to live the good life, even at personal cost, from those who seek to satisfy the self without regard for others or for the Divine.

There are two types of ethics: personal ethics and social ethics. Personal ethics are those moral actions expected from individuals. Social ethics are the ethics of groups of people. Some moralists argue that the personal ethics of the individual are the only kind of ethics. Ethics are the same whether an individual belong to a group or not. However, those who claim that there are two types of ethics argue that ethics in a group are different from ethics as an individual. For example, those who argue that there is only one type of ethic say that joining the military or the police does not make the use of violence moral, while the latter say that it is morally justified for members of such organizations to use violence. Being a member of the organization changes the moral status of the police or military for ethicists who adopt this position.

Discussions of ethics have generated rules for living. Among all the things that humans do some things involve ethics while other activities do not. Mores, manners and morals all develop rules for human behavior in different societies. However, mores and manners do not have moral force, even if many people act as though they do.

## MORAL DISCOURSE

Moral discourse is conducted at different levels. The simplest level is the level of moral judgments. Suppose at this level a moralist advances the claim that "abortion is wrong." If the moral judgment were to elicit a reply from an interlocutor, it might simply be "why?" The justification for the claim that abortion is wrong would advance the moral discussion to the level of moral philosophy in which the assertion could be made "because it's murder."

Quite often moral discourse breaks down at the level of moral judgment or moral philosophy. Partisan exchanges quickly become heated verbal conflicts with little if any light shed on the subject of the morality of abortion. If the moral discourse is to advance then it would need to move to the third level, which is the level of ethics. At this level questions and moral claims become more general and abstract.

Moral discourse at the ethical level has the possibility of advancing moral understanding. Moral judgments at this level can develop moral judgments that are well supported by adequate reasons. At the ethics level of moral discourse questions such as, "What is murder?" could be answered by "homicide." This answer is imprecise because any killing of human beings is a homicide whether the killing is intentional or accidental.

It is rare (if it has ever existed) for a political system not to allow for the justified use of force for its police forces or to specify the rules of engagement in military actions. Pacifists would hold such acts to be murder, but most people would see such use of violence as justified. Therefore it would be reasonable for the skeptical interlocutor to seek a precise definition of homicide in the matter of the death of a fetus.

In a search for precision in the definition of homicide the interlocutor could ask the moralist a question seeking qualifications of the definition: "Is any homicide a murder?" The moralist could reply that a fetus is a human being.

The skeptical interlocutor could then ask, "What is a human being?" "Is a fetus a human in actuality or merely potentially?" Many more questions could be raised to explore fully the ethics of abortion or any other moral issue.

The highest level of moral discourse is in the area of meta-ethics. This level is universal and cross-cultural. In this area investigations are conducted into how different systems of ethics handle different questions. Comparisons and contrasts are made between Hindu, Christian, Jewish, Muslim, Buddhist, naturalistic, or rationalistic systems of ethics such as the professional ethics of physicians.

The levels of moral discourse are supplied moral language from the experiences of real life situations occurring in historical contexts. This is why moral philosophy like political philosophy is called a practical discipline. Ethics deals with practical matters and not with the merely abstract. The question, "How ought we to live?" occurs in the business of life.

Ethics is also a normative discipline as are logic and aesthetics and logic. These three disciplines seek to understand what is good, true, and beautiful. To do so judgments have to be made about the values that are represented in goodness, truth, and beauty. This creates a problem known as the is-ought problem. Ethics decisions require the combining of fact and moral principles; however, moral principles come from different sources from those of facts.

Judgments of facts are made in real life situations where the data of life exists in a local setting. Consequently there is a context in which moral action takes place and it includes the facts of the situation, the inward attitudes of the moral actor, the principles that guide the decision, and the consequences of the action (or non-action).

## MORAL DECISION MAKING

Moral decision making means acting upon the basis of some kind of principle in the midst of a set of facts. The principle may be something such as love or the golden rule or a deontological maxim such as Immanuel Kant's categorical imperative, which says that humans are to act only on the maxim that they can will that the action will be a universal law. Sometimes the moral rule is stated as a law such as "Thou shalt not bear false witness."

Moral decision making may be based upon the individual's highest good (*summum bonum*). Numerous goods are offered as the highest good for which people should strive. These include pleasure (hedonism), money, fame (actors), power (Machiavelli), conquest, honor (warriors), sex, happiness, the glory of God or the will of God, the good of the nation, the party, the society, the tribe and others.

Ethical decisions can be based upon the good will of a person. However, good intentions may not produce good consequences, because individual acts may be morally sound but have greater consequences than is generally recognized. Instead of basing ethics on rules or a *summum bonum* some moral philosophy is based upon the consequences. Acts are judged by whether the consequences are good or bad. Sometimes the consequences are all likely to be bad. However, consequences may be unevenly distributed.

Moral feelings are varied and signal the presence of moral situations that require moral judgments. The five basic feelings—joy, love, anger, fear, or grief—can signal that one is in the presence of one or more ethic events. For example, anger is a signal that a person is experiencing injustice. Feelings of fairness or unfairness are feelings that arise with experiences of injustice. They create anger or moral outrage. They can also evoke feelings of moral disgust or contempt which are feelings of moral inferiority or superiority.

**ETHICAL THEORIES**

The emotive theory of ethics denies the reality of ethics. It claims that ethics is just a report of someone's feelings. The epistemology of logical positivists and other strict empiricists has been used to argue that moral claims are simply reports of liking or disliking something because all that can be known are feelings. This position reduces ethics to mere matters of taste. Cannibalism, Nazi atrocities, or other heinous acts are in this ethical theory reports of subjective preferences.

Strict determinists such as Clarence Darrow have argued that there is no reality to ethics. For there to be moral actions there must be free will with the power to choose between options. Darrow and other determinists deny free will and therefore ethical responsibility. Darrow argued this successfully in the Leopold and Loeb case in his summation to the jury. Most people who understand the claims of Emotivists and Determinists reject these positions. Most moralists believe that except for a few poor souls, most people have free will and moral responsibility for their actions. Ethics is a rational activity. It separates humans from animals. Cats kill birds or mice because it is their nature to do so. Animals mate in response to instinctive drives. Humans may kill, mate or do other activities but it is expected that their behavior will be guided by reason.

Among ethical theories hedonism has been widespread. Hedonism comes from *hedone*, which is the Greek word for pleasure. Hedonists argue that the *summum bonum* of life is to maximize pleasure and to minimize pain. The ancient Cyrenaics and the Epicureans were hedonists. In the case of the Cyrenaics the goal was to maximize gross bodily pleasure in orgies of food, alcohol and sex in an "eat, drink, and be merry, for tomorrow we die" approach to life. For the Cyrenaics all pleasures are equal. In contrast, Epicurus sought qualitative pleasures. He also sought to avoid pain, so his ethic was to gain pleasure after avoiding pain. The Cyrenaics and the Epicureans were both practitioners of an individual ethic of pleasure. Their personal ethic denied any social responsibility. In contrast, utilitarianism is a social ethics. It asks, "What's the greatest good for the greatest number of people?"

Jeremy Bentham argued that people are born under two sovereign masters: pleasure and pain. They spend their lives maximizing pleasure and minimizing pain. He then developed a calculus of pleasure for guiding public decision-making. His calculus of pleasure was a quantitative approach to the pleasure gained by people when faced with group decisions. He sought to measure seven criteria for his calculus of pleasure-pain to judge what ought to be done.

These criteria were the "intensity," or how strong were the pleasures and pains; the duration of the pleasure or pain experience—that is, how long it will last; the certainty, or how likely the pleasure is to occur; propinquity, how near at hand is the pleasure; fecundity, or the characteristic or ability of something to produce still further pleasures; purity, its freedom from ensuing pains; and the extent of the pleasure, that is, the number of people affected by it.

Using the calculus of pleasure-pain Bentham thought that it would be straightforward to decide what would be the greatest good for the greatest number of people. All that was needed would be decided by compiling how much pleasure or happiness was generated versus how much pain would be suffered if a tax policy were enacted or some other decision were made.

Aristotle wrote about ethics in his book *Ethics*, and he developed a teleological ethic with happiness as its goal. Jefferson's "pursuit of happiness" in the Declaration of Independence is expressing this goal. He also advocated following a golden mean between the extremes of ethical positions—moderation is a virtue.

Ethics that stress the virtue of the moral actor can be faced with the problem that many words are vague. Terms such as *courage* do not have a clearly defined cutoff. This creates the possibility of vague moral statements that are neither determinately true nor determinately false. For example, courage is a virtue but the brave man looks rash compared to the cowardly man; and the brave man looks cowardly compared to the rash man.

A final difference in ethical positions is that between relativists and objectivists. For relativists, ethics are personal standards that vary from individual to individual. There are ethical standards but they are subjective. Ethical standards depend upon the choices of individuals or of societies. For example, in answer to the question, "Is abortion wrong?" the relativist would say it is a matter of the individual person, or that it varies from society to society. Relativists often claim that one opinion is always as good as another, and that when two people disagree, it can never be determined whose position is more reasonable to hold. Contradiction between principles is not a virtue for relativists.

Objective ethics are those such as the Ten Commandments written on stone. The moral law may not be liked by someone but it is not a matter of subjective choice as to its existence. Like the laws of the Romans that came to be written on a stone pillar, they are in the public as standards that can be disobeyed or ignored but their objective existence cannot be denied.

Relativistic ethical claims such as the claim that justice is a matter of personal choice has to counter the fact that in order to argue against a group or individual who have imposed a moral rule the claim that it is "unfair" is an appeal to an objective standard.

## ETHICS IN STEM CELL DEBATES

Stem cell research is new area of scientific endeavor. As a new area of biological and medical research, it entered the policy arenas of America where vigorous ongoing debates about abortion were being conducted. Many of the alleged ethical judgments concerning stem cell research have been political positions that seek to prevent even the least quarter to opponents in the stem cell debates. In the case of stem cell research, ethical judgments are usually made on the grounds that the use of embryonic stem cell material from abortions is moral or not moral.

The basis of the moral judgment is usually that the use of an aborted fetus is moral or it is not moral. When the embryos in question are from unwanted embryos supplied by fertility clinics the facts are different from those involving aborted fetuses. Arguments have been advanced that using in vitro embryos is morally permissible because it is the work of the scientific community and not simple the deeds of private individuals.

Arguments have been made about when is a fetus a human person. The claim that it is one at conception even in cases of in vitro fertilization require the combining of principles derived from revelation with some biological facts.

Widespread disagreement with this position means that it may be justified belief for its advocates but it has not been morally persuasive to others. Some moralists such as Peter Singer have argued that in vitro embryos are not sentient beings. The embryo has no consciousness, therefore it does not qualify as human.

Some supporters of fetal embryonic stem cell research have argued on the basis of the consequences. To discard the stem cells of an aborted fetus would be wasteful (negative consequence) while to use them could lead to medical breakthroughs (positive consequence). Others have argued on a utilitarian basis. The pain suffered by an embryo, especially in vitro, is insignificant compared to the pleasure that will be experienced by those who regain health from the scientific discoveries of the research. A calculus of pleasure and pain would land on the side of pleasure as the greatest good for society.

Opposition to stem cell research is based on Biblical exegesis and moral theology that is far from universally accepted. However, this ethical position is objective in the sense that it is derived from objective ethical sources such as the Ten Commandments.

Ethics in the stem cell debates, like ethics in general, is made difficult because of disputes over the nature of what is good or ethical, what is human, the nature of the human condition, and how to live. Rapid scientific advances have created new sets of facts. Stem cells were unknown until recently and now the problem has become finding moral ways to advance knowledge and to live as good persons who apply this knowledge.

**SEE ALSO:** Advocacy; Moral Status of Embryo.

**BIBLIOGRAPHY.** Laura Black, *Stem Cell Debate: The Ethics and Science Behind the Research* (Enslow Publishers, Inc., 2006); Simon Blackburn, *Being Good: A Short Introduction to Ethics* (Oxford University Press, 2003); Roger H. Crook, *Introduction to Christian Ethics* (Prentice-Hall, 2006); S. Cromwell Crawford, *Hindu Bioethics for the Twenty-First Century* (State University of New York, 2003); Fred Feldman, *Introduction to Ethics* (McGraw-Hill, 1998); David Guinn, ed., *Handbook of Bioethics and Religion* (Oxford University Press, 2006); Suzanne Holland, Karen Lebacqz, and Laurie Zoloth, eds., *The Human Embryonic Stem Cell Debate: Science, Ethics, and Public Policy* (MIT Press, 2001); D. Keown, *Buddhism and Bioethics* (Macmillan, 1995); Louis Newman, *An Introduction to Jewish Ethics* (Prentice-Hall, 2004); John F. Peppin, Mark J. Cherry, and Ana Iltis, *Religious Perspectives in Bioethics* (Tayor & Francis, 2004); Fred Rosner, *Contemporary Biomedical Ethical Issues and Jewish Law* (KTAV Publishing House, 2007); Gerald J. Williams, *Short Introduction to Ethics* (University Press of America, 1998).

Andrew J. Waskey
Dalton State College

# European Consortium for Stem Cell Research—EuroStemCell

**THE EUROSTEMCELL CONSORTIUM** brings together sixteen partners, integrating a broad range of disciplines and combining the expertise of the best laboratories in Europe. The centers involved are all international leaders in their respective fields, and collectively provide the skills and technologies necessary for groundbreaking stem cell research. The collaborative activities of the consortium are laying the groundwork for taking stem cell technology to the clinic in the form of well characterized cell lines and a solid pre-clinical skills and knowledge base.

EuroStemCell, the European Consortium for Stem Cell Research, most recently has produced promising results for treating the debilitating and often fatal genetic disorder of muscular dystrophy (MD). Researchers from the San Raffaele Scientific Institute in Milan, Italy, led by Dr. Giulio Cossu, have been studying the most common form of the disease, known as Duchenne muscular dystrophy. They discovered that the mesoangioblast muscle stem cell, present in the walls of blood vessels, produced encouraging results when injected in mice. They took mesoangioblast stem cells from the blood vessels of dogs with the mutation, corrected it using gene therapy, and re-injected the modified stem cells.

They also repeated the procedure with cells from healthy dogs, using drugs to prevent immune rejection. Both treatment procedures resulted in the increased production of dystrophin, though the injection of the donor stem cells yielded the most encouraging results. Repeated doses of cells

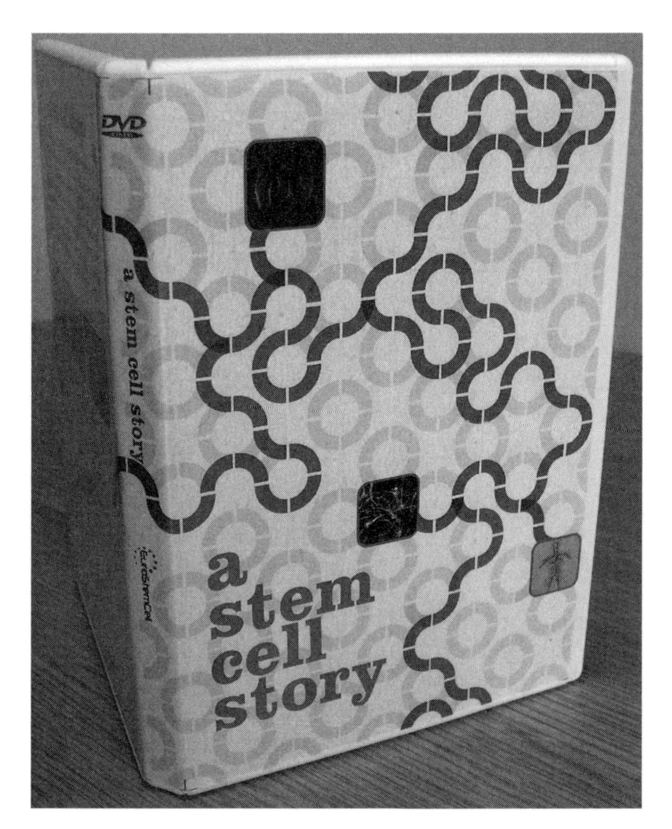


*EuroStemCell, which published this educational DVD, has dedicated considerable resources to public outreach.*

from the healthy dogs restored muscle function in four of five dystrophic dogs.

In their experiment, researchers found that stem cells successfully established themselves in the host tissue, allowing for the production of dystrophin, offsetting the effects of muscular dystrophy. The injected stem cells not only produced dystrophin in the affected leg, but in other areas of the body as well, including respiratory muscles, leading researchers to believe that they are on the right track to finding an effective treatment for MD sufferers.

EuroStemCell's research program is organized into eight work packages on specific areas of stem cell research, supported by six flagship projects that span the work package areas. Five work packages focus on the fundamental biology of stem cells.

The focus of the Identification and Isolation of Stem Cells work packages is to identify, isolate and undertake comparative characterization of stem cells for tissues of major clinical importance: neural stem cells for brain repair; mesodermal stem cells for giving rise to blood cells and muscular tissue; epithelial stem cells for skin replacement and for generation of thymus and other epithelial organs.

The purpose of the third work package, Lineage Analysis and Differentiation Potential, is to determine the normal routes a stem cell takes when differentiating into specialized cells and contributing to tissues. Analyzing these lineages will highlight the intermediate cell types generated by stem cells, as well as their locations, migratory routes and cellular environments in normal individuals. This is an important source of information for the isolation, culture and differentiation of stem cells in the laboratory, and is therefore crucial if stem cells are to be used for stem cell regenerative therapies and drug discovery.

The Self-renewal and Up-Scaling work package aims to analyze the factors that control stem cell self-renewal (the ability of a stem cell to make copies of itself indefinitely) and use this information to define the conditions and procedures that will be required for the generation of expanded and clinically acceptable resources for cell therapies. The Control of Differentiation work package aims to develop tools that allow the reproducible generation of stem cell populations capable of efficient and directed differentiation into all specialized cell types necessary for tissue repair.

A sixth work package, Applications in Neurological Disease, will test the ability of transplanted stem cells and cell lines, generated in work packages one, three, and four, and derived from endogenous neural stem cells, to differentiate into therapeutically relevant cell types for the treatment of Parkinson's Disease, stroke and myelin diseases using animal models.

Work package seven, Applications in Muscle Repair and Neuromuscular Disease, will test the ability of stem cells and cell lines, generated in the other work packages, for their capacity to contribute to skeletal muscle, using mouse models for muscular dystrophy. The goal of an eighth work package, Epidermal Repair, is to use animal models to improve the techniques for grafting cultured epidermis and optimize the conditions for recreating hair follicles, sweat and sebaceous glands in the skin of human burns victims.

### FLAGSHIP PROJECTS

The Generation of Antibodies for Stem Cell Identification project seeks to widen the range of antibodies available in stem cell community and characterize their utility for identifying sub-populations of cells during differentiation. The project will take advantage of existing efforts among partner institutions to generate antibodies and apply them to the stem cell research.

The Development of a Prototype European Stem Cell Database and Stem Cell Registry project will establish a stem cell database (Stem DB) containing a wide range of information about stem cells—from basic biology to clinical applications. The data will be derived from new findings generated by the EuroStemCell consortium and existing published data.

A third flagship project, the Forum for Ethics and Societal Issues Related to Stem Cell Research, will consider a range of topical issues relating to stem cell research. The work will be presented in a series of workshops, involving participants from both EuroStemCell and the EU Framework 5 EuroStem ethics project. The workshops will not only identify and analyze issues but also come up with suggestions as to how they are to be handled and relate these proposals to current regulations in various countries where the research is carried out.

The Stem Cell Bioinformatics project will facilitate comparative analysis of the stem cell molecular profiling data generated in the other EuroStemCell work packages, and foster bioinformatics collaborations among different participating groups. A Clinical Roadmap project aims to generate a statement on the steps necessary in developing clinical applications from stem cells. Clinicians, basic scientists, bio-industry representatives and ethicists will be engaged in this process through a series of workshops focused on neurological, neuromuscular and skin disorders

The final flagship project involves public engagement and outreach to create a climate of open and informed debate, as it is important that practicing scientists are encouraged to participate in outreach activities, and are equipped with the necessary skill sets. EuroStemCell has dedicated considerable resources to developing a provocative, forward looking public engagement and outreach program.

**SEE ALSO:** France; Germany; International Society for Stem Cell Research; International Stem Cell Forum; Italy; United Kingdom.

**BIBLIOGRAPHY.** EuroStemCell, www.eurostemcell.org (cited November 2007); Institute for Stem Cell Research, www.iscr.ed.ac.uk (cited November 2007); StemCellResearchNews.com, www.stemcellresearchnews.com (cited November 2007).

Fernando Herrera
University of California, San Diego

## Experimental Models

**EXPERIMENTAL MODELS HELP** researchers understand the developmental and function of a biological process. A model system in biological research refers to anything that scientists use to recreate aspects of a disease or any biological process.

The study of a biological process has made intensive use of experimental models, as performing such work in human is difficult for experimental, practical, and ethical reasons. A model can be a cell living in a dish. Or it can be used the animal models that have long played an important role in biology are both invertebrates (e.g., Drosophila, Aplysia) and vertebrates (e.g., Zebrafish, rodents, non-human primates), as well as mutant and transgenic animals that have revolutionized scientists' ability to characterize normal, abnormal, and restorative development.

Stem cells can be clinically beneficial through a range of mechanism-encapsulated in the idea of therapeutic plasticity. The field of stem cell biology and regenerative medicine is rapidly moving toward translation to clinical practice, and in doing so has become even more dependent on animal donors and hosts for generating cellular reagents and assaying their potential therapeutic efficacy in models of human disease. Advances in cell culture technologies have revealed a remarkable plasticity of stem cells from embryonic and adult tissues, and transplantation models are now needed to test the ability of these cells to protect at-risk cells and replace cells lost to injury or disease. Stem cells can be applied to two basic experimental models. First, preliminary experiments are performed using cultured stem cells grown in dishes. These cells come from human tissue samples or from model organisms such as mice or rats. Second, refined potential stem cell therapies are tested in animal models, such as mice, rats, and non-human primates, before being used in clinical trials.

The process of developing a potential therapy starts out as a testable idea based on initial research findings. This idea must be followed up with rigorous research and testing in the lab using different experimental models, which can take years of works. Even if the therapy looks great in lab experiments, it will become a viable treatment only after it is proven safe and effective in human clinical trials.

The first step is to establish an experimental model- a laboratory-based scenario that stimulates that way a stem cell therapy might work in humans. To be useful, an experimental model must possess these features: (1) it must accurately reflect the biology of human stem cells; (2) it must be reproducible, allowing experiments to be credibly repeated; and (3) it must be time effective, allowing experiments to be completed, analyzed and repeated within a reasonable time period.

Several issues need to be considered to establish the best experimental model using stem cells for understanding developmental and function of a biological process: (1) To discover the best stem or progenitor cell in vitro protocols for isolating, expanding, and priming these cells to facilitate their massive propagation into just the right type of stem cells, and (2) To establish the best animal models of human disease and injury, using both small and large animals, for testing new regenerative medicine therapeutics.

## APPLICATIONS OF STEM CELLS AS FOR EXPERIMENTAL DISEASE MODELS IN VITRO

Although many common diseases can be modeled in rodents, in many cases there animal models do not faithfully reproduce the human syndrome at either the molecular or anatomical levels. Species differences between rodents and humans might be one reason for clinical failures—rodent cells are differentially vulnerable to human transgenes and toxins compared with human cells. Human stem cells represent a renewable source of tissue that can generate target tissues. Therefore, these cells are a valuable tool of experimental disease models in vitro.

Recent remarkable advances allow us to control growth and differentiation of human stem cells that are derived from embryos, fetal, or the adult tissue. Human stem cells can be induced to differentiate into physiologically active and presumably functional cells, which occur through well-defined stages that involve waves of proliferation and maturation that are coordinated through temporal patterning in the developing tissues. These cells can be held in culture for many weeks or months for further maturation if required. Furthermore, the generation of human stem cell lines that carry mutations conferring predisposition to certain diseases will supply valuable research tools for studying by which processes the disease arise and potentially lead to the development of new therapeutic strategies.

## STRATEGIES FOR DISEASE MODELING IN STEM CELLS

Several strategies can be used to introduce the gene of interest into stem cells and their progeny - the introduction of mutations by viral infections, homologous recombination, nucleus transfer from the affected patients own cells, or by prenatal diagnostics. These cells could then be differentiated into the afflicted cell type and used to study the onset and progression of the disease, screen for new drugs, and test new therapies. For example, generation of pancreatic beta cells from human embryonic stem cells that carry particular maturity-onset diabetes of the young mutation could help towards a better understanding of the development of the disease and facilitate discovery of a cure. In neurodegenerative diseases, the ability to generate large number of defined neural derivatives raises the prospect of developing in vitro disease models as reported in recent studies of human embryonic stem cells-derived neurons examining toxicity in Parkinson's disease, Amyotrophic lateral sclerosis (ALS), Huntington's disease, and multiple sclerosis.

Most of stem cells including human embryonic and fetal stem cells can be transduced with viral vectors that carry specific mutations in a disease-causing gene of interest. Adeno-associated virus (AAV), and lenti- and retroviral vectors can be used for this purpose. Adeno-associated virus and lentiviral vectors infect dividing and non-dividing cells, whereas retroviral vectors infect only dividing cells. Cultures of infected cells that express the gene of interest can then be expanded. The transgene can be expressed through differentiation, allowing the examination of the effects of the mutant proteins in post-mitotic cells. Stable transgene expression can be achieved through transgene incorporation into the genome. The culture can also be enriched for the infected cells suing selection markers such as antibiotic resistance. However, the viral transduction to deliver mutant genes to cells has limitations. For example, the rates of infection are heterogenous and insertion into the genome is random.

Homologous recombination allows site specific insertion of a gene and has been used to generate transgenic lines from mouse embryonic stem cells. This technique has recently been show to work in human embryonic stem cells, although the recombination rates are low. The power of this technique is clear, as target genes can be inserted into know parts of the human genome without the risk of disrupting areas that are crucial for normal cell function. As technology advances, it might be also possible to use homologous recombination in fetal and adult stem cells.

In addition to genetic manipulation of normal stem cell cultures, it might be also useful to isolate stem or progenitor cells from embryos or postmortem fetal tissue that carries mutations linked to specific diseases. The advantage of this approach is that the insertion site and copy number of the mutation is identical to the normal situation in humans. Although this tissue is rare and appropriate clinical screening is required for its identification, large number of cells can be obtained following in vitro expansion from a single tissue source. One limitation of this approach is that if the mutation is very severe, it might not be possible to passage the cells that carry it and the cell lines might not be fully renewable.

At present, most embryonic stem cell lines have been derived from excess embryos that are collected from couples who undergo in vitro fertilization but that are no longer required. Therefore, it is impossible to ignore the associated ethical and political issues even if we use stem cells only for experimental models. Furthermore, most of what the research community knows about the nature and behaviors of stem cells comes from in vitro studies of these cells, subjecting them to growth factor and other morphogenetic or toxic molecule concoctions that attempt to mimic as possible growth condition in vivo. But many of events that investigations observe and attempt to characterize in a dish are not perfect as they occur in life because the cells are exposed to nonphysiological amounts of potent growth factors, cytokines, and morphogens that have profound effects on their choices to divide or differentiate along a particular line. Even so, recent studies using human stem cells achieve a rather impressive level of recapitulating many of the differentiation cascades that lead to the generation of normal cell lineage diversity as it evolves in vivo.

## EXPERIMENTAL MODELS TO UNDERSTAND THE BIOLOGY OF STEM CELLS

After the refinement of the in vitro models of different stem cell populations to generate cells that are homogenous as possible, it is feasible to use the results of in vitro studies for in vivo experimental

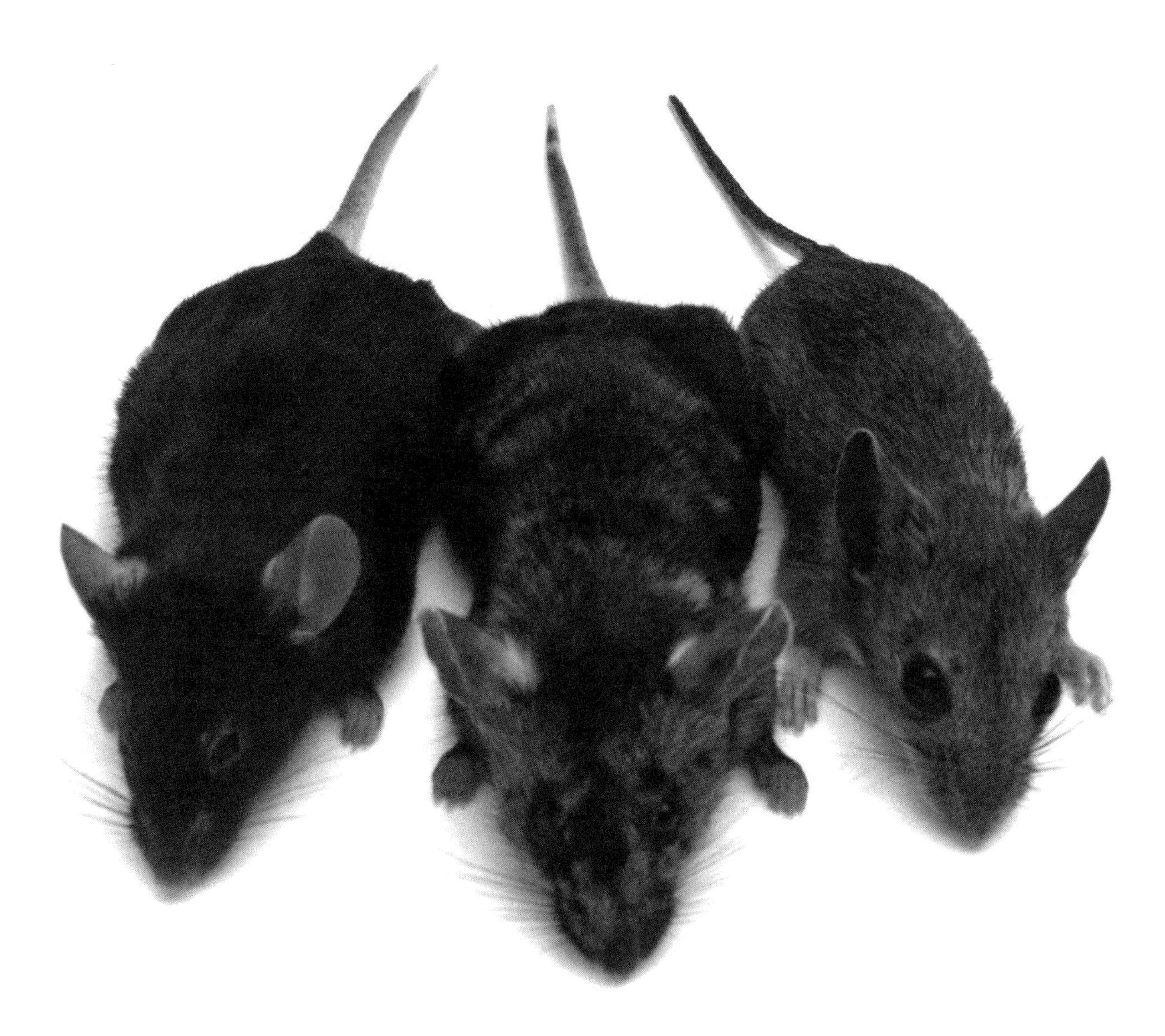

*From left:* Mus musculus *(house mouse); chimera, a genetic fusion of a house and wood mouse; and* Apodemus sylvaticus *(wood mouse). Both small and large animals are used for testing new regenerative medicine therapeutics.*

models for transplantation. Stem cell therapies involve more than simply transplanting cells into the body and waiting for them to go to work. A successful stem cell therapy requires an understanding of how transplanted cells work, combined with a reliable experiment model to enduring that the stem cells perform the desired action in the body. Whether stem cells survive, and whether they can still be transplanted after manipulation will have to be tested in experimental models. Regardless of the mechanism of action of any putative intervention (cellular or pharmacological), there is a need to demonstrate pathological and functional recovery in appropriate experimental models.

Several important issues remain to be resolved before delivery of functional cell population in vivo can be accomplished, including the type and number of cells to be delivered, site of engraftment, prevention of abnormal tissue formation (e.g. teratoma) due to contamination of the graft with remaining undifferentiated cells, and donor/recipient compatibility and graft rejection. Allogeneic transplantation of stem cell-derived cells will require immunosuppression in order to avoid graft-versus-host disease.

On a final note, recent advances suggest that patient-derived inducible pluripotent stem (iPS) cells may use as different strategies of avoiding this problem in the near future. The major advantage of using tissue-specific stem cells and iPS cells is that the patient's own cells can be expanded in culture and then re-introduced into the patient without immune rejection.

**SEE ALSO:** Clinical Trials Worldwide; Differentiation, In Vitro and In Vivo; Human ES Cell Isolation.

**BIBLIOGRAPHY.** A.J. Joannides and S. Chandran, "Human Embryonic Stem Cells: An Experimental and Therapeutic Resource for Neurological Disease," *Journal of the Neurological Sciences* (v. 265/1-2, October 2007); Dennis A. Steindler, "Stem Cells, Regenerative Medicine, and Animal Models of Disease," *ILAR Journal* (v. 48/4, 2007); Gianvito Martino & Stefano Pluchino, "The Therapeutic Potential of Neural Stem cells", Nature Reviews Neuroscience (v. 7/5, May 2006); Henrik Semb, "Human Embryonic Stem Cells: Origin, Properties and Applications," *APMIS* (v. 113/11–12, November–December 2005); Nicolas Legrand, Kees Weijer, and Hergen Spits, "Experimental Models to Study Development and Function of the Human Immune System In Vivo," *The Journal of Immunology* (v. 176, October 2005); Rebekah J. Jakel, Bernard L. Schneider, and Clive N. Svendsen, "Using Human Neural Stem Cells to Model Neurological Disease," *Nature Reviews Genetics* (v. 5/2, February 2004).

Masatoshi Suzuki
University of Wisconsin, Madison

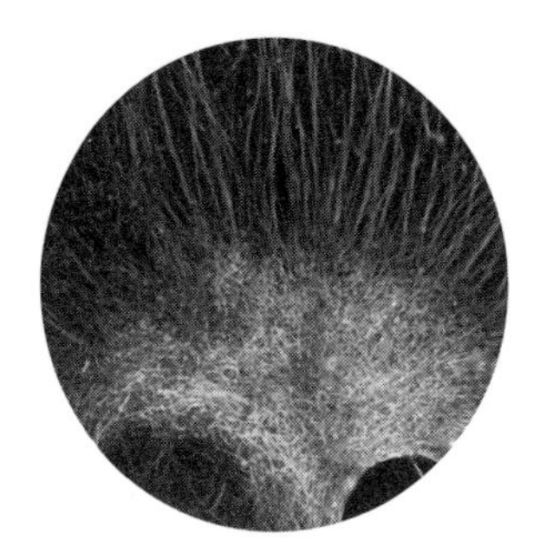

# F

## Federal Government Policies

**SINCE THE ISOLATION** of human embryonic stem cells by Dr. James Thomson in 1998, the federal government of the United States has struggled to create a standard human stem cell research policy. Much of the stem cell research debate is influenced by the competing moral and ethical arguments that continue to shape U.S. governmental policy in this scientific arena. Federal stem cell policy has wide implications and is not just limited to the stem cell research field. Much of the debate regarding stem cell research addresses the status of human embryos that are used in research.

With the advent of in vitro fertilization techniques and their growing use during the 1980s, the federal government became concerned with developing regulations for biotechnologies that use human embryos or embryonic tissue. Significant ethical and moral concerns arose over the potential for abuse of newly developed biotechnologies, and rising concern among many religious groups over the potential for fertilized embryos, viewed by many as sacred human lives, to be discarded and other ethical concerns led the federal government to consider and ultimately adopt comprehensive legislation. This legislation effectively banned federal funding of research conducted on human embryos. The Dickey Amendment, passed by Congress in 1995 and signed by President William Clinton in 1996, expressly forbade all federal funding for the creation of human embryos for the purpose of research or for any research that would result in the destruction of a human embryo. Since its passage, the amendment has been included in all of the U.S. Department of Health and Human Services, Department of Labor and the Department of Education appropriations, ensuring that the Dickey policy remains law.

The isolation of human embryonic stem cells in 1998 by Thomson represented an enormous new concern in the bioethics debate that was already raging. Politicians and government agencies struggled to create a uniform policy that adequately addressed issues raised by a concerned public. Because of the relative youth of the stem cell field, uniformity in scientific information was often not readily available or presented to the public.

Many of the original concerns discussed in regulating novel technologies such as in vitro fertilization surfaced again in the federal stem cell policy debate. Many conservative religious groups strongly argued that federal support of embryonic stem cell research would result in the destruction of many more human embryos and decrease the value of human life. Other groups also renewed concerns over the possible abuse of embryo manipulating technologies. It is important to note that many of these groups did not object to research conducted on adult human stem cells.

In contrast, many scientific groups argued that broad federal support for this relatively young field was necessary. Scientific groups touted the potential of stem cell research to yield potential cures to intractable illnesses, which warranted thorough consideration by the public. Many scientific and some business groups also argued that stringent regulation of stem cell research could stifle the field and damage the ability of the United States to maintain a leading role in a promising new scientific area.

## CLINTON ADMINISTRATION PROPOSALS

In 1999 the National Bioethics Advisory Commission, which directly advised President Clinton, recommended federal legislation to permit harvesting of human embryonic stem cells from embryos that were "left over" from in vitro fertilization treatments. However, the panel explicitly noted that this option should only be available in the case that the harvesting of embryonic stem cells would not be the proximate cause of the destruction of the human embryo. By adding this restriction, the advisory commission hoped to maintain compliance with the Dickey Amendment, which had been previously signed into law by President Clinton.

The suggestions of the National Bioethics Advisory Commission were taken under advisement; however, a policy decision on the federal level was not made at this time, as the Clinton administration was drawing to a close. Much of the regulation of the stem cell field would be determined and administered by the next U.S. president, George W. Bush.

## FEDERAL FUNDING GUIDELINES

After taking office, President George W. Bush was faced with the task of developing a comprehensive policy to regulate federal funding of stem cell research projects. The policy established by President Bush outlines a number of criteria that allow for federal funding in a limited number of circumstances. The current policies of the U.S. federal government do not restrict or limit federal funding of human adult stem cell research programs, with the most stringent regulation reserved for research regarding human embryonic stem cells.

President Bush's policy implemented across all relevant federal agencies, such as the National Institutes of Health, establishes three primary criteria for the use of federal funds in embryonic stem cell research. The first criterion establishes that federal funds that are sought for embryonic stem cell research must be reserved for research that uses embryonic stem cell lines derived or isolated before 9:00 P.M., Eastern Standard Time, on August 9, 2001. The second criterion establishes that the embryonic stem cells that are being used in the course of research must have been derived from an embryo that was originally created for reproductive purposes but was no longer needed.

The final criterion directs that the egg and related embryonic stem cells extracted for research purposes must have been obtained with the full consent of the donor without any financial incentives. On the basis of these criteria, the National Institutes of Health have identified 71 individual stem cell lines developed from genetically different blastocysts (an early stage of embryonic development) that may be used in research and that receive federal funding. However, only 21 lines are considered viable.

## OTHER FEDERAL GUIDELINES

Although a comprehensive set of criteria and conditions exist that must be met for research groups to obtain federal funding, federal regulation and guidelines overseeing privately funded stem cell research are significantly less stringent. However, standard regulations still apply to all forms of stem cell research conducted within the United States. All of the standard regulations that are applied to research regarding human specimens are also applied to research that uses human subjects or introduces stem cells into human subjects.

The National Academies, which comprises four separate scientific institutions, advises Congress on issues of federal policy as it relates to stem cell research. The National Academies have developed a series of guidelines for all stem cell research to promote ethical research. The academies recommend that each institution that conducts stem cell research create an oversight board to monitor stem cell as well as embryonic stem cell research. The academies also recommend strict guidelines regarding the process of obtaining consent from the donors of oocytes for the creation of embryonic stem cell lines.

In addition, the National Academies have responded to recent concern that both private and publicly funded research endeavors may seek to create chimeras by introducing human embryonic stem cells into the blastocysts of other primates or animals, sparking widespread bioethical concern. At present, the National Academies recommends against performing chimera research. However, strong calls continue for the federal government to directly ban this research outright in the interest of preventing a myriad of ethical concerns.

## ADULT STEM CELL RESEARCH

President George W. Bush has also outlined a series of policy statements and an executive order that increase the emphasis that is placed by the federal government on adult stem cell research. Executive Order 13435, signed by President Bush on June 20, 2007, directs the National Institutes of Health to pursue and fund research that uses adult human stem cells. The order also calls for the secretary of the National Institutes of Health to issue a report to the president each year regarding progress that has been made in the adult stem cell research field while specifically outlining the adult stem cell research funded by the National Institutes of Health. This executive order emphasizes the Bush administration's policy of encouraging additional research into adult stem cells as a potential alternative to embryonic stem cell research.

Many scientific groups object to the added emphasis that is placed on adult stem cell research, feeling that this emphasis detracts from embryonic stem cell research, which may have greater therapeutic potential.

## PUBLIC PERCEPTION

Gradually, public perception has begun to shift in regard to stem cell research. In the 2004 presidential election, Republican candidate George W. Bush, as well as several Democratic candidates, sparred over the issue of stem cell research, which became a charged and controversial issue during the campaign. Stem cell research has also received additional media coverage and the backing of a number of high-profile celebrities.

Following the 2004 death of Christopher Reeve, a famous actor crippled by a horse riding accident in 1995, stem cell research lobbying efforts gained additional traction. Christopher Reeve had been an outspoken advocate for increased federal funding and support of embryonic stem cell research, which is viewed as a potential source of cures for spinal cord injuries and related neurological diseases. Nancy Reagan, former first lady of the United States, also continues to be an outspoken advocate for federal funding of embryonic stem cell research. Following the death of her husband former President Ronald Reagan in 2004, Nancy Reagan's support of stem cell research was widely publicized. Nancy Reagan has also been joined by other celebrities including Michael J. Fox, a famous actor who suffers from Parkinson's disease.

Increased lobbying in support of federal funding of embryonic stem cell research and media attention may lead to shifts in public perception as well, which could affect federal policies in the long term.

## NEW POLICY CONSIDERATIONS

With the perception of increased public support for embryonic stem cell research, several legislative proposals have been crafted that would revise federal policy. The 109th and 110th Congresses have taken up the issue of embryonic stem cell research and stem cell research funding extensively. In the early days of the 110th Congress, the Stem Cell Research Enhancement Act of 2007 (H.R. 3) was successfully passed by both the House of Representatives and the Senate. The legislation called for the lifting of President Bush's restriction of federal funding for research only on stem cells lines isolated before August 9, 2001. This legislation allowed federal funding for research conducted with other embryonic stem cell lines. However, the legislation also contained explicit provisions allowing use of only those embryos that were left over from in vitro fertility treatments and donated freely without financial incentive. Although the Stem Cell Research Enhancement Act of 2007 successfully passed both houses of Congress, President Bush vetoed the bill on June 20, 2007, shortly after issuing another executive order encouraging federal funding of stem cell research that did not involve the destruction of human embryos.

As international regulation and standards are being further developed in this area, United States policy makers are taking them into consideration. There is a strong concern among many that the United States risks falling behind in stem cell research as the result of an overly stringent policy. Conversely, there are fears that if the United States pursues a national stem cell research policy that is too lax, it will lose moral leadership by being viewed as pursuing a policy devaluing human life.

The issue of federal stem cell research policies, and in particular federal embryonic stem cell research funding, is widely anticipated to be an important issue in the presidential election of 2008. The next elected U.S. president and Congress will have significant implications for the future direction of U.S. federal regulation and funding of stem cell research.

**SEE ALSO:** Cells, Adult; Cells, Embryonic; Christopher Reeve Foundation; Michael J. Fox Foundation; Presidential Campaigns; Stem Cells, Bush Ruling; United States.

**BIBLIOGRAPHY.** "Fact Sheet: Embryonic Stem Cell Research," August 9, 2001, www.whitehouse.gov (cited January 2008); George W. Bush, "Remarks on Stem Cell Research," August 9, 2001, www.whitehouse.gov (cited January 2008); Antonio Regalado and David P. Hamilton, "How a University's Patents May Limit Stem Cell Research," *Wall Street Journal*, July 18, 2006; Sheryl Gay Stolberg and David E. Sanger, "Bush Aides Seek Compromise on Embryonic Cell Research," *New York Times*, July 4, 2001.

John S. Kuo
University of Wisconsin

# Feeder/Feeder-Free Culture

**THE CHARACTERISTICS OF** stem cells are self-renewal (ability to divide indefinitely without differentiating), maintaining a full diploid karyotype, generating any tissue when introduced into an embryo, and colonizing the germ lines of recipient embryos. It is difficult to grow stem cells in culture because of the spontaneity of differentiation. Stem cells must be cultured on a medium that provides signals for maintaining the undifferentiated state or they will proliferate and differentiate without control. The culture, manipulation, and characterization of embryonic stem cells, embryonic germ cells, and adult stem cells in vitro require a mix of nutrients, hormones, growth factors, and blood serum.

Human embryonic stem cells derived from an inner cell mass of blastocysts have the pluripotency to form all three embryonic germ layers; some scientists prefer the term totipotency, because it means the cell can produce any cell in the body, though the suggestion of totality could also be misleading because an individual stem cell has not been shown to be capable of producing an embryo. Traditional culture techniques using mouse fibroblast cells are fine for research but are unsuitable when the stem cell line is intended for human clinical use because of the potential to introduce animal pathogens into the treatment.

Established protocols using a wide range of materials (some available that have been specifically created for embryonic stem cell culturing) and a variety of chemical/biological substrates allow researchers to grow stem cells in vitro. These culture techniques usually include mimicking the in vivo environment in a laboratory by adding molecular components similar to those found naturally within the stem cell niches of the body.

## FEEDER CULTURE

The first step in using a feeder culture is growing the feeder cells or using a prepared formula available from a variety of suppliers. Feeder cells—often mouse (mitotically inactive primary mouse embryonic fibroblasts) or human fibroblasts—are used in culture protocols to keep the stem cells from differentiating. The feeder cells provide secreted factors (many of which have not been identified), extracellular matrix, and cellular contact to keep the stem cells from differentiating and to maintain the normal karyotype. Researchers plate embryonic stem cells onto feeder layers. A limitation of working with feeder cells is cell overcrowding between the feeder cells and the embryonic stem cell colonies. An additional key factor in using feeder cells is to ensure that the density of the feeder cell is sufficient for the delivery of the right amount of factors to maintain the cells in an undifferentiated state without depleting nutrients in the coculture environment, and therefore diminishing the capacity of growth of stem cell colonies.

A Japanese patent has been filed for the use of an immobilized notch ligand protein as a feeder for culturing stem cells. The Notch pathway plays an important role in in vivo stem cell niches of the hematopoietic system, gut, mammary gland, and muscles. The patent calls for using a notch ligand protein on a human cell membrane to maintain the stem cells in an undifferentiated state. The hope is that using this type of feeder will allow the stem cells to be used for cell transplantation and genetic therapy. Other possible feeders to be used for stem cell culturing include human fetal muscle and skin, adult fallopian tube epithelium, and human fibroblasts from foreskin, skin, endometrial, embryo and placenta, and breast parenchyma cells.

## FEEDER-FREE CULTURE

In order to culture cells in the absence of a feeder cell layer, coating the culture plate with a permissive substrate is necessary. The substrate provides important adhesion and contact dependent factors necessary to maintaining undifferentiated cell cultures. Mouse embryonic stem cells grow without feeder cells in a supplement of leukemia-inhibiting factor (LIF) to maintain symmetric division and inhibit differentiation. Human cells do not respond to LIF in the same way. To use human embryonic stem cells for clinical therapy, the culture medium for growing and differentiating stem cells needs to be able to provide the nutrients and necessary factors without the possibility of transferring animal or human viruses to the stem cells. A feeder-free culture system is designed to keep the stem cells from differentiating while protecting the stem cells from direct contact with the feeder in an effort to prevent cross-contamination or passing nonhuman pathogens into the stem cells.

Research is progressing with the development of a variety of protocols. For example, increasing the dose of basic fibroblast growth feeder in a serum-free culture, altering the concentration of serum replacement supplements, changing the concentration of growth factors and other nutrients, or using different permissive substrates (e.g., fibronectin) will allow human embryonic stem cells to grow without differentiation, for prolonged periods of culturing and to maintain the pluripotency and normal karyotype of the stem cells. Furthermore, a feeder-free culture system allows for reducing the exposure of growing cells to animal viruses.

A possible substrate for feeder-free culturing is Matrigel (a trade-name protein mixture from BD Biosciences derived from mouse tumor cells; contains laminin and collagen as well), which can be used in a thin layer or as a three-dimensional gel. The gel is appropriate for maintaining undifferentiated embryonic stem cells. Laminins are derived from the basal lamina and are glycoproteins creating the structural scaffold in tissues.

**SEE ALSO:** Cells, Embryonic; Cells, Mouse (Embryonic); Methods of Growing Cells.

**BIBLIOGRAPHY.** M. Amit, C. Shariki, V. Margulets, and J. Itskovitz-Eldor, "Feeder Layer- and Serum-Free Culture of Human Embryonic Stem Cells," *Biology of Reproduction* (v.70/3, 2004); George Q. Daley, "Simplifying hESC Culture," *Blood* (v.105/12, 2005); Louise A. Hyslop, et al., "Examples of Improved Feeders and Feeder-Free Methods for Derivation of Human Embryonic Stem Cells," *Expert Reviews in Molecular Medicine* (v.7/19, 2005).

Lyn Michaud
Independent Scholar

# Florida

**THERE IS MUCH** controversy today about whether stem cell research must be confined to adult stem cells only and whether ethically, adult stem cells are preferred over the embryonic stem cells. Different groups are concerned about the topic of stem cell research with regard to the viability, survival, and protection of the embryo; the cloning issue; federal funding; and the consent of donor. Cloning is also opposed by religious organizations as well.

In Florida, stem cell research has gained an adequate amount of public attention through the media and has been the subject of public meetings by government agencies. Stem cell research has been supported and funded by many private companies and authorities, but the National Institutes of Health holds the largest source of funds. Embryonic stem cell research has been supported by a number of U.S. Senators and Representatives who have been resisting abortion on religious grounds.

Most of them are accepting of it in the medical research field, however, and also agree that, as long as the embryo is not implanted in a mother's womb, it is not going to develop into a human being. On August 9, 2001, however, President George W. Bush announced that research on human embryonic stem cells will be funded only if it meets approved standards.

In October 2005, Senator Ron Klein (D-Boca Raton) and Representative Franklin Sands (D-Weston) cosponsored the "Florida Better Quality of Life and Biomedical Research Act" to allocate $15 million of state funds a year for a decade towards human embryonic stem cell research. The bill died the following year in the Committee on Commerce and Consumer Services.

In January 2007, Rep. Anitere Flores (R-Miami) filed a bill in that would allocate $20 million to adult stem cell research; however, the bill would not have allowed for embryonic stem cell research. Also in January, the Governor Charlie Christ announced that he would not back human embryonic stem cell research, but recommended that the state legislature spend $20 million on adult stem cell research. Rep. Flores's bill died in May 2007.

In March 2007, Senator Mike Hardipolos (R-Indialantic) filed a bill in the Florida state Senate calling for $20 million in adult stem cell research while prohibiting research on embryonic stem cells, which also died in the Committee on Health and Human Services Appropriations.

The stem cell issue will be debated again in Florida because of the state supreme court and the leadership of another moderate Republican governor. The issue will be revisited as the Florida Supreme Court has allowed two initiatives to be placed on the ballot for November 2008: one requiring the state to support embryonic stem cell research and the other prohibiting state money for research that "involves the destruction of a live human embryo." In Florida, there are a number of organizations working on political and social levels. Their main goal is to promote awareness in people about the issues regarding stem cell research, its benefit in the field of medicine, and its therapeutic role. Ethically, morally, and politically, human embryonic stem cells are important and are a sensitive topic for discussion. In addition to ethical issues, some scientists also are not supporting embryonic stem cell research, because of the risk of teratoma (tumor) formation from these cells. There is no concrete proof showing that embryonic stem cells are capable of treating a disease.

The adult stem cells, like the hematopoietic stem cells, which are involved in formation of blood cells in bone marrow, presently are the only type of stem cells frequently used in the treatment of human diseases. Adult stem cells are capable of producing a variety of cells and tissues and are

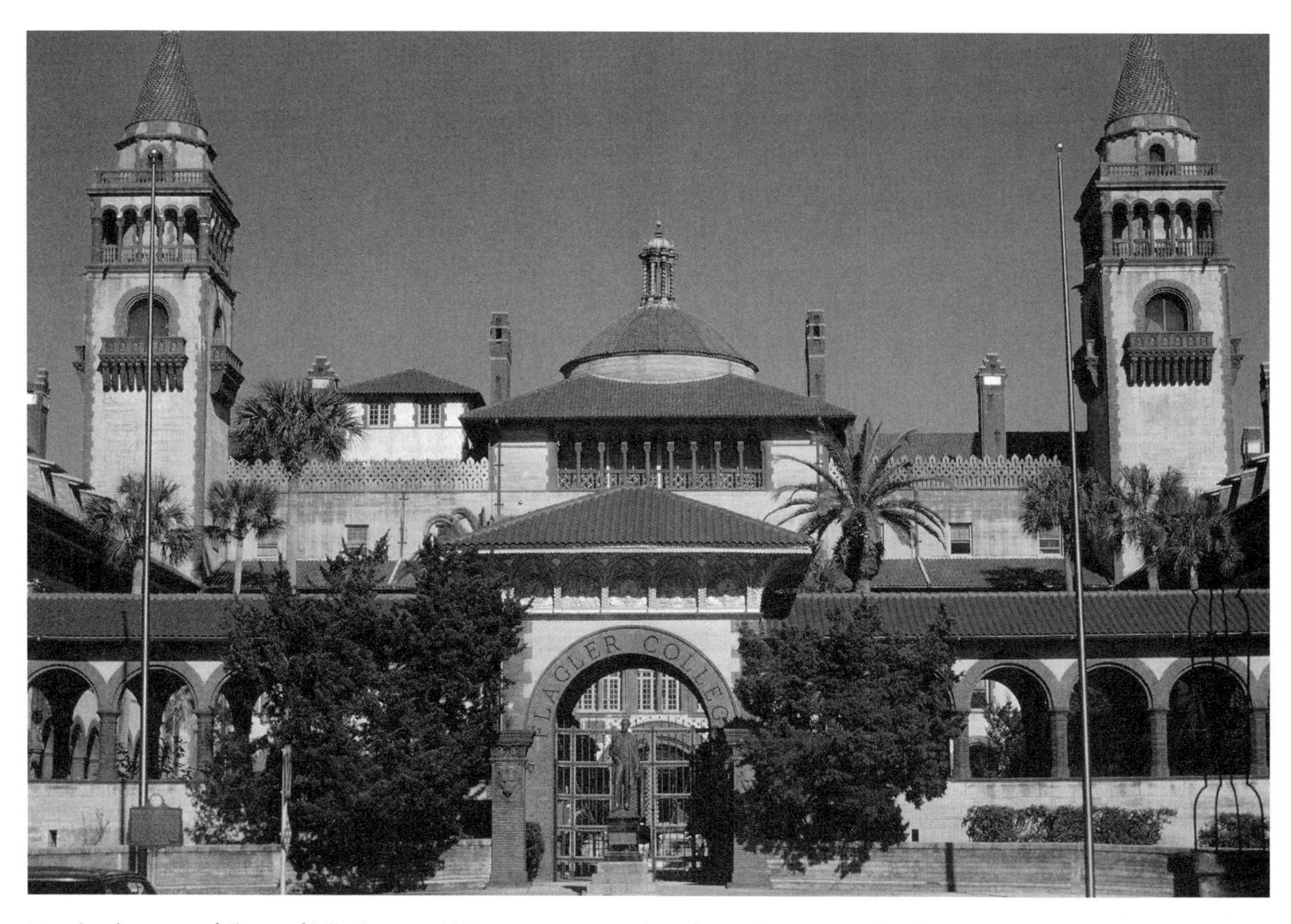

*Despite the recent failures of bills that would have spent as much as $20 million in state funds on adult stem cell research, universities in Florida are continuing their work toward developing treatments using adult stem cells.*

often present in only minute quantities to be isolated. However, the capacity of embryonic stem cells to divide is far beyond that of adult stem cells. Much of the stem cell research being conducted at various universities in Florida uses adult stem cells, particularly those derived from the bone marrow. For example, the University of Florida College of Medicine Adult Stem Cell Engineering and Therapeutic Core focuses on developing therapies for various kinds of cancer and other brain disorders using adult stem cells. Additionally, researchers at the University of Central Florida are investigating using bone marrow derived adult stem cells for treatments for Alzheimer's disease and other brain ailments. Finally, the Miller School of Medicine at the University of Miami Interdisciplinary Stem Cell Institute aims to use stem cell technology and basic science research to develop regenerative medicine therapies useful for patients.

**SEE ALSO:** Cells, Embryonic; Cloning; Federal Government Policies; Stem Cells, Bush Ruling.

**BIBLIOGRAPHY.** Florida Cures, www.floridacures.com (cited December 2007); Florida Family Policy Council, www.florida4family.org (cited December 2007); "Florida May Vote on Stem Cells," www.bioethics.net (cited December 2007); Stem Cell News, "Florida State University Researcher's Device Provides a Major Boost to Adult Stem Cell Research," www.stemcellnews.com (cited December 2007).

G. Ishaq Khan
Dow University of Health Sciences

# Fluorescence-Activated Cell Sorting

**FLUORESCENCE-ACTIVATED CELL SORTING,** frequently referred to as FACS, allows for isolation (sorting) or enumeration (analysis) of different populations of cells and molecules based on user-defined characteristics. FACS is based on the light-scattering properties of cells as well as the detection of user-defined fluorescent markers.

First, forward scatter and side scatter of normal light are used to determine cell size and complexity, respectively. The larger the cell, the more forward scatter there is, and the more complex the cell (i.e., a cell undergoing division or apoptosis, or with more vacuoles, etc.), the higher the side scatter. Second, fluorescent markers are used to delineate specific populations of cells within the whole population. Up to 32 different markers can be simultaneously detected, although it is far more common to use two to six markers. These markers are user defined and based on the experimental questions being asked. One can observe differences in a molecule on the surface of a cell, determining whether that cell is activated or not, the nature of the DNA content of the cell, whether that cell is undergoing cellular division or death (via necrosis or apoptosis), the phenotypic cell markers, the percentages of cells within a particular subset of cells, and so on.

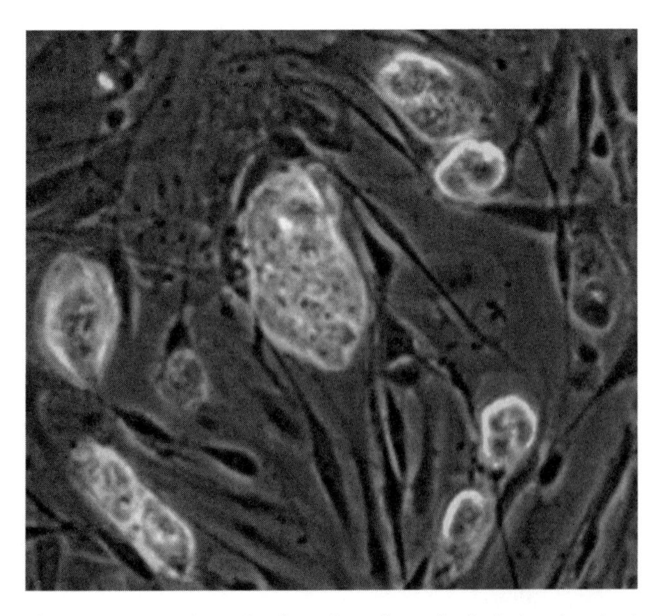

*Fluorescence-activated cell sorting allows for isolation (sorting) or enumeration (analysis) of different populations of cells.*

FACS machines contain one or more lasers, which excite the fluorescently tagged markers and cause emissions in distinct, specified ranges. The machine can then visualize individual cells as they are passed within the laser beams in a fluid stream, at a rate of up to tens of thousands of events per second, and determine fluorescence emission of each marker that may be on that cell. After the cell has passed through the laser field and the emission pattern of that cell has been collected and stored, the machine determines whether it falls within the user-defined collection parameters and uses an electrical field to either positively or negatively charge the fluid drop; the drop is then designated to one of up to three tubes on the basis of charge (positive, negative, and none). A variety of machines exist from different manufacturers, with the ability to enumerate cells or isolate (sort) populations of cells on the basis of a specific user set parameters. On the basis of the ability of the machine, even rare positive events (less than 1 in 10,000) can be isolated.

One of the first methods to determine and isolate populations of stem cells was side population (SP) analysis. This analysis on a FACS machine is based on the ability of stem cells to efflux a DNA labeling dye termed Hoechst 33342, part of the Hoescht dye family, at two wavelengths. This SP of cells is able to efflux or "kick out" the Hoechst dyes at a faster rate than that of more mature cells within the population and is a unique marker of many stem cell populations, including those isolated from bone marrow (hematopoietic stem cells), embryos (embryonic stem cells), and tumors (cancer stem cells). Using a FACS machine with sorting capabilities, SPs can be captured and isolated for further characterization. Although SP isolation leads to the selection of cells capable of self-renewal, considered stem cells, there is no specific marker selection via this method. Thus, the determination of cell populations based on cell markers is frequently performed in conjunction with SP characterization and isolation.

A second use of FACS for stem cell research is the determination of populations on the basis of various cell surface and intracellular markers. Each type of cell in an organism has a unique set of molecules on its surface. These molecules, termed *markers*, are involved in many cellular processes, including specific movement of cells, cellular division, activation of various cellular processes, induction of cell death, and so on. Although a specific set of markers on a cell define the cell to a subset population, the markers themselves can be redundant. Thus, although two different cells may have marker 1 (i.e., CD34, which is involved in cell–cell adhesion), it is the presence or absence of markers 2 (c-kit, a receptor involved in cellular signaling controlling cell survival, proliferation, and differentiation) and 3 (Sca-1, which is involved in cellular self-renewal) that define the cells as residing within different populations.

Markers specific for stem cells are dependent on the origin of the stem cells themselves, whereas hematopoietic (origin for all blood cells) stem cells are CD34+, Sca-1+, c-kit+, and CD43+; skeletal muscle stem cells are CD34+/–, Sca-1+, c-kit–, and CD43–. In addition, cells with stem cell–like self-renewal capabilities have been discovered in many cancers. These "cancer stem cells," although expressing markers for specific cell lineages of tumor origin, such as breast, colon, or brain, also express markers specific for stem cell lineage. It is thought that these cancer stem cells arise from mutations within normal stem cells and that cancer arises and is sustained from such mutated normal stem cells. Thus, breast cancer stem cells are EpCam+ (involved in cellular adhesion), CD44+ (involved in cell–cell interactions, adhesion, and migration), and CD24- (involved in cell adhesion). Colon cancer stem cells, meanwhile, are Epcam+, CD44+, and CD133+ (unknown function), and brain cancer (glioblastoma) stem cells are CD133+ and nestin+ (intracellular filament protein of nerve cells), although recent reports document CD133– cancer stem cell populations for both colon and brain cancer. Thus, FACS is an integral part of stem cell research, allowing for not only isolation of stem cell populations but also characterization of these stem cells.

**SEE ALSO:** Cancer; Cell Sorting.

**BIBLIOGRAPHY.** Margaret Goodell, et al., "Isolation and Functional Properties of Murine Hematopoietic Stem Cells that Are Replicating In Vivo," *Journal of Experimental Medicine* (v.183, 1996); Margaret Goodell, et al., "Dye Efflux Studies Suggest that Hematopoietic Stem Cells Expressing Low or Undetectable Levels of CD34 Antigen Exist in Multiple Species," *Nature Medicine* (v.3/12, 1997); Emanuela Gussoni, et al., "Dystrophin Expression in the *mdx* Mouse Restored by Stem Cell Transplantation," *Nature* (v.401, 1999).

Cathie G. Miller
Henry Ford Health System

# Fragile X Syndrome

**FRAGILE X SYNDROME** (FXS) is the most common inherited cause of mental disability. Although the precise number of people with this disorder is unknown, the Centers for Disease Control and Prevention has estimated that 1 in 4,000 males and 1 in 6,000 females have FXS. FXS is caused by the absence or dysfunction of a protein called the Fragile X mental retardation protein (FMRP). FMRP is essential to the nervous system because it is necessary for proper nerve maturation and for forming efficient nerve connections in developing embryos. The absence of FMRP in FXS patients is caused by a change, or mutation, in the Fragile X Mental Retardation 1 gene, FMR1. The FMR1 gene is responsible for producing the FMRP protein at the correct time during embryonic development. Currently, no cure exists for FXS. However, research on stem cells from humans, mice, and flies has helped us understand how the disease develops and may lead to improved treatment options.

The symptoms of FXS can vary widely, with boys often more affected than girls. FXS most commonly affects intelligence, learning, physical appearance, social interactions, speech, and the senses. The intellectual disabilities in FXS patients range from mild learning disabilities to severe mental retardation. The physical symptoms of FXS are often undetectable in children; however, some teens and adults with FXS have long ears, faces, and jaws. Some patients have connective tissue defects, which cause flat feet, extendable joints, balance problems, and non–life-threatening heart murmurs.

About 20 percent of FXS patients are prone to seizures. Furthermore, autism-like behaviors (i.e., flapping hands, self-biting, repetitive actions, and walking on the toes) are also frequently observed in FXS children. Children with FXS may also have behavioral challenges that cause them to be extremely anxious in new social situations. Attention deficit disorder (ADD)/attention deficit hyperactivity disorder (ADHD) as well as autism are both common in FXS patients. Boys with FXS usually have some speech language problems. Most begin using words later in childhood than their unaffected peers. Speech problems may range from enunciation, stuttering, omitting parts of words, and misunderstanding tone of voice. FXS patients may also have difficulty comprehending body language. Finally, FXS patients can be extremely sensitive to sensory stimulation (e.g., bright light, loud noises, or skin sensitivity). Some children with FXS avoid being touched and have trouble making eye contact.

The symptoms of FXS can be reduced and/or eliminated with treatment. Because developmental defects cause many of the symptoms, physicians believe that the earlier FXS is diagnosed, the more the patient can learn, and the better the outcome. Since FXS affects so many aspects of personal development, many types of treatment are used. Despite their mental disabilities, FXS patients are capable of learning. Through special educational programs FXS children can progress in school, learn independence, and become employed as adults. Heart murmurs can be monitored by a physician, seizures treated with medication, and balance problems addressed with physical therapy. Speech therapy can improve speech impediments and help patients communicate, while behavioral therapy can help children cope with stress induced by social situations and sensory sensitivity.

## INHERITANCE

The FMR1 gene is located on the X chromosome, one of the chromosomes that determine an individual's sex. For this reason, FXS is a sex-linked disease that affects boys more than girls. All genetic material (DNA) in humans is located in two pairs of 23 chromosomes. An individual inherits half of their DNA from their mother (23 chromosomes) and half from their father (another 23 chromosomes). Twenty-two out of the 23 pairs of chromosomes are identical. The nonidentical pair of chromosomes determines the sex of the individual: these are the X and the Y-chromosomes.

A woman has two X chromosomes, one that was passed from her mother and the other from her father. A man has one X chromosome and one Y chromosome; the X was inherited from his mother and the Y from his father. A male who inherits a defective FMR1 gene will have FXS, because his only X chromosome will have the mutated gene. A woman who inherits one defective FMR1 gene may not be as severely affected by FXS because she has a second X chromosome that contains a normal FMR1 gene.

The defect in the FMR1 gene that causes FXS is caused by an abnormally long stretch of DNA at the beginning of the FMR1 gene. DNA is made up of four types of molecular building blocks, or nucleotides, called adenine (A), guanine (G), cytosine (C), and thymine. The beginning of a normal FMR1 gene typically has between 6 and 45 repeats of the nucleotides CGG. In contrast, people with FXS have over 200 CGG repeats. This large number of repeats causes the gene to be turned off during the development of a fetus, ultimately causing a deficiency in the FMRP protein. Without FMRP, the nervous system in the fetus fails to develop properly.

Some people have a higher than normal number of CGG repeats in their FMR1 gene (55–200 repeats), but do not have FXS. People with this in-between number of repeats have the Fragile X premutation, but do not have FXS because their FMR1 gene still works. However, people with FMR1 premutations are considered to be carriers of FXS because they can have children with FXS. Carrier men will pass the premutation to all of their daughters and none of their sons. Carrier women with one FMR1 premutation have a 50 percent chance of passing the permutation to her children. The FMR1 premutation is unstable and is prone to further, albeit inconsistent, expansion when passed from one generation to the next. Thus, the FMR1 premutation can be passed down within families for generations before any child inherits a full mutation and is affected by FXS.

### STEM CELL RESEARCH

Since FMR1 mutations affect the early development of neurons during fetal formation, scientists studying FXS need to understand how the FMR1 gene works in the pre-nerve cells of a fetus. These pre-nerve cells are called neuronal stem cells or embryonic stem cells. By studying the embryonic stem cells derived from mice, flies, and humans, scientists have begun to understand how the FMR1 gene is important for nerve maturation. Furthermore, studies have found that a decrease in FMRP protein ultimately alters nerve cell signaling and may affect how nerves work together in the brain to learn and create memories. Drugs could possibly block these aberrant signaling events and improve the learning capability of FXS patients.

Stem cells derived from animals have limited research potential because they lack the repeat sequences at the beginning of the FMR1 gene. As a result, these models are inadequate for scientists who want to study how and why the extended repeats turn off the FMR1 gene. Recently, scientists have developed human embryonic stem cells with the FMR1 gene defect. Studies of these cells have shown that the FMR1 gene is still functional in the earliest stages of the embryo and is shut off later during development. By understanding how and why the FMR1 gene gets turned off, scientist may be able to reverse this event in embryos with the FXS mutation.

**SEE ALSO:** Cells, Embryonic; Cells, Neural; Down Syndrome.

**BIBLIOGRAPHY.** Maija Castren, "Differentiation of Neuronal Cells in Fragile X Syndrome," *Cell Cycle* (July 2006); Centers for Disease Control and Prevention, Department of Health and Human Services, "Single Gene Disorders and Disability (SGDD)—Fragile X Syndrome," www.cdc.gov (cited December 2007); Rachel Eiges, et al., "Developmental Study of Fragile X Syndrome Using Human Embryonic Stem Cells Derived from Preimplantation Genetically Diagnosed Embryos," *Cell Stem Cell* (November 2007); Fragile X Research Foundation, "About Fragile X—Cause," www.fraxa.org (cited December 2007); National Institute of Health, National Institute of Child Health and Human Development, "Fragile X Syndrome," www.nichd.nih.gov (cited December 2007).

Renee C. Ireton
University of Washington

# France

**THE EUROPEAN UNION** agreed with Great Britain's regulations except on the creation of embryos: Article 18 of the Council of Europe Convention on Human Rights and Biomedicine prohibits creation of human embryos for research purposes. Therapeutic cloning is illegal in Germany, Austria, Portugal, Ireland, Norway, and Poland. The Netherlands, which is politically liberal, included a ban in 2003. The Council of Europe—comprising 15 European Union member states and more than 40 countries, including Russia and Turkey—adopted a Convention on Biomedicine that prohibits the creation of embryos for research purposes. Stem cell research in France is able to progress as a result of government support with appropriate legislation and funding, strong scientific research foundation, public support of biomedical research, and international cooperative relationships and partnerships.

Human embryonic stem cell research is permitted under the Bioethics Law approved in February

2006. The guidelines under this legislation require five-year licenses for the import of human embryonic stem cell lines derived from leftover embryos created for in vitro fertilization, and the law allows French-based researchers to also create stem cell lines from embryos created for in vitro fertilization in France. Researchers may develop research proposals and carry out approved research under the jurisdiction of the Biomedicine Agency, looking to them for authorization and to ensure compliance. For embryos to be used for research, consent must be received from the persons for whom the embryos were created. However, French law prohibits the creation of human embryos specifically for research including procurement of human embryonic stem cells, and also prohibits reproductive and therapeutic cloning.

The French National Institute for Health and Medical Research (INSERM) was established in 1964, taking over the work of the French National Institute of Hygiene. The work of INSERM falls under the joint auspices of the Ministry of Health and the Ministry of Higher Education and Research. The mission of this public agency is to ensure cooperation and collaboration among scientists in all fields related to human health by advancing knowledge and clinical therapies through the formation of National Research Programs begun in 2004 in cardiovascular diseases, diabetes, bone and joint diseases, human nutrition, imagery, and alcohol.

Involving basic, clinical, therapeutic, and public health research, National Research Programs are organized by three groups: a steering committee (made up of experts in the area of interest) to determine the scope of research and request proposals, the Strategic Orientation Committee (made up of stakeholders who choose to be involved in helping develop, support, and evaluate the program's research), and the Scientific Council (made up of international experts selected by the steering committee), to choose research projects for funding including those for stem cell research.

To fulfill this mission, the institute has worked in close partnership with other public or private research institutions and care centers such as hospitals. Today, the majority (85 percent) of INSERM's more than 300 research laboratories are housed within university hospital or cancer treatment centers, with the others being located on the research campuses of the CNRS (French scientific research institute) or of the Pasteur and Curie Institutes.

The Pasteur Institute, located in Paris, was founded in 1887 with international funding for Louis Pasteur's work and the study of infectious diseases. The Pasteur Institute remains at the forefront of microbiology, immunology, and molecular biology and is a EuroStemCell partner. A research team at the institute was one of the first European groups to investigate teratomas and discovered that a single cell could differentiate into a variety of cell types. For this genetic research, Andre L. Woff, Francois Jacob, and Jacques Monod won a Nobel prize in 1965.

## AGENCE DE LA BIOMÉDECINE

The French Biomedicine Agency is a public agency under the jurisdiction of the Ministry of Health and Solidarity (the governmental body responsible for all aspects of health and social welfare) to oversee transplants of organs, tissues, and cells; procreation; embryology; and human genetics for safety, quality, and ethical and legal responsibilities. The agency authorizes, monitors, and controls the clinical and research activities related to reproduction, genetics, transplants, and the therapeutic use of stem cells. In addition, the agency provides information for regulatory or legislative action and increases public awareness information regarding human organ, tissue, and cell donation and sperm and ovule donation.

The agency is headed by a director general, working with a board of directors (representing government, public health, and private experts) and the orientation council of advisors. Representatives on the orientation council include science, medicine, and social science professionals and representatives from diverse stakeholders to ensure that policies meet medical, scientific, legal, and ethical standards and to evaluate research proposals for compliance with these standards before approval.

As part of its oversight activities, the agency ensures safe transplantation by maintaining a list of donors and those people needing transplants. The agency also is responsible for safe and quality fertility management of the creation of embryos for implantation and genetic testing of embryos.

A primary goal of the agency in relation to stem cell research is establishing a national registry of human embryos and embryonic cells (for tracking purposes, while ensuring individual anonymity), with the cooperation of authorized organizations, to collect and maintain information on the biological material held.

The French Biomedicine Agency is responsible for authorizing and ensuring compliance of research on human embryos and human embryonic stem cells (hES). The agency began authorization of research on human embryos and embryonic stem cells in 2006 and took oversight for the 40 research authorizations on imported embryonic stem cell lines made by temporary arrangement from September 2004 to February 2006. Stem cell research has been approved for a trial period of five years, at which time the agency will evaluate the results and consider extension of authorization. A second independent evaluation will be completed by the parliamentary office for the evaluation of scientific and technological choices. These two evaluations will be used by parliament in reexamining bioethics law provisions.

Appropriate authorization by the French Biomedicine Agency allows researchers to create and work on hES from spare in vitro–conceived embryos and on cell lines imported from other countries (in compliance with legal and ethical guidelines and with the transaction completed within 12 months after authorization). Donation with written consent (and reapproval after three months) is required from parents allowing the embryo to be used for research purposes. Although French law allows for the procurement of hES from extra embryos for research related to medical treatment and without availability of alternative options, the law prohibits human embryo creation for the specific purpose of research or procuring hES.

## OTHER AGENCY ACTIVITIES

The authorization procedure by the agency to evaluate research protocols from French scientific teams requires proposals to be submitted to the director general during established submission periods. The proposals will be reviewed by scientific experts, and the orientation council will review the expert reports to determine approval or denial of the research proposal and forward it to the director general for a final decision. Both decision and orientation council verdicts will be forwarded to the ministers for health and research. The ministers may then request reconsideration of denied proposals and suspend or cancel authorization on scientific, legal, or ethical grounds.

Once a research proposal has been authorized, the Biomedicine Agency must monitor and control the research. Annual reports prepared by the researchers are submitted to the agency to provide information on research progress, and at the end of the authorized research, a final report will be submitted to the agency for examination. The agency is also authorized to ensure research compliance by inspection (including inspecting storage of embryonic stem cells to ensure quality and safety), and if any violations are found, the authorized researcher will be given an opportunity to correct the issue or provide a reason for noncompliance. The director general of the agency may suspend (for three months) research for violations of laws, regulations, or the conditions of the authorization. The orientation council is then notified and may withdraw the research authorization. Modifications to the authorized research must be submitted for evaluation before work may proceed and must follow the same authorization process.

The Biomedicine Agency also provides information regarding agency activities to the government and public for a better understanding of evolving technology and scientific discovery, with the purpose of promoting appropriate legislative/regulatory action and international cooperation in public health interest.

The agency is also active internationally for support overseas (in Morocco, Tunisia, Vietnam, and Bulgaria) by providing expertise (especially in tissue and organ transplant) and medical teams at the disposal of the other countries. Funding is provided by the Ministry of Foreign Affairs.

**SEE ALSO:** Cells, Embryonic; Clinical Trials (Adult Cells); European Consortium for Stem Cell Research—EuroStemCell; International Laws; Regulations Overview; United States.

**BIBLIOGRAPHY.** Agence de la biomédecine, "Publication of the Decree Relating to Research on Human Embryos and Embryonic Stem Cells" (Press Release Saint-Denis, February 7, 2006); "About the Agence de la biomédecine," www.agence-biomedicine.fr (cited November 2007); Ministry of Health and Social Affairs, "Stem Cell Research Fact Sheet," www.sweden.gov.se (cited June 2004); ScanBalt, "Organization," www.scanbalt.org (cited November 2007).

Lyn Michaud
Independent Scholar

# Fuchs, Elaine

**ELAINE FUCHS IS** the Rebecca C. Lancefield Professor of Mammalian Cell Biology and Development at Rockefeller University in New York City. She is also a research investigator for the Howard Hughes Medical Institute. Fuchs was raised in suburban Chicago, where a semirural childhood of farms and exposure to nature stimulated her interest in science, as did members of her family. Her father was a geochemist who worked at Argonne National Laboratories. His specialty was meteorites. She also had an aunt who worked at the laboratories as a biologist, and her sister is a neurosurgeon.

Fuchs graduated in 1972 from the University of Illinois with a bachelor's of science degree and the highest distinction in the chemical sciences. Her undergraduate thesis was in physical chemistry and her research topic was the electrodiffusion of nickel through quartz. She chose the University of Illinois instead of the University of Chicago because her father, aunt, and sister were all graduates of the University of Chicago, and she wanted to be different.

After graduation, Fuchs was selected to go to Uganda with the Peace Corps. She had wanted to go to Chile, where President Allende, a liberal democratic Marxist, was making changes in the organization of the economy and social structure that were to provoke a revolution by anti-Marxists. Ultimately, she went to neither Uganda nor Chile but did travel in India, Nepal, Guatemala, Mexico, Peru, Bolivia, Ecuador, Turkey, Greece, and Egypt. She was also concerned at this time with the issues of social justice being promoted by the feminist movement, which was the next step in her political development, following participation in protests against American participation in the Vietnam War in her undergraduate days.

Princeton University hosted Fuchs as a graduate student while she worked on her doctoral degree in biochemistry. She worked with Charles Gilvarg and had to contend with misogynistic attitudes from her mentor, but eventually proved her worth. Her specific research topics were on changes in bacterial cell walls during sporulation. The formation of spores after encystment is a special action of some bacteria. It enables them to produce dormant forms of the bacterium that enhances their chances for survival in harsh or adverse environmental conditions. The specific bacterium she studied was *Bacillus megaterium*.

In 1977 Fuchs moved to the Massachusetts Institute of Technology (MIT) to do her postdoctoral studies. At MIT, Fuchs worked in the laboratory run by Howard Green, an opportunity she had sought in order to be a part of Green's pioneering work on mammalian stem cell biology. The goal was to move from bacteria to humans, so that her research could be medically useful. Fuchs credits her work at MIT with giving her a solid grounding in cell biology. In addition, the contacts she made with fellow postdoctoral researchers created an exciting and stimulating atmosphere.

Her research at MIT was investigating the mechanisms that underlie the balance between growth and differentiation in epidermal keratinocytes. Human epidermal keratinocyte cells are cells that are isolated from the normal human neonatal foreskin of adult skin. They can be cryopreserved at the end of a primary culture. In addition, they can be used in a culture encouraged to propagate into 16 doublings. Human karatinocytes can be used as an in vitro model for dermal toxicology tests. These tests can be used to screen new skin products for toxicity or other problems. They can also be used for developing substitutes for the dermal layer of the skin. There are other applications that include using them to study human skin development, differentiation, and cellular aspects of skin disease.

The study of epidermal keratinocytes continued to attract Fuchs even after she joined the University of Chicago staff in 1980. She served as Amgen Professor of Molecular Genetics and Cell Biology and as an Investigator of the Howard Hughes Medical Institute. In 2002 she returned to New York City to serve at Rockefeller University.

Fuchs is now seeking to identify and characterize keratin genes. Her basic research goal is to understand the transcriptional mechanisms that underlie gene expression and differentiation. Both gene expression and differentiation are part of the growth of the epidermis and of hair follicles. Her research seeks to understand the role played by Wnt and BMP signaling in skin. Wnt proteins constitute a family of genes and signaling molecules. They regulate cell-to-cell interactions during embryogenesis. Research has suggested that they are linked to cancer. When mutated in mouse tissue, they have developed significant defects. On the surface of a cell, Wnt proteins bind to receptors of the Fizzled and LRP families.

Some studies have revealed the probable pathway of Wnt action. They use cytoplasmic relay components to send a signal that is transduced to beta-catenin. The beta-catenin acts as a transcriptional coactivator because it is able to associate with the Tcf-LEF family of transcription molecules. Wnt signaling is a regulator of self-renewal in normal stem cells and has been found in both hematopoietic systems and in the epidermis. The Wnt mechanism has been suspected of playing a role in the rise of many types of epithelial cancers. The study of Wnt and BMP signaling in skin is also important because mechanical or other kinds of injuries to the skin are a common occurrence. However, they are also involved in arthritis. Wnt and BMP signals also have been observed in adult human articular cartilage following a mechanical injury.

Fuchs's research involves identifying and describing the keratin genes. The exact focus of her current research is on the role plenipotentiary stem cells play in skin. By examining epithelial morphogenesis, her research seeks to understand how external cues are transmitted as signals to evoke changes in the transcription of cytoskeletal architecture of the epidermis. These studies are making connections between normal cells and the processes that mutate into human diseases of the skin, genetic disorders, or proinflammatory disorders.

Fuchs has pioneered some reverse genetics approaches. These approaches make it possible to assess protein functions. The assessment of protein functions provides information on their role in the development of diseases. By focusing on epidermal cells, Fuchs has been able to become a leader in the study of skin stem cells. This has brought new knowledge of the role of epidermal cells in the development of hair as well as human skin.

Fuchs is a winner of the Dickson Prize in Medicine (2004), among many other awards, and is recognized as a world-class stem cell researcher. She is married to a fellow academic, David Hanson, and has continued to shape her concerns for ethics in science and a better order in the world. She is known for promoting women in science. Her scientific-social concerns are to promote scientific humanism—the power of knowledge in service of human betterment.

**SEE ALSO:** Cells, Adult; Rockefeller University.

**BIBLIOGRAPHY.** H. Nguyen, M. Rendl, and E. Fuchs, "Tcf3 Governs Stem Cell Features and Represses Cell Fate Determination in Skin," *Cell* (v.127/1, 2006).

Andrew J. Waskey
Dalton State College

# Funding for IVF

**THE IN VITRO** fertilization (IVF) procedure was first developed in 1975 in England by Dr. Robert Edwards (an embryologist) and Dr. Patrick Steptoe (a gynecologist). The physician team developed the concept and began research in 1971, and the first IVF baby, Louise Brown, was born in 1978. The procedure itself involves the surgical removal of the eggs from the woman's ovary after the woman has been given ovulation-induction medications so that her body makes multiple eggs. Once retrieved, the eggs and sperm are mixed in a Petri dish so that fertilization can occur. Once fertilized, the embryos are placed within the woman's uterus so implantation can occur. IVF accounts for less than 5 percent of all infertility treatments in the United States.

The IVF procedure was first introduced in the United States in 1981. It is estimated that between 1985 and 2000, the procedure resulted in 139,000 births. With the addition of other technological advances, such as gamete intrafallopian transfer (GIFT), ZIFT (zygote intrafallopian transfer), and combined procedures, that number rose to 300,000 births by 2002. The use of GIFT and ZIFT increases the cost of IVF but accounts for less than 1 percent of all IVF cycles in the United States.

The IVF procedure was initially developed for women who had tubal factors that made pregnancy impossible. Worldwide, 80 million couples have infertility issues. In the United States, tubal factors are the third highest indication for use of IVF (10 percent). The first two diagnoses are male factor (16 percent) and diminished ovarian functioning (12 percent), which is most commonly associated with advanced maternal age.

IVF success is related to both the diagnosis and maternal age. Women less than 35 years of age are much more likely to achieve a live birth (37 percent), and women over the age of 42 years have the lowest success rates (10 percent). Older women, therefore, on average have more IVF attempts than younger women, thus increasing the cost significantly. Older women on average also have 3.3 embryos transferred compared with 2.1 embryos for younger women (under the age of 35).

IVF has not evolved without criticism. The procedures have both ethical and economic implications, and IVF has been responsible for a dramatic rise in multifetal pregnancies since the 1980s. In 2002 more than 130,000 infants were born of multifetal pregnancies within the United States. Since 1980, there has been a 65 percent increase in twin gestations and a 500 percent increase in triplet and higher-order multifetal pregnancies. The use of ovulation induction agents and assisted reproductive technology (ART) increases the risk of a multifetal pregnancy by 25 percent. This phenomena has occurred globally as a result of IVF and ART technologies.

## COST

The average cost of an IVF cycle in the United States is $12,400. This cost typically does not include ovulation-induction medications, which are used in 99 percent of all IVF cycles in the United States. Older women have higher medication expenditures than younger women, and the cost of IVF and ART accounts for 0.03 percent of healthcare expenditures within the United States annually. These numbers do not take into account other related costs, such as time off work, disability from pregnancy complications (which occur more commonly with IVF-obtained pregnancies), high-risk-pregnancy costs, and costs related to the disproportionate share of perinatal morbidity and mortality related to IVF pregnancies, specifically multifetal pregnancies. Costs related to prematurity, low birth weight, and very low birth weights are higher for multifetal gestations. In addition, higher-order multiples are more likely to result in infants that have long-term mental and physical handicaps. These costs can be insurmountable.

Cost analyses have been performed to examine the economic differences in the number of embryos transferred. From an economic standpoint, transferring three embryos is the least expensive route in the short term because a pregnancy is more likely to occur, thus reducing the need for additional IVF cycles (cost related directly to the IVF procedure itself). Although transferring fewer embryos increases short-term cost because of the need for repeated procedures, transferring a single embryo actually decreases the long-term cost because these pregnancies are less likely to have as many complications. IVF-related long-term costs are directly related to the number of fetuses carried during the pregnancy. Even pregnancies in which fetuses die or are selectively reduced (a voluntary termination of one or more fetuses), the complication rates remain higher than in a pregnancy that was initially a singleton pregnancy.

Multiple gestations also are associated with higher levels of neonatal and pediatric care than singleton gestations. Singleton gestations that are conceived via IVF have higher complication rates than naturally achieved pregnancies, and in addition, singleton children born as a result of IVF have higher postneonatal hospitalization costs than naturally conceived singleton children. Children conceived through IVF also have higher congenital abnormalities, which appear to be related to the severity of the couple's infertility status. Singleton pregnancies achieved via IVF are more likely to have medical conditions that drive up economic costs. Higher rates of gestational hypertension, placenta previa, preterm labor, caesarean birth, preterm birth, and low birth weight occur in women who conceive a single fetus via IVF. Mothers who conceive a single fetus via IVF are also more likely to be hospitalized during the pregnancy than are women who conceive naturally.

## FUNDING

Funding for IVF in the United States is at the discretion of individual insurance companies. Researchers have concluded that insurance companies that cover ART technologies only see a negligible increase in the monthly cost in per member expenditures. Most insurance carriers do not cover the IVF procedure, although 14 states currently have laws that require insurers to either wholly cover or cover some form of infertility diagnosis and treatment. These states include Arkansas, California, Connecticut, Hawaii, Illinois, Maryland, Massachusetts, Montana, New Jersey, New York, Ohio, Rhode Island, Texas, and West Virginia. The extent of coverage and what specific procedures are covered, however, varies greatly from state to state. Interestingly, states that mandate coverage of IVF procedures have lower multifetal pregnancy rates when compared with states that do not mandate coverage of IVF procedures.

The United States is one of the few industrialized countries that does not offer IVF coverage through the government. In Europe, Denmark leads the European nations, with the highest number of funded cycles annually: 2,031 cycles performed for every 1 million inhabitants. Austria and Macedonia perform the least procedures, with 602 and 186 performed, respectively. Worldwide, Israel leads with the most IVF cycles performed annually, at 3,263 procedures per 1 million inhabitants. Countries that perform the fewest covered IVF cycles are those countries from the former Soviet Union and countries within the Middle East or Latin America. Other countries that perform more than 1,000 cycles per 1 million inhabitants include France, Germany, Great Britain, Finland, Cyprus, Australia, Slovenia, Iceland, Sweden, Belgium, Norway, and the Netherlands.

Developing countries typically do not have access to IVF procedures. In many of these countries, infertility is caused by a tubal factor resulting from sexually transmitted infections, unsafe abortion, and postpartum uterine infection from substandard healthcare facilities. In many of these countries, infertility carries a social stigma of shame, isolation, economic deprivation, and violence. There are some researchers who advocate for unmedicated IVF cycles in Africa and Latin America.

Globally, differing laws can have a huge effect on factors related to costs associated with IVF. In Italy, a new law was passed that allowed the transfer of more than three embryos during an IVF cycle. The passage of this law has led to a significant increases in triplet birth rates, which has in turn driven up healthcare expenditures.

IVF is a costly procedure, the long-term financial costs of which are often overlooked in cost-analysis studies. Both singleton and multifetal pregnancies that result from IVF have risk factors that may make expenditures higher than traditional estimates.

**SEE ALSO:** International Laws; In Vitro Fertilization.

**BIBLIOGRAPHY.** Peter R. Brinsden, *In Vitro Fertilization and Assisted Reproduction* (Parthenon, 1999); Gary N. Clarke, "A.R.T. and History, 1678–1978," *Human Reproduction* (v.21, 2006); Richard G. Edwards, "IVF and the History of Stem Cells," *Nature* (v.413, 2001); Richard G. Edwards, "Changing Genetic World of IVF, Stem Cells and PGD. A. Early Methods in Research," *Reproductive BioMedicine Online* (v.11, 2005).

Michele R. Davidson
George Mason University

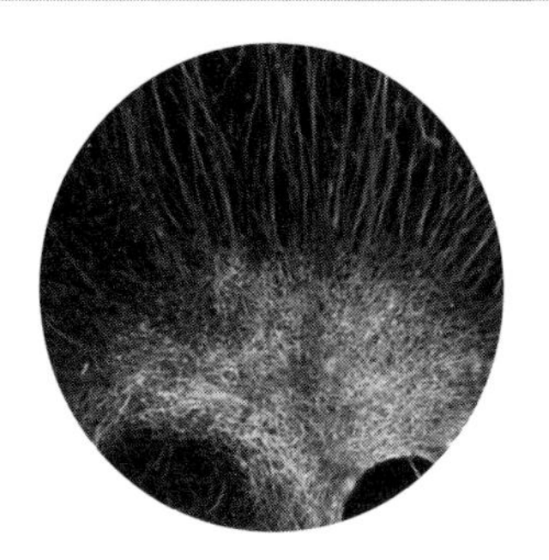

# G

## Gage, Fred

**FRED H. "RUSTY"** Gage is based at the Salk Institute in La Jolla, California, where he is a professor in the laboratory of genetics. His work has concentrated on the adult central nervous system. His major discovery has been that stem cells exist within the brain and that these can develop into brain cells, owing to certain stimuli. He has shown that exercise and environmental stimulation do contribute brain cell growth. This is contrary to the scientific orthodoxy of previous generations and it has eliminated that barrier to scientific research. Gage's work is seeking to understand the methodology by which this function happens. Once understood, this could lead to replacing or enhancing brain and spinal cord tissues that have been lost or damaged by neurodegenerative disease or by trauma. With their discovery, Fred Gage and his lab team have opened up the whole new field of central nervous system (CNS) gene therapy.

Neurons or brain cells do not divide, as other cells do. So, science has always contended that a person is born with about 100 billion neurons and that the human brain retains that same number, less any cells that may die off over a lifetime. With the discovery of the development of new neurons in the brains of adult songbirds, in the mid-1980s, a new controversy arose in neuroscience. This was the idea of neurogenesis or neuron creation in the adult brain. Some central questions were how and why this neuron birth occurs in the adult brain, and if this occurs in birds, than does this also occur in mammals and in humans.

Laboratory work performed by Gage and his colleagues has demonstrated that people can grow new nerve cells. They have found small populations of immature nerve cells existing among mature cells. These occur because of neurogenesis. The goal of Gage's research is to understand the mechanism(s) for stimulating the neurogenesis process, or to try to answer the question of how immature nerve cells in the adult brains of mammals experience stimulation to become mature functioning nerve cells in the spinal cord and brain.

Research has shown that physical exercise is a stimulant. Gage and his research colleagues have found that physical exercise can promote the growth of new brain cells in the hippocampus. Located on the inside of the medial temporal lobe of the brain, the hippocampus plays a part in the making of new memories. A part of the limbic system, it is an important factor in the making of long-term memory and spatial navigation. Two hippocampi are found in mammals and in humans. The shape of the hippocampus resembles the shape of a sea horse, for which it is named. Also important in the stimulation of new brain cell growth are the enriching environmental experiences of a mammalian subject. Both exercise and stimulating experiences enhance new brain growth.

## RESEARCH

The next issue was to confirm neurogenesis. The research was two fold. With the application of the molecule BrdU, Georg Kuhn led the research using immunocytochemistry, combined with confocal microscopy and quantitative stereology to make the measurement of neurogenesis. This provided one conformation. The second was a double-blind study using the mice in the lab. Lab mice live in little mouse cages in the lab. In Gage's study they kept one-half of the adult mice in the small cages and put the other half into a big complex stimulating environment with ample exercise and let them stay there for 45 days. Then, within the second set of mice, they found a very big change in the numbers of neurons in the hippocampus. These results where published in their paper in *Nature* in 1997.

The next question would be does this phenomenon occur in primates, and then in human? This research would require fresh human brain tissue. Some of the laboratory physicians went back to their own countries and participated in clinical trials in order to obtain fresh tissue. They would send brain sections back to San Diego to be worked on, and this is how Gage's lab discovered that neurogenesis occurs in humans.

## FURTHER RESEARCH

The goal of the research is to study the process of neurogenesis and find the underlying cellular and molecular mechanisms. It is anticipated that knowledge in this area will provide ways to repair aged or damaged brain cells. The repair of damaged brain cells could be of immense help to patients who suffer dementia from diseases such as Parkinson's or Alzheimer's. In addition, spinal cord injuries can also be theoretically repaired. Gage and his colleagues have demonstrated that because stem cells persist in the dentate gyrus, a part of the hippocampus, they can give rise to new neurons. The development of new neurons in a scientific experiment is proof that neurogenesis occurs in humans.

The brain and the central nervous system have the capacity for self-repair. Gage's lab, working in this field of neurogenesis, hopes to discover and understand how this occurs normally and to learn about the molecular, cellular, and environmental factors that control it. With this type of knowledge they may be able to activate and amplify the existing cell-repair process within the human body, rather than engineering from the outside and then transplanting cells. Beyond his research Gage has worked to expand methods of private and public funding. Gage, Irving Weissman of Stanford University, and David Anderson cofounded StemCells, Inc. (Nasdaq: STEM). They and other scientists sit on a Scientific Advisory Board, which directs the company.

## HONORS

Among the numerous awards and honors presented to Fred Gage have been membership as a fellow in the National Academy of Sciences, fellow in the Institute of Medicine of the National Academy of Sciences, fellow of the American Academy of Arts and Sciences, Bristol-Myers Squibb Neuroscience Research Award (1987), IPSEN Prize in Neuronal Plasticity (1990), Charles A. Dana Award for Pioneering Achievements in Health and Education (1993), Christopher Reeve Research Medal (1997), Max Planck Research Prize (1999), and the Robert J. and Claire Pasarow Foundation Award (1999).

In 2001 Gage served as president of the Society for Neuroscience and was the Vi and John Adler Professor on Age-Related Neurodegenerative Diseases. In 2002 he won the MetLife Award for Medical Research, and in 2003, he won a German prize, the Klaus Joachim Zulch-Preis, which was awarded through the Max Planck Society. He is a member of the Science Advisory Board of the Genetics Policy Institute.

**SEE ALSO:** California; Cells, Adult; Salk Institute; StemCells, Inc.

**BIBLIOGRAPHY.** Fred H. Gage and Yves Christen, *Isolation, Characterization and Utilization of CNS Stem Cells* (Springer-Verlag, 1997); Fred H. Gage, Gerd Kempermann, and Hungjun Song, eds., *Adult Neurogenesis* (Cold Spring Harbor Laboratory, 2007); Michael E. Selzer, Pamela W. Duncan, Fred H. Gage, and Leonardo G. Cohen, eds., *Textbook of Neural Repair and Rehabilitation, Volume 2: Medical Neurorehabilitation* (Cambridge University Press, 2006); I. M. Verma, *Regenerative Medicine* (National Academies Press, 2003).

Andrew J. Waskey
Dalton State College

# Gearhart, John

**DR. JOHN GEARHART** is a leading scientist in human genetics and an advocate for embryonic stem cell research. His numerous accolades include an induction in 1999 into the Academy of Achievement, a nonprofit museum of living history located in Washington, D.C. Gearhart works on stem cells derived from fetal tissue yet actively supports federal funding for embryonic stem cells. His chief argument in favor of using fetal tissue from abortion clinics is that this tissue would be discarded otherwise. At present, when he obtains tissue for research, there is no contact between the donating woman, who has signed a consent form, and the researchers. The woman is not financially rewarded in any way, nor is anyone involved in the transfer process.

Gearhart grew up in Girard College, an orphanage in Philadelphia, Pennsylvania, which he entered at the age of 6 years and left between the ages of 16 and 17 years. His father had died in a car accident, and his mother consequently placed John and one of his brothers into the all-male orphanage, which had been established in 1848 to raise and educate boys. Gearhart lived at the orphanage until he moved to Pennsylvania State University after graduation.

Although initially intending to study horticulture, Gearhart quickly developed a passion for human genetics. His first goal was to be a pomologist—an expert in growing apples, peaches, and pears. At the time, the way to improve on these fruits was through breeding. Unsatisfied with the time commitment dedicated to one fruit tree, Gearhart turned to flowers, which could show the results of selective breeding much more rapidly.

It did not take long for Gearhart's attentions to turn to animal genetics. He wanted to study humans, but the resources were not available in those years; therefore, he started with the fruit fly and continued with the mouse until he reached Johns Hopkins University School of Medicine, where he could finally study human genetics. In the field of human genetics, a significant portion of Gearhart's work has been on the cellular and molecular mechanisms of the genetic mutation causing Down syndrome (trisomy 21).

Gearhart first attended Pennsylvania State University, earning a bachelor's of science in biological science in 1964. From there, Gearhart moved to the University of New Hampshire (UNH) to obtain a master's degree in genetics in 1966. At UNH, Gearhart became a self-proclaimed expert on lilacs, as New Hampshire is "the lilac state."

From UNH, Gearhart moved to a leading genetics institute: Cornell University in Ithaca, New York. At Cornell, in 1970, Gearhart earned his doctoral degree in genetics, development, and embryology. He then held positions at the Institute for Cancer Research in Philadelphia and the University of Maryland in Baltimore before settling down at Hopkins in 1980. Ten years later, Gearhart joined the Medical Genetics Center in addition to the Center for Reproductive Biology.

At Hopkins, Gearhart has served as professor of comparative medicine, gynecology and obstetrics, physiology, and population dynamics on the medical campus, as well as at the Bloomberg School of Public Health, where he is professor of biochemistry and molecular biology. As of early 2008, he serves in the department of gynecology and obstetrics as director of research and director of the developmental genetics division.

Much of his research has focused on the manner in which genes regulate the formation of tissues and embryos. For over 20 years, he has researched the causes of mental retardation and other birth defects. The isolation of the stem cells of mice enabled him to attack a difficult challenge, the isolation and culturing of human stem cells.

Gearhart, working with his team, was the first scientist to isolate human pluripotent stem cells in 1998, retrieving his stem cells from the developing gonads of aborted fetuses. During his research, Gearhart's team successfully identified and isolated the stem cells and maintained them in a nutritive environment where they continued reproducing without differentiating. These cells were characterized to be similar to embryonic germ cells derived from the gonadal ridge and to embryonic stem cells derived from the inner cell mass. The achievement may profoundly impact drug development and transplant therapy, and supports the possibility of growing human tissues in the laboratory to replenish failing organs. The stem cells that Gearhart uses are pluripotent, meaning they have the ability to differentiate into multiple cell types; however, and importantly, they are not totipotent, which would mean that they have the ability to differentiate into a living, independent organism.

Gearhart has been an advocate of federal funding for further embryonic stem cell research. He believes that the possible future benefits of human stem cell research warrant the support of the national government.

**SEE ALSO:** Cells, Embryonic; Cells, Fetal; Cloning; Differentiation, In Vitro and In Vivo; Federal Government Policies; Johns Hopkins University.

**BIBLIOGRAPHY.** Academy of Achievement, "From Orphan to Eminent Scientist," www.achievement.org (cited February 2008); M. Bellomo, *The Stem Cell Divide: The Facts, the Fiction, and the Fear Driving the Greatest Scientific, Political and Religious Debate of Our Time* (AMACOM/American Management Association, 2006); C. B. Cohen, *Renewing the Stuff of Life: Stem Cells, Ethics, and Public Policy* (Oxford University Press, 2007); C. Fox, *Cell of Cells: The Global Race to Capture and Control the Stem Cell* (Norton, 2007); S. Lewis, *Arrowsmith* (Buccaneer, 1982); K. R. Monroe, R. Miller, and J. Tobis, eds., *Fundamentals of the Stem Cell Debate: The Scientific, Religious, Ethical, and Political Issues* (University of California Press, 2007); M. Ruse and C. A. Pynes, eds., *The Stem Cell Controversy: Debating the Issues (Contemporary Issues)* (Prometheus, 2006).

Claudia Winograd
University of Illinois, Urbana-Champaign

# Genetics Policy Institute

**THE GENETICS POLICY** Institute (GPI) is a nonprofit education and advocacy organization whose primary purpose is to defend the rights of researchers to engage in stem cell research and the rights of patients to benefit from therapies developed through stem cell research. GPI is located in the United States, with headquarters in Wellington, Florida, and an office in Washington, D.C., but conducts research, education and policy activities on a worldwide scale.

The origins of GPI lie in the Clonaid trial of 2002, in which Bernard Siegel, J.D., founder and executive director of GPI, played a key role in exposing Clonaid as a fraud. Clonaid, a U.S. company associated with the Raëlian Movement headquartered in Montreal, CA, claimed to have produced a human clone that they called "Baby Eve" for a childless couple, but were unable to produce the alleged child or provide any DNA evidence that they had in fact created a human clone. Siegel's involvement with this case motivated him to found GPI in order to help establish a legal distinction between therapeutic cloning (supported by GPI) and reproductive cloning (opposed by GPI, as by most researchers and practitioners involved in therapeutic cloning research and practice). GPI has since expanded its scope to include public policy in all areas of stem cell research on an international level.

GPI is a leader in the "pro-cures" movement, which advocates for ethical stem cell research that may lead to treatment for human disease and injury, and provides a counterpoint to organizations that seek to unduly restrict or prohibit such research. GPI seeks to remove barriers to research (including funding restrictions) and practice in regenerative medicine, and to that end regularly monitors global laws and regulations concerning stem cell research. GPI was the principal organizer of a global coalition that successfully opposed a United Nations treaty that would have banned somatic cell nuclear transfer (therapeutic cloning) throughout the world.

GPI disseminates information about therapeutic cloning through press releases, publications, a speaker's bureau, scientific conferences, and its Web site. In June 2004 GPI organized a scientific conference, "Human Cloning in All Its Aspects" at the United Nations. GPI organizes an annual stem cell summit in partnership with academic institutions such as Stanford University and the Harvard Stem Cell Institute: In September 2008 GPI will present the World Stem Cell Summit in Madison, Wisconsin, in collaboration with the University of Wisconsin Stem Cell and Regenerative Medicine Center and WiCell Institute, an affiliate of the University of Wisconsin that hosts the National Stem Cell Bank. The Student Society for Stem Cell Research (SSSCR), founded in August 2003, is a network of more than 2,500 students in 15 countries sponsored by the GPI. SSSCR engages in advocacy, education and direct action in support of stem cell research and includes member from the undergraduate to the doctoral level.

**SEE ALSO:** Cloning; United States.

**BIBLIOGRAPHY.** GPI: The Voice of the Stem Cell Community, www.genpol.org (cited May 2008); Student Society for Stem Cell Research, stemcellrsch.org (cited May 2008).

Sarah Boslaugh
BJC HealthCare

# Georgia

**GEORGIA HAS AN** impressive academic and clinical research history in biomedical science. In 1998 physicians at Children's Healthcare of Atlanta (in partnership with Emory University) performed the first allogenic umbilical cord blood stem cell transplant on a child for sickle cell disease, resulting in a cure. To attract technology industry professionals, the Georgia Research Alliance creates a collaborative network of researchers. Georgia promotes nonembryonic stem cell and related research, and researchers are performing work on National Institutes of Health–approved human embryonic stem cells to discover treatments for human disease.

No federal legislation in the United States regulates stem cell research except the executive order to not allow federal funding for embryonic stem cell research in cell lines created after August 9, 2001; each state is responsible for determining policy, regulation, and funding. Georgia legislators considered and failed to pass bills in 2006 and 2007 regarding umbilical cord blood banking and stem cell research on nonembryonic sourced stem cells.

Georgia's current policy comes from an April 14, 2006, executive order to create the Governor's Commission for New Born Umbilical Cord Blood Research and Medical Treatment to establish statewide cord blood banking networks and promote nonembryonic stem cell research, though not providing state funding for this research. Public funding is available through competitive grants from federal sources, such as the National Institutes of Health, and state research funds, as well as private foundations and biotech companies.

The Georgia Research Alliance is a private, nonprofit corporation begun in 1990 to enhance Georgia's economy through collaboration by academia, business, and government to encourage technology research and development by attracting top scientists and fostering new business development. Funding is provided by the state, universities, and private sources. The alliance's four areas of focus include eminent scholars, research laboratories and equipment, national centers for research and innovation, and technology transfer.

The research universities affiliated with the alliance that have researchers focused on stem cell research include the University of Georgia, the Medical College of Georgia, Emory University, Clark Atlanta University, and the Georgia Institute of Technology. With past investments of over $400 million, the alliance has attracted over 50 eminent scholars, 17 of whom specialize in stem cell research.

## INSTITUTIONS

The Regenerative Bioscience Center at the University of Georgia conducts research on National Institutes of Health–approved human stem cell lines for translation into clinical therapy to alleviate human diseases. The center promotes cross-discipline and multi-institutional research within the Georgia Research Alliance with the Georgia Institute of Technology, Georgia State, the Medical College of Georgia, and Emory University. The center increases knowledge, facility, and technology resources to gain external funding. In addition to research, the center provides education to national/international researchers, graduate and undergraduate classes taught by the faculty, and high school students interested in biomedical science careers through the young scholars program.

The Human Embryonic Stem Cell Workshop at the University of Georgia includes four days of hands-on laboratory education and lectures for participants to learn about innovations and the techniques for working with human embryonic stem cell lines. The laboratory portion includes how to propagate, maintain, and cryopreserve undifferentiated stem cells, as well as differentiation techniques using feeders and karyotyping of stem cells. Human Embryonic Stem Cells Symposia are held in conjunction with the workshop to discuss the latest news in stem cell research, tissue engineering, and clinical applications for treating human disease.

Steven Stice, director of the center and professor at the University of Georgia, in collaboration with the U.S. Naval Research Laboratory, created a kit containing neural cells grown from human embryonic stem cells to detect a broad spectrum of chemical weapons. The device is designed to detect changes in cell activity.

The Stem Cell/Restorative Program at the Medical College of Georgia uses adult stem cells for the treatment of brain injuries. The current studies are in animal models, with the hope of translating them into clinical therapy for adults and children with cerebral palsy and stroke, using adult stem cells.

The Parker H. Petit Institute for Bioengineering and Bioscience opened at the Georgia Institute of Technology in 1995. Researchers at the institute enjoy collaborative relationships across academic disciplines. The institute fosters partnerships or multiple-university research in regenerative medicine and stem cell research.

The Center for the Engineering of Living Tissues, established in 1998, has a mission to find innovations using tissue engineering to develop medical implants and address issues relating to organ/tissue transplant. The center partners the Georgia Institute of Technology and the Emory University School of Medicine, forming a team made up of members of both universities.

The Biomedical Research and Training Program is multidisciplinary, involving graduate and undergraduate programs in the biological sciences, chemistry, computer science, and physics. One of Clark Atlanta University's researchers is an eminent scholar in the Georgia Research Alliance and performs stem cell research regarding the proliferation, differentiation, and control of human reproductive cells.

Emory University in Atlanta has roots dating back to the 1830s as a teaching institution. Today, Emory offers undergraduate and graduate courses and has a medical school. Educational and research preparation and opportunities are available through the graduate division of biological and biomedical sciences and the biochemistry and cell and developmental biology program.

**SEE ALSO:** Cells, Embryonic; University of Georgia.

**BIBLIOGRAPHY.** Biomedical and Health Sciences Institute, "Regenerative Bioscience Center," www.biomed.uga.edu (cited November 2007); Emory University, "Cell & Developmental Biology Program," www.emory.edu (cited November 2007); Georgia Research Alliance, "About," www.gra.org (cited November 2007); University of Georgia, www.uga.edu (cited November 2007).

Lyn Michaud
Independent Scholar

# Germany

**GERMANY REMAINS AT** the forefront of stem cell research, with a strong foundation in academics and private/commercial business. The country maintains sensitivity for protecting human dignity, and research is carefully regulated with appropriate legislation and funding. Stem cell researchers benefit from networking relationships within the country, with the Stem Cell Network of North Rhine Westphalia and through regional relationships through the ScanBalt organization to enhance biotechnology within the Nordic and Baltic Sea region, as well as European and international affiliations.

The embryo protection law prevents the derivation of new stem cell lines because the technique destroys the embryo. A recent ruling by members of Germany's lower house of parliament passed an amendment to this law allowing scientists to import embryonic stem cells created before May 1, 2007, in order to allow German scientists to keep pace with the rest of the scientific world. Research on human embryonic stem cells may proceed under the Stem Cell Act of 2002, using only imported stem cell lines created before January 1, 2002. Funding for stem cell research is provided by the German Research Foundation and through other public entities and private foundations and companies.

The Stem Cell Network of North Rhine Westphalia was founded with a dual focus on biomedical research and socio-ethico-legal considerations. The network puts together cross-discipline experts in science, medicine, religion, philosophy, sociology, and law for research in embryonic-sourced stem cells. Funding by the state of North Rhine–Westphalia amounted to $80,000 in 2007 and $75,000 in 2006 for joint projects with interdisciplinary participation.

The projects funded included studies of endothelial precursor calls for tissue engineering treatment, pluripotent and multipotent human stem cell microRNA expansion, controlling germ cell differentiation, controlling osteoprogenitor cells, human embryonic stem cell cardio myocyte selection and immunologic properties for use in animal mouse model, culturing human somatic periodontal stem cells as therapy for periodontitis, magnetic resonance imaging hematopoietic stem/progenitor cells for cell migration, and differentiation in vitro with smart contrast agents.

## INSTITUTIONS

The Fraunhofer Technology Center was established in 1999 and is a central point of contact for research and development for national and global researchers. The Fraunhofer Institute is a member of the Fraunhofer Alliance of Life Sciences, and in 2004, it established the cell differential and cell technology group at University of Lübeck to focus on medical use of adult stem cells including isolation, differentiation, and growth of stem cells for regenerative medicine. The institute maintains a permit to import human embryonic stem cells.

Funding for the institute comes from public and commercial research and development contracts. In 2007 the institute employed 213 scientific and technical professions, including 32 research fellows, along with support staff. The money is used to translate fundamental science innovation to practical information application. The institute provides services in consulting, feasibility studies, prototype development, testing, and manufacturing engineering and support within the Saar, Brandenburg, and Schleswig-Holstein regions.

The Dresden University of Technology is a teaching and research university with English-lan-

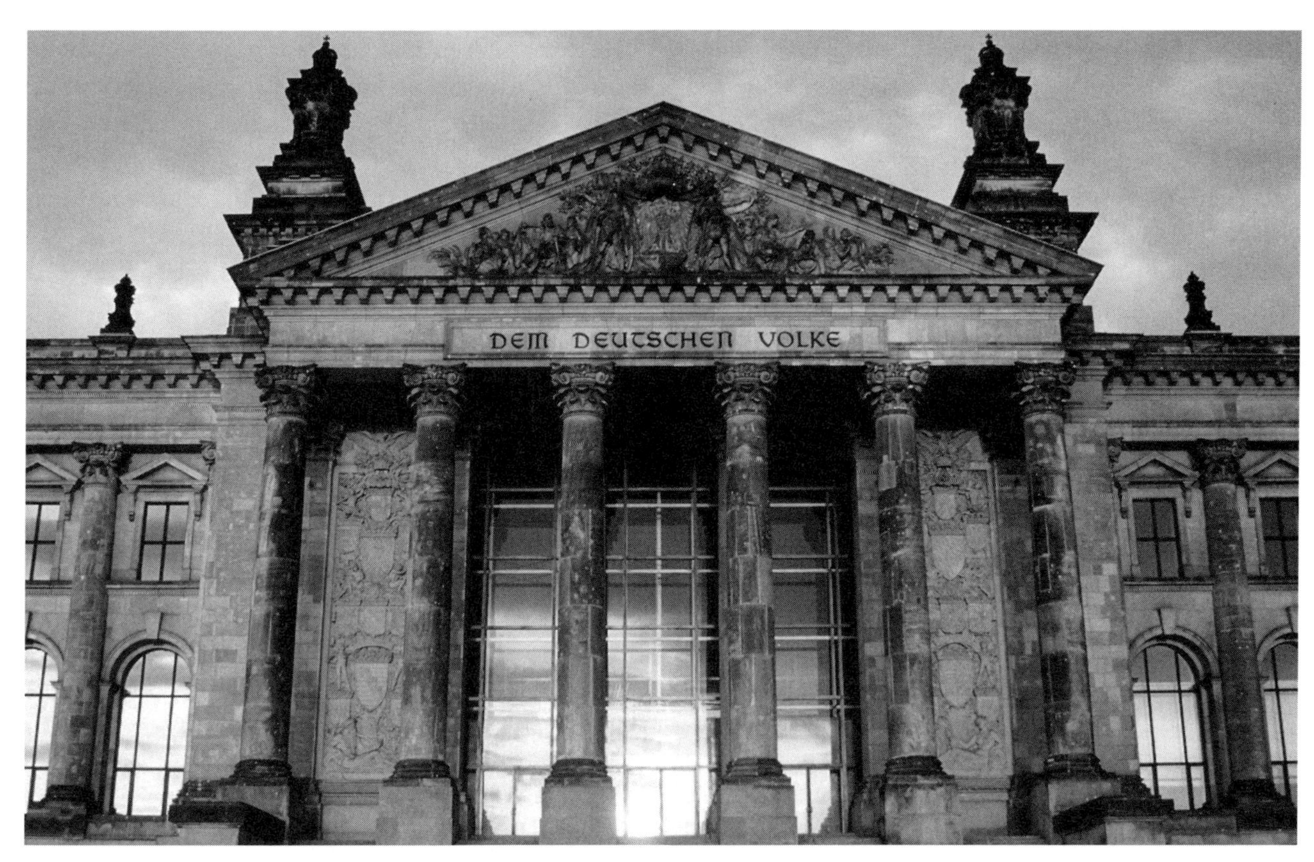


*A recent ruling by members of Germany's lower house of parliament allows German scientists to import embryonic stem cells created before May 1, 2007.*

guage programs enrolling graduate students from 30 countries. The school combines the concepts of fundamental science with translations of the technology into regenerative medicine and bioengineering. The university established the Research Center for Regenerative Therapies in 2006 through funding by the German Research Foundation; it was expanded with the establishment of From Cells to Tissues to Therapies, Cluster of Excellence, supported by the federal government. The center's research is performed through a network of over 70 laboratories in Dresden, including industry partners working toward a mission of developing regenerative therapies for human disease based on basic research in understanding developmental and growth processes. The center currently uses hematological stem cells in transplants. Research is focused on understanding stem cell physiology in animal models for diabetes and neurodegenerative, bone/cartilage, and cardiovascular diseases.

The biotechnological center supports research and education in molecular bioengineering. The center's basic and preclinical research labs opened in 2000 to host research groups dedicated to genetics, proteomics, biophysics, cellular machines, tissue engineering, and bioinformatics. The center's laboratories are situated for maximum networking opportunities, with biotech businesses housed in the same building as well a proximity to the Max Planck School for Molecular Cell Biology and Bioengineering and the Center for Regenerative Therapies.

The International Max-Planck Institute established the Max Planck Institute of Molecular Cell Biology and Genetics in 2001 as a research school for molecular cell biology and bioengineering, molecular cell biology, bioengineering, developmental biology, genetics, biophysics, neurobiology, and bioinformatics. The school provides a cross-discipline approach, with fundamental research and translation into regenerative medicine and applied bioengineering and with the Dresden University of Technology. Students accepted in the school are also affiliated with the Dresden International Graduate School of Biomedicine and Engineering in one of three international doctoral programs: cell and developmental biology, regenerative medicine and nanobiotechnology, and biophysics and bioengineering.

The Max Bergmann Center of Biomaterials is also affiliated with the Dresden University of Technology. The center was established in 2002 with the mission of creating biological material for use by university and commercial researchers.

Heinrich Heine University, located in Dusseldorf, was founded in 1907 to train physicians and is now home to the departments of medicine, science, economics, law, and philosophy. Biomedical research at the center is funded by the German Research Foundation, and current projects in the live sciences include cardiovascular medicine, clinical hematology, neuroscience, aging, biochemistry, and developmental biology. The university also acts as a biotech company incubator with successes including Qiagen and Rhein-Biotech.

The Third Spring School on Regenerative Medicine combines a conference for international scientists to share opinions and experience using stem cells with one week's practical methodology for working with stem cells. The cross-discipline approach is intended to provide a complete picture of the stem cell differentiation process and translation therapeutic application in creating artificial organ tissue and cells for transplant to treat human disease.

### COLLABORATION

Germany maintains international collaborations and networks in the area of stem cell research including the International Stem Cell Forum and the EuroStemCell Project. In addition, Germany is a member of ScanBalt, an organization based in Copenhagen, Denmark, to mediate and coordinate education, research, and development in biotech and life sciences within the Scandinavian and Baltic Sea region. The members are able to overcome country size restraints to become globally competitive in stem cell research as a region. ScanBalt maintains a virtual campus via the Internet to provide members with up-to-date listings of courses, lectures, job openings, ongoing research projects, and requests for proposals from funding agencies.

**SEE ALSO:** Bonn University; Cells, Embryonic; European Consortium for Stem Cell Research—EuroStemCell; International Laws; International Society for Stem Cell Research; International Stem Cell Forum; Stem Cell Network of North Rhine.

**BIBLIOGRAPHY.** Dresden Center for Regenerative Therapy, www.crt-dresden.de (cited November 2007); Fraunhofer Institute, "Profile," www.ibmt.fraunhofer.de (cited November 2007); Regenerative Medicine-Rostock Medical, www.unirostock.de (cited November 2007); ScanBalt, www.scanbalt.org (cited November 2007); Stem Cell Network of North Rhine Westphalia, Germany, Stemmzellen.nrw.de (cited November 2007); CellNet.Org, cellnet.org (cited November 2007).

LYN MICHAUD
INDEPENDENT SCHOLAR

# Germ Layers (Mesoderm, Ectoderm, Endoderm)

**ONE OF THE** earliest embryonic stages after the fertilized egg implants into the uterine wall is the gastrula, when the fertilized egg has gone through several divisions and the cells can be classified into three groups that have first begun to show differentiated characteristics. These groups are called germ layers and represent some of the first lineage specific stem cells in embryonic development. These differentiated cells can be grouped into three types, which are layered across the gastrula. Each layer, called a germ layer, will eventually become certain types of tissues in the adult. These layers are the endoderm and ectoderm, and in between them the mesoderm.

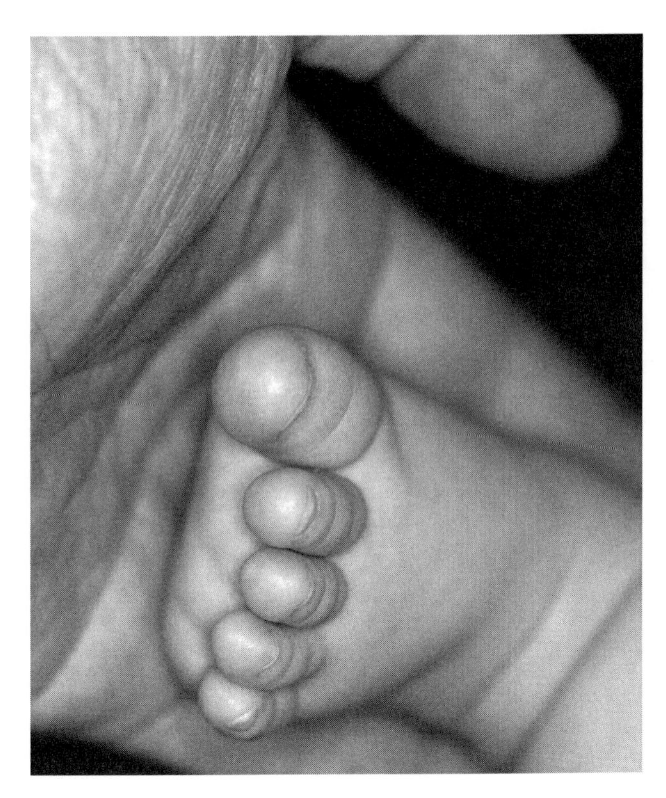

*The ectoderm, the outermost of the three germ cell layers, eventually develops into the epidermis and hair.*

The endoderm is so called because it is in the innermost layer of the three germ layers. It eventually becomes many of our "internal linings," such as cells lining most of the gastrointestinal tract as well as those cells lining the lungs, liver, pancreas, all other glands opening into the gastrointestinal tract, and some other organs such as the upper urogenital tract and female vagina. Additionally, the endoderm cells give rise to the colon, stomach, intestines, lungs, liver, and pancreas.

The ectoderm, or outermost layer of germ cells, eventually becomes our "outer lining" in the form of epidermis (outermost skin layer) and hair. The ectoderm is also the precursor to mammary glands and the central and peripheral nervous systems.

Finally, the layer in between the endoderm and the ectoderm is called the mesoderm. The mesoderm will develop into everything else—the dermis of the skin, the heart, our musculature, urogenital system, bones, and bone marrow and therefore blood. The mesoderm is the germ layer that distinguishes evolutionarily higher life forms from lower life forms with radial body symmetry. The mesoderm allows higher life forms to have an internal body cavity in which the organs can reside, protected from the movements and shocks of the outer body layers by fluids and connective tissue.

Because of the enormous ability of these germ layers to differentiate into a vast variety of organs and tissues, they attract much attention from scientists looking to determine how it is that humans develop. In stem cell jargon, a pluripotent stem cell is one that can become any of the three germ layers. Multipotent stem cells may give rise to lineages restricted to one dermal layer, or even one lineage within a dermal layer. For example, it should be possible to derive a mesoderm stem cell and guide its differentiation into a new bone such as a femur for a patient with a birth defect, or to develop new bone marrow for a patient with lymphoma. If these lineages could be reliably produced from human embryonic stem cells or induced pluripotent stem cells, they would represent an important source of tissue for both understanding development and potentially for new cell based therapies.

Germ layer cells are not the same cell population as germ cells. The term *germ cell* refers to the reproductive cells, or gametes, in the reproductive organs. For example, human germ cells are eggs and sperm.

**SEE ALSO:** Bone Marrow Transplants; Cancer; Cells, Developing; Cells, Embryonic; Developmental Biology; Human ES Cell Isolation; Lineages; Liver.

**BIBLIOGRAPHY.** M. Bellomo, *The Stem Cell Divide: the Facts, the Fiction, and the Fear Driving the Greatest Scientific, Political and Religious Debate of Our Time* (AMACOM/American Management Association, 2006); J. M. W. Slack, *From Egg to Embryo: Regional Specification in Early Development (Developmental and Cell Biology Series)* (Cambridge University Press, 1991); National Institutes of Health Web site for Stem Cell Information, stemcells.nih.gov (cited May 2008).

Claudia Winograd
University of Illinois, Urbana-Champaign

# Geron Corporation

**THE GERON CORPORATION** is a biopharmaceutical company located in Menlo Park, California. Geron was founded in 1990 by Dr. Michael West with a mission to research cellular mechanisms of aging and to advance the study of telomerase. The name Geron comes from the Greek meaning "old man."

In 1995 West approached Dr. James Thomson at the University of Wisconsin, Madison, with an offer to provide funding for Thomson's research to isolate stem cells from six-day-old embryos left over from in vitro fertilization. Of the 36 embryos the University of Wisconsin team used, 14 developed to the blastocyst stage, and from these embryos, the inner cell mass was used to establish five human cell lines, two of which were female and three of which were male.

In 1996 West approached Dr. John Gearhart at Johns Hopkins University with an offer to provide funding for Dr. Gearhart's research to isolate primordial germ cells from the gonadal ridge of 8–12-week-old aborted fetuses. Both research teams receiving Geron funding generated pluripotent cells capable of generating all three layers (ectoderm, mesoderm, and endoderm) of body cells. Both teams were published in scientific journals within days of each other. During this same time frame, Geron established an agreement with Roslin BioMed in Scotland for their cloning technology, with plans for making transplantable cells for individual patients. Michael West left Geron in 1998.

Under the leadership of Dr. Thomas B. Okama, Geron continues with the mission to develop therapeutic products to treat cancer, spinal cord injury, heart failure, diabetes, and HIV/AIDS. To meet this goal, Geron collaborates with researchers around the world to advance embryonic stem cell technology for therapeutic application in treating human disease by improving the culture and growth under conditions capable of commercial manufacture and to develop purification methods for differentiated cells as well as genetic modification enhancement. In addition, Geron remains active in the research on telomerase, with possible clinical applications as a diagnostic marker for cancer screening and for patient treatment and monitoring.

## CURRENT RESEARCH

Geron's current research (along with the research of collaborators) includes animal model testing of six different therapeutic cell types (neural cells for spinal cord injury and Parkinson's disease, cardiomyocytes for heart disease, pancreatic islet ß cells for diabetes, osteoblasts for osteoporosis, chondrocytes for osteoarthritis, and hematopoietic cells for blood diseases and to prevent immune rejection of the other cell types). These cells are derived from human embryonic stem cells, and preliminary positive results have shown evidence of engrafting or functional improvement in treated animals.

The telomerase inhibitors have been developed, including for use as an anticancer drug and a cancer vaccine that target the enzyme telomerase. Preclinical trials have shown the anticancer drug to be active against cancer stem cells in patients with multiple myeloma, multiple types of breast cancer, advanced prostate cancer, chronic lymphocytic leukemia, and solid tumors and has shown a synergistic effect when combined with radiation therapy in mice bearing human breast cancer. The U.S. Food and Drug Administration gave the go-ahead to initiate clinical testing of the telomerase vaccine in patients with acute myelogenous leukemia. Early clinical testing of the telomerase inhibitor drug includes testing for safety and tolerability.

In addition, the company is developing human embryonic stem cell therapies. One cell therapy is targeted toward treating spinal cord injury; the preclinical studies for spinal cord injury show cell survival in both mild and moderate lesion sites and remyelination in more severe injuries and a lack of impairment of spontaneous recovery in mildly injured rats. Another cell therapy is targeted toward treating patients with myocardial disease. Cardiomyocytes that differentiated from human embryonic stem cells have survived, engrafted, and prevented heart failure when transplanted into an infracted rat heart. Geron researchers and collaborators have also developed an improved method of deriving islet cells from human embryonic stem cells that secrete insulin and glucagons and have the confirmed genetic markers for islet cells.

In collaboration with the University of California, Los Angeles, and the Biotechnology Research Corporation of Hong Kong, Geron has determined that small molecule telomerase activators enhance the functional activity of immune cells from HIV/AIDS donors. The activators increase proliferation of cytotoxic T-cells and improve their inhibition capability against the virus in HIV-positive donors and enhance antiviral activity of cytotoxic T-cells.

Geron holds more than 60 patents and maintains intellectual property licenses or ownership for inventions and technology necessary for work in stem cell research. The proprietary methods grow, maintain and scale up undifferentiated human embryonic stem cells in a chemically defined culture medium in preparation for differentiation into cells that can be used therapeutically.

A 2002 agreement between Geron and the University of Wisconsin gave Geron exclusive rights to the differentiated neural cells, cardiomyocytes, and pancreatic cells derived from embryonic stem cells for therapeutic application. Geron maintains nine cell lines: five cell lines derived from University of Wisconsin, Madison, cells, two cell lines derived at the University of California, San Francisco, and two lines cloned from one of the University of Wisconsin lines.

Because of potential ethical issues arising from research on human embryos, Geron formed an ethics board early on to determine guidelines by which research and development of therapies for clinical application could proceed. The Geron Ethics Board invited public individuals to provide input and discussion on the ethical issues related to human embryonic stem cell research. In establishing guidelines for the ethical development of therapies derived from human embryonic stem cell research, the Geron Ethics Board considered the inherent value of the research against personhood, justice, aging and death, and the processes related to the research, including the origin of the embryos and conception. The final recommendations can be summed up by researchers ensuring that the research will reduce human suffering while maintaining the dignity and value of the embryo.

Researchers from Geron have been published in numerous scientific and clinical publications including but not limited to the *Journal of Neuroscience*, *Experimental Neurology*, *Circulation Research*, *Blood*, *Cancer Journal*, *Fertility and Sterility*, *Nature Biotechnology*, *Cloning and Stem Cells*, *Human Embryonic Stem Cells*, *Developmental Dynamics*, *Stem Cells*, *Glia*, *Stem Cells and Development*, *Cell Transplantation*, and the *Journal of Experimental Medicine*.

**SEE ALSO:** California; Cells, Embryonic; Cells, Sources of; Gearhart, John; Johns Hopkins University; University of Wisconsin, Madison.

**BIBLIOGRAPHY.** Geron Corporation, *Milestones* (Geron, 2006); Geron Corporation, www.geron.com (cited November 2007); Thomas B. Okama, "Human Embryonic Stem Cells: A Primer on the Technology and its Medical Applications," in *The Human Embryonic Stem Cell Debate: Science, Ethics, and Public Policy* (Bradford/MIT Press, 2001); Ann B. Parson, *The Proteus Effect: Stem Cells and Their Promise for Medicine* (Joseph Henry, 2004).

Lyn Michaud
Independent Scholar

# Goldman, Steven A.

**STEVEN A. GOLDMAN** is a stem cell researcher at the University of Rochester. He was previously at Cornell in the Division of Cell and Gene Therapy as the chief of the division. He also held the Glenn-Zutes Chair in Biology of the Aging Brain and was a professor of neurology, neurosurgery, and pediatrics. Goldman graduated summa cum laude with a bachelor's degree in biology and psychology from the University of Pennsylvania in 1978. In 1983 he completed a medical degree at Cornell University Medical College. However, instead of entering medical practice, he undertook studies for a doctoral degree. He completed his second doctorate in cellular neurobiology at Rockefeller University in 1984.

After completing his formal education, Goldman began the practice of medicine with a residency at the Cornell Medical Center in New York Hospital and Memorial Sloan Kettering Cancer Center in Medicine from 1984 to 1985. He then did a second residency in neurology from 1985 to 1988 and was chief resident in neurology from 1987 to 1988. Earning degrees has allowed Goldman to become certified as a physician. He is certified as a diplomate by the National Board of Medical Examiners (1985), with medical licensure by the State of New York (1985), and as a neurologist by the Board of Certification in Neurology, American Academy of Neurology and Psychiatry (1989). Goldman has many NIH grants and has been awarded a number of honors during his productive career.

## CAREER AND HONORS

Goldman's career has been a series of upwardly mobile places of service in neurology. From 1988 to 1992, he was an assistant professor of neurology and an assistant attending neurologist at the New York Hospital–Cornell University Medical Center. From 1992 until 1997, he served as associate professor of neurology and neuroscience at the New York Hospital–Cornell University Medical Center. In 1997 he was granted tenure as associate professor of neurology and neuroscience at the New York Hospital–Cornell University Medical Center. Goldman has a unique combination of both clinical and scientific skills that has kept him at the front of biomedical research in the stem cell field for many years.

From 1997 until 2001, Goldman served as professor of neurology and neuroscience at Cornell University Medical College. In addition, he was senior attending neurologist at New York Presbyterian Hospital. From 2001 until 2003, he was Nathan Cummings Professor of Neurology and Neuroscience at Cornell University Medical College. From 2003 until this writing, he has been adjunct professor of neurology at the Weill Medical College of Cornell University.

Goldman has been the recipient of many awards and fellowships. He was a Benjamin Franklin National Scholar, University of Pennsylvania, 1974–78; a Senatorial Scholar, State of Pennsylvania, 1974–78, and a Mayor's Scholar, City of Philadelphia, 1974–78. He was elected into Phi Beta Kappa at the University of Pennsylvania (1977) and was a Medical Scientist Training Program trainee, U.S. Public Health Service (1978–84), a Grass Foundation Fellowship winner (1978), and a Cornell Scholar in Biomedical Science (1988–91). He was given a clinical investigator development award from the National Institutes of Health (NIH)/National Institute of Neurological Disorders and Stroke (NINDS) for two years (1988–93), a FIRST Award from the NIH/NINDS for five years (1992–97), an Irma T. Hirschl Career Scientist Award for four years (1993–97), and a Jacob Javits Neuroscience Investigator Award from the National Institute of Neurological Disorders for seven years (2002–09).

## PROFESSIONAL SERVICE

There are a number of medical and scientific societies to which Goldman belongs. These include the American Society for Clinical Investigation (elected 2001), American Neurological Association (elected 1995), American Academy of Neurology, American Society for Cell Biology, American Society for Gene Therapy, Association for Nervous and Mental Diseases, and American Association for the Advancement of Science Society for Neuroscience.

Government service rendered by Goldman is extensive. It includes service on the NIH/NINDS Broad agency/RFP 96-07 review panel, NINDS Neuro-B2 review committee (1997), NINDS/Small Business Innovative Research review committee (1998), NINDS Neural Stem Cell Advisory Committee (1999), NINDS Special Emphasis Panel ZNS1-L01 (2000), U.S. Food and Drug Administration Stem Cell/Biological Response Modifiers Advisory Committee (2000), National Heart, Lung, and Blood Institute Scientific Review Group (SRG; Stem Cell Plasticity) (2001), NINDS Molecular, Cellular, and Developmental Neurosciences (MDCN) 7

(2001), NINDS MDCN6 (2002), National Institute of Mental Health SRG (2002), NINDS MDCN6 (2003), NINDS SRG (2003), National Institute on Aging SRG (2004).

Professional society and foundation service by Goldman includes acting as a neurobiology of disease workshop coordinator for the Society for Neuroscience (2002), participating in the Neural Disorders Committee of the American Society for Gene Therapy (2001–05), serving on the executive committee of the New York Academy of Medicine/Ellsberg Neurosurgery fellowship (2001–05), and being annual meeting president for the Association for Nervous and Mental Diseases in 2001. Goldman also has served as a member of the Children's Neurobiological Solutions scientific advisory board and as a grant reviewer for the Wellcome Trust, the Volkswagen Foundation, the Israel–U.S. Binational Trust, the National Multiple Sclerosis Society, and the Christopher Reeve Paralysis Foundation.

Goldman, as a top specialist, has served as a consultant or an adviser for several organizations. His work as a consultant or adviser includes service with Merck Inc. (2003), the Merck Neuroscience Research Labs, Q Therapeutics (2003), Aventis Pharmaceuticals (2001–03), and Neuronyx Inc. (2001–02).

## CURRENT RESEARCH

Current projects being conducted by Goldman and his colleagues are extensive and include research into human oligodendrocyte progenitor molecular biology, human neural stem cell and progenitor gene expression and differential signaling, tumor stem and progenitor cells of the human central nervous system, induced neurogenesis in neurodegenerative disease, progenitor cell–based myelination of congenitally dysmyelinated brain, relationship between angiogenesis and neurogenesis in the adult canary, regulation of astrocytosis from endogenous progenitors, and neural induction and therapeutic use of human ES cells.

Goldman is particularly recognized for his excellent contributions to the field of stem cell science. He has developed novel ways to isolate specific types of adult neural progenitor cells from human biopsy brain samples that involves sorting the cells using genetic markers, and then proving the cells can integrate and function within the living rodent brain. This work is paving the way for clinical trials using stem cells to treat diseases such as Parkinson's and Multiple Sclerosis.

**SEE ALSO:** Gage, Fred; New York; Weill-Cornell Medical College.

**BIBLIOGRAPHY.** Steven A. Goldman, "Glia as Neural Progenitor Cells," *Trends Neuroscience* (v.26, 2003); Steven A. Goldman, "Disease Targets and Strategies for the Therapeutic Modulation of Endogenous Neural Stem and Progenitor Cells," *Clinical Pharmacology and Therapeutics* (v.82/4, 2007); Steven A. Goldman, "Neurogenesis in the Adult Songbird: A Model for Inducible Striatal Neuronal Addition," *Adult Neurogenesis* (Cold Spring Harbor Laboratory, 2008); Steven A. Goldman and M. S. Windrem, "Cell Replacement Therapy in Neurological Disease," *Philosophical Transactions of the Royal Society of London B Biological Sciences* (v.361/1473, 2006); Steven A. Goldman, et al., "Progenitor Cell-Based Myelination as a Model for Cell-Based Therapy of the Central Nervous System," *Ernst Schering Research Foundation Workshop* (v.60, 2006); Steven A. Goldman and F. J. Sim, "Neural Progenitor Cells of the Adult Brain," *Novartis Foundation Symposium* (v.265, 2005); H. M. Keyoung and Steven A. Goldman, "Glial Progenitor-Based Repair of Demyelinating Neurological Diseases," *Neurosurgery Clinics of North America* (v.18, 2007); F. J. Sim and Steven A. Goldman, "White Matter Progenitor Cells Reside in an Oligodendrogenic Niche," *Ernst Schering Research Foundation Workshop* (v.53, 2005).

Andrew J. Waskey
Dalton State College

# Gut Stem Cells

**THE GUT IS** a common term for the intestinal part of the gastrointestinal tract, which is the pathway by which food enters the body, is processed for digestion of nutrients, and remnants exit the body. The gastrointestinal tract is therefore from the mouth to the anus. The cells lining the gastrointestinal tract, especially those cells lining the intestine, are constantly sloughing off and being replaced by new ones. This process is important to absorption of nutrients as well as to defense against invading microbes that enter the system through the gut. In order to replace the lost cells, a population of gut stem cells lines the gastrointestinal tract. These cells are studied in numerous laboratories because they are maintained throughout adulthood and consistently produce viable gut cells. In some diseases, these stem cells are lost; additionally, scientists are investigating ways to reintroduce stem cells therapeutically.

An important stem cell population for a gastrointestinal disease is the pancreatic stem cell population in diabetes. There has been evidence in animal models that transplanting pancreatic stem cells from a healthy animal into a diabetic animal can reintroduce insulin-producing cells into the recipient animal. Such a transplantation may someday be used to cure type 1 diabetes mellitus, where the patient's immune system attacks and destroys his or her own insulin-producing cells.

In the intestine, stem cells reside in a niche called the intestinal crypt. The intestine is not a smooth surface; rather, the lining is made of multiple finger-like projections called villi that increase the surface area of the intestine to better absorb nutrients. At the base of these projections lies the crypt. Stem cells in the crypt divide into more stem cells and partially differentiated gut epithelial cells. As the stem cells continue to divide, the older cells are pushed up toward the tips of the villi; as these cells migrate up and out, they develop into mature intestinal cells, of which there are several types. Once a cell reaches the top of a villus, it is sloughed off, to be replaced by a new cell.

The stem cell population in the intestinal crypts has only recently been investigated in detail, because until recently the technology was not available to find these stem cells. Researchers investigate the molecular and genetic mechanisms behind intestinal stem cell renewal and differentiation. It is hoped that a better understanding of intestinal stem cells can lead to therapeutics whereby a person's own intestinal stem cells, donated stem cells from another gastrointestinal tract, or even hematopoietic stem cells can be used to treat gastrointestinal diseases such as inflammatory bowel disease, Crohn's disease, and others.

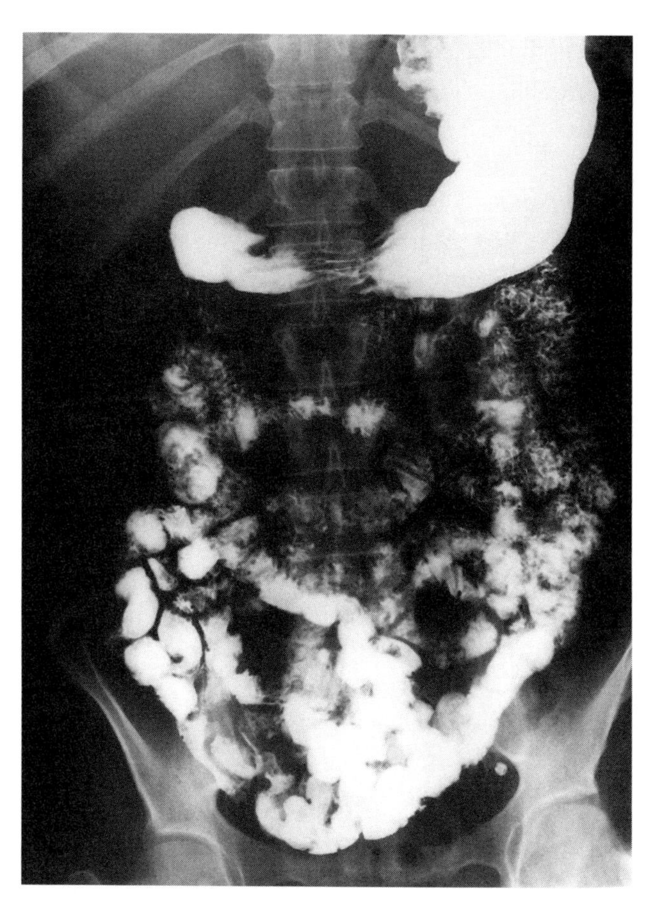

*Gut stem cells lining the gastrointestinal tract are often studied because they consistently produce new cells in adults.*

**SEE ALSO:** Diabetes; Markers of Stemness; Microenvironment and Immune Issues.

**BIBLIOGRAPHY.** A. Al-Toma and C. J. Mulder, "Review Article: Stem Cell Transplantation for the Treatment of Gastrointestinal Diseases—Current Applications and Future Perspectives," *Alimentary Pharmacology & Therapeutics* (December 2007); M. Bjerknes and

H. Cheng, "Gastrointestinal Stem Cells II. Intestinal Stem Cells," *American Journal of Physiology Gastrointestinal and Liver Physiology* (September 2005); M. Brittan and N. A. Wright, "The Gastrointestinal Stem Cell," *Cell Proliferation* (February 2004); B. Soria, F. J. Bedoya, and F. Martin, "Gastrointestinal Stem Cells I. Pancreatic Stem Cells," *American Journal of Physiology Gastrointestinal and Liver Physiology* (August 2005); T. H. Yen and N. A. Wright, "The Gastrointestinal Tract Stem Cell Niche," *Stem Cell Reviews* (September 2006).

Claudia Winograd
University of Illinois, Urbana-Champaign

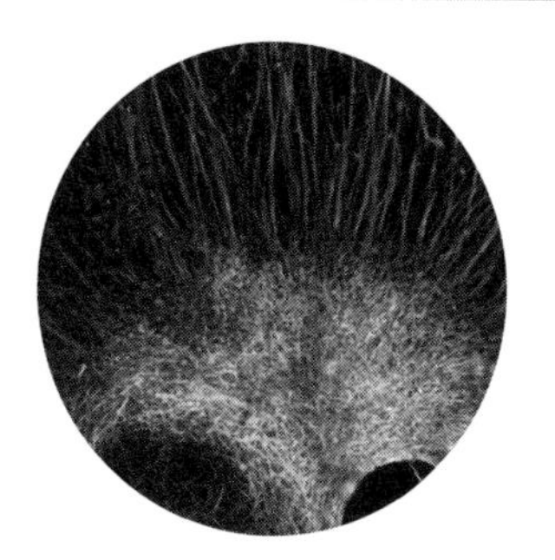

# H

## Harvard University

**HARVARD UNIVERSITY, FOUNDED** in 1636, is a private university located in Cambridge, Massachusetts, and is the oldest institution of higher learning in the United States. It is a member of the Ivy League. Recently, Harvard University opened the Harvard Stem Cell Institute (HSCI), a body committed to translating stem cell research in the laboratory into the clinic as quickly as possible in an attempt to treat disease. Harvard supports research primarily in developing new therapies for disease (e.g., diabetes, cardiovascular disease, and cancer). In fact, HSCI identifies itself as a "scientific collaborative established to fulfill the promise of stem cell biology as the basis for cures and treatments for a wide range of chronic medical conditions." HSCI states that at present, no embryonic stem cells (ES) have been used to treat diseases in humans, although research on these ES shows great potential. "Stem cell-based therapies are already in widespread clinical use, in the form of bone marrow and cord blood transplants."

The Harvard community consists of the university, the medical school, and 18 research institutions and hospitals, making it one of the world's largest concentrations of biomedical researchers. HSCI is aware of the importance of interdisciplinarity in this novel field of science; therefore, it is devoted to the virtue of community. HSCI works closely with its allies: Beth Israel Deaconess Medical Center, Howard Hughes Medical Institute, Brigham and Women's Hospital, Massachusetts General Hospital, Children's Hospital Boston, Joslin Diabetes Center, the Forsyth Institute, McLean Hospital, the Schepens Eye Research Institute, and the Immune Disease Institute, among other institutions from around the world. Harvard also incorporates nearly every department into its stem cell research: the John F. Kennedy School of Government, Harvard School of Public Health, Harvard Law School, Harvard Divinity School, Harvard Business School, Harvard Medical School, Radcliffe Institute for Advanced Study, and Harvard University.

HSCI states that it is currently "supported primarily by private philanthropic donations," which allows it to support a spectrum of research activities that could not otherwise be supported by sources such as the National Institutes of Health. The HSCI has created a unique fusion of professional institutions to address societal issues regarding stem cell research, ranging from legal and political issues to economic and ethical concerns; this interdisciplinary approach has permitted a unique synthesis of the institution's resources and its collaborators.

## PROGRAMS

As of October 2007, HSCI focuses on basic research and clinical translation in five principal disease areas: cancer, diabetes, nervous system diseases, blood diseases, and cardiovascular disease. Studies suggest that

> In the United States alone it has been estimated that as many as 100 million people suffer from diseases that could be amenable to stem cell–based therapies.

As a consequence, the mission of HSCI is to encompass basic research on all aspects of stem cell biology, with an emphasis on improving human health. In addition to the five major disease areas listed here, faculty members at HSCI have expanded their works to include research in muscle, kidney, skin, reproductive, and liver and gastrointestinal tract diseases.

HSCI has training opportunities for nearly all members of the academic community: undergraduates, graduates, and postdoctoral students. Undergraduate students interested in gaining laboratory experience may review the principal investigators' and faculty members' profiles to determine in which laboratory he or she would like to work; students are then encouraged to inquire directly to those researchers. An undergraduate summer research intern program is also available for students who are interested in participating in stem cell research in an HSCI-affiliated laboratory.

Although there is not a separate graduate training program in HSCI, students interested in stem cell research should apply to an existing program at one of the Harvard graduate schools and then contact a research adviser in a stem cell research lab. More information regarding the M.D./Ph.D. program, postdoctoral opportunities, and research-training fellowships are available online.

The most promising, but most controversial, stem cell work is research involving human embryonic stem (ES) cells. ES cells suggest extreme promise in the future of medicine and diseases treatment and therapy because of the potential of the ES cells to develop into any cell in the body. In more recent years, ethical issues surrounding the use of human ES cell research has been at the forefront of science, religion, and politics; ethics is also at the forefront of HSCI.

The Harvard Stem Cell Research Committee was established to review proposals by Harvard scientists to work on human ES cells. The committee examines the proposals to distinguish which projects will qualify for federal funding under the policies announced by President George W. Bush, who limited federal funding of stem cell research, and which projects will not. The committee consists of faculty from several schools, including Harvard Medical School, the John F. Kennedy School of Government, the Harvard School of Public Health, and the Faculty of Arts and Sciences. According to former Harvard Provost Steven Hyman, "The committee's review and recommendations ensure that human ES research at Harvard is conducted according to the highest ethical standards." The research committee must examine each case independently, reviewing local, state, and federal laws, and make decisions based on the merit of the proposal. Research involving human subjects must be reviewed by one of Harvard's institutional review boards as well, which ensures that the work meets federal guidelines related to research on humans.

## ETHICS

Scientists have been aware of the existence of stem cells for nearly a century; only within the past decade (late 1990s), however, were human ES cells first cultivated in the research laboratory. Along with the technological and scientific advancements made and therapeutic potential involved, there has also been a magnification of the sociopolitical controversy surrounding the issue of the use of ES cells. The stem cell is important for science because the cells are undifferentiated, meaning that they do not yet have a specific physiological function; the ES cell may also be referred to as pluripotent, meaning that they are able to differentiate into all derivatives of the primary germ layers: mesoderm, endoderm, and ectoderm. When certain conditions are induced in the body or in the laboratory, the stem cell begins to develop into specialized tissues and organs. Stem cells are also unique in their ability to self-renew, or to divide and give rise to more stem cells. The unique plasticity of ES cells has suggested new prospects for regenerative medicine and tissue replacement. To date, no approved medical treatments have been derived from ES cell research, however.

Some organs in humans contain stem cells that operate throughout the adult life and that contribute to the repair and maintenance of those organs; not every organ contains stem cells. Adult stem cells have restricted developmental capability; for example, the adult stem cell is only able to give rise to certain cell types, and their capacity to reproduce and proliferate is limited. ES, in contrast, can divide indefinitely and can differentiate into nearly every cell of the body. Researchers are excited about the potential of the ES cells to differentiate into any kind of tissue in the body; this capability implies that there is great potential for the effective treatment of a spectrum of diseases ranging from tissue damage, to organ failure and diabetes.

The debate surrounding the use of human embryonic tissue derives from the fact that the cells are derived from the inner cell mass of an embryo in its early stage, known as a blastocyst. For many years, the only way to derive the ES stem cells is to destroy the blastocyst-stage embryo. Human embryos reach the blastocyst stage within about five days postfertilization; the blastocyst consists of roughly 75–150 cells during this stage. Many individuals are opposed to the destruction of the embryo because they consider the blastocyst to be biologically and morally comparable to a human individual.

## POTENTIAL

More recently, however, the scientific journal *Nature* published a letter by Dr. Robert Lanza, medical director of Advanced Cell Technology, which stated that his team had discovered a method of extracting ES stem cells without actually destroying the embryo.

According to the HSCI, the human ES lines created at Harvard are derived from frozen embryos left over after in vitro fertilization treatment. Harvard researchers hope to derive ES stem cells by somatic cell nuclear transfer in the near future. Somatic cell nuclear transfers, or "therapeutic cloning," involve the transfer of a nucleus from a donor cell (such as a skin cell) to an unfertilized egg. The injected egg will induce division, and when it reaches a mass of a few hundred cells, ES stem cells that are genetically identical to the original donor cell can be derived. No fertilization would occur during this procedure, and because the mass is not implanted into a uterus, pregnancy is not necessary.

This technique has great therapeutic promise because the resulting stem cells could be transplanted into the original donor and would not suffer from rejection, as the donor would recognize the stem cells as "self." As a result, effective transplantations could occur without the problems of rejection that often occur with transplants from unrelated donors. HSCI also states that the somatic cell nuclear transfer could be useful in studying the basis of human disease and synthesizing and discovering new drugs for effective treatment.

HSCI recognizes that stem cells represent a unique opportunity and challenge. HSCI was created to achieve excellence in stem cell research. Harvard is distinguished from other institutions in that it encompasses not just one discipline, department, or school, but many. HSCI realizes that "clinical and laboratory scientists must engage with those attuned to the political, societal and ethical implications of the research" and that "the excessively politicized and emotional debate engendered by stem cell research requires a champion institution whose tradition of rational deliberation can balance the voices of opinion with a strong counterweight of exceptional science." Harvard realizes the importance of interdisciplinarity and diversity; with its tradition of excellence, its diversity of expertise, and its exceptional academic community, Harvard is unquestionably one of the world's leading centers for stem cell research.

**SEE ALSO:** Cells, Adult; Cells, Embryonic; Federal Government Policies; Lanza, Robert; Nuclear Transfer, Somatic.

**BIBLIOGRAPHY.** Harvard Stem Cell Institute, www.hsci.harvard.edu (cited November 2007); Alvin Powell, "From the Laboratory to the Patient," *Harvard Gazette* (April 22, 2004); Alvin Powell, "Vigilant Eyes Oversee Stem Cell Research," *Harvard Gazette* (April 22, 2004); H. Semb, "Human Embryonic Stem Cells: Origin, Properties and Applications," *Acta Pathologica, Microbiologica, et Immunologica Scandinavica* (v.113, 2005); I. Wilmut et al., "Somatic Cell Nuclear Transfer," *Nature* (v.419/6907, 2002).

Krishna Subhash Vyas
University of Kentucky

# Hawaii

**HAWAII HAS A** growing biomedicine industry that is important to the state's economy and to researchers performing fundamental research on stem cells. Progress is possible through appropriate legislation and public funding. As no federal legislation in the United States regulates stem cell research (except by an executive order to not allow federal funding to be used for embryonic stem cell research except on human embryonic stem cell lines created before August 9, 2001), each state is responsible for determining policy and funding for stem cell research. In 2007 Hawaii approved H.B. No. 364 to establish stem cell research policy and form an institute for regenerative medicine at the University of Hawaii.

The institute is assigned the goals of supporting stem cell and related research, translating innovation into clinical therapies through development and clinical trials, and establishing appropriate regulation and oversight. The state will benefit monetarily from royalties, patents, and licensing fees from the institute's discoveries and innovations. Funding provided to the institute is not to be used for human reproductive cloning.

The bill permits derivation of human embryonic stem cells and somatic cell nuclear transfer, as well as research on human embryonic stem and germ cells and human adult stem cells. This research requires institutional board review to consider ethical and medical implications. Excess embryos from in vitro fertilization may be donated by the parents with informed consent and the understanding that their confidentiality is to be maintained. The bill bans the sale of embryonic or fetal tissue directly, though handling fees are permissible.

To support stem cell and other biomedical research, the state offers high technology investment tax credits; other funding must be applied for through various sources such as the National Institutes of Health and private grant and foundation money, though there is extensive competition.

The Kaka'ako Biomedical Park in Honolulu is home to the University of Hawaii's John A. Burns School of Medicine, including an academic building and a research building. The complex is located near Waterfront Park and has views of Waikiki and Diamond Head. The park is meant to attract biotech companies for economic growth by increasing jobs and expanding the tax base. One such company located at Kaka'ako is Tissue Genesis, Inc. The company was established in 2001 to research bioengineering to create vascular and musculoskeletal tissue and cell therapies for regenerative medicine with the hope of using a patient's own cells.

## RESEARCHERS

The John A. Burns School of Medicine was founded in 1965. The school's mission is to train biomedical and allied health professionals in addition to physicians. Among the 14 departments are the departments of biochemistry, physiology and reproductive biology, and cell and molecular biology. The school also has centers on aging and clinical research and an Institute for Biogenesis Research.

Research at the University of Hawaii relating to stem cells includes work by the cell and molecular biology department (offering undergraduate and graduate courses and a broad range of research opportunities in cell differentiation in early development, DNA structure of germ cells and somatic cells, germ cells, and cloning).

Research at the Cardiovascular Research Center is being done to identify genetic mutations in mice leading to abnormal skin cell (keratinocyte) stem cell differentiation, genetic links to cardiovascular disease, and a study to determine the relationship between white blood cells and the replenishing of brain neural stem sells. Research by the Institute for Biogenesis Research includes studies on assisted fertilization and cloning, cell aging, and rejuvenescence.

**SEE ALSO:** Cells, Embryonic; Cloning; Stem Cells, Bush Ruling.

**BIBLIOGRAPHY.** House of Representatives, 24th Legislature, 2007, H.B. No. 364; John A. Burns School of Medicine, jabsom.hawaii.edu/jabsom (cited November 2007); University of Hawaii, "Cell and Molecular Biology Department," www.hawaii.edu/cmb (cited November 2007); Tissue Genesis Inc., "Highlights," www.tissuegenesis.com (cited November 2007).

Lyn Michaud
Independent Scholar

# Heart

**CARDIOVASCULAR DISEASE IS** a leading cause of morbidity and mortality in the United States and other developed nations. The term *cardiovascular disease* refers to any pathology of the heart and blood vessels, whether in larger vessels such as arteries and veins, or in microvasculature. A common form of cardiovascular disease is atherosclerosis, or narrowing of the arteries due to buildup of fatty deposits in the blood vessel lining. If a deposit, or plaque, breaks off it can travel through the vasculature until lodging somewhere, interrupting blood flow to the downstream tissues. When a blockage occurs in the heart, a part of the heart is temporarily deprived of vital oxygen, and a myocardial infarction occurs, more commonly known as a heart attack. The lack of oxygen results in necrosis or death of the heart muscle affected and permanent scarring. For severely affected patients the only recourse is heart transplantation. However, this is a draconian measure and there are only a limited number of hearts available. Even if a person survives a heart attack, there will often be lasting damage without recovery.

Current research into stem cell biology offers the potential of either replacing damaged heart tissue or perhaps modifying and protecting tissue from ongoing death. In either case there may be some chance of restoring some heart function, or indeed bringing the heart back to its original condition. In late 2006, three teams of researchers discovered cardiovascular stem cells in mouse embryos. These cells were stem cells that had differentiated enough to have cardiovascular character, but could still differentiate further into various types of cardiac tissue. The three teams were based at the Massachusetts General Hospital in Boston, the Mount Sinai School of Medicine in New York, and the Children's Hospital in Boston; they were led by Dr. Kenneth Chien, Dr. Gordon Keller, and Dr. Stuart Orkin, respectively. Continuing research will investigate the presence of these stem cells in human embryonic tissue, and their potential for adult therapeutics. In this case the hope is that endogenous heart progenitor or stem cells may be recruited to repair damaged heart tissue, if more is known of their biology.

Another potential avenue for research is the collection and expansion of myoblasts, or muscle stem cells, from adult skeletal muscle. Scientists are investigating the factors that induce differentiation of adult myoblasts into various muscle tissues. The three types of muscle are skeletal, smooth, and cardiac. If scientists discovered how to guide myoblasts to produce cardiac muscle cells, these new cells could be surgically introduced into hearts of patients who have suffered from heart attacks. The goal would be to establish new heart muscle that had been lost due to the heart attack. However, this avenue of research has met many problems, the most serious of which is that the myoblasts do not survive well after transplantation and are not able to repair or integrate into the damaged tissue. Interestingly, adult mesenchymal cells appear to be able to home into the damaged heart and have clinically relevant effects. In a recent series of papers, patients with heart disease received transplants of mesenchymal cells. In one report there was some indication of recovery, but in two others there were no differences between treated and nontreated patients. The mechanism by which the adult mesenchymal cells induce functional effects remains elusive. However, they do not seem to survive in the heart tissue itself, but rather have an acute anti-inflammatory effect and then die. This anti-inflammatory effect of the mesenchymal cells may also be important for modulating functional recovery in a number of other diseases including stroke and ALS. In April 2007 a group of scientists led by Sir Magdi Yacoub at Imperial College London in the United Kingdom reported their ability to grow a heart valve from stem cells derived from adult bone marrow. While of great interest, it may take several years to determine the clinical implications of this research.

Human embryonic stem cells also hold great hope for being able to make all types of cardiac tissues—namely heart valves, heart muscle, or endothelial cells that line the heart and its vasculature. However, challenges remain including the derivation of populations of heart cell precursors that can engraft and produce functional muscle, and elimination of the potential formation of teratomas within the heart due to a few remaining pluripotent cells developing within the transplant. Much work is currently underway around the world to deal with these issues.

Until recently, while the American Heart Association (AHA) supports scientific research into adult stem cells and guided differentiation of these cells into cardiac cells, it has not supported studies on embryonic and fetal stem cells. However, the advent of human induced pluripotent stem cells may now allow researchers to investigate how heart cells can be produced using AHA funding.

Finally, although repairing the damaged heart is the goal for much stem cell work, there are two other major areas of research. First, the development of human embryonic stem cells into heart tissues may be able to inform us of how the heart arises and thus give insight into the various developmental deficits in heart formation. Second, as human embryonic stem cells can give rise to limitless numbers of beating muscle cells in the dish, these may be used to screen various drugs for side effects. This is important, as one of the major problems with producing new drugs for humans is that they often interfere with heart function. This can now be tested in the dish before moving forward in expensive drug development programs.

**SEE ALSO:** Cells, Adult; Cells, Embryonic; Cells, Fetal; Cells, Human; Cells, Mouse (Embryonic); Children's Hospital Boston; Differentiation, In Vitro and In Vivo; Keller, Gordon; Massachusetts; Massachusetts General Hospital; Mount Sinai School of Medicine; New York; Orkin, Stuart; Tissue Culture; United Kingdom.

**BIBLIOGRAPHY.** American Heart Association, www.americanheart.org (cited January 2008); N. Dib, D. A. Taylor, and E. B. Diethrich, *Stem Cell Therapy and Tissue Engineering for Cardiovascular Repair: From Basic Research to Clinical Applications* (Springer, 2005); M. Yacoub, "Viewpoint: Heart Valve Engineering. Interview by James Butcher," *Circulation* (August 21, 2007).

Claudia Winograd
University of Illinois, Urbana-Champaign

# Heart Attack

**HEART ATTACK, OR** acute myocardial infarction (AMI), is one of the most common medical conditions found in daily practice and is still the major cause of death in most countries. AMI is classified under ischemic heart diseases (IHD), which group also includes conditions such as angina pectoris and heart failure.

The main pathophysiological mechanism involved in IHD is the imbalance between the demand and supply of oxygen to the cardiac tissues. This imbalance generally begins with the atherosclerosis (deposition of lipids on the vascular endothelium) of coronary arteries and later leads to the formation of thrombus inside the coronary vessels (the rupture of the unstable atheretomous plaque, platelet aggregation, activation of the coagulation cascade, and fibrin deposition). Although angina pectoris is usually short lasting and results from temporary disorders of coronary blood circulation, AMI is the result of the thromboembolic obstruction of the coronary vessels when the body's endogenous anticoagulant system is unable to liquidize the formed thrombus.

Because of prolonged hypoxia, the myocardial cells involved undergo necrotic changes, and the area immediately surrounding the necrotic area shows an inflammatory reaction. Later, a scar replaces the area of necrosis.

In the acute period of AMI, the area of necrosis is pale in color, in contrast to the remaining myocardium, and is surrounded by a zone of hyperemia. Early microscopic changes include the formation of coagulative necrosis (cell death) with the loss of nuclei of the myocardiocytes and the infiltration of the neighboring tissue by neutrophils, lymphocytes, and macrophages. In subsequent stages of development, connective tissue can be seen, replacing the zone of necrosis.

## RISK FACTORS AND CLINICAL FEATURES

Risk factors for AMI are the same as those of IHD and include factors such as older age, male sex, smoking, diabetes mellitus, hyperlipidemia (high levels of lipids in blood), and obesity.

AMI may present with a variety of clinical symptoms, and they depend on the localization of the infarct. The typical signs include retrosternal chest pain (pressing or compressing character) radiating to the left or right arm, shoulder, jaw, or back that usually lasts for 20 minutes or more. Dyspnea and palpitations frequently accompany chest pain. Other signs, such as pain in the abdomen, nausea, and vomiting (mimicking heartburn), syncope (temporary loss of consciousness), diaphoresis (excessive sweating), anxiety, and palpitations are not uncommon. Often in hypertensives and people with diabetes mellitus there may be an absence of a very bright clinical picture, and AMI may present with only generalized weakness or mild discomfort in the chest.

## INVESTIGATION AND DIAGNOSIS

Out of the several myocardial markers, troponin 1 and creatine kinase MB fraction are the most specific. The increase in the level of these myocardial markers tells us about the possible injury of cardiomyocytes. Although nonspecific, a common blood count shows an increase in the white blood count, which reaches a peak in the third or fourth day and then stays elevated for about a week. The erythrocyte sedimentation rate is usually elevated for over a week.

An electrocardiogram (ECG) to determine AMI depends on multiple factors, such as the part of the myocardium affected in the process of necrosis, the extent of the myocardial thickness damage, and the stage of AMI. Depending on the thickness of the myocardial damage, AMIs are divided into Q-dependant or total-thickness MI, in which we see a deep Q wave in the ECG, and Q-independent or partial-thickness MI, without the deep Q wave. Other signs seen in the acute period include the well-known ST elevation, negative T wave, and reciprocal changes in opposite leads. The area of the myocardium affected, and hence the affection of the corresponding coronary artery, is evaluated by monitoring typical ECG changes in different ECG leads. Other additional methods of diagnosis often used for diagnosis of AMI are echocardiography of the heart, myocardial perfusion imaging, and coronary angiography.

The World Health Organization diagnostic criteria explain the presence several of the following criteria for the diagnosis of AMI: ischemic type of chest pain lasting more than 20 minutes, rising of the myocardial markers of necrosis, and typical ECG changes.

## TREATMENT OPTIONS

Medical care includes the prescription of antiplatelet drugs (aspirin), thrombolytic therapy (tissue plasminogen activator), beta blockers (metoprolol), anticoagulant medications (heparin), and angiotensin-converting enzyme inhibitors (Captopril).

Two surgical care options for AMI are percutaneous coronary intervention (PCI) and coronary artery bypass grafting—the main surgical choices for AMI. Interestingly, PCI is becoming a major treatment option for early-diagnosed AMI patients because of its high efficacy and success rates, which are equivalent or even higher than traditional thrombolytic therapy. Percutaneous coronary intervention includes the location of the thrombosed coronary artery by an angiogram and its subsequent dilation by balloon angioplasty and intracoronary stenting.

Novel treatment options includes stem cell therapy, in vitro engineered cardiac tissue, which is later implanted in vivo, and polymeric left ventricular restraints for treatment of possible heart failure. These new treatment modalities have emerged as possible alternatives for heart transplantation for the treatment of damaged myocardium and are at different stages of experimentation and clinical trials.

## STEM CELLS AND AMI

The use of endogenous or exogenous progenitor cells in cardiology has been a much-debated issue over the years. Interestingly, in the former half of the last century, the heart was considered a terminally differentiated postmitotic organ, which means that the cardiomyocytes are incapable of further division following injury. With the development of electron microscopy, immunohistochemistry, and other superior methods of investigation, however, this theory was contradicted and a new theory, proving the opposite, was taken into consideration.

With the fast development in the field of stem cell research, the application of stem cell technology in treatment of IHD is gaining major interest. As we know, human stem cells can be broadly classified into embryonic (developing from the embryo) and adult stem cells (present in different adult tissues). Examples of adult stem cells used in cardiology are hemopoietic stem cells and cardiac progenitor cells.

The following classes of stem cell therapies have been discussed through the previous years, and although each class has its own advantages and disadvantages, and some of them are successfully being incorporated into diverse clinical trials showing tremendous promise in future medicine, at present, they are not a part of the standard treatment protocol for AMI patients.

Historically, embryonic stem cells (ESCs) were the first kind of stem cell treatment proposal that included the most primitive kind of human cells derived from the developing blastocysts. Although initial researches showed promise in the use of ESCs for treatment of a variety of medical conditions, still the actual use of ESCs in clinical practice is limited. This is both because of their ability to produce teratomas and malignant carcinomas, their ability to cause tissue rejection and other adverse effects, and the maelstrom of ethical and legal questions.

Mesenchymal stem cells (MSCs), derived from the bone marrow, differentiate into different kinds of tissues including chondrocytes, myocytes, and so on. Their use in AMI is explained by their ability to concentrate into injured tissues and the subsequent differentiation and maturation into cardiomyocytes. Human trials are being conducted with MSCs at different research laboratories, but results are too early to claim its role in cardiac regeneration.

## ADULT BONE MARROW–DERIVED CELLS

Interest in adult bone marrow–derived cells (BMCs) has escalated in recent years because of their properties of neovascularization and angiogenesis, which in turn is an effective way to repair damage tissue by providing necessary nutrients and oxygen supply. Interestingly, the use of autologous BMCs also decreases the chances of tissue rejection and bypasses the ethical and legal questions concerned with the use of ESCs.

The mechanism of action of direct BMC implantation into the injured myocardium has a dual explanation. Some scientists believe that the BMCs never differentiate into cardiomyocytes, but just fuse with the existing heart cells, but others emphasize the possible transdifferentiation of BMCs into cardiomyocytes.

## CARDIAC PROGENITOR CELLS

A more recently described population of cells discovered in rodent and human hearts is the so-called cardiac progenitor cell. In experimental rat models, these cells have been isolated and proven to be multipotent, with the ability to differentiate into endothelial cells, myocardial cells, and smooth muscle cells when injected into an infracted heart.

These resident cells are very specific for the heart, and hence, are a potential replacement for all the above-mentioned stem cell therapies, but their lower numbers in the adult heart poses a limitation to their isolation, culture, and utilization.

**SEE ALSO:** Cells, Adult; Cells, Embryonic; Heart.

**BIBLIOGRAPHY.** Samer Garas and A. Maziar Zafari, "Myocardial Infarction," www.emedicine.com (cited November 2007); Dina Gould Halme and David A. Kessler, "FDA Regulation of Stem-Cell-Based Therapies," *New England Journal of Medicine* (v.355, 2006); José Marín-Gracía and Michael J. Goldenthal, "Applications of Stem Cells in Cardiology: Where We Are and Where We Are Going" *Current Stem Cell Research and Therapy* (v.1, 2006).

Rahul Pandit
St. Petersburg State Medical Academy

# Homologous Recombination

**HOMOLOGOUS RECOMBINATION IS** a process by which exchange of genetic material occurs between two DNA strands, resulting in genetic recombination. This process occurs naturally in organisms and is also used as a powerful tool in genetic engineering. During meiosis in eukaryotes, homologous recombination occurs in chromosomal crossover, resulting in shuffling of genetic material. It also occurs during repair of damaged DNA in organisms by using genetic material from a homologous chromosome.

The nuclei of cells in our body contain chromosomes that carry the genetic material and occur in pairs—one each from the father and one from the mother. Chromosomes in actuality are tightly packed DNA strands. The variations existing in the population are the result of the exchange of DNA sequences between chromosomes producing a variety of combinations. Exchange of genetic material occurs between a pair of identical (homologous) chromosomes, producing recombinant DNA. This process is called homologous recombination. It can also be initiated artificially by the introduction of DNA sequences into the cell. The foreign DNA sequence is similar to the target gene and is flanked by sequences identical to the ones upstream and downstream of the target gene's locus. The cell recognizes these identical sequences as homologues, and exchange can occur between these sequences. The target gene is swapped with the artificial DNA, which is inactive and serves only as a marker. Thus, the function of the gene is eliminated, or "knocked out."

There are vast applications of homologous recombination in mouse genetics. Gene targeting in cells is done by homologous recombination to create recombinant DNA and genetically modified organisms. In mouse genetics, this method is used to target specific alleles in the mouse embryonic stem cells. Artificial genetic material similar to the target gene is introduced into the nucleus of the embryonic stem cell, which represses the target gene by the process of homologous recombination. Thus, the functions of individual genes can be studied. More than 10,000 mouse genes have been knocked out (inactivated) with the help of gene targeting, which has produced more than 500 different mouse models of human disorders, including cancer, diabetes, cardiovascular diseases, and neurological disorders. Groundbreaking work was done on homologous recombination in mouse stem cells by Mario Capecchi, Martin Evans, and Oliver Smithies, for which they were awarded the Nobel Prize in 2007.

## KNOCKOUT MICE

Homologous recombination is one of the most important technologies used in mouse genetics. It can be used to specifically modify any gene in mammalian cells. These modifications or mutations can be activated at any point, at any time, in any specific cell or organ in an adult, or even developing, animal. For these modifications to be inherited embryonic stem cells are required, which are pluripotent cells. These cells are extracted from early mouse embryos and are cultured easily in artificial conditions. Embryonic stem cells can be modified genetically by the help of homologous recombination. Artificial DNA sequences can be introduced into stem cells by retroviruses or any other vector.

This genetic material is then incorporated into the chromosomes by the process of homologous recombination. These mutant cells are then injected into mouse embryos and implanted in surrogate mothers. Mice produced from these embryos are known as *knockout mice*. These mice are genetically modified and thus may exhibit phenotypical modifications, which provide important clues to the function of specific genes. In this manner, a *knock in mouse* can also be produced by homologous recombination. Knock in mice are produced when an artificial gene is integrated into a locus on a chromosome by homologous recombination. When a human gene is introduced into a cell, this produces a humanized mouse.

Homologous recombination is the method of choice when it is required that a specific allele be replaced by an engineered DNA sequence without affecting any other locus in the genome. To do this, one must know the DNA sequence to be targeted and also the DNA sequences upstream and downstream from the locus. The next step is to design and produce a DNA construct that would replace the target gene. This engineered construct can be either functional (different alleles) or nonfunctional (genetic markers). The artificial DNA contains flanking sequences, in addition to the target locus, that are identical to those upstream and downstream from the target locus. Negative selection markers may also be added to the vector (flanking sequences), whereas positive selection markers are only added at the targeted locus.

The DNA construct is introduced into the cells that contain target gene of interest. The engineered construct aligns with the target locus, and recombination takes place between the homologous (identical) sequences. This results in the incorporation of an artificial DNA sequence into the chromosomes, and the gene of interest is relocated into the original DNA construct. The foreign DNA cannot replicate and is eventually lost from the cell, but the modified chromosome replicates as usual with its new addition. Antibiotics are added to the growth medium to allow positive selection of cells that have successfully undergone recombination. The positive section marker (antibiotic-resistance allele) is incorporated into the genome of cells undergoing homologous recombination. In case there is recombination of sequences other than the desired ones, the negative marker is also taken up, thus ensuring the death of those cells.

Cells having recombinant chromosomes are injected into blastocysts, which are implanted into mice and carried to term. The mouse pups born in this manner contain both modified and nonmodified tissue and thus are not complete knockout mice. Breeding of these mice is done over several generations until a pair of true knockout mice (homologous knockouts) is isolated. Knockout mice allow researchers to establish the role of a gene by observing an individual lacking that gene completely.

## APPLICATIONS

Homologous recombination and gene targeting are one of the most important tools available to geneticists. The physiology of mammals can be studied in great depth and at a much broader aspect through the use of these methods. Knockout mice can provide information about a vast array of human genes because humans and mice share many similar genes. These mouse models give a better understanding of what is the role of similar genes in human disorders. More than 10,000 genes (almost half the whole mammalian genome) have been studied with the help of this technology.

Gene targeting has shed light on the role of many genes in fetal development and also helped in understanding the causes of several human congenital disorders. The involvement of genes in mammalian organ development and establishment of body plan has been studied thoroughly. Knockout mice have helped in studying and modeling different human diseases. Mouse models have been developed for several different human disorders such as cystic fibrosis, thalassemia, hypertension, diabetes, arthritis, atherosclerosis, cancer, Parkinson's disease, and many more. They also provide a platform on which drug therapies can be developed and tested.

There are limitations to homologous recombination and gene targeting. About 15 percent of the knockouts prevent the development of altered embryos into adult mice. Thus, the functions of those genes cannot be studied to the full extent, and their roles in human health cannot be established. In some cases, the genes play different roles in embryological stages and adulthood. Furthermore, knocking out a gene may not produce any phenotypical change, and the changes observed in mouse models may be quite different from those observed in humans when the same gene is inactivated in both. Despite the drawbacks, homologous recombination has proved to be one of the most effective means for studying gene function in living animals and has been dispersed to all fields of health sciences. It is developing into a vast pool of knowledge that will help in treatment and prevention of human diseases.

**SEE ALSO:** Cells, Mouse (Embryonic); Mouse ES Cell Isolation; Nuclear Reprogramming.

**BIBLIOGRAPHY.** Hemin R. Chin and Steven O. Moldin, *Methods in Genomic Neuroscience* (CRC Press, 2001); National Human Genome Research Institute, "Knockout Mice," www.genome.gov/12514551; Lee M. Silver, *Mouse Genetics: Concepts and Applications* (Oxford University Press, 1995).

Aun Raza
National University of Science and Technology

## Human Embryonic Stem Cells

**EMBRYONIC STEM CELLS** derived from preimplantation embryos are undifferentiated cells capable of differentiation into derivatives of all three embryonic germ layers. These cells are also capable of self-renewal and have an almost unlimited developmental potential.

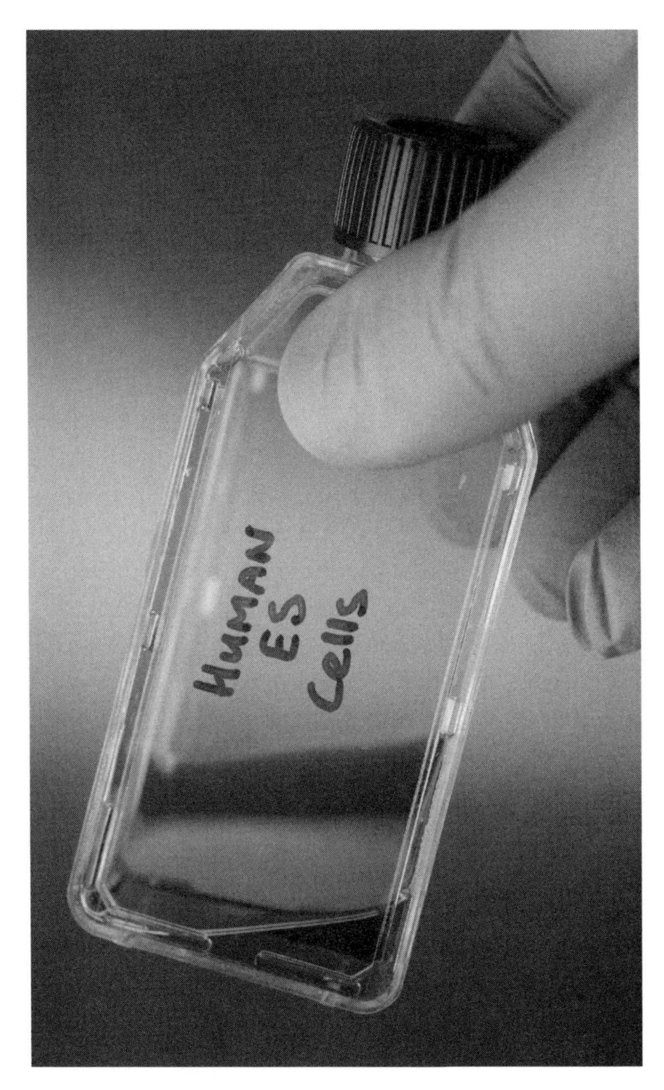


*Embryonic stem cells are derived from the inner cell mass of a preimplantation blastocyst about five days postfertilization.*

During the last decade, there has been ongoing research into the isolation of inner cell mass (ICM), as it is useful in establishing embryonic stem cell lines, which in turn have the ability to develop into most of the specialized cells in the human body, including blood, skin, muscle, and nerve cells. They also have the capacity to divide and proliferate almost indefinitely in culture.

The method for establishing a human embryonic stem cell line comprises the following steps:

isolate cells of an ICM from an isolated blastocyst stage embryo by creating an aperture in the blastocyst stage embryo by laser ablation, and remove cells of the ICM from the blastocyst stage embryo through the aperture; culture the cells of the ICM in the presence of an embryonic stem cell medium and an inactivated feeder layer to produce ICM-derived masses; and culture the ICM-derived masses to produce an isolated human embryonic stem cell line.

Human ES cell lines are derived from the embryos produced by in vitro fertilization, a process in which oocytes and sperm are placed together to allow fertilization to take place in a culture dish. ES cells are derived from the ICM of the preimplantation blastocyst approximately five days postfertilization. After a human oocyte is fertilized in vitro by a sperm, it forms a zygote. The zygote undergoes a series of cleavage, and by day five the cavity of the blastocyst is completed. The ICM begins to separate from the outer cells, which become the trophectoderm that surrounds the blastocyst. This represents the first observable sign of differentiation in the embryo.

The ICMs have the potential to generate any cell type of the body, but only before implantation. If the ICM is removed from its normal embryonic environment and cultured under appropriate conditions, the ICM-derived cells can continue to proliferate and replicate themselves indefinitely and still maintain the developmental potential to form any cell type of the body. Day five blastocysts are, therefore, used to derive ES cell cultures. They consist of 200–250 cells, and the trophectoderm must be removed from these cells to derive ES cell cultures. This is done either by microsurgery or immunosurgery. Immunosurgery is a process in which antibodies attacking the trophectoderm help break it down, thus freeing the ICM. These pluripotent ICM-derived cells are ES cells.

The ability to isolate ES cells from blastocysts and grow them in culture seems to depend in large part on the integrity and condition of the blastocyst from which the cells are derived. In short, the blastocyst that is large and has distinct ICMs tends to yield ES cells most efficiently. Several methods have been used for isolation of ICM for the establishment of embryonic stem cell lines.

## NATURAL HATCHING OF THE BLASTOCYST

The natural hatching of the blastocyst is a procedure in which a blastocyst is allowed to hatch naturally after being planted on the feeder layer. Hatching takes place on day six. The ICM develops an outgrowth, which is removed mechanically and then grown for establishing ES cell lines.

This process also presents some disadvantages. These are that in given culture conditions, trophectoderm cells proliferate very fast, which suppresses the outgrowth of ICM; removing the outgrowth of the ICM mechanically may lead to a chance of isolating trophectoderm cells; and in humans, the percentage of the blastocysts hatching spontaneously is very low.

## MICROSURGERY AND IMMUNOSURGERY

In microsurgery, the ICM is isolated by mechanical aspiration. The blastocyst is held by the holding pipette, using a micromanipulator system, and is positioned in such a way that the ICM is at the nine o'clock position. The ICM is aspirated using a beveled shape biopsy needle and is inserted into the blastocoel cavity.

This procedure also presents some disadvantages. First, the possibility of isolating the complete ICM is low, and many times, cells are disintegrated. Second, it is a very tedious procedure and may cause severe damage to the embryo.

Immunosurgery is a commonly used procedure to isolate ICM. In this procedure, the zona pellucida of the blastocyst is removed by exposing the blastocyst either to acid tyrode solution or pronase enzyme solution. This then is exposed to human surface antibody for about 30 minutes to one hour. This is followed by exposure of the embryos to guinea pig complement to lyse the trophectoderm. The complement-mediated lysed trophectoderm cells are then removed from ICM by repeated mechanical pipetting with a finely drawn Pasteur pipette.

This method has the following disadvantages. First, the embryo is exposed for a long time to acid tyrode or pronase, causing deleterious effects on the embryo and thereby reducing the viability of embryos proper. Second, it is a time-consuming procedure, taking about 1.5 to 2.0 hours. Third, the yield of ICM per blastocyst is low. Fourth, critical storage conditions are required for antibody and complement used in the process. Finally, it involves the risk of transmission of viruses and bacteria of animal origin to humans, as animal-derived antibodies and complement are used in the process. In this process, two animal sera are used. One is rabbit antihuman antiserum, and the other is guinea pig complement sera.

To simplify the procedure of ICM isolation and make it safe, scientists have invented a novel method of isolation of the ICM, using a noncontact laser, wherein the use of animal-based antisera and complements have been eliminated. At present, lasers are being investigated as tools to aid fertilization and in assisted hatching. Recently, an infrared 1.48-µm diode laser beam focused through a microscope objective was shown to allow rapid, easy, and nontouch microdrilling of mouse and human zona pellucida, and a high degree of accuracy was maintained under conventional culture conditions.

This invention involves the isolation of ICM, using a laser ablation technique, without undergoing the cumbersome procedure of immunosurgery. Hence, using this invention, animal-derived antibodies or sera are eliminated and the procedure is made safe, simple, rapid, and commercially viable. This invention obviates the shortcomings associated with the conventional methods of isolation of ICM, and the ICM isolated by this invention is found to be intact, with no destruction or damage to the cells. The invention thus provides a quick, reliable, and noninvasive method for isolation of ICM. It also completely ruptures the trophectoderm, thereby minimizing the contamination of ICM and thus ensuring the purity of ICM.

ICM cells, once derived, are grown in culture. Human ES cells are grown on a feeder layer of mouse embryonic fibroblasts and require the presence of basic fibroblast growth factor (bFGF or FGF-2). In these conditions, human ES cells show remarkable proliferative capacity and stability in long-term culture and have the capacity to differentiate into cell types from all three germ layers. A feeder-free human ES cell culture system has been developed in which human ES cells are grown on a protein matrix (mouse matrigel or laminin) in a bFGF-containing medium that has been previously conditioned by coculture with fibroblasts. Without optimal culture conditions or genetic manipulation, embryonic stem cells rapidly differentiate.

Human ES cells may offer exciting new possibilities for transplantation medicine: Because ES cells have the developmental potential to give rise to all adult cell types, any disease resulting from the failure of specific cell types would be potentially treatable through the transplantation of differentiated cells derived from ES cells. Human ES cells also can be used to study early events in human development. In addition, such cells could be used to explore the effects of chromosomal abnormalities in early development. Human ES cells could also be used to test candidate therapeutic drugs and to screen potential toxins, as well as to develop new methods for genetic engineering. Because ES cells are immortal cell lines, they could be genetically manipulated before differentiation either to reduce immunogenicity or to give them new properties to combat specific diseases. Because of the range of diseases potentially treatable by this approach, elucidating the basic mechanisms controlling the differentiation of human ES cells has dramatic clinical significance.

**SEE ALSO:** Cells, Embryonic; Cells, Human; Mouse ES Cell Isolation.

**BIBLIOGRAPHY.** "Explore Stem Cells," www.explorestemcells.co.uk (cited November 2007); National Institutes of Health, "Stem Cell Information," stemcells.nih.gov (cited November 2007).

Sana Fatima Asad
National University of Science and Technology

# Huntington's Disease

**HUNTINGTON'S DISEASE IS** a hereditary type of chorea, which is a neurological condition that is associated with involuntary and irregular movements caused by movements of various muscle groups. It is a fatal disease and had no known cure before the development of certain stem cell treatments. The disease is named after the American doctor George Huntington, who first described the condition in detail in 1872. In fact, most variables of the disease—type and severity of symptoms, age at which onset occurs, effect on lifestyle—can vary considerably. However, it is most commonly observed as becoming manifest in patients between the ages of 30 and 50 years.

It was discovered in 1993 that Huntington's disease is caused by a single gene. A person with one parent who has the gene has a 50 percent chance of inheriting the faulty gene, and if that happens, it is certain that the disease will manifest itself during the lifetime of the patient, except in the case of an early death. Early possible symptoms include short-term memory lapse, behavior change, uncontrolled movement (mild), and clumsiness. As the disease develops, more severe involuntary movement takes place, as well as the loss of communication skills and other effects caused by these symptoms.

These symptoms, especially as they become more severe, can be very distressing, both for the patient and for carers and loved ones. The patient is likely to suffer additional psychological issues including depression and mood swings, which make care provision more trying. A range of medical assistance is likely to be required to deal with the secondary effects of the disease (e.g., psychological counselors, nutritionists, and occupational therapists) in addition to dealing with the root cause. In cases in which the presence of the gene in a family is not known, then it can take some time before the reason for the symptoms becomes clear. Where the presence of the gene is known in the family, then there is an effective test to determine whether it is present in an individual. Embryos are tested for the presence of the gene in some countries before use in in vitro fertilization treatments.

## STEM CELL TECHNOLOGIES

Scientists in the United States, United Kingdom, and South Korea, among other countries, are actively involved in using stem cell technologies to try to develop an effective treatment for Huntington's disease. In the United States, for example, the private company StemCells Inc. has entered into a joint venture with the High Q Foundation with a view to developing more accurate models of the disease and, hence, develop a means of combating it. In the United Kingdom, ReNeuron Group PLC signed a similar agreement with Angel Biotechnology Holdings PLC to produce a master cell bank that can then be used to tackle the disease.

The high level of technical skills required in this industry, together with the need for highly equipped laboratories and specialized equipment, means that individual companies or university departments are highly unlikely to be able to deploy all the needed resources individually. As a consequence, joint ventures and contract agreements are required to enable organizations to bring together the necessary combination of resources required to approach particular projects. It also, of course, helps to explain the high cost of potential treatments because commercial companies need to recover the expenses they incur in mobilizing all of those resources, and inevitably, all organizations have a need to show a profit for their work. Given how many research projects fail to produce viable, marketable treatments of one sort or another, this means that the ones that do need to show a profit also need to cover the costs of failed projects. This has the unfortunate effect of making treatments effectively beyond the reach of all but the richest societies.

However, early results from a number of rodent experiments suggest that the use of stem cells might be effective in reversing the effects of damage to brain cells. Work at Seoul National University, for example, suggests that injected human neural stem cells can migrate into a striatal lesion and result in long-term return of functionality in atrophied cells. Transplants of fetal striatal tissue have been performed in a number of human patients in the United States. Although these cells have not shown outright adverse effects, positive results have been mixed. Therefore, development of effective human testing will require more time.

It may take more than a decade before a possible treatment becomes available on a market basis. The length of time involved and the effect that such a wait might have on patients convinces many people that they should try to become involved in clinical trials of new treatments. There may be practical difficulties with organizing the attendance of such a trial, and there is no guarantee that the treatment will lead to an improvement. Indeed, there may be negative consequences and adverse effects, with the psychological effects possibly being the worst of all to handle. Even so, becoming part of a clinical trial probably represents the best chance for a patient to obtain a possible effective treatment at an early date.

**SEE ALSO:** Cells, Human; StemCells, Inc.

**BIBLIOGRAPHY.** Huntington Project, www.huntingtonproject.org (cited November 2007); Huntington's Disease Clinical Research at University College London, hdresearch.ucl.ac.uk (cited November 2007); "ReNeuron: Stem Cell Company Signs Manufacturing Contract for Huntington Disease Line," *Mental Health Business Week* (March 11, 2006); "Seoul National University Hospital; Intravenous Neural Stem Cells Induce Functional Recovery in Huntington Disease," *Mental Health Business Week* (September 3, 2005); "Stem Cell Innovations and High Q Foundation Collaborate to Develop Novel Models of Huntington's Disease," *Business Wire* (June 25, 2007).

John Walsh
Shinawatra University

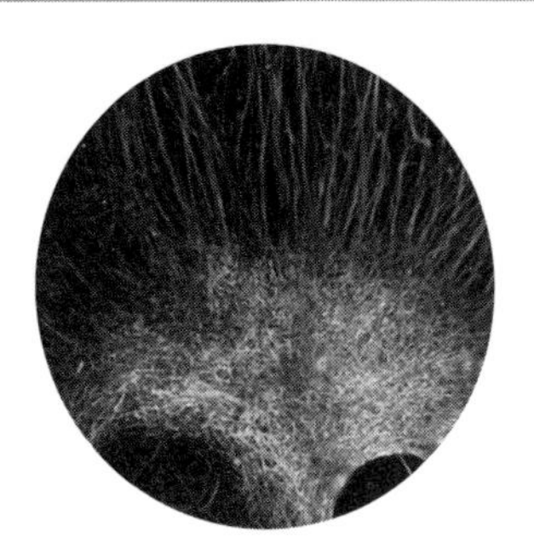

# I

## Idaho

**IDAHO HAS A** strong academic foundation for biomedical research and works in collaboration with regional and national organizations to perform basic research and clinical trials using adult stem cells for cancer treatment.

As no federal legislation in the United States regulates stem cell research (except by an executive order to not allow federal funding to be used for embryonic stem cell research except on human embryonic stem cell lines created before August 9, 2001), each state is responsible for determining policy and funding for stem cell research. Idaho has no clear position on stem cell research, making it an allowable and unregulated activity. Public and private funding is available through competitive grant funding, but no money is dedicated by the state for stem cell research.

Mountain States Tumor Institute at St. Luke's in Boise has been treating cancer for over 50 years. The institute provides treatment at 12 locations in Idaho and Oregon. In addition to treatment and prevention activities, the institute participates in national clinical trials. Current research participation through the National Cancer Institute to collect data includes using stem cell transplants to allow high-dose chemotherapy to be used for increased efficacy in killing cancer cells in multiple myeloma or primary systemic amyloidosis and in patients with progressive or recurrent Hodgkin's lymphoma.

The University of Idaho in Moscow is a four-year public university conferring bachelor's, master's, doctoral, and professional degrees in a variety of disciplines including medicine, biology, engineering, math, and physical sciences. A researcher in the Department of Microbiology, Molecular Biology, and Biochemistry is collaborating with the National Human Neural Stem Cell Resource to research the interaction of human cytomegalovirus with cells in the developing fetal brain. The National Human Neural Stem Cell Resource has a mission to expand research on neural stem cells nationally. The Molecular Biology Core Facility at the University of Idaho was established in 1995 with funding from the National Institutes of Health for teaching, consulting, and research collaboration. Services are available to researchers throughout the university system in Idaho and within the region.

The Center for Reproductive Biology is located at the University of Washington and was established in 1999. The center is a collaborative effort with the University of Idaho that began in 1989 with discussion on collaborative research projects. The center's mission is to improve the possibility of grant funding, improve research collaboration, and combine education and research opportunities for students.

To meet its goals, the center has developed core laboratories for the centralization of cross-discipline research with researchers at both Washington State University and the University of Idaho. This is an organized research unit that integrates the investigators throughout the universities. The molecular cytogenetics core provides karyotyping on established human cell line and human clinical samples, stores established cell lines, and provides growing cultures or fixed cell pellets to researchers. The histology core provides tissue preparation, immunohistochemistry, and in situ hybridization to researchers. The assay core analyzes hormone (i.e., steroids and gonadotropin) levels in the animals exposed to endocrine disruptors. The toxicology core studies toxins and metabolites in tissue and biological fluids. The transgenic core procures cost-effective transgenic and knockout mice for researchers. The molecular biology core performs DNA and protein sequencing and oligonucleotide and peptide synthesis. The genomics core provides bioinformatics support. Finally, the proteomics core separates proteins from cell mixtures and identifies proteins found to be up- or down-regulated in response to particular stimulus, disease, or treatment of interest to determine the fundamental biological processes and function.

University of Idaho Research Park, located in Post Falls, is focused on bringing together academia, researchers, and the technology industry to enhance the economy through collaboration. The participants network to promote the region for business development. The 125-acre research park is within 20 miles of Spokane, Washington, and is 10 miles from the University of Idaho in Coeur d'Alene.

**SEE ALSO:** Cells, Embryonic; University of Washington/Hutchinson Cancer Center.

**BIBLIOGRAPHY.** Center for Reproductive Biology, "About Us," www.crb.wsu.edu (cited November 2007); Mountain States Cancer Center, "About Us," www.stlukesonline.org (cited November 2007); National Human Neural Stem Cell Resource, "Collaborators," www.nhnscr.org (cited November 2007); National Institutes of Health, "Clinical Trials," www.clinicaltrials.gov (cited November 2007); University of Idaho Research Park, www.uirp.com (cited November 2007).

Lyn Michaud
Independent Scholar

# Illinois

**THE SEEDS OF** public funding for stem cell research in Illinois were planted in the early to mid-2000s. However, attempts in Illinois in 2004 to pass legislation publicly funding stem cell research were unsuccessful, and the measure died in the Illinois Senate. In 2005 Illinois's next attempt at funding stem cell research did not even get called to a vote. In fact, Illinois's first successful policy to support stem cell research did not come from the state legislature at all.

In July 2005 the Illinois Regenerative Medicine Institute (IRMI) was founded by an executive order from Governor Rod Blagojevich. His order set up the IRMI as a program under the Illinois Department of Public Health (IDPH). This made Illinois the first state in the Midwest and the fourth in the country to allocate public funds to stem cell research; New Jersey, California, and Connecticut were the three states that preceded Illinois in this commitment. These four states were quickly joined by several others, adding to the national support for publicly funded stem cell research. It was specified in Governor Blagojevich's executive order that the newly established IRMI would give no money to any research involving human cloning. The sale and purchase of embryonic tissue for research was also prohibited under this order, and parameters were set regarding the latest time period that blastocyst cells could be harvested.

In 2006 IRMI handed out its first set of grants, distributing 10 awards that totaled $10 million for research projects working with adult, cord blood, and embryonic stem cells. Grants were reviewed by the panel established by the IDPH, consisting of two bioethicists and six medical personnel from around the world. Grants were awarded for projects such as research to develop replacement blood vessels, eliminating the need for graft harvesting. Other awards were given to research developing treatments for ischemic stroke, muscular dystrophy, and neurodegenerative diseases.

Later in the year, Governor Blagojevich distributed another $5 million, in seven separate grants, to public universities in Illinois to further the cause of stem cell research. It had been proposed that the 2007 budget include more money for research, which would be total $100 million over five years. However, the legislative bodies had not yet acted on this proposal; therefore, the governor responded by distributing the extra $5 million in 2006.

Although Illinois only recently started providing public funding for stem cell–related projects, private institutions have been supporting such research in Illinois since the early 1990s. For example, Children's Memorial Hospital in Chicago started a program in 1992 that concentrates on pediatric stem cell transplantation. Since its inception, the program has performed over 700 transplants to treat cancers, blood disorders, immune deficiencies, and metabolic disorders. Dr. Morris Kletzel is the director of this program. A similar program at the University of Illinois in Chicago has performed 50 transplants per year since 1997. These treatments, here referred to as stem cell transplants, are also commonly known as bone marrow transplants, in which autologous stem cells are harvested directly from bone marrow.

Illinois's most recent legislation was signed into effect in August 2007. Senate Bill 4 was sponsored by State Senator Jeffrey M. Schoenberg and State Representative Tom Cross and was signed into effect by Governor Rod Blagojevich; it took effect on January 1, 2008. The bill permits researchers to receive state funds for embryonic stem cell research. As with the grants distributed in 2006, Senate Bill 4 prohibits money from being used in research related to human cloning. Again, the IDPH will use the IRMI to distribute research funding.

**SEE ALSO:** *Individual U.S. State Articles*; Biotechnology, History of; Clinical Trials Within U.S.: Batten Disease; Clinical Trials Within U.S.: Blind Process; Clinical Trials Within U.S.: Cancer; Clinical Trials Within U.S.: Heart Disease; Clinical Trials Within U.S.: Peripheral Vascular Disease; Clinical Trials Within U.S.: Skin Transplants (Burns); Clinical Trials Within U.S.: Spinal Cord Injury; Clinical Trials Within U.S.: Traumatic Brain Injury; Ethics; Federal Government Policies; Moral Status of Embryo; Special Interest/Lobby Groups; United States.

**BIBLIOGRAPHY.** Children's Memorial Hospital Stem Cell Transplant Program, www.childrensmemorial.org/depts/stemcell (cited January 2008); Illinois Regenerative Medicine Institute, www.idph.state.il.us/irmi (cited January 2008).

John S. Kuo
University of Wisconsin

# India

**IN SEPTEMBER 2006** India's first stem cell transplant center was opened in Chennai, Tamil Nadu, by a private company called LifeCell, in collaboration with United States–based Cryo-Cell Inc. This center marks another milestone in Indian efforts to stay on top of this burgeoning medical trend without getting entangled in ethical controversies.

The medical and economic potential of stem cell research has long been recognized, and measures are slowly being put in place to establish India as a reliable supplier of stem cell–related resources. Guidelines regulating stem cell therapy and research have been set in place, and efforts have begun toward establishing a national network of stem cell researchers and research centers.

Indian research in stem cells includes work in both embryonic and adult stem cells and basic science, as well as clinical research. This differs from policies in some other countries that permit the use of only adult stem cells. In addition, it is legal for human stem cells to be obtained from aborted fetuses and in vitro fertilization clinics, as well as from adult tissues, after obtaining informed consent and institutional review board approval. However, the creation of embryos for the sole purpose of harvesting stem cells is forbidden.

Work with stem cells has been continuing for over 20 years in certain medical centers in the country, including cord blood and bone marrow–derived hematopoietic stem cells in hospitals in New Delhi, Mumbai, and Vellore. Worldwide, old techniques have been refined and new ones developed, and new uses have been discovered for these cells. This advent of new technology and ideas has had an effect on Indian stem cell research as well. Projects involving the use of limbal, hematopoietic, embryonic, neural, islet, liver, and bone marrow–derived stem cells and involving preservative agents for stem cells have been awarded grants by various government agencies over the past few years.

The principal funding agencies have been the Indian Council of Medical Research and the Department of Biotechnology of India's Ministry of Science and Technology. These agencies have also been instrumental in the establishment of guidelines and regulations for the use of stem cells in practice and research and in charting the course of future stem cell research in the country.

## NATIONAL INITIATIVE

One of the main difficulties faced by stem cell researchers in India has been the lack of resources for large-scale studies, as most research groups were fragmented. Plans for a nationwide stem cell research initiative were put forward in 2005 by the Department of Biotechnology. One of the initiative's primary aims is to bring together privately and publicly funded stem cell research groups in and around a city to form stem cell city clusters. These clusters were envisioned with the expectation that they would permit a pooling of resources from both privately and publicly funded stem cell research institutes, as well as encourage interactions between basic science researchers and clinicians.

Another effort toward promoting stem cell research in India involves the establishment of specialized centers for research and therapy using stem cells. The chief objective of these centers is to promote multidisciplinary research to address clinical issues. In 2005 the Department of Biotechnology announced that it would support medical schools or institutions interested in establishing specialized centers for cell-based therapy. These centers will be provided a grant for a maximum of 10 years—an initial period of five years that can later be renewed for a further five.

During the first two years, the centers are expected to concentrate on preclinical research such as standardization of laboratory methods, the formulation of standard operating procedures, safety monitoring, data monitoring, and so on. They are also expected to conduct preclinical studies to help obtain clearance from the Drug Controller General of India (DCGI; the body that regulates the testing and marketing of new drugs or procedures in India) for future clinical trials. By the third year, all preclinical studies should be completed and clinical studies started.

The formulation of standard operating procedures, evaluation of study proposals for research projects, and evaluation of data are to be carried out by a Task Force for Stem Cell Research and the subcommittees constituted by it. Because the driving force of this program is benefit to the patient, all applicants for the grant are required to conduct research that can provide a translation of basic science research to clinically applicable studies. They must provide detailed descriptions of safety monitoring and data monitoring programs along with their research proposals. These centers are also required to organize annual meetings between the investigators involved to facilitate a regular exchange of information.

## ETHICAL CONTROVERSIES

Certain controversies in the past raised the issue of a lack of ethical oversight. In one instance, Indian researchers in the Institute of Immunohematology, a center of the Indian Council of Medical Research (ICMR), were accused by other researchers in the country of violating India's policy of rejecting the conduct of clinical trials of unproven procedures or treatments developed outside India when they are conducted exclusively on Indian patients.

In another instance, a Delhi-based fertility specialist created a furor when she claimed to have used embryonic stem cells for the treatment of different diseases and injuries in around 100 patients. Although several of her patients claimed that her therapy had caused dramatic improvements, the lack of any preliminary studies (to determine possible adverse effects or to prove efficacy) and of a standard operating procedure ignited several protests against what was viewed as indiscriminate use of an as yet inadequately researched technique. Other researchers feared that the legislatorial backlash would be so severe as to cripple stem cell research in the country.

Unlike in the United States, embryonic stem cell research is legal in India. There are no or few public debates about abortion, which is also legal across the country, raising the issue of India being a source of stem cells. In an effort to avoid exploitation and unethical behavior, the country is tightening regulations on embryonic stem cell research. Until the advent of these enforceable rules (based on the Indian Council of Medical Research's guidelines), stem cell research in India was a rapidly burgeoning but uncontrollable trend. With these rules, it is envisaged that research may be more effectively regulated.

## GUIDELINES

The ICMR published, in 2006, the National Guidelines for Stem Cell Research and Therapy. These guidelines deal with the following topics: the mechanisms for review and monitoring; classifications and definitions of stem cell lines; classification of areas of stem cell research into permissible, restricted, and prohibited; clinical uses of umbilical cord blood and research using fetal cells or placenta; derivation of human embryonic stem cell lines, the procurement of materials for their generation, and their banking and distribution; the responsibility and accountability of the researcher; the use of stem cells for therapeutic purposes; rules governing international collaboration; and the commercialization of stem cell research and patent issues arising from it.

These guidelines also express the need for two regulatory committees for stem cell research: a National Apex Committee for Stem Cell Research and Therapy (NAC-SCRT) and an Institution Committee for Stem Cell Research and Therapy (IC-SCRT). These committees require that the autonomy of donors of material for research purposes be preserved by such methods as a prohibition of financial or other enticements for the donation of human oocytes, sperm or embryos, or human somatic cells.

In the case of women seeking infertility treatment, the attending physician and the investigator intending to use the human embryonic stem cells should not be the same person, to avoid coercion; the consent of donors of supernumerary embryos should be procured at least 24 hours in advance and not at the time of donation; and the donors should be informed of their right to withdraw consent up until the time the blastocyst is actually used in the derivation of cell lines. The guidelines also stipulate that any profit made from the commercialization of intellectual property rights be shared with the community that contributed, directly or indirectly, to it.

## RESTRICTIONS

ICMR's National Guidelines for Stem Cell Research and Therapy categorize stem cell research and therapeutic procedures into three categories: permissible, restricted, and prohibited. The permissible areas of research and therapy, all carried out with the prior approval of the IC-SCRT or the DCGI, include

> in-vitro and in-vivo studies on established cell lines from any type of stem cell; in-vivo studies on any non-primate experimental animals using fetal/adult somatic stem cells from any organ provided appropriate consent is obtained from the donor; establishment of new human embry-

onic stem cell lines from spare embryos after obtaining prior donor consent; establishment of umbilical cord stem cell banks; processing of cells for clinical trials.

The restricted areas of research include

creation of a human zygote with the specific aim of deriving a human embryonic stem cell line for any purpose; clinical trials sponsored by multinationals involving stem cell products imported from abroad (they will require prior approval of the NAC-SCRT); research involving the introduction of human embryonic stem cells, human embryonic germ cells or human somatic cells into animals at an embryonic or fetal stage of development; studies on chimeras; research in which the identity of the donors of the cells from which the human embryonic stem cells were derived may become known to the investigator.

The prohibited areas of research include

any research related to human germ line genetic engineering or reproductive cloning; any in-vitro culture of an intact human embryo beyond fourteen days; transfer of human blastocysts generated in the laboratory into a human or non-human uterus; any research involving implantation in-utero of a human embryo after in-vitro manipulation.

The guidelines also prohibit breeding of animals into which human stem cells have been introduced and the nonautologous donation of stem cells.

**SEE ALSO:** Cells, Embryonic; Human Embryonic Stem Cells; Lineages; United States.

**BIBLIOGRAPHY.** D. Balasubramanian, "Stem Cell Research and Applications in India—The Current Scene and a Roadmap for the Future," *Stem Cell Research, From Bench to Bedside. Proceedings of the Eleventh Annual Symposium* (Ranbaxy Science Foundation, 2007); Department of Biotechnology, Ministry of Science and Technology, "Support for Establishment of Specialised Centres for Cell-Based Therapy," *Current Science* (v.89.1, 2005); Ganapati Mudur, "Indian Researchers Accused of Violating Ethical Guidelines," *British Medical Journal* (v.330, 2005); G. S. Mudur, "Stem Cell March, Minus Checks—Lack of Research Rules Allows Doctors to Do as They Like," *The Telegraph, Calcutta* (November 17, 2005); T. V. Padma, "India Plans National Stem Cell Initiative," www.scidev.net (cited January 2005).

Azara Singh
Christian Medical College

# Indiana

**INDIANA IS WORKING** to establish itself as a leader in nonembryonic stem cell research to avoid the conflicts associated with embryonic stem cell research. Thus, researchers have supportive legislation and funding, as well as public support, with a goal of improving the economy in the biotechnology sector.

As no federal legislation in the United States regulates stem cell research (except by an executive order to not allow federal funding to be used for embryonic stem cell research except on human embryonic stem cell lines created before August 9, 2001), each state is responsible for determining policy and funding for stem cell research. In Indiana, stem cell research is permitted on adult stem cells and fetal stem cells if consent is received from the biological parent. Indiana prohibits research on human embryonic stem cells in accordance with Indiana code 31-20-2, regarding embryos from assisted reproduction. The law also prohibits the sale of oocytes, zygotes, embryos, and fetuses.

In 2007 the Indiana legislature also approved the establishment of an Adult Stem Cell Research Center at Indiana University and gave the Indiana University School of Medicine approval to administer the center, including appointing a director and accepting income from donations, gifts, and so on, to be used to support the center's activities.

BioCrossroads is a development organization to enhance economic growth in the life sciences. The organization provides money and support to business start-ups and established businesses in biotechnology by providing networking and collaboration opportunities among Indiana's various academic, clinical, and industry institutions. Money is available through the Indiana Future Fund and the Indiana Seed Fund

Other services provided by BioCrossroads include the Indiana Health Information Exchange, which facilitates the sharing of clinical information among healthcare providers and other healthcare entities, and the Translational Research Initiative partnership with Indiana University, which leverages resources in promoting life science research to gain national and private grant funding.

### RESEARCH ACTIVITIES

Indiana University–Purdue University in Indianapolis was founded in 1969. The university offers bachelor's, master's, doctoral, and professional degrees in a variety of disciplines including medicine, biology, engineering, math, and physical sciences. The university is home to the Indiana University School of Medicine.

The Adult Stem Cell Research Center to be established at Indiana University will fall under the purview of the School of Medicine to encourage collaboration among all of Indiana's stem cell researchers. Research being done or completed by the university includes the discovery of cells that control the creation of endothelial cells and investigating the possibility of using these cells for medical treatment for circulation problems in the extremities, for heart disease, and for repair of blood vessels, and to use adult stem cells to alleviate diseases secondary to increasing age,

The Emerging Technology Center in Indianapolis allows the university to assist business startups using discoveries made by researchers at the university. EndGenitor Technologies Inc. is one such firm and has capitalized on the research performed by university professors. The start-up company intends to develop and market test kits for researchers to test samples for endothelial stem and progenitor cells.

The Indiana Cord Blood Bank collects, preserves, and stores cord blood as a source of adult stem cells for use in blood transplants for treating blood diseases and cancers, anemia, inherited metabolic disorders, and immune system deficiencies.

The Bindley Bioscience Center opened in 2005 through funding provided by a Purdue alumnus to integrate the life sciences and engineering departments for cross-discipline research at the university. The speciality of the center is basic research with a focus on translating this research to clinical application for testing, diagnosis, and treating human disease, including tissue engineering for use in regenerative medicine.

**SEE ALSO:** Alabama; California; Cells, Embryonic; United States.

**BIBLIOGRAPHY.** BioCrossroads, "Mission and Initiatives," www.biocrossroads.com (cited November 2007); Indiana Legislature, 115th General Assembly, "Senate Bill No. 203," www.in.gov (cited November 2007); Indiana Legislature, "Adult Stem Cell Research Center," www.in.gov (cited November 2007); Indiana University School of Medicine, www.medicine.indiana.edu (cited November 2007); Purdue University, "Bindley Bioscience Center," www.purdue.edu (cited November 2007).

Lyn Michaud
Independent Scholar

# Indiana University

**THE INDIANA UNIVERSITY** system consists of eight regional campuses offering undergraduate, graduate, and professional programs in a variety of academic disciplines including medicine, biology, engineering, math, and physical sciences. Although the flagship undergraduate university campus is located in Bloomington, the medical school and medical research is located in Indianapolis. In agreement with Indiana's law regarding stem cell research, Indiana University's stem cell research focuses on adult-source stem cells.

In 2007 the Indiana legislature approved the establishment of, and appropriated $50,000 for, an Adult Stem Cell Research Center at Indiana University. The legislature gave the Indiana University School of Medicine approval to administer the center, including appointing a director and accepting income from donations, gifts, and so on, to be used to support the center's activities. The center will be tasked with providing an assessment of the status and future of adult stem cell research and with devising a strategy for Indiana University to attract and retain adult stem cell research scientists.

## INDIANA UNIVERSITY SCHOOL OF MEDICINE

The Indiana University School of Medicine was established in 1903 and has established itself as a research center for both basic and clinical research. A highlight in its adult stem cell research includes an early clinical trial using stem cell injections for treating peripheral artery disease (clogging atherosclerosis and hardening of arteries) to demonstrate the safety of using stem cells for blood vessel growth and wound healing, as the stem cells/progenitor cells targeted the lining of the blood vessel. With additional research, the team hopes to find a therapy to restore adequate stem cells in patients with heart disease or at risk for heart disease so that the body will be able to repair or replace damaged blood vessels and prevent the progression of heart disease.

Using a patient's own stem cells from bone marrow could reduce the complications associated with such a transplant. Research is currently focused on the regeneration of limbs/digits, cardiovascular system, musculoskeletal system, neural/endocrine system, biomaterials and chemical biology, bioinformatics and systems biology, and cancer.

The Melvin and Bren Simon Cancer Center, founded in 1992 and renamed in 2006, part of the School of Medicine. The center provides patient care, education, and research opportunities. Research is focused on improving cancer care with gene therapy trials for testicular cancer, brain tumors, genetic diseases, and other disorders.

## RESEARCH CENTERS

The Center for Regenerative Biology and Medicine was established in 2001 through a grant from the state of Indiana's 21st Century Research and Technology Fund. It is a multidisciplinary collaboration between the university's School of Science and the School of Medicine. The center's research is coordinated through multiple academic disciplines, including the basic science behind the development of cells/tissue/organs and the regeneration capabilities of plants and animals for translation into human clinical therapies to repair damaged or diseased tissue.

The center has nine organized research programs: regeneration of appendages, blood, heart, musculoskeletal, neural, endocrine, plant, and cancer, as well as the basic science of biomaterials and chemical biology and of bioinformatics and systems biology, and a focus on bioethical issues associated with the field of regenerative science and medicine.

In addition to research, the center offers graduate-level education leading to master's and doctoral degrees in regenerative biology and medicine with a cross discipline approach.

## CELL THERAPY PRODUCTS

The Emerging Technology Center helps researchers translate basic science innovations into clinical/commercial applications by assisting with new business development, including developing business plans and arranging financing.

One example of the center's success is EndGenitor Technologies, founded by two physicians at the Indiana University School of Medicine, who discovered endothelial stem cells/progenitor cells by comparing adult blood cells with infant umbilical cords to create cell therapy products for treating extremities circulation problems/heart disease and problems with blood vessels and circulation, as well as for treating chronic problems associated with aging. The physicians are owners in the company and continued to teach at the university after hiring a chief executive officer and support staff.

In the short term, the company will produce test kits for researchers to use for detecting the presence of endothelial stem and progenitor cells or as a research tool for testing a compound's ability to block the growth of blood vessels and tumor growth, or for compounds that promote growth or repair of blood vessels.

The Indiana University Center for Bioethics was established in 2001 to research and educate the university and the public about the social, ethical, and legal issues associated with science, health, and research. The stem cell study group focuses on the social, ethical, legal, and policy issues relating to human embryonic stem cells.

The Biomechanics and Biomaterials Research Center fosters interdisciplinary research across several medical and engineering disciplines. The center promotes research in biological mechanics, biomaterials design and synthesis, transplants/implants, and tissue engineering.

### STEM CELL BANK

Indiana's General Biotechnology is an umbilical stem cell bank founded in 2007 after a postdoctoral student from Indiana University studied how to improve cord blood processing. The company accepts, cryopreserves, and stores these cells to meet the growing demand for stem cells used in blood and bone marrow transplants, as well as other procedures, with hope for expansion to include adipose cells for use in bone/cartilage repair and stem cells for veterinary use.

**SEE ALSO:** Cells, Adult; Cells, Embryonic; Indiana.

**BIBLIOGRAPHY.** Indiana Legislature, 115th General Assembly, "Senate Bill No. 203," www.in.gov (cited November 2007); Indiana Legislature, "Adult Stem Cell Research Center," www.in.gov (cited November 2007); Indiana University Bone Marrow and Stem Cell Transplantation Program, www.cancer.edu (cited November 2007); Indiana University School of Medicine, www.medicine.indiana.edu (cited November 2007); Indiana University Simon Cancer Center, "Clinical Trials," www.iucc.iu.edu (cited November 2007).

Lyn Michaud
Independent Scholar

# Induced Pluripotent Stem Cells

**IN STEM CELL** jargon, a totipotent stem cell is one that arises very early in development and is capable of generating both extra embryonic (e.g., placenta) and embryonic tissues. In humans these totipotent stem cells are only found during the first few divisions of the fertilized egg. From the inner cell mass, pluripotent stem cells can be isolated that are able to produce any cells within the body. Until very recently, these could only be isolated from early embryos. However, a new technique pioneered by a group in Japan now allows pluripotent stem cells to be generated from adult cells within the body. This work was based on the idea that any cell in the body can be "reprogrammed" to a more primitive state, and was first proven through the cloning of Dolly the sheep. The term for these new reprogrammed pluripotent cells is *induced pluripotent stem cells.*

The power of induced pluripotent stem (IPS) cells is that they do not require the destruction of embryos and they may one day be produced from the patient's own adult cells, allowing the generation of perfectly matched tissues for transplantation therapies. However, in some cases where there is a genetic disease, the IPS cells may have the same deficit. Pluripotent stem cells were first induced in murine cells in the year 2006 and in human cells one year later. Thus the technology is still quite new and much research is still warranted. To date, in all characteristics the IPS cells resemble true pluripotent stem cells in all respects tested.

To induce a pluripotent stem cell, scientists introduce specific pluripotency genes into non-pluripotent cells, such as fibroblasts. These pluripotentcy genes include two very important transcription factors known to maintain mouse and human embryonic stem cells in a primitive state—Oct-4 and Sox-2. Fibroblasts are cells that produce and secrete the fibrous extracellular matrix that holds cells together in the body. The vector to introduce these genes into a non-pluripotent cell is called a retrovirus. The retrovirus does not have any viral

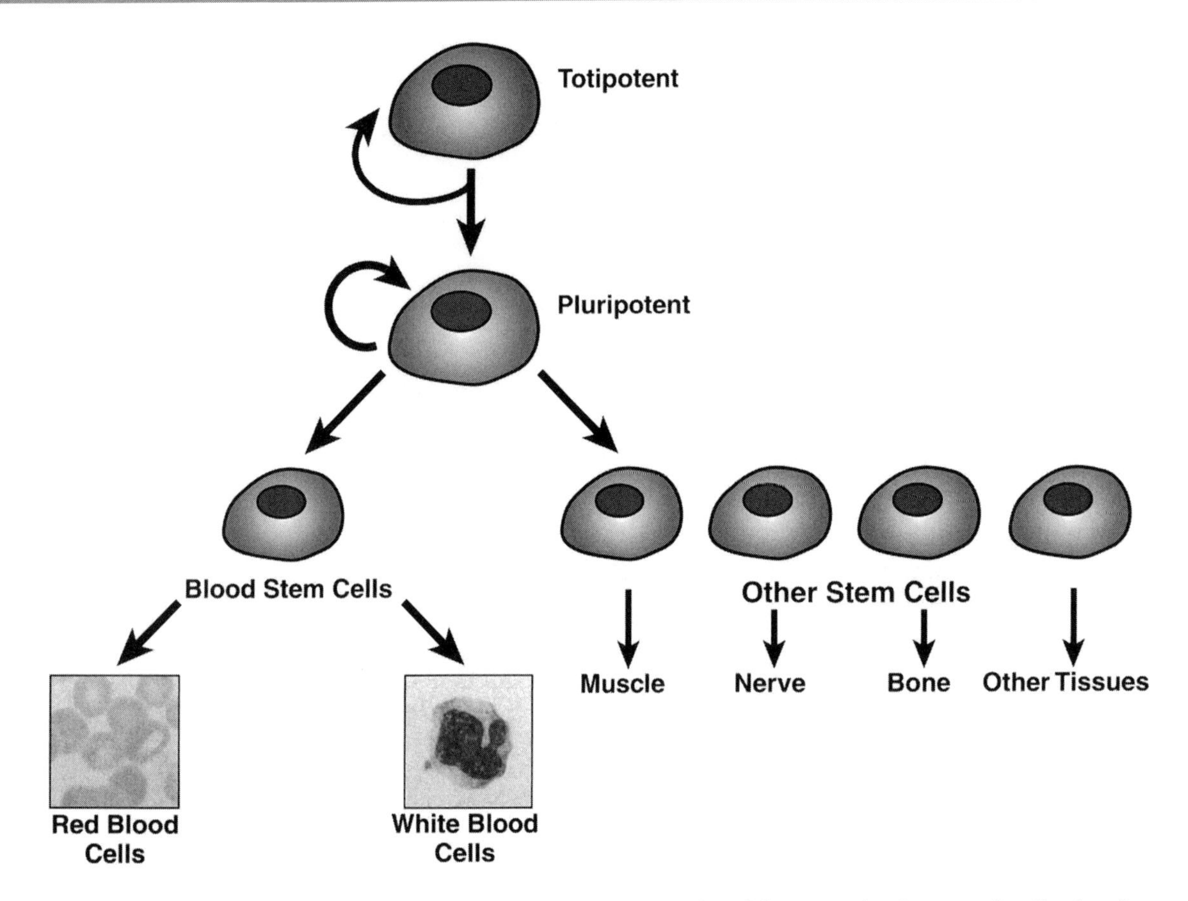


*Hierarchy of stem cells. Induced pluripotent stem cells may one day be produced from a patient's own cells, allowing the generation of perfectly matched tissues for transplantation therapies.*

capacity except that it can enter the cells easily and the genes it carries are thus accessible to the cell.

The first research laboratory to show induction of pluripotent stem cells in the mouse was a Japanese group led by Dr. Shinya Yamanaka at Kyoto University. This work was performed in mouse cells and published in 2006. In 2007 the Yamanaka group and other independent American labs showed a more advanced technique for inducing mouse pluripotent stem cells. However, one of the introduced genes (cMyc) caused cancer one-fifth of the time when the IPS cells were introduced into test mice. The Yamanaka group then developed IPS cells without using this gene and the resulting mice did not develop cancer. Later that year, the same group at Kyoto University, and independently a group led by Dr. James Thomson at the University of Wisconsin, Madison, created IPS cells from human fibroblasts. The two groups used overlapping sets of genes, in particular both Oct-4 and Sox-2.

Now that researchers have the capability to induce pluripotent stem cells from adult differentiated cells, the next steps are to improve on the techniques (perhaps not have the new genes inserted into the genome), as well as to learn what drives the pluripotent stem cells to differentiate in particular ways. Given the immense regenerative potential of these pluripotent stem cells, it will be imperative to understand each milestone in the differentiation process for a particular organ or tissue type in order to use the IPS cells in stem cell therapy.

**SEE ALSO:** Cancer; Cells, Adult; Cells, Embryonic; Cells, Mouse (Embryonic); Cells, Sources of; Japan; Kyoto University; National Institutes of Health; University of Wisconsin, Madison; WiCell.

**BIBLIOGRAPHY.** M. Bellomo, *The Stem Cell Divide: the Facts, the Fiction, and the Fear Driving the Greatest Scientific, Political and Religious Debate of Our Time* (AMACOM/American Management Association, 2006); R. I. Freshney, G. N. Stacey, and J. M. Auerbach, *Culture of Human Stem Cells (Culture of Specialized Cells)* (Wiley-Liss, 2007); J. F. Loring, *Human Stem Cell Manual: A Laboratory Guide* (Academic Press, 2007); M. Nakagawa, M. Koyanagi, and K. Tanabe, et al., "Generation of Induced Pluripotent Stem Cells without Myc from Mouse and Human Fibroblasts," *Nature Biotechnology* (January, 2008); National Institutes of Health, stemcells.nih.gov (cited May 2008); N. Swaminathan, "Stem Cells—This Time Without the Cancer," *Scientific American* (November 30, 2007); K. Takahashi, K. Tanabe, and M. Ohnuki, et al., "Induction of Pluripotent Stem Cells from Adult Human Fibroblasts by Defined Factors," *Cell* (November 30, 2007); J. Yu, M. A. Vodyanik, and K. Smugo-Otto, et al., "Induced Pluripotent Stem Cell Lines Derived from Human Somatic Cells," *Science* (December 21, 2007).

Claudia Winograd
University of Illinois, Urbana-Champaign

# International Laws

**INTERNATIONAL LAW AND** the regulation of stem cell research, particularly embryonic stem cell research, has been a difficult and contentious issue for nations and international organizations. Many different perspectives exist, within nations and within individual cultures, that have differing views and interpretations of stem cell research and its ethical effects. A truly comprehensive set of international regulations is still under development and may continue to be debated for many years. Many of the current regulations that are being devised by the international community arise from the nations that have been most influential in the stem cell research field. In addition, other policy concerns and the desire to gain a competitive edge in the stem cell research field at the expense of other countries have slowed progress on developing a unified international system for regulating stem cell research.

Approaches to the regulation of stem cell research vary widely from nation to nation. Some countries have enacted strict bans, whereas other countries have provided financial support for stem cell research.

## AFRICA AND ASIA

Throughout the continent of Africa, there are at this time very few explicit pieces of legislation regulating embryonic stem cell research. The only nation in Africa to have substantial stem cell research legislation is South Africa.

At present, South African policy allows for the use of unused embryos remaining from in vitro fertilization techniques in research and also for the creation of embryos for research purposes. In general, many African nations are viewed as having friendly policies toward embryonic stem cell research, with little regulation being the norm.

Several Asian nations also have entered the stem cell research arena as influential players. Many Asian nations do not have explicit stem cell research regulations at this time, with some exceptions. Legislation in both China and Singapore establishes specific laws that allow for the use of embryonic stem cells derived from unused embryos created from in vitro fertilization, and also for embryos that are created for the specific purpose of research.

The government of Singapore has made stem cell research, and in particular embryonic stem cell research, a national priority. It has specifically created Biopolis—a new research complex dedicated to advancing biomedical research, through legislation and financial subsidies. To date, Singapore has invested over $3 billion in establishing the biomedical and stem cell research infrastructure in Biopolis.

The efforts of the government of Singapore created a loose regulatory environment, and the nation's subsidy and encouragement of stem cell research have alarmed other governments. There is a perception that Singapore's national policies, focusing on advancing stem cell research, are attracting many scientists from other nations like the United States, thereby increasing Singapore's standing in this research frontier compared with other nations.

## EUROPEAN UNION AND RUSSIA

The European Union (EU) as a whole remains split on the issue of stem cell research. A number of countries within the EU have enacted various levels of restrictions on human embryonic stem cell research, including Austria, Germany, Ireland, Italy, and Portugal. In contrast, other EU nations such as Sweden, Finland, Belgium, the Netherlands, Denmark, and the United Kingdom allow embryonic stem cell research within their borders.

The United Kingdom has established a series of embryonic stem cell research policies that allow for the destruction of human embryos for embryonic stem cell research under the conditions that the embryonic stem cell research is undertaken because it could increase knowledge about human development, knowledge regarding serious diseases, or the potential to apply knowledge to the treatment of serious diseases.

Legislation passed in Russia created a stem cell research climate that allows the use of embryonic stem cells derived from eggs left over from in vitro fertilization, and also from eggs that are used explicitly to create embryos for research. This policy is one of the least restrictive within Europe and Asia. There is also concern that many of the regulatory policies and the lack of sufficient enforcement mechanisms within Russia could lead to international difficulties.

There are currently many different businesses in the country that offer injections of embryonic and adult stem cells to patients on a questionable scientific basis. Concern has been expressed that, at this stage, this type of therapy is unsafe and could be dangerous to a patient's health. There is also concern that because of lax regulation and weak enforcement efforts, the potential for unethical stem cell research to occur is greatly increased in Russia.

## AUSTRALIA AND THE UNITED STATES

Australia has adopted a number of policies that are viewed as being less restrictive to stem cell research, and particularly embryonic stem cell research. Among these policies is an allowance for the use of existing embryonic stem cell lines in research, as well as the ability to create new lines from unused embryos remaining from in vitro fertilization treatments. However, Australian law clearly lays out restrictions on the creation of embryos for research purposes, outlawing the creation of any embryo for purposes that are solely research driven.

The United States has failed to develop a comprehensive stem cell policy. Individual states have taken up the issue and have developed varying policies that cover a broad spectrum of stem cell regulatory issues. The federal government has prohibited research funding for use in research that uses embryonic stem cell lines derived after August 9, 2001. The federal government has also established clear policies that ban the creation of an embryo for the explicit purpose of scientific research.

## IMPORTANCE OF INTERNATIONAL REGULATION

International research cooperation in the field of stem cell biology will likely only enhance the future development of stem cell therapies. However, disparate regulatory structures that vary from country to country may have the effect of significantly damaging efforts at international scientific collaboration. Disparate regulation and a lack of international cooperation could fuel competition, with potentially dangerous consequences. There is concern in the scientific community that competition between nations could damage the ethical integrity of the stem cell research field.

Increasingly, calls for international regulation are also based on efforts to maintain the integrity of scientific research. The Hwang Woo-Suk incident greatly increased this impetus. Hwang Woo-Suk was a prestigious South Korean scientist who was previously involved in cloning research and who subsequently entered stem cell research. Hwang Woo-Suk claimed to successfully use somatic cell transfer cloning techniques to create 11 discrete embryonic stem cell lines by combining somatic human DNA with donated embryos. His reports were viewed as a breakthrough in possibly developing individualized patient therapy using autologous stem cells. His results were previously viewed as improbable, given the complexity of higher-primate genetics. Naturally, it was important that the validity of Hwang Woo-Suk's claims be verified in the process of standard scientific investigation.

Unfortunately, Hwang Woo-Suk's research group and other labs were unable to reproduce any significant verifying data. As a result, Hwang Woo-Suk, one of the most recognized and important researchers in South Korea, was dismissed from his academic and scientific positions. International regulation has been encouraged to increase research transparency and also to facilitate cooperation between nations in an effort to reduce scientific fraud.

One of the most significant and fundamental reasons for the creation of an international regulatory regime arises from moral and ethical concerns. The issue of embryonic stem cell research has widely split world opinion on the basis of moral and ethical systems. Some nations have acted to ban substantial embryonic stem cell research on the basis of ethical, moral, and religious grounds, whereas other nations have cited these same grounds as a basis for proceeding with extensive embryonic stem cell research.

## THE VATICAN

The Vatican, which directs the Roman Catholic Church and its doctrines, has strongly called for international regulation. The Catholic Church called for a ban on all research that involves the destruction or use of human embryos. The Vatican believes that a human embryo has the potential to become a person, and that a fertilized embryo represents human life. Therefore, the conduct of research on human embryos would degrade the sanctity of human life.

Even more important, the Catholic Church argues that the destruction of human embryos for the purpose of scientific research would be tantamount to murder. As a result, the Catholic Church believes that stem cell research ought to be prohibited under all circumstances in which an embryo may be harmed, out of respect for the life of the embryo and the inviolability of the individual. Given this stance, the potential benefits of stem cell research or therapies are outweighed by the necessity of protecting and affording each individual human the same rights and inviolability.

This view of stem cell research, grounded in a religious and moral tradition, has held significant sway on the international stage as a result of the Roman Catholic Church's representation of up to one sixth of the world's population. Many other religious groups also share the viewpoint espoused by the Vatican and have been vocal on a global scale in terms of their opposition to stem cell—and particularly embryonic stem cell—research.

Many groups counter the arguments that are provided by the Vatican by asserting a different definition of human life, which allows embryos to be considered as biological material rather than sentient human beings. Other groups contend that the potential benefits of stem cell research outweigh the harm that it could cause to embryos, and that the potential therapies that might result would benefit a far greater number of people. Still others argue that even Catholic theology cannot be defined so narrowly and that there may be a basis for support of stem cell research even within Catholic tradition.

## THE UNITED NATIONS

The United Nations (UN) is often viewed as a major organization that formulates international regulations. It is the role of the UN to mediate a policy that addresses the concerns of both proponents and opponents of stem cell research. At this point, the UN is continuing to attempt to develop a policy regarding stem cell research. Conflicts between individual member states and ideological differences have delayed the establishment of a uniform policy.

Although the UN has failed to reach agreement on specific stem cell regulations, it has established a series of guiding principles in the Universal Declaration on the Human Genome and Human Rights, many of which principles are applicable to stem cell research. This declaration was developed by the UN Educational, Scientific, and Cultural Organization (UNESCO) in 1997 and subsequently adopted by the UN General Assembly in 1998. Since this declaration was adopted by the full UN body, this document is now viewed as a crucial component of international human rights law, which seeks to protect the rights and liberties of all people. The declaration contains a number of fundamental statements that affect stem cell research, other emerging biotechnologies, and research fields.

One of the primary tenets of the declaration is the universal ban on human reproductive cloning, which is viewed as a violation of human rights and dignity. In the eyes of many scientists, the ban also serves as an important declaration for what it does not forbid. This declaration specifically outlaws reproductive cloning and leaves the issues of therapeutic or research cloning open for future debate.

The use of therapeutic cloning is viewed by many embryonic stem cell researchers as an important technology because of its potential to overcome graft-host rejection. In many cases, if embryonic stem cells were implanted into a human patient with a normally functioning immune system, the embryonic stem cells would be recognized as foreign and targeted for destruction. Through therapeutic cloning, the intention is to use somatic cell transfer techniques to create embryos as a source of embryonic stem cells that are genetically matched to the patient, to prevent rejection.

This technology also raises a series of ethical concerns and has become another locus of debate regarding how an embryo should be viewed in moral and ethical terms. However, the lack of a UN stance on this type of cloning could provide international flexibility regarding such technology. A number of countries have begun to move to either ban or to functionally allow this type of cloning for stem cell research purposes within their territory.

## WHO AND OTHER INTERNATIONAL BODIES

The World Health Organization (WHO) has also taken up the issue of bioethics and stem cell research. WHO has developed a number of consensus statements that were agreed on by member states, including statements that pertain to genetic technology and to basic research guidelines, such as the necessity of obtaining informed consent. However, WHO lacks significant regulatory power and the ability to enforce regulatory decisions. In addition, the majority of the work that has been accomplished by WHO is consensus building and concerns a statement of global principles rather than specific regulations.

To provide guidance to the entire international community, a group of scientists representing 14 different nations gathered at Cambridge, England, to establish basic guidelines for stem cell research that could be applied internationally. This group was called the Hinxton Group and continues to refine international guidelines and directives today. The Hinxton Group, however, does not have any enforcement powers. Rather, the group provides voluntary guidelines and mechanisms. There is hope from the members of the group that its regulations will be enforceable to some degree with the cooperation of scientific peer review and publications. As the field of international stem cell research expands, and particularly in the wake of a number of controversies regarding fraudulent research, there is a perception that journals may be willing to begin enforcing these regulations in an attempt to maintain the integrity of such scientific research.

The Hinxton Group developed a consensus statement that outlines the overall regulatory structure and mission of the group. The Hinxton Group recognizes the enormous potential that exists for stem cell research to improve society and the incredible medical benefits that may be possible with future research. At the same time, the group encourages regulation of the stem cell research field because of bioethical concerns. The group seeks to establish guidelines and regulations that are sensitive to cultural differences between countries and that allow for close regulation while providing the kind of flexibility that is important in new research fields. The general consensus the Hinxton Group has reached also includes specific provisions that enumerate the rights of scientists to travel out of their own countries and conduct research that may not be permissible in their home country but is ethical and permissible in the country in which the research is being conducted. The Hinxton Group holds that these individual scientists should not be subjected to prejudice or legal action for this decision.

The group has also developed a consensus calling for the creation of an international embryonic stem cell line bank. In the interest of cooperative scientific research, the group believes that this bank should be maintained by an international organization and that cells from this bank should be provided to researchers without bias as to nationality for the purpose of ethical research.

A number of other international bodies that were created primarily as partnerships between stem cell researchers also exist. The International Society of Stem Cell Research is one of these groups that is highly respected and expected to lead in developing international stem cell research guidelines. The aim of the International Society of Stem Cell Research is to facilitate contact and cooperation between stem cell researchers on an international level.

## PROBLEMS OF INTERNATIONAL REGULATION

The international regulation of stem cell research and international laws regarding stem cell research face a number of serious challenges. One of the primary challenges that these laws, guidelines, and regulations faces is the absence of viable enforcement mechanisms. The Hinxton Group, UN, WHO, and the International Society for Stem Cell Research currently have no enforcing powers for any generated regulations.

There is also the significant issue of international dissent. With the polarization of the stem cell research field on moral and ethical grounds, it is increasingly difficult for nations to reach a consensus on some of the more difficult aspects of stem cell field, such as the use or creation of human embryos for research. Because of the ideologies that underlie many of these positions, countries are unwilling to compromise and seek to maintain their own moral and ethical interpretations of stem cell research. International and supranational bodies also face difficult ethical and moral decisions when attempting to enumerate code that incorporates and respects disparate moral and religious systems throughout the world.

There are also many economic incentives that could encourage individual countries to cheat or refuse to enforce international laws and regulations in their respective scientific communities. Because of the competitive nature of the stem cell research field, many nations are pursuing policies that provide limited regulation to encourage research investment within their country, giving them an edge in the stem cell field. These countries will likely be very reluctant to join any substantive international regulatory regimen out of fear that their programs will be targeted. In particular, many developing nations have hailed stem cell research as an opportunity to enter the biomedical field and compete effectively against nations that are already advanced in traditional scientific fields. Efforts to regulate these nations extensively may spark angry responses if their economic growth or competitiveness were threatened.

As stem cell research advances, the pressure to develop a comprehensive international regimen will only escalate. The importance of international regulation will also continue to increase as transnational and international cooperation swells to higher levels. Future regulations and international laws must take into account many different viewpoints and allow for the flexibility to continue advancing research in stem cell biology and technology to improve the human condition.

**SEE ALSO:** Cells, Adult; Cells, Embryonic; Cells, Human; Clinical Trials Worldwide; International Society for Stem Cell Research.

**BIBLIOGRAPHY.** M. Bellomo, *The Stem Cell Divide: The Facts, the Fiction, and the Fear Driving the Greatest Scientific, Political and Religious Debate of Our Time* (AMACOM/American Management Association,

2006); C. B. Cohen, *Renewing the Stuff of Life: Stem Cells, Ethics, and Public Policy* (Oxford University Press, 2007); C. Fox, *Cell of Cells: The Global Race to Capture and Control the Stem Cell* (Norton, 2007); K. R. Monroe, R. Miller, and J. Tobis, eds., *Fundamentals of the Stem Cell Debate: The Scientific, Religious, Ethical, and Political Issues* (University of California Press, 2007); M. Ruse and C. A. Pynes, eds., *The Stem Cell Controversy: Debating the Issues (Contemporary Issues)* (Prometheus Books, 2006).

John S. Kuo
University of Wisconsin

# International Society for Stem Cell Research

**THE INTERNATIONAL SOCIETY** for Stem Cell Research (ISSCR) defines itself as "an independent, nonprofit organization established to promote and foster the exchange and dissemination of information and ideas relating to stem cells, to encourage the general field of research involving stem cells and to promote professional and public education in all areas of stem cell research and application."

The ISSCR has several committees, which serve a variety of functions for the institution itself. Committees range from finance to ethics and from public policy to public education and government affairs.

The ISSCR annual meeting is an opportunity for individuals to learn about novel research in all areas of stem cell science. The meeting provides a forum for scientists to discuss and present their research as well as for participants in the arenas of academia, industry, and government to discuss the special issues that stem cell science raises in their fields.

**SEE ALSO:** International Laws.

**BIBLIOGRAPHY.** International Society for Stem Cell Research, www.isscr.org (cited November 2007).

Krishna Subhash Vyas
University of Kentucky

# International Stem Cell Forum

**THE INTERNATIONAL STEM CELL FORUM** (ISCF) was established in 2003 by 21 funded research organizations from all over the world. The first stem cell advance occurred in the United States in 1957, when an intravenous bone marrow transplant was performed on a cancer patient receiving radiation and chemotherapy. The first technique that germinated embryonic stem cells occurred in the United States in 1992. In the last decade, the advancement of stem cell research has materialized quite rapidly. With these rapid advances, a global community has emerged and come together to form the ISCF.

Collaborating countries include Spain, Finland, the United States, Australia, Canada, China, the Czech Republic, Germany, France, Israel, Italy, the United Kingdom, the Netherlands, South Korea, and Sweden. The primary goal of the organization is to encourage global collaboration and funding for stem cell research. The organization aims to promote best practice guidelines with regard to all aspects of stem cell research by accelerating developments within this new and dynamic field. The organization is guided by a steering committee that consists of a panel of international experts.

The initial members consisted of nine funding agencies whose primary mission was speed up the rate of developments within the field of stem cell research. Today, that number has more than doubled. Because the agencies basically used the same technologies and scientific process, they banded together to standardize future developments that would maintain stem cell lines. The collaborative body identified areas in which collaboration would benefit all members. These included the sharing of research from multidisciplinary perspectives and different nations, sharing of research and protocols to reduce expenditures related to duplication of resources, joint training, identification of and plans to eliminate research gaps, identification of funding sources, identification of ethical issues, and management related to issues involving intellectual property.

The organization works in a collaborative manner to establish as many human embryonic stem cell isolates as possible. There are two parts to the initiative. Extensive and complex studies of these cell isolates were performed in 17 laboratories in 11 different countries throughout the world. This work focused on identifying the different stem cells and determining whether the different lines shared any commonalities. These discoveries resulted in two international workshops that were held in the United States and that disseminated the findings of the data. The second initiative is currently in process and involves comparing the different culture media in the human embryonic stem cells to see whether genetic changes occur after a certain length of time. This phase is currently in the data collection stage.

The ISCF routinely identifies projects of interest for the organization. As stem cell research and advances continue to grow, ethical and legal aspects will continue to rise. The ISCF currently has an Ethics Working Party that reviews ethical policies of countries throughout the world that engage in stem cell research and use stem cell technology. The group is currently working to draft an ethical document that addresses country-specific ethical issues within the field.

Intellectual property rights is another heated topic within stem cell research. As research developments are made, regulations regarding intellectual property are in increasing need. This global document will assist in developing guidelines that will prevent researchers from infringing on existing patents and help protect stem cell research intellectual property. The International Stem Cell Initiative is another working group that is attempting to standardize criteria involving human embryonic stem cell lines by working with various laboratories throughout the world. The number of stem cell banks has increased in number globally. The International Stem Cell Banking Initiative seeks to support current stem cell banks and to assist with the development of new banks throughout the world.

The world's stem cell lines are reported to various registries that serve as the record keepers of all known stem cell lines. There are three international banks that are used by the organization including the ISCF registry, the UK Stem Cell Registry, and the U.S. National Institutes of Health registry. As new lines are discovered, researchers report these findings to various registries. The primary purpose of the registries is to create immediate access to scientists throughout the world so that there is smooth dissemination of research advances as they occur.

**SEE ALSO:** Cells, Embryonic; International Laws.

**BIBLIOGRAPHY.** The International Stem Cell Forum, www.stemcellforum.org (cited November 2007).

Michele R. Davidson
George Mason University

# In Vitro Fertilization

**IN VITRO FERTILIZATION** (IVF) involves the combination of an unfertilized oocyte and spermatozoa in a Petri dish to allow fertilization to occur. Subsequent cleavage of the newly formed zygote can be supported in vitro by various culture conditions. Transfer of embryos into the uterus has resulted in pregnancy and live births in many mammalian species. Embryos cultured to the blastocyst stage have provided a source for embryonic stem cells. Embryonic stem cells have the capacity to renew and to differentiate into many cells of the body, a term known as potency. Therefore, in vitro fertilization provides a clinical application for infertility issues as well as a research avenue to understand early development.

Although the process of reproduction has been of interest to both science and philosophy since Aristotle's time, the first example of in vitro fertilization was shown by Lazaro Spallanzani (1729–99) when he demonstrated that tadpoles only developed if oocytes came into contact with

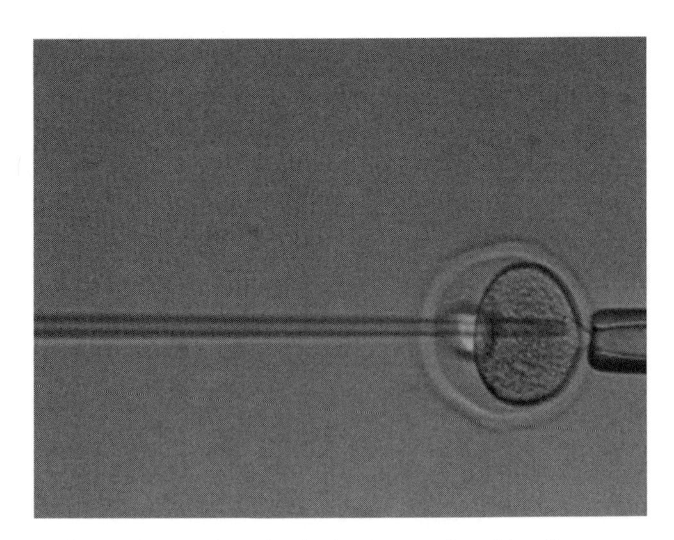

*In vitro embryo culture has helped researchers identify markers associated with pluripotency, such as Oct-4.*

semen. Much later, Yanagimachi and Chang (1963) reported the fertilization of hamster oocytes with capacitated sperm which prefaced the successes in human in vitro fertilization. The first live birth from human in vitro fertilization was in 1978, by Patrick Steptoe and Robert Edwards in the United Kingdom. Since then, the in vitro fertilization procedure has become a routine treatment option for patients dealing with infertility.

## PROCEDURE

The first step in the in vitro fertilization process involves the superovulation of the female. In current paradigms, this entails the down-regulation of gonadotrophic-releasing hormone from the hypothalamus which suppresses the anterior pituitary from secreting the gonadotrophins: follicle stimulating hormone and luteinizing hormone. This results in a temporary state of hypogonadotrophic hypogonadism. Once this state is reached, gonadotrophin stimulation can begin by the administration of follicle stimulating hormone to induce follicle growth in the ovaries. During this time, follicle growth is monitored via ultrasound and by peripheral blood levels of estradiol.

Once follicle size and estradiol levels have reached the desirable size and levels, respectively, human chorionic gonadotrophin is given for ovulation induction. Ovulation in normal cycles is preceded by a surge in luteinizing hormone. Since the β-subunit of human chorionic gonadotrophin is similar to that of luteinizing hormone, human chorionic gonadotrophin is often used in lieu of luteinizing hormone. Once ovulation has been induced, oocyte collection is scheduled to occur within 36 hours postinjection. This 36-hour window is critical because during this time, the oocytes within the follicles will reinitiate meiosis II and will progress to metaphase II.

During oocyte collection, semen will be obtained by masturbation and will be processed typically by gradient centrifugation to remove the seminal plasma and debris. Next, the oocytes and sperm will be combined in a Petri dish to undergo fertilization. An alternative approach is to perform intracytoplasmic sperm injection where an isolated sperm cell is injected into each oocyte. This helps the sperm bypass the zona pellucida of the oocyte and results in high rates of fertilization. Successful fertilization is evidenced by the appearance of two pronuclei in the oocyte at approximately 16–18 hours postinsemination. The pronuclei are said to come into syngamy where the nucleus from the oocyte comes into close proximity with the nucleus from the spermatocyte.

Once fertilization has been achieved, the zygote begins cleavage divisions. The embryo will divide from one to two cells and then two to four, and so forth, but will remain the same size within the confines of the zona pellucida. The first cleavage divisions of the embryo are under posttranscriptional maternal control. The metabolic driving force comes from pyruvate and lactate in the culture media. At the four to eight cell stage, zygotic gene activation or embryonic genome activation occurs and all subsequent cleavage divisions are supported by the embryo's own protein production. By the eight to ten cell stage, the embryo will undergo compaction and form a morula. From the eight cell stage and on, the metabolic activity of the embryo requires glucose to grow.

For these changes in embryo metabolism, sequential media has been developed and is widely used for embryo culturing today. Culturing with sequential media entails placing the embryos in lactate and pyruvate-rich media for the first two days of in vitro culture and then switching to a glucose-rich media from days three to six of culture. Compaction is characterized by an increased number of adhesion and gap junctions. Cells become morphologically indistinguishable and begin to polarize. The morula stage is the last time in development the embryo exhibits totipotency or the ability to differentiate into all cell types. Formation of the blastocyst is the first differentiation event the embryo will undergo and occurs between days five and six in vitro.

The first differentiated structure that appears is the trophectoderm, which consists of the cells that line the outer layer of the blastocyst and will form the chorionic placental structures during embryo implantation. The blastocyst contains a fluid filled cavity and will increase in size. The inner cell mass consists of cells that will form the embryo proper, and is also the source of embryonic stem cells. These cells are pluripotent and will form the three germ layers during gastrulation.

## CLINICAL AND RESEARCH APPLICATIONS

Human in vitro fertilization was initially used to help women with infertility due to obstructed fallopian tubes. It has evolved and is now used for many couples struggling with various infertility issues, including male factor infertility and poor ovarian response. In addition to its clinical applications, in vitro fertilization is widely used in the research world. Although much work has been done in the rabbit and mouse models, advances in genetic and microscopic technology have allowed for many investigations into human development.

One of the main techniques currently used is preimplantation genetic diagnosis. This technology was initially intended to be used in the prevention of birth of babies with disabilities by combining in vitro fertilization with the injection of stem cells to repair damaged tissues. What evolved was a method in which micromanipulation is used to remove one to two blastomeres from the eight cell embryo without detriment to the embryo. With this cell(s), genetic testing can be performed to detect chromosomal abnormalities via fluorescent in situ hybridization and karyotyping or single gene disorders via the polymerase chain reaction. With this valuable genetic information, transfer of a healthy embryo to the mother can follow, eliminating the possibility of carrying an inherited disease to the next generation.

In non-human research applications, the micromanipulation technique is commonly used in the formation of chimeric animals where cells from the inner cell mass of one embryo are excised and injected back into a different embryo resulting in an animal with two genetically distinct cell populations. From chimeric animals, the pluripotency of the cells injected are tested. This revealed the great potential that embryonic stem cells have to differentiate into most cells of the body. In addition, adult stem cells can be tested and have proven to be multipotent where stem cells from the blood or nerve lineages are capable of differentiating into numerous body tissues.

In vitro embryo culture has also proven to be a useful research tool in the identification of markers associated with pluripotency and the undifferentiated state, as well as lineage determination and terminal differentiation. A good example is that of Oct-4, a marker of pluripotency that is found in the developing embryo throughout the preimplantation period and also maintains embryonic stem cells in the undifferentiated state. Other genes involved in maintaining the undifferentiated state are Nanog and Sox-2.

Recently, a great deal of research has involved the identification of various differentiation pathways stem cells can follow to form the desired tissue. These pathways include the induction of pathways leading to neuronal, hematopoietic, and cardiac lineages, just to name a few. With the use of in vitro fertilization and embryo culture, not only can early embryogenesis be studied but events occurring during human gastrulation can also be identified. The isolation and culture of stem cells provides a common platform for this research. Multidisciplinary, collaborative efforts will unveil the great potential that stem cells provide in early developmental research.

**SEE ALSO:** Cells, Embryonic; Cells, Sources of; Egg Donation; Funding for IVF; Human Embryonic Stem Cells; Lineages.

**BIBLIOGRAPHY.** Peter R. Brinsden, *In Vitro Fertilization and Assisted Reproduction* (Parthenon, 1999); Gary N. Clarke, "A.R.T. and History, 1678–1978" *Human Reproduction* (v.21, 2006); Richard G. Edwards, "IVF and the History of Stem Cells," *Nature* (v.413, 2001); Richard G. Edwards, "Changing Genetic World of IVF, Stem Cells and PGD. A. Early Methods in Research," *RBM Online* (v.11, 2005).

Maria Giakoumopoulos
University of Wisconsin, Madison

# Iowa

**STEM CELLS GIVE** rise to many different cell types that make up an organism. They can be classified according to their origin as embryonic stem cells, fetal stem cells, or adult stem cells. Embryonic stem cells are harvested through in vitro extraction of the inner cell mass of a blastocyst, the earliest stage following fertilization, when the embryo consists of only a few cells.

Fetal stem cells are collected from various regions of the fetus later in development. As such, fetal cells are partially differentiated at the time of harvest and are therefore more limited in their ability to give rise to tissues in the body compared to embryonic stem cells. Adult stem cells are harvested from an individual any time after birth and maintain their ability to differentiate into a few specialized cell types related to the tissue from which they were harvested.

As stem cells can differentiate into specialized tissues both in vitro and in vivo, they are a desirable instrument for cellular therapies. Stem cells have opened up novel avenues for disease control, tissue engineering, and organ transplantation. However, they are accompanied by several moral and ethical considerations. The delicate nature by which these cells are procured has, since their discovery, attracted the attention and scrutiny of scientists, physicians, ethicists, politicians, and media.

In 2002 a bill was passed banning somatic cell nuclear transfer for either reproductive or therapeutic cloning. In 2007, the Iowa General Assembly and newly elected Governor Chet Culver passed a bill allowing for therapeutic cloning within the state making Iowa one of the few U.S. states to take a progressive stand on this debate and allow the advancement of stem cell use and research. The new bill aims to

> ensure that Iowa patients have access to stem cell therapies and cures and that Iowa researchers may conduct stem cell research and develop therapies and cures in the state, and to prohibit human reproductive cloning.

In line with the bill's aims, scientists within Iowa are currently conducting research aimed at controlling and analyzing the outcomes and behavior of stem cells in therapeutic treatments through in vitro and clinical practices.

In vitro characterization and manipulation are the gateways of stem cell research. Scientists must understand stem cell developmental transitions and how to control their differentiation to specific cell fates. Current examples of in vitro research include analysis of disease processes in relation to endogenous stem cell populations and communication. For example, differentiation of submucosal gland tissue within the lung is an important contributor to several hypersecretory lung disease processes, including chronic bronchitis, asthma, and cystic fibrosis. Analysis of a putative adult stem cell compartment within the airway epithelium has resulted in the identification of molecular markers for signaling pathways that regulate stem cell phenotypes and their ability to differentiate into submucosal tissue following airway injury.

In addition to analyzing the behavior of stem cell differentiation, Iowa's researchers are also trying to develop microenvironments that will allow precise control over the role of stem cells in tissue repair and growth. This includes the differentiation of postnatal stem cells into multipotential neural stem cells. These studies have shown that adult neural stem cells maintain the potential to differentiate into functional neurons with the morphological and functional properties of mature central nervous system neurons. This finding was confirmed when tetanus toxin, a toxin that targets neurons with high specificity, retained its specificity toward these stem cell–derived neurons.

In separate in vitro studies, directional growth and differentiation of adult rat hippocampal progenitor cells are being analyzed on micropatterned polymer substrates. Chemical modification of these cells leads to controlled cell alignment and adaptation of neuronal morphology. A three-dimensional substrate can be used to guide cell–cell interactions and further aid in controlling neural stem cell differentiation for guided nerve regeneration.

Controlled growth is also being achieved by studying a type 2 transmembrane protein (LIGHT). This protein was originally identified because of its contributing role in T-cell regulation and dendritic cell maturation. It is now being used to regulate stem cell proliferation and differentiation. Initial results indicate that LIGHT induces differentiation and overrides many of the other factors guiding or inhibiting stem cell behavior.

In clinical studies, investigations are evaluating the effects of stem cell transplantation on various physiological processes. Researchers have identified the major complications associated with transplantation of unrelated umbilical cord blood in patients with Shwachman-Diamond syndrome (SDS), a disorder characterized by pancreatic deficiency and variable neutrophil populations. Graft-versus-host-disease has been a challenging issue. However, it has been found that unrelated umbilical cord blood, in the absence of a matched family member, is a beneficial alternative stem cell source for SDS patients undergoing hematopoietic stem cell transplantation.

In other adverse effect–related research, cognitive and psychiatric status in hematopoietic stem cell transplantation patients shortly before and after transplant is being analyzed. Iowa researchers have found that before transplant, participants showed mild impairments on several neuropsychological measures. After transplant, however, improvements were observed on depression/anxiety scores and neuropsychological measures.

For stem cells to realize their clinical promise, researchers must not only attempt to analyze the events controlling stem cell behavior but also determine the outcomes and adverse effects one might face during and after stem cell therapy. The magnitude and diversity of stem cell research within the state of Iowa shows that all of these areas are being addressed for the safety and progression of current and future stem cell–based treatments of disease.

**SEE ALSO:** Cells, Adult; Cells, Embryonic.

**BIBLIOGRAPHY.** L. J. Beglinger, et al., "Neuropsychological and Psychiatric Functioning Pre- and Post-hematopoietic Stem Cell Transplantation in Adult Cancer Patients: A Preliminary Study," *Journal of the International Neuropsychological Society* (v.13/1, 2007); J. Bolkcom, ed., Iowa Stem Cell Research and Cures Initiative, Senate File 162, 2007; S. Bonde and N. Zavazava, "Immunogenicity and Engraftment of Mouse Embryonic Stem Cells in Allogeneic Recipients," *Stem Cells* (v.24/10, 2006); E. B. Kelly, *Stem Cells* (Greenwood, 2006); X. M. Liu, R. R. Driskell, and J. F. Engelhardt, "Airway Glandular Development and Stem Cells," *Current Topics in Developmental Biology* (v.64, 2004); J. B. Recknor, D. S. Sakaguchi, and S. K. Mallapragada, "Directed Growth and Selective Differentiation of Neural Progenitor Cells on Micropatterned Polymer Substrates," *Biomaterials* (v.27/22, 2006); E. W. Rowe, et al., "Development of Functional Neurons from Postnatal Stem Cells In Vitro," *Stem Cells* (v.23/8, 2005); S. Ryang, "Does It Have to Be hESC? A Note on War, Embryo, and the Disabled," *Anthropological Quarterly* (v.79/3, 2006); R. Vibhakar, et al., "Successful Unrelated Umbilical Cord Blood Transplantation in Children with Shwachman-Diamond Syndrome," *Bone Marrow Transplantation* (v.36/10, 2005); G. M. Zou, J. J. Chen, and J. Ni, "LIGHT Induces Differentiation of Mouse Embryonic Stem Cells Associated with Activation of ERK5," *Oncogene* (v.25/3, 2006).

Megan E. Pearce
Aliasger K. Salem
University of Iowa

# Iran

**THE ISLAMIC REPUBLIC** of Iran is a Middle Eastern country with an ancient and prestigious history and a present marked by the presence of considerable resources of oil and gas that buttress its status and power in the modern world. It is bordered by Afghanistan and Pakistan to the east, the Persian Gulf to the south, Iraq and Turkey to the west, and the former Soviet Republics of Armenia, Azerbaijan, and Turkmenistan to the north, in addition to the Caspian Sea. Most of the country consists of mountain ranges surrounding the central plain, with much of the land more than 1,500 feet above sea level.

The country is ethnically diverse, including Turkic peoples, Aryans, Kurds, and the Bakhtyari people, together with Assyrians, Arabs, and Jewish people. The linguistic situation is similarly complex. Iran is believed to have one of the largest reserves of oil in the world, and this resource represents its principal revenue-earning export. This export has helped make Iran a medium-income country. The total land area is a little over 636,000 square miles, and the population exceeds 70 million people. The capital city is Tehran.

Although Iran (previously known as Persia) became a proud member of the Islamic world early on, it retained a number of cultural institutions that stressed its independence, including the use of the Farsi language and the solar calendar. Most Iranians follow the Shi'ite version of Islam, but the country has a long (and occasionally broken) tradition of tolerance for other religions, including ancient indigenous religions such as Mazdaism and Zoroastrianism. During the 20th century, Iran suffered repeatedly from external interference by colonial powers aimed at controlling the oil reserves that were becoming increasingly important in the world market. This included the unjust extraction of resources from the country and the propping up of a royal family increasingly viewed as decadent and oppressive.

In 1979 an Islamic Revolution led by Ayatollah Khomeini spearheaded a postcolonial revival of Islam as means of state governance. Subsequently, Iran has been governed by a complex amalgam of religious and sectarian interests, which represent the often-contradictory nature of the country. American foreign policy in the 21st century has led to influential groups in Iran seeking to upgrade its military defences by developing nuclear weapons. Iranian influence has grown considerably in the region as a result of the American-led war in Iraq.

Iranian attitudes toward stem cell research appear to bear out an understanding of Iran and Iranians as being a complex and occasionally contradictory country and people. Iran has a long and proud history of scientific research and exposition dating back more than 2,000 years and encompassing the Dark Ages, when Islamic scientists were among the most advanced in the world. That tradition has been revived in the modern age, but in general terms, only in those cases where a religious imprimatur can be obtained for the field and means of research. This approval is not easily obtained, and in any case, there is no single religious voice that commands the attention of all the faithful. The result is that Iranian scientists must constantly be alert to changing opinions or thoughts in terms of their own research interests and in the way they interact with each other. Women, notably, must obey strict dress codes in public and are subject to constant monitoring of their behavior.

Because scientific research often necessitates close teamwork, male and female scientists may find themselves faced with critical scrutiny of their actions. Other problems exist with respect to the restrictions placed on Iranian scientists wishing to travel to international conferences or participate in international collaborative research projects, and it has proved problematic to invite some scientists to visit Iran, notwithstanding the legendary hospitality of the Iranian people.

This external pressure has persuaded many Iranian scientists and academics to migrate elsewhere, either to enable other countries to benefit from their work or to take less-skilled employment. Salaries for scientists in Iran are comparatively low. The Royan Institute plays an important role in promoting international links and research collaboration. The institute is located in Tehran and houses the principal research in the country in terms of both infertility and stem cells.

However, in terms of stem cell research in particular, a crucial interpretation of Islamic law and tradition has been that life does not begin until three months after conception. Human cells of fetuses less than three months old are, therefore, available for experimentation without any ethical issues intruding. As a consequence, experimentation is taking place in a wide range of fields, from tackling heart disease to the cloning of sheep.

The relevant announcement was made in 2002 by Ayatollah Ali Khamenei, considered to be the supreme religious leader of the country. The Ayatollah praised research on surplus embryos created as part of fertility experiments as a lofty mission that could help Iran and the Islamic world reclaim its position as a globally important player. The result has been that scientists have had freedom to conduct experiments that are rather envied by many in the United States, for example, where comparable research has been precluded by the interventions of conservative and influential religious figures. Concrete results of the Iranian research are only just emerging because of the length of time the peer-reviewing process takes in academic publication and because there is a need for improvement to the ability of international scientists to verify the results of Iranian science. Outstanding claims include the successful cloning of a still-living sheep and the use of bone marrow cells to repair the cornea.

Success in promoting Iranian science, in stem cells as elsewhere, has been used by some governing elites as a means of boosting national pride and militarism through the nuclear program. Scientists themselves tend to prefer to maintain the principles of scientific progress in their work and would rather it were not intermingled with political issues, although of course, there are some exceptions to this rule. However, in the modern world, the politicization of science is difficult to avoid.

**SEE ALSO:** International Laws; Regulations Overview.

**BIBLIOGRAPHY.** Ali Ansari, *Modern Iran*, 2nd ed. (Longman, 2007); Anne Barnard, "Iran Looks to Science as Source of Pride," *Boston Globe* (August 22, 2006); Afshin Molavi, *The Soul of Iran: A Nation's Journey to Freedom*, rev. ed. (Norton, 2005); Royan Institute, www.royaninstitute.org/cmsen (cited November 2007); LeRoy Walters, "Human Embryonic Stem Cell Research: An Intercultural Perspective," *Kennedy Institute of Ethics Journal* (v.14/1, 2004).

John Walsh
Shinawatra University

# Israel

**ISRAEL IS A** leading country in both adult and embryonic stem cell research as a result of having laws supportive of stem cell research that are derived from Judaic laws on healing and saving lives, funding from various public and private sources, and strong academic and clinical research institutions and professionals dedicated to advancing technology and improving patient outcomes. Israel has been active in stem cell research and involved in many breakthroughs in the discovery of human embryonic stem cell lines and maintaining stem cell lines for availability to researchers around the world; their stem cells are listed in the National Institutes of Health registry as qualifying for federally funded research. In 2001 a research team directed the differentiation of cultured embryonic cells in beta cells of the pancreas to make and secrete insulin.

## LAWS, REGULATION, AND FUNDING

Israel is progressive regarding stem cell research, though for political reasons, they may abstain from voting on such issues in the United Nations. Public discussion of stem cell research is rare, with some media presentation and debate at the Knesset (Israeli's Parliament) Science and Technology committee when lawmaking is discussed.

Israeli law allows for the procurement of human embryonic stem cells from early-stage embryos left over from assisted reproduction (in vitro fertilization) and for the creation of human embryos, including cloned embryos, for research. The Human Cloning and Genetic Manipulation law has been in effect since 1998 and remains in effect until March 2009. It prohibits reproductive cloning or genetic manipulation of embryos to be used in in vitro fertilization.

Funding for research includes grants from the Ministry of Science, the Israel Science Foundation, research and development arrangements with other countries including Australia, grants, and private funding.

## ORGANIZATIONS

The Israeli Stem Cell Research Forum was formed in 2005 and is administered by the Israeli Ministry of Health. The forum's mission is to advance the translation of fundamental stem cell research into clinical applications, including in the area of regenerative medicine. Regenerative medicine relies on controlling cell development to grow healthy tissues using cell-based therapy to improve organ function in diseased or injured organs and tissues, instead of drugs or devices.

The Cell Therapy Consortium is a networking body with the intent of translating research into commercial products. The consortium is divided into three groups. The adult stem cell group focuses on isolating and growing stem cells from various blood sources. The embryonic stem cell group creates clinically usable human embryonic stem cell lines. The tools development group uses applied research and development to move scientific breakthroughs into usable therapies. Included under the auspices of the consortium are some of Israel's biotech companies working with blood, bone, heart, and nerve cells.

The Israeli Consortium Bereshit (Genesis) for Cell Therapy was formed to allow cell therapy companies in Israel to provide stem cell technologies and products—including stem cell lines—to researchers around the world. The Israeli Stem Cell Society is a networking body established to promote collaboration for stem cell researchers internationally in the vast number of fields related to stem cell research, including developmental biology, functional genetics, and clinical professionals. The society makes its home at the Technicon.

## RESEARCHERS

The Technicon, located in Haifa, was formed in 1924. The university offers academic studies in science, engineering, and medicine, as well as related academic disciplines, in an environment that fosters innovation and professional ethics. The Technicon is home to a medical school: The Bruce Rappaport Faculty of Medicine began in 1969 and was incorporated into Technicon in 1971 with a vision of joining clinical practice and technological development. The school meets this goal through affiliations with eight hospitals and the scientific community. The medical school has received a number of international prizes and grants including the 2001 Albert Lasker Award for Basic Medical Research for the discovery of ubiquitin for protein degradation. In addition, the medical school enables international cooperation with other globally recognized entities such as the Coriell Institute in New Jersey, Johns Hopkins University School of Medicine in Maryland, and Cleveland Clinic Foundation in Ohio.

Technicon's role in stem cell research includes Dr. Itskovitz's collaboration with Dr. James Thomson at the University of Wisconsin, Madison, in the discovery of human embryonic stem cell lines. Current stem cell research at Technicon includes generating new stem cell lines and methods, performing regenerative therapy using tissue engineering to grow new tissue, and the use of stem cell–based treatment for diabetes. Technicon's facilities include a stem cell research center and a tissue engineering center. The tissue engineering center uses technology to produce new tissue by combining cells and materials to induce growth and differentiation. By combining the expertise of fundamental science with engineering and medicine, the Technicon is able to translate scientific innovation into an enhanced quality of life during the treatment of human disease.

The Hadassah Human Embryonic Stem Cell Research Center was founded in 2003 at the

Goldyne Savad Institute of Gene Therapy to collaborate with the Department of Obstetrics and Gynecology there. The facilities include an assisted reproduction facility that acts as a source of embryos and a Current Good Manufacturing Production facility to create products to be used in clinical trials. The center has received approval from the Israeli Ministry of Health Supreme Ethical Committee to develop new cell lines without using animal products for use in human transplant.

The center's focus is developing technologies for the use of stem cells in transplant and cell-based therapy to treat human disease. In addition to research, the Stem Cell Research Center plays a role in supporting and encouraging other researchers in Israel to participate in stem cell research. Hadassah has a long history of success with stem cells including the first documentation of inducing differentiation of stem cells into muscle and nerve cells through culturing techniques.

Researchers at Hadassah have identified a possible shortcoming of the stem cell lines currently in use: Most of the cell lines were established for research purposes and not for clinical use. This is especially true for cell lines developed using co-culture techniques with mouse cells leading to the possibility of pathogenic cross-over into humans. Therefore, researchers at the center intend to develop cell lines for clinic trials, improve the techniques of stem cell expansion, develop pure differentiated cells and use them in animal models, modify the cells genetically for cell-based therapy, improve safety of the cells used in clinical therapy, and solve the problem of transplant rejection. For cells to be used in a clinical setting, they need to be enriched for one cell type and to have developed methods for creating and proliferating single cell types.

The researchers used animal model transplantation in mice to show improved function of the organ. For stem cells to be used for gene therapy, the stem cell must reach the target tissue and then be able to express the characteristics of the cells needed for repair. Researchers also hope to solve the problem of immune rejection by using somatic cells' nuclear transfer (therapeutic cloning) to grow stem cells identical to the patient's to prevent rejection.

Hadassah's work in collaboration with the Department of Endocrinology and Neurology focuses on using stem cells to treat diabetes and Parkinson's disease and with the Department of Neurology to use stem cells for treating multiple sclerosis. In meeting the goal of promoting stem cell research in Israel, Hadassah serves as a national center for collaborative research and provides cells and culture material as well as technical assistance to Israeli researchers and to scientists internationally.

The Weizmann Institute of Science, located in Rehovot, was founded in 1934 and in 1949 was named in honor of Chaim Weizmann. The school offers education in the scientific disciplines of biology, biochemistry, chemistry, physics, and math and computer science. At the institute, in the 1960s, Leo Sachs was the first scientist to demonstrate stem cell growth in culture.

**SEE ALSO:** Australia; Cells, Adult; Cells, Embryonic; Coriell Institute; Lasker Foundation; Thomson, James.

**BIBLIOGRAPHY.** Hadassah Human Embryonic Stem Cell Research Center, www.hadassah.org.il (cited August 2007); International Conference on Signal Processing, Communications and Networking, "Global Regulation of Human Embryonic Stem Cell Research and Oocyte Donation," www.stemcellconsortium.org (cited August 2007); Weizmann Institute of Science, "At a Glance," www.weizmann.ac.il (cited August 2007).

Lyn Michaud
Independent Scholar

# Italy

**ITALIAN STEM CELL** research is currently receiving contributions from different research groups, mainly connected to public and private universities and to university hospitals from all over the country. The funding of stem cell research in Italy relies principally on public financial support. Some funds are directly granted by the Ministry of Research, which partially sustains stem cell projects, but the major funding comes from the Ministry of Health, which distributes funds among those groups that have applied through a specifically appointed committee. A total of 7.5 million Euros were provided in 2003–05.

## RESEARCH

The most relevant results of Italian stem cell research come from the San Raffaele Stem Cells Research Institute, directed by Giulio Cossu and Angelo Vescovi. Founded in 2000 at the San Raffaele Hospital in Milan, the Stem Cells Research Institute is composed of different research subgroups, which mainly concentrate on the pathophysiology of skeletal muscle development, neural stem cells, and cellular therapy for type 1 diabetes.

Type 1 diabetes mellitus has long been considered an autoimmune disease, in which pancreatic beta cells are progressively destroyed by selective and largely ignored immune mechanisms. Ezio Bonifacio, director of the Pancreatic Islet Transplantation Program at San Raffaele, is working on type 1 diabetes immunology and recently focused on the employment of mesenchymal stem cells (MSCs) as a possible means for restoring lost beta cells. The pathways involved in MSC migration to pancreatic islets have been investigated by Bonifacio and colleagues, who provided evidence that bone marrow MSCs are attracted by pancreatic islets, both in vitro and in vivo, through a specific set of chemokine receptors, whose characterization may play a role in future therapeutic applications.

Cossu and colleagues contributed to the identification of skeletal muscle progenitors, further defined as mesoangioblasts, as they derive from blood vessels. These cells are believed to give rise to part of the skeletal muscles during embryonic and fetal life, and their use in preclinical studies has been greeted with optimism. In 2006 Cossu published an article in *Nature* indicating that an intraarterial injection of mesoangioblast stem cells can ameliorate muscle function in dogs with an experimental model of Duchenne's syndrome, qualifying these cells to be possible candidates for regenerative therapy. Cossu currently coordinates an MSC project funded by the European Commission, aiming at the identification of cell therapy protocols that hopefully could be implemented as therapeutic options for many neuromuscular diseases in the near future.

Angelo Vescovi's team is an internationally renowned research group that focuses on neural stem cell pathophysiology: the group's findings about adult human brain neurogenesis are presently contributing to a full characterization of adult neural stem cells, which could soon lead to the development of a cellular therapy for many different neurological disorders. Together with Martino Gianvito, head of the neuroimmunology unit at San Raffaele Hospital, Vescovi demonstrated the effectiveness of adult neural stem cell administration in a mouse model of multiple sclerosis, in which an active remyelinization process has been documented as being sustained by stem cells.

Even the University of Milan is working on projects related to neural stem cells: Elena Cattaneo, head of the Stem Cell Biology Laboratory, is involved in the recognition of the factors influencing neural stem cell differentiation, and particularly of the mechanisms responsible for Huntington's disease, an inherited neurodegenerative disorder striking people around 30–40 years of age that is characterized by the preferential loss of cortical and striatal neurons, leading to progressive neurological deterioration. The total absence of any effective treatment is leading Cattaneo's team to figure out any molecular target that could become suitable for drug design.

Stem cell research also is carried out at the Higher Health Institute. Cesare Peschle holds the office of director of the Hematology, Oncology, and Molecular Medicine Department and is presently supervising different research lines, mainly involving the use of hematopoietic stem cells for cardiovascular regenerative applications or the use of MSCs as a potential source of bone and muscular regeneration.

Gianluigi Condorelli, Professor of Medicine at La Sapienza University in Rome, is presently collaborating with the Higher Health Institute and the University of San Diego in different research lines concerning cardiovascular applications of stem cell research. He studied different molecular aspects of cardiac hypertrophy and heart failure and tested, in preclinical studies, the employment of low doses of human cord blood progenitors in ischemic limbs. Mice treated with a low quantity of these CD34+ cells demonstrated neovascularization, and possibly a recovery of muscular tissue in previously ischemized limbs, encouraging further studies on this protocol.

Condorelli has also been involved in myocardial regeneration research: He participated in a cardiac cell study issued in collaboration with San Raffaele Hospital, in which 10 patients with refractory angina were treated with direct intramyocardial administration of autologous bone marrow, with good results in terms of myocardial perfusion, clinical symptoms, and quality of life, which appeared significantly ameliorated after a 12-month follow-up.

Murine embryonic stem cells (MESC) have been used by Giuseppe Novelli, Professor of Genetics at Tor Vergata University in Rome, as a model for gene therapy. Novelli's group published encouraging results about the possibility of modifying MESCs's genome with small DNA fragments. If the target stem cell bears a mutation, it can be modified with this technique and prospectively used as a therapy for patients suffering from genetic diseases. Novelli studied cystic fibrosis, using the small-fragment homologous replacement method, contributing to assessing the preclinical efficacy of this method in changing advantageously mutations involved in human disease.

## ITALIAN STEM CELL POLICY

Italian policy toward stem cell research is regulated by a law issued in 2004 after a long debate. The Italian law (no. 40/2004), which disciplines assisted reproduction, actually prohibits all human embryo investigation: Any sort of research project based on human ovocytes, sperm, or embryo manipulation is considered illegal. After the approval of this law, however, a group of Italian members of parliament tried to abolish it, promoting a referendum, but the Italian Constitutional Court ruled in favor of an amendment of the law, rather than a complete abolition. Italian public opinion remains divided between two main positions. On one side, the Science and Life Committee position essentially reflected the Catholic and pro-life point of view, assuming that the embryo is a human being and consequently needs to be protected.

On the other, the Referendum Promoting Committee brought together some illustrious Italian scientists such as Umberto Veronesi, who was personally involved in the campaign, and claimed that the amendment of the law would restore freedom of research in Italy. After months of fierce debate, the referendum took place in June 2005, but the law remained unmodified, as a quorum of 50 percent plus one of all the voters was not reached. At the present time, the law remains in force, although part of public opinion remains dissatisfied with the present bill and because of the restrictive rules regarding assisted fertility.

To overcome the moral debate relating to human embryo research in Italy, the use of a particular technique called somatic cell nuclear transfer has been suggested many times in the past, first by the Nobel laureate Renato Dulbecco in 2000, when he had been appointed chief of an ad hoc committee by the Minister of Health.

This method represents a line of research for which Italian scientists made considerable efforts, as the sole use of adult stem cells is not considered appropriate to all contexts of research, and the exploitation of embryonic stem cells produced abroad, although not manifestly prohibited by Italian laws, is very expensive. The process consists of the replacement of the nucleus of an unfertilized human egg cell with another nucleus gathered from a patient's somatic cell. As a result, a valuable source of stem cells can be obtained without using of human embryos. Unfortunately, a sharp dissent was then voiced by the Catholics, as a violation of human dignity was nevertheless seen in such practice.

Meanwhile, new techniques are emerging and being progressively perfected, and embryo-sparing technologies to derive embryonic stem cells without sacrificing the entire embryo might soon provide a valuable and controversy-free embryonic stem cell source.

**SEE ALSO:** Cells, Embryonic; Cloning; European Consortium for Stem Cell Research—EuroStemCell; Human Embryonic Stem Cells; Huntington's Disease; Nuclear Transfer, Somatic; Regulations Overview; Religion, Catholic; Vescovi, Angelo.

**BIBLIOGRAPHY.** Fondazione San Raffaele, "Stem Cells Research Institute Home Page," www.sanraffaele.org/EN_home (cited December 2007); Laboratory of Stem Cell Biology, University of Milan, users.unimi.it/~spharm/cattaneo (cited December 2007).

David James Pinato
Eastern Piedmont University
School of Medicine

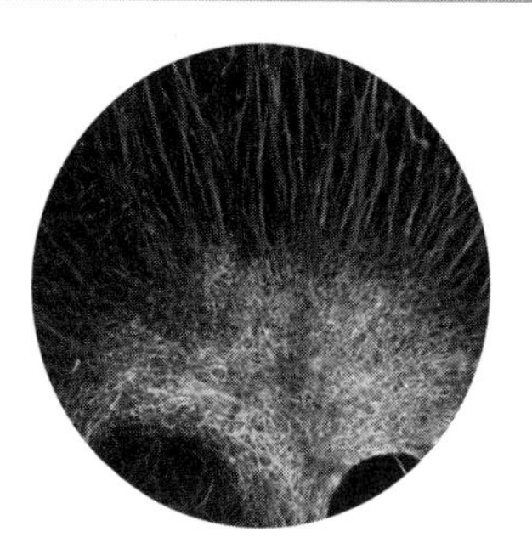

# J

## Jaenisch, Rudolf

**RUDOLF JAENISCH IS** a member of the Whitehead Institute and Professor of Biology at Massachusetts Institute of Technology (Cambridge, MA). Jaenisch's long and impressive career has focused mainly on epigenetic mechanisms in cells. The study of epigenetics relates to understanding how environmental factors surrounding the cell alters gene expression without changing the DNA sequence and what impact this has on the function and development of a cell. To do this Jaenisch has used a range of tools including stem cells, genetically altered mice and cloning techniques.

Jaenisch was born in 1942 in Germany. Jaenisch enrolled in a medical program and pursued additional research opportunities in a leading German laboratory of P. H. Hofschneider where he produced some seminal work studying bacteriophages. He did the rest of his clinical training in Germany and then a post doctoral fellowship in the United States with Arnold Levine at Princeton. Focusing on the virus SV40 and the mechanisms of cancer, Jaenisch moved towards using mice as models for cancer and became fascinated with how and why certain types of cells may be susceptible to getting cancer. Working with the notable developmental biologist Beatrice Mintz, he soon added early embryo development to his list of interests. After starting his own lab at the Salk Institute in California, Jaenisch began collaborating with Paul Berg and others to develop novel ways to detect viral DNA within infected mice. This led to the idea of transgenic animals and finally cloning. A brief time spent back in Germany was followed by his final move to the Whitehead Institute where his work moved to epigenetics and the study of how DNA methylation could control gene expression.

Jaenisch was impressed by the creation of the first cloned animal—Dolly the sheep by Ian Wilmut using somatic cell nuclear transfer. He set out to try to understand how a fully differentiated nucleus from and adult cell could be "reprogrammed" by the egg's cytoplasm. He thought this was the most pure form of epigenetics, and by studying signals involved with this reprogramming it may be possible to better understand biology in general. However, he was also well aware that many clones he produced were not perfect and had developmental or adult problems. One of his goals is to understand why these problems exist and how to fix them. His most recent work has included some seminal papers on induced pluripotent stem (iPS) cells. In an amazing paper he took skin fibroblasts from an adult mouse with sickle cell anemia, an inherited disease, generated iPS cells from them, repaired the defective gene in these cells, differentiated the newly corrected cells into a blood lineage, and cured the same mouse of the disease through bone marrow transplantation. This stands as a testament to his amazing scientific and technical skills and his ability to keep on top of the most exciting discoveries with high quality papers.

Jaenisch's awards include the Peter Gruber prize in Genetics (2001), the Robert Koch Prize for Excellence in Scientific Achievement (2002), and the Charles Rodolphe Bruphacher Foundation Cancer Award (2003). In 2003, Jaenisch was elected to the National Academy of Sciences.

**SEE ALSO:** Massachusetts Institute of Technology; Salk Institute; Somatic Cell Nuclear Transfer; Whitehead Institute; Wilmut, Ian.

**BIBLIOGRAPHY.** J. Hanna, M. Wernig, S. Markoulaki, C. W. Sun, A. Meissner, J. P. Cassady, C. Beard, T. Brambrink, L. C. Wu, T. M. Townes, and R. Jaenisch. "Treatment of Sickle Cell Anemia Mouse Model With iPS Cells Generated From Autologous Skin," *Science*. (Deccember 21, 2007).

Clive Svendsen
Allison Ebert
University of Wisconsin, Madison

# Japan

**STEM CELL RESEARCH** in Japan has lagged behind other countries, such as the United States. Because the government did not approve the establishment of embryonic stem cells in Japan for a long time, Japanese researchers imported stem cells from other countries. From bioethical points of view, derivation and use of human embryonic stem cells have been limited to basic research for the present. Therefore, carrying out clinical research applying human embryonic stem cells or cells originated from these stem cells to the human body has been prohibited, as has utilization of these cells in medicine and in related fields. However, the government recently decided to formulate a strategic, prioritized science and technology budget that is in line with resource-allocation policies focused on innovation creation, including stem cell research.

In 2002 two major initiatives were taken in Japan to create centers that will work with and advance the stem cell research in the country, one at Kyoto University and the other at the RIKEN Institute facility in Kobe. At Kyoto University, a plan to create embryonic stem cells from fertilized eggs left unused from fertility treatments was approved in March 2003 by the government panel under the Ministry of Education, Culture, Sports, Science, and Technology. The approval was the first in Japan related to research on human embryonic stem cells. The second initiative was the Center for Developmental Biology in Kobe—an initiative of RIKEN, Japan's Institute of Physical and Chemical Research. Not only these two initiatives but other institutes such as Keio University School of Medicine (Tokyo), Osaka University Medical School (Osaka), and Mitsubishi Kagaku Institute (Tokyo) have been supported by increasing funding and political support and have been recognized as global stem cell research centers. Many important articles have been published by Japanese researchers at these institutions. Some critics have expressed fears that the government's short-term goals will hold back research. However, the next generation will prove crucial with regard to what role Japan will play in stem cell research.

## GUIDELINES AND RESTRICTIONS

In Japan, the establishment and use of human embryonic stem cell lines must be performed in conformity with the 2001 Guidelines for Derivation and Utilization of Human Embryonic Stem Cells of the Ministry of Education, Culture, Sports, Science, and Technology, after approval by the institutional review board. To date, the government approved proposals by two research institutes to establish human ES cell lines: the Institute for Frontier Medical Sciences, Kyoto University, and the National Research Institute for Child Health and Development, Tokyo. The first group, located at Kyoto University, was organized by Norio Nakatsuji and engaged their project in 2003. Nakatsuji was known earlier for the study of monkey stem cells. Surplus frozen human embryos, donated by consenting couples, were used to establish human embryonic stem cell lines. At present, they provide three human ES cell lines, corded khES-1 (established in August 2003) and khES-2 and khES-3 (both established in November 2003).

In November 2000, the Ministry of Education, Culture, Sports, Science, and Technology established the first guidelines to regulate human cloning techniques and manipulation of human embryos in the Act on Regulation of Human Cloning Techniques. This law describes, first, the prohibition of transferring human cloning embryos (including a human stomatic nuclear transfer embryo, human–animal hybrid embryo, human–animal clone embryo, or human–animal chimeric embryo), and second, establishment guidelines on the handling of specified embryos by the Minister of Education, Culture, Sports, Science, and Technology. In the supplementary provisions of this act, it indicates that the government needs to review this act on the basis of the results of study by the Council for Science and Technology Policy and others on how human fertilized embryos should be handled and should take necessary measures based on the results of the review.

On the basis of the Report on Human Embryo Research Focusing on the Human Embryonic Stem Cells, the Guidelines for Derivation and Utilization of Human Embryonic Stem Cells were established in September 2001 by the Ministry of Education, Culture, Sports, Science, and Technology. The guidelines attempted to appropriately promote research on human embryonic stem cells by providing fundamental rules to be observed from bioethical points of view. This publication indicated that deviation and use of human embryonic stem cells shall always be carried out appropriately in accordance with the guidelines and shall be limited to basic research for the present. Therefore, the following activities should not be carried out under the guidelines: clinical research applying human embryonic stem cells or cells originated from them to the human body, and use of these cells in medicine and related fields.

## STEM CELL RESEARCH INSTITUTIONS

Although the environment surrounding stem cell research is still tough, the numbers of institutions and researchers studying stem cells have been increased gradually. For using human embryonic stem cells in basic researches, a total of 43 proposals have been registered with the Ministry of Education, Culture, Sports, Science, and Technology. The listed institutions include the University of Tokyo (the Institute of Medical Sciences and Graduate School of Medicine and Faculty of Medicine), Kyoto University (Institute for Frontier Medical Sciences and Graduate School of Medicine and Faculty of Medicine), Keio University (School of Medicine), Shinshu University (Graduate School of Medicine), Gifu University (School of Medicine), and RIKEN Center for Developmental Biology.

In August 2006 Kazutoshi Takahashi and Shinya Yamanaka, Japanese stem cell researchers in the Institute for Frontier Medical Sciences, Kyoto University, reported in *Cell* on a quartet of genes, *Oct3/4*, *Sox2*, *c-Myc*, and *Klf4*, that caused cultured mouse skin cells to behave remarkably like embryonic stem cells. They named their stem cells as induced pluripotent stem cells (iPS Cells). In November 2007 Yamanaka published an article in *Cell* indicating that they had succeeded in inducing pluripotent stem cells from adult human fibroblasts, using a similar method as in their mouse study. James Thomson, a pioneering University of Wisconsin molecular biologist, also reported similar success in *Science*.

Although the risk of tumorigenesis resulting from overexpression of a protooncogene c-myc and retroviral gene transfer remains to be determined, it is possible now to produce a stem cell from almost any other human cell instead of using embryos as needed previously, using this novel concept that originated from Japan. Just after Yamanaka's discovery, the Japanese government announced it would increase the strategic budget for stem cell research to enter the stem cell research race. Although stem cell research in Japan has lagged behind other countries, this new discovery will boost stem cell research.

**SEE ALSO:** Japan Human Cell Society; Kyoto University; Okano, Hideyuki; Thomson, James.

**BIBLIOGRAPHY.** Bureau of Science and Technology policy, Cabinet Office, Government of Japan, "Science and Technology Policy, Council for Science and Technology Policy," www8.cao.go.jp (cited June 2007); Center for Developmental Biology, "RIKEN Center for Developmental Biology (RIKEN CDB)," www.cdb.riken.jp (cited October 2007); "Japan Joins Global Research Race, Domestic Stem-Cell Creation Approved," *Japan Times* (March 28, 2007); Kyoto University, "Institute for Frontier Medical Sciences, Kyoto University," www.frontier.kyoto-u.ac.jp (cited November 2007); Minister of Education and Science in Japan, "Guidelines to the Law Concerning Regulation Relating to Human Cloning Techniques and Other Similar Techniques" (December 2001); Ministry of Education, Culture, Sports, Science, and Technology, "The Guidelines for Derivation and Utilization of Human Embryonic Stem Cells," www.mext.go.jp, September 2001 (cited November 2007); National Institutes of Health, "International Stem Cell Research," stemcells.nih.gov (cited November 2007); Kazutoshi Takahashi, et al., "Induction of Pluripotent Stem Cells from Adult Human Fibroblasts by Defined Factors," *Cell* (v.131, 2007); Kazutoshi Takahashi and Shinya Yamanaka, "Induction of Pluripotent Stem Cells from Mouse Embryonic and Adult Fibroblast Cultures by Defined Factors," *Cell* (v.126/4, 2006); University of Minnesota Medical School, "Stem Cell Policy: Stem Cell Research Center," www.mbbnet.umn.edu (cited November 2007); Junying Yu, et al, "Induced Pluripotent Stem Cell Lines Derived from Human Somatic Cells," *Science* (v.318, 2007).

Masatoshi Suzuki
University of Wisconsin, Madison

# Japan Human Cell Society

**THE JAPAN HUMAN** Cell Society (Nihon Hito Saibou Gakkai) is a Japanese professional society for basic scientists and physicians whose research is focused on the study of human cells. The Japan Human Cell Society, originally established in 1983 as the Human Cell Research Meeting (Nihonn Hito Saibou Kennkyu-kai), is open to a growing number of people earnestly seeking the establishment of an institution allowing the comprehensive presentation of research findings and exchange of opinions by persons in various fields in Japan, and the publication of a technical journal relating to human cells. At present, this society has 600 members around the world.

The society publishes a bimonthly peer-reviewed journal—*Human Cell*—that is widely regarded as one of the preeminent journals in the field. This official journal of the Japan Human Cell Society was first published in 1998. In 1990, this research meeting further evolved into the Japan Human Cell Society, and *Human Cell* was reborn as the official journal of this society. This publication was registered in Index Medius and PubMed starting in 1992. An editorial branch office for this publication was opened in the United States in 2004. Twenty volumes of *Human Cell* had been published by December 2007.

*Human Cell* publishes original research articles of studies using human cells, embryonic stem cells derived from animals, or regenerative medicine using animal cells. One of the characteristics of this journal is the large number of papers it contains on cell line derivation. The journal serves as a forum for international research on all aspects of human cell biology and related disciplines, in addition to showcasing the research activities of the society. Papers in any of the following categories will be considered: research articles, rapid communications, reviews, and letters to the editor. The current editor-in-chief is Isamu Ishiwata, from the Ishiwata Obstetric and Gynecologic Hospital, Mito, Ibaraki, Japan.

**SEE ALSO:** Japan; Kyoto University.

**BIBLIOGRAPHY.** Blackwell Publishing, *Human Cell*, www.blackwellpublishing.com (cited November 2007); Isamu Ishikawa, "Towards Enrichment of *Human Cell*," *Human Cell* (v. 19/1, 2006); Japan Human Cell Society, "The Japan Human Cell Society," jhcs.umin.jp (cited November 2007); University Hospital Information Network, "The Japan Human Cell Society," center.umin.ac.jp (cited November 2007).

Masatoshi Suzuki
University of Wisconsin, Madison

# Johns Hopkins University

**JOHNS HOPKINS UNIVERSITY** (1876) is a private university located in Baltimore, Maryland. Johns Hopkins offers both undergraduate and graduate programs and was the first university in the United States to emphasize research in education. The mission of Hopkins is "The encouragement of research . . . and the advancement of individual scholars, who by their excellence will advance the sciences they pursue, and the society where they dwell." Johns Hopkins, in fact, was a model for most large research universities throughout the United States.

The university boasts 32 Nobel laureates and is academically strong in every discipline, from art history to biomedical engineering to international studies to romantic languages.

Johns Hopkins used $1.44 billion in science, medical, and engineering research in the 2005 fiscal year, which made it the leading U.S. academic institution in research and development spending. The National Science Foundation ranked Johns Hopkins as number one on the list of institutions receiving federally funded research and development, which for Johns Hopkins amounted to over $1.2 billion. Research at Johns Hopkins on stem cells is supported by the National Institutes of Health (NIH), healthcare organizations, partnerships with corporations, and private donors.

At Johns Hopkins, undergraduate students are expected and encouraged to become involved with undergraduate research. In this respect, some undergraduate students have the opportunity to work alongside graduate students, postdoctoral fellows, and leading professionals in science to study stem cells in a laboratory setting. Johns Hopkins is also renowned for its academic healthcare centers and its graduate schools of medicine, public health, and international studies. The Johns Hopkins Hospital was ranked as the top hospital in the United States in the *U.S. News and World Report* annual ranking of American hospitals for the 17th year in a row; the medical school ranked second in the nation.

## CURRENT STEM CELL RESEARCH

Johns Hopkins explains in its publications that one of the greatest discoveries made in medicine was the potential of a single, undifferentiated cell; Johns Hopkins has noted in several instances that the use of a single, undifferentiated cell could be used in the future to address disease, pain, and cancer. The university, along with other organizations and institutions, also realizes that stem cell research raises ethical concerns and that policy and politics on stem cell research must be carefully regulated and balanced by science and medicine. Researchers at Johns Hopkins, and around the globe, are excited about the potential of the stem cell and the prospects of its use as a medical therapy in the future.

John Gearhart of Johns Hopkins discovered that a type of pluripotent stem cell could be isolated from human gonadal tissues in 1998. This stem cell (the embryonic germ cell) seemed similar to human embryonic stem cells discovered in the same year by Dr. James Thomson at the University of Wisconsin, Madison. However, over the years the embryonic germ cell has not gained widespread use in the scientific community.

Johns Hopkins believes that the use of stem cells for the promotion of human health and lifestyle should be the focus of biomedical experimentation and understanding. Hopkins supports the use of the somatic cell nuclear transferring

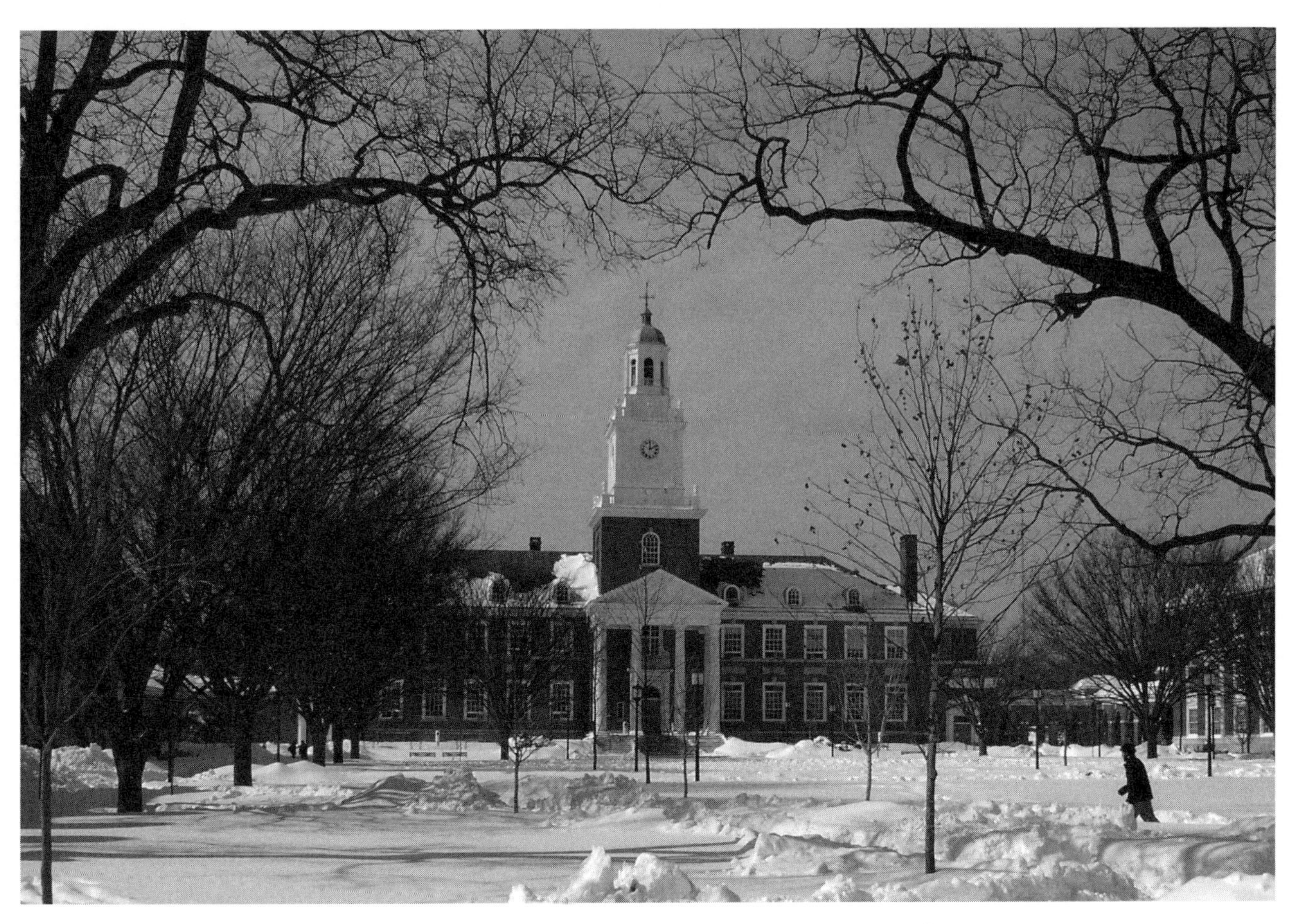

*As the leader among U.S. academic institutions in research and development spending, with $1.44 billion in science, medical, and engineering research in 2005 alone, Johns Hopkins is poised to become a major force in the world of stem cell research.*

technique (research cloning) to produce stem cell lines that are genetically identical to the parent cell; the stem cell lines, although controversial for some, give researchers a tool that will allow them to understand the development and progression of the cell and of disease and to predict what sorts of therapies could be used to treat disease and injury.

The use of somatic cell nuclear transfer could also reduce the possibility that a body would reject the transplantation. Reproductive cloning, however, is strongly opposed by the institution. Reproductive cloning can be defined as the use of biomedical technology and somatic cell nuclear transfer for the purpose of cloning a human being.

**SEE ALSO:** Clinical Trials Within U.S.: Blind Process; Federal Government Policies; Regulations Overview; United States.

**BIBLIOGRAPHY.** L. Cheng, et al., "Human Adult Marrow Cells Support Prolonged Expansion of Human Embryonic Stem Cells in Culture," *Stem Cells* (v.21, 2003); J. D. Gearhart, "New Potential for Human Embryonic Germ Cells," *Science* (v.282, 1999); D. Solter and J. D. Gearhart, "Putting Stem Cells to Work," *Science* (v.283, 1999); Johns Hopkins University, "A Brief History of JHU," webapps.jhu.edu (cited August 2007).

Krishna Subhash Vyas
University of Kentucky

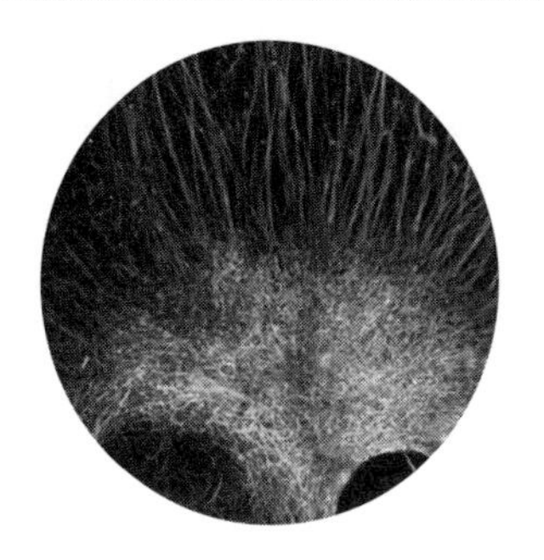

# K

## Kansas

**KANSAS BECAME THE** 34th state of the United States in 1861 and occupies the exact center of the landmass of the continental United States. It has a total area of just over 82,000 square miles and is bordered by Nebraska, Missouri, Oklahoma, and Colorado. The capital city is Topeka, although both Wichita and Kansas City are now larger and more populous urban areas. The total population of the state is more than two and a half million. The name Kansas derives from the name of the Native Americans who were previously in occupation of the land. A number of Native Americans were relocated to what is now Kansas when settlers elsewhere wished to acquire the land on which they lived. For a period, Kansas, together with Nebraska, was intended to be a form of large-scale Indian reservation, but the continued demand for land and other resources meant that settlers continued to enter the state, and the reservation plan was abandoned.

Kansas was caught between the North and the South during the American Civil War, and the state was a battleground for rival political ideologies, which, in some ways, it has remained subsequently. Lying on the Great Plains, and specifically on the westward-rising landscape, Kansas has come to represent not just the geographical center of the country but also its moral and political center. Although Republican Senator Sam Brownback is a long-standing and rather outspoken opponent of embryonic stem cell research, for example, the Kansas State University–based Midwest Institute for Comparative Stem Cell Biology has been pursuing a range of research issues in the field of stem cells based on the use of umbilical cord material, which is free of ethical controversy.

Kansas has a well-developed tertiary education sector, which provides many opportunities for joint research projects and networking. Research output is linked to entrepreneurial opportunities through the National Institute for Strategic Technology Acquisition and Commercialization and the Kansas State University Research Fund.

Kansas has been a traditionally Republican state, although demographic and economic changes in urban areas in particular have changed the political complexion of the state overall. Political conservatism of the Kansan type is not customarily opposed to scientific progress such as that represented by stem cell research. However, in recent years, factions within the Republican Party have endeavored, with electoral success, to equate narrowly defined moral

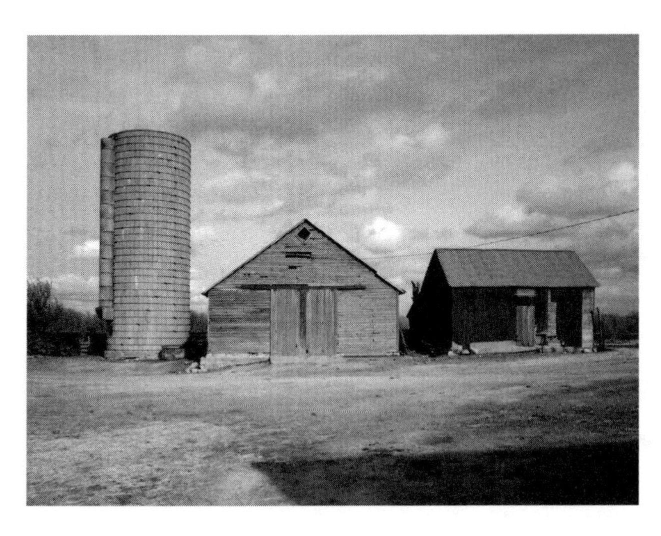

*Throughout history, technology has helped Kansans with such problems as grasshopper infestations and unproductive land.*

issues with a broader conservative world view as a means of persuading people to vote against their own economic interests. Stem cell research and, in particular, embryonic stem cell research has been seized on in this regard as the kind of high-profile and emotive issue that can be used to label people representing alternative political ideals as being immoral and unsuitable for office. The rhetoric surrounding stem cell research is in contrast with the actual process of scientific progress, which is bringing tangible benefits to many.

A survey conducted in 2006 found that an overwhelming majority of Kansas residents (nearly 2-to-1) favored supporting stem cell research using both embryonic and adult stem cells. Furthermore, most Kansas residents opposed a ban on somatic cell nuclear transfer (SCNT) and favored allowing scientists to use donated embryos from in vitro fertilization clinics. A bill proposed by the Kansas state legislature would criminalize SCNT with the intention of preventing reproductive cloning, but at the expense of therapeutic cloning. Therefore, the generation of new embryonic stem cell lines would be outlawed as well.

**SEE ALSO:** *Individual U.S. State Articles*; Biotechnology, History of; Clinical Trials Within U.S.: Batten Disease; Clinical Trials Within U.S.: Blind Process; Clinical Trials Within U.S.: Cancer; Clinical Trials Within U.S.: Heart Disease; Clinical Trials Within U.S.: Peripheral Vascular Disease; Clinical Trials Within U.S.: Skin Transplants (Burns); Clinical Trials Within U.S.: Spinal Cord Injury; Clinical Trials Within U.S.: Traumatic Brain Injury; Ethics; Federal Government Policies; Moral Status of Embryo; Special Interest/Lobby Groups; United States.

**BIBLIOGRAPHY.** Kansas University Medical Center, www.kumc.edu/stemcell/toolkit2.html (cited June 2008); Midwest Institute for Comparative Stem Cell Biology, www.vet.ksu.edu/research/stemcell (cited November 2007); Craig Miner, *Kansas: The History of the Sunflower State, 1854–2000* (U. Press of Kansas, 2005).

John Walsh
Shinawatra University

# Keller, Gordon

**GORDON M. KELLER** is the senior scientist in the Division of Stem Cell and Developmental Biology at the Ontario Cancer Institute. He is also the director of the McEwen Centre for Regenerative Medicine and works at the MaRS Center in the Toronto Medical Discovery Tower in Canada. He also holds the Canada Research Chair in embryonic stem biology.

Keller's research interests are in the areas of lineage-specific differentiation of embryonic stem (ES) cells in culture; development of hematopoietic, vascular, and cardiac lineages from ES cells; commitment of ES cells to endoderm-derived lineages; and growth and differentiation of human embryonic stem cells. More specifically, Keller is focused on a research program that is seeking to define and to describe fully the essentials of the process of embryonic development. He is seeking to understand the early events that are part of the process of the establishment, growth, and maturation of the embryonic hematopoietic and vascular system.

Hematopoiesis is the process that results in the formation of blood cellular components. The cells involved are multipotent because they have the ability to become a number of different types of cells. They are not, however, germ cells, which are part of the reproductive process. Specifically, any type of cell found in the blood system can be made from the multipotent hematopoietic cells. The rate of production of cells in the blood system is at a relatively high rate, so great numbers of these cells are continually being made.

Identifying and understanding the earliest blood cell precursors of the hematopoietic system will aid in the development of treatments. There are also endothelial precursors involved. These precursors form the vascular system, and develop into structures known as blood islands. These islands can be found in the yolk sac of the mouse embryo and develop after 7.5 days of gestation.

The development of hematopoietic and endothelial lineages in near simultaneity in the blood islands is a kind of scientific platform. From it, Keller has hypothesized that both of these lineages are developing from a progenitor cell that has issued a series of commands for development. The progenitor cell is called the hemangioblast. Understanding the nature of the hemangioblast is very important because doing so will answer questions about the early stages of lineage commitment.

Studying mouse embryos before blood island development is an important part of the current research. It is extremely difficult to gain access to the mouse embryo at fewer than seven days because there are just a few cells available. To study the very early events, Keller has developed a model that is based on the in vitro potential of ES cells.

Keller and others have found that as ES cells differentiate in cultures, they generate colonies that have been labeled embryoid bodies (EBs). These bodies consist of the precursors from multiple lineages, including those of the hematopoietic and vascular systems. From earlier studies, it is known that as the embryo develops, it establishes both the hematopoietic and the endothelial lineages. What happens within the EB parallels the kinetics of development as well as the differential gene expression patterns.

As Keller has used the embryonic stem cell differentiation model, he has found a novel precursor. It develops very early in the EBs and then displays a unique power to generate cells. The cells it generates are of both the hematopoietic and endothelial lineages. This novel precursor has been found by Keller to have the characteristics of the hypothetical hemangioblast. It surely represents the earliest of the hematopoietic and endothelial precursor cells that have been described.

During his investigations, Keller and his associates have used a subtractive hybridization method. The method is used between closely staged populations. The aim has been to identify genes that are involved in the development of the hemangioblast, from which there is the subsequent generation of hematopoietic and endothelial progeny.

Keller's subtractive hybridization method has successfully isolated a number of new genes. These are expressed at the stage of hemangioblasts. In addition, they are found in the embryonic hematopoietic and endothelial stages. These stages are ones in which lineages of isolated EBs are found.

The current focus of Keller's laboratory is to define the functions of the genes that have been identified. The next step is to map their role in the development of hematopoiesis and vascular biology.

Keller is president of the International Society for Stem Cell Research (ISSCR). In 2005, as president of the society, he addressed an open letter to the president of Italy, Romano Prodi, and to the ministers of the Italian Republic. The letter supported Italian Minister of Research and University Fabio Mussi's decision to withdraw from the European Union's Ethical Declaration against Human Embryonic Stem Cell Research as an ethical act supported by the ISSCR.

**SEE ALSO:** Canadian Stem Cell Network; Cells, Embryonic; International Society for Stem Cell Research.

**BIBLIOGRAPHY.** S. L. D'Souza, A. G. Elefanty, and Gordon Keller, "SCL/Tal-1 Is Essential for Hematopoietic Commitment of the Hemangioblast," *Blood* (v.105/10, 2005); H. J. Fehling, et al., "Tracking Mesoderm Induction and Its Specification to the Hemangioblast," *Development* (v.130/17, 2003); Gordon Keller,

"Embryonic Stem Cell Differentiation: Emergence of a New Era," *Biology and Genes Development* (v.19/10, 2005); Gordon M. Keller and Paul M. Wassarman, *Differentiation of Embryonic Stem Cells* (Elsevier Academic, 2003); H. T. Ku, et al., "Committing Embryonic Stem Cells to Early Endocrine Pancreas In Vitro," *Stem Cells* (v.22/7, 2004); A. Kubo, et al., "The Homeobox Gene HEX Regulates Proliferation and Differentiation of Blood," *Blood* (v.105/12, 2005); A. Kubo, et al., "Development of Definitive Endoderm from Embryonic Stem Cells in Culture," *Development* (v.131/7, 2004); G. Lacaud, et al., "Haploinsufficiency of Runx1 Results in the Acceleration of Mesodermal," *Blood* (v.103/3, 2004); G. Lacaud, Gordon Keller, and V. Kouskoff, "Tracking Mesoderm Formation and Specification to the Hemangioblast in Trends," *Cardiovascular Medicine* (v.14/8, 2004); J. G. Lieber, et al., "The In Vitro Production and Characterization of Neutrophils from Embryonic Blood," *Blood* (v.103/3, 2004); R. Martin, et al., "SCL Interacts with VEGF to Suppress Apoptosis at the Onset of Development," *Development* (v.131/3, 2004); D. Mohn, et al., "Mouse Mix Gene Is Activated Early during Differentiation of ES and F9 Stem," *Development Dynamics* (v.226/3, 2003).

Andrew J. Waskey
Dalton State College

# Kentucky

**KENTUCKY IS THE** 26th largest state by population and the 37th largest by land area in the United States. The state has two major research universities, the University of Kentucky and the University of Louisville. These two universities jointly control in excess of $400 million in federal research funding. In 1994 the state of Kentucky established a spinal cord and head injury research trust funded by surcharges on traffic citations. This research trust fund has greatly bolstered support for researchers in Kentucky to develop stem cell–based treatments for traumatic and degenerative neurological illnesses. Research at the University of Kentucky has focused on the relationship of stem cells to hematological malignancies. At the University of Louisville, stem cell research has focused on stem cell–based therapy for spinal cord injury and on methods of extracting and modifying stem cells from adult organisms.

## UNIVERSITY OF KENTUCKY

At the University of Kentucky, age-related changes in adult stem cells have been studied extensively. Dr. Gary Van Zant's stem cell research group has demonstrated that some characteristics of aging may be the consequence of stem cell dysfunction. Specific findings include a correlation between DNA fidelity in mouse hematopoietic stem cells and mean life expectancy. In related research, Van Zant and his colleagues at the University of Kentucky have been instrumental in demonstrating that hematological malignancies may be caused by changes in the response of stem cells to growth factor or by errors in stem cell DNA repair.

Marrow stem cell research has also demonstrated that bone marrow stem cells from older donors may have errant homing mechanisms, possibly as a result of age-related changes. Therefore, a bone marrow transplant from an older individual is less likely to be successful even if the stem cells appear healthy. The relationship of stem cells to hematological cancers might mean that treatment failure of leukemias and lymphomas could be in part a result of the treatment response of differentiated cancer cells, without a commensurate response in the cancer stem cells that are available to repopulate the tumor.

In addition, Van Zant's laboratory has also identified and mapped a stem cell gene *Latexin*, which is instrumental in determining the number of adult stem cells in the body (particularly in the bone marrow). It may be possible to exploit the properties of this gene and reduce recovery time following chemotherapy as well as increase the number of viable cells following bone marrow transplant. The Latexin protein may also increase stem cells in umbilical cord blood to a level sufficient for transplant therapy in adult patients.

The universities of Kentucky and Louisville are both participating in the Osiris phase 3 clinical trial, "Evaluation of Prochymal Adult Human Stem Cells for Treatment-Resistant Moderate to Severe Crohn's Disease." Crohn's disease is a debilitating gastrointestinal disorder with a hypothesized autoimmune etiology, but no truly effective cures. This study is one of the first phase 3 clinical trials involving stem cells. In this therapy, adult human stem cells obtained from healthy volunteers are modified by a proprietary method and infused into Crohn's patients who failed conventional treatment methods. The trial is placebo controlled. These modified adult stem cells are hypothesized to have an immunosuppressive effect that could improve Crohn's symptoms and disease course. The study director, Dr. Jane Onken, is based at Duke University in North Carolina.

## UNIVERSITY OF LOUISVILLE

In 2005 researchers in Dr. Fred Roisen's lab at the University of Louisville demonstrated partial recovery of spinal cord–injured rats following a form of stem cell therapy. The research of Roisen's group has focused on glial-restricted precursors, a type of partially differentiated neural stem cell that can further differentiate into the support cells of the nervous system—astrocytes or oligodendrocytes. These researchers were prompted to study possible therapy with oligodendrocytes because of findings of nerve demyelination after spinal cord injury.

In Roisen's 2005 study, glial precursor cells modified by gene therapy were injected into the spinal cords of rats that had suffered an experimentally induced spinal cord injury. Rats that received the combination gene/stem cell treatment showed statistically significant improvement in limb function and spinal cord impulse conduction, whereas control animals that received no therapy or either the gene or stem cell therapy alone demonstrated no significant improvement. Postmortem examination of the treated spinal cords demonstrated that stem cells had migrated into the spinal cord and formed myelin-producing oligodendrocytes.

In response to federal limitations on the available funding sources for embryonic stem cell research, some Kentucky scientists have sought to obtain nonembryonic stem cell lines that display characteristics similar to those demonstrated by embryonic stem cells.

The research group of Dr. Mariusz Ratajczak at the University of Louisville has explored the use of progenitor cells from the olfactory neurosensory endothelium as a possible source for cells that display many of the properties common to embryonic stem cells. These cells, obtainable from endoscopic sinus surgery, demonstrate an almost unlimited capacity for replication and, when isolated in culture, express proteins such as nestin that are characteristically found in neural stem cells. The tendency of these olfactory neurosensory progenitor cells to differentiate into neurons of specific types can be enhanced by specific signaling molecules. Under the influence of exogenous signaling, differentiation into myelin and dopamine-producing cells have both been demonstrated. These characteristics could eventually be used in designing experimental therapies for Parkinson's disease or multiple sclerosis.

Ratajczak's group at the University of Louisville has also demonstrated that a particular population of adult hematopoietic stem cells may have properties that are similar to those of embryonic stem cells. These cells, which are present in small numbers in adult bone marrow, are termed *very small embryonic-like cells*, or VSELs. Although rare in adult marrow, Louisville researchers have demonstrated that VSELs can be grown in vitro once they are isolated from a murine source. Once amplified by culture, these cell populations can be manipulated in traditional ways with growth factors to differentiate into various cell lines such as cardiac cells, neurons, and pancreatic cells.

Kentucky currently has no laws banning or encouraging embryonic stem cell research. Kentucky legislators have proposed a ballot measure for the 2008 election that would provide state constitutional protection for conducting stem cell research. Similar ballot measures were first proposed in Missouri. Kentucky state legislators have discussed methods for allocating state funds for embryonic stems cell research similar to the popularly approved California stem cell research initiative.

**SEE ALSO:** *Individual U.S. State Articles*; Biotechnology, History of; Clinical Trials Within U.S.: Batten Disease; Clinical Trials Within U.S.: Blind Process; Clinical Trials Within U.S.: Cancer; Clinical Trials Within U.S.: Heart Disease; Clinical Trials Within U.S.: Peripheral Vascular Disease; Clinical Trials Within U.S.: Skin Transplants (Burns); Clinical Trials Within U.S.: Spinal Cord Injury; Clinical Trials Within U.S.: Traumatic Brain Injury; Ethics; Federal Government Policies; Moral Status of Embryo; Special Interest/Lobby Groups; United States.

**BIBLIOGRAPHY.** Y. Liang, et al., "The Quantitative Trait Gene Latexin Influences the Size of the Hematopoietic Stem Cell Population in Mice," *Nature Genetics* (v.39/2, 2007); C. T. Marshall, et al., "The Therapeutic Potential of Human Olfactory-Derived Stem Cells," *Histology and Histopathology* (v.21/6, 2006); "Missouri's Stem Cell Ballot Measure Too Close to Call," *USA Today,* November 8, 2006, www.usatoday.com, (cited November 2007); University of Kentucky, uky .edu (cited November 2007); University of Louisville, louisville.edu (cited November 2007).

John S. Kuo
University of Wisconsin

# Korea, South

**SOUTH KOREA HAS** made stem cell research headlines several times, thanks both to the use of cord blood cells in treating spinal cord injury and to the research fraud scandal of Hwang Woo-Suk. Similar to many other Asian nations, South Korea is more permissive of embryonic human stem cell research than most Western countries. This difference in attitude is often credited to the fact that Asian countries lack a history of abortion debates, which in the Western world have put a premium on unborn human life and have underscored the beliefs of at least some Christian Westerners that life begins at conception or during gestation. Though South Korea has been subject to diligent Christian missions, especially in the years since the Korean War, its philosophical and moral heritage remains fundamentally Confucian.

Though Confucius does not in his writings specify the moment at which life begins, any more than the Bible does, Confucian tradition holds that life—personhood, humanity, selfhood—begins at birth. Personhood requires the presence of a psyche, a mind, an awareness of some sort; the Western Christian idea of a soul that resides in the unborn fetus is a foreign one to most Confucians, and the embryo does not have the special mystique for them that it seems to have for so many Westerners. This is not to say that it is treated casually or that South Koreans support human embryonic stem cell research unanimously.

On November 25, 2004, a team of researchers from Chosun University, Seoul National University, and the Seoul Cord Blood Bank reported the successful transplant of multipotent adult stem cells isolated from umbilical cord blood. The recipient of the cells (Hwang Mi-Soon, age 37 at the time) was a spinal cord injury patient who subsequently recovered her mobility and ability to walk after 19 years in a wheelchair. Within two weeks, she was able to move her hips; two weeks after that, she was walking with the assistance of a walker. Magnetic resonance imaging and computed tomography scans showed regeneration of the spinal cord, though Western commentators warned that the recovery could be coincidental.

Not long after the Hwang Mi-Soon case, South Korea published its Bioethics and Biosafety Act, which went into effect on January 1, 2005. The act set out guidelines for Korean human embryo stem cell research as follows: human cloning is prohibited; producing embryos for anything other than the purpose of pregnancy is likewise prohibited (in other words, there is a ban on "embryo farms" producing embryos for research or other purposes); embryos that have been stored for more than five years may only be used for research on contraception, infertility, the cure of rare or incurable disease (as decreed by the president), or other research that has been approved by the president and the Bioethics Committee, and in such cases, research may only be conducted on embryos in which embryological primitive streaks have not yet appeared; and somatic cell nucleus transfer shall not be conducted except in the course of research to cure rare diseases or those as yet incurable by other means.

## SCANDAL

The proscription against cloning was in part a response to the work of Hwang Woo-Suk, a South Korean medical researcher who had just had a study published in the journal *Science*, claiming to have produced human embryonic stem cells through cloning. A veterinarian who went into scientific research in the hopes of producing a superior cow, he first captured media attention in 1999, at the age of 46, when he announced he had created a cloned dairy cow he named Yeongrong-i, the fifth successful cow clone. Amid the media flurry, which reintensified two months later when he announced he had also produced Jin-i, the first clone of a Korean cow, it was noted that although he was very communicative with the media, he produced no scientific evidence of his claims. Still, Hwang was considered a scientific hero of sorts in South Korea.

Over the next five years, Hwang continued to work in bovine medicine and genetics, claiming that he had produced a cow resistant or immune to bovine spongiform encephalopathy (mad cow disease), another claim that has not been verified. Then, in a February 2004 press announcement preceding the publication of his article in the March 12 issue of *Science*, Hwang claimed that he had created an embryonic stem cell through somatic nuclear transfer—the first cloned human stem cell—using 242 eggs and somatic cells from a single female donor. A year later, a further paper claimed that he had produced 11 human embryonic stem cells using 185 eggs and somatic cells from a variety of different patients, which in of itself constituted a major breakthrough above and beyond the achievement of cloning.

Only two months after that announcement, Hwang's team announced the first successful dog clone, an Afghan hound named Snuppy (for *SNU*—Seoul National University, Hwang's employer—plus *puppy*). Snuppy was carried to term by a Labrador Retriever in a project in which 1,095 embryos were transplanted into 123 dogs. Of the three pregnancies that resulted, one ended in spontaneous miscarriage and two were carried to term—the other clone died of pneumonia as a puppy. The dog brought SNU and Hwang inevitable prestige on top of his previous accomplishments, and he was appointed head of the World Stem Cell Hub. Then, however, Hwang's stories started to unravel.

First, in late 2005, University of Pittsburgh researcher Gerald Schatten announced the end of his collaboration with Hwang, citing concerns about egg donations involved in the research, and asked *Science* to remove his name from the Hwang papers. (*Science* refused, on the basis of its official policy on such matters.) Days later, another Hwang collaborator, Roh Sung-il, held a press conference to announce that, unbeknownst to Hwang, he had purchased eggs from women for $1,400 each. Hwang resigned from his post but maintained his innocence. The Ministry of Health argued that because no commercial interest had been furthered, no ethical breach had been made in the exchange of eggs for money. Media attention to the matter was received unfavorably by a South Korean public that considered Hwang a national hero, and many women came forward volunteering to donate their eggs to his research in the future.

Meanwhile, Seoul National University took a close look at Hwang's work and soon concluded that—although Snuppy was a genuine clone—all of Hwang's human stem cell work was fraudulent and fabricated. None of the stem cells he claimed to have cloned could be matched to patient DNA; his study had been supplied with 2,061 eggs, not 185, and he had himself distributed the donation forms of which he claimed to be unaware; and parthenogenetic process had not been ruled out as a source of the 2004 stem cell. *Science* retracted his two articles on January 11, 2006, and the next day Hwang held a press conference, blaming other members of his team for deceiving him, alleging theft, sabotage, and a conspiracy. He claimed that the technology for human cloning existed, that he possessed it, and that if given six months, he could reproduce his results. A week later, he claimed that two of his stem cell lines had been switched without his knowledge.

Hwang resigned his position at the university but had his resignation held until the university's investigation could conclude, at which point his employment was terminated; he was indicted shortly after for fraud, violation of bioethics law, and embezzling research funds. In retrospect, it seems possible that his cloned cow claims were false as well. The sad thing is that his grandiose claims overshadowed his real accomplishments: the creation of Snuppy and the possibly accidental discovery of a method of parthenogenesis that can be used to create genetically matched stem cells.

Hwang remains a popular figure in his country, with many supporters claiming he was wrongfully persecuted. In the meantime, the depth of his deception has caused a flurry of activity among bioethicists and policy makers and has fed the fear that although Asia may have a great deal to contribute in the field of stem cell research, the lax regulations that allow this research to be conducted also enable the possibility of science-damaging scandals such as this one.

**SEE ALSO:** Cells, Sources of; Cloning; Egg Donation; International Laws; Methods of Growing Cells; Moral Status of Embryo; Parthogenesis.

**BIBLIOGRAPHY.** "Disgraced Korean Cloning Scientist Indicted," *New York Times*, May 12, 2006; W. S. Hwang, et al., "Evidence of a Pluripotent Human Embryonic Stem Cell Line Derived from a Cloned Blastocyst," *Science* (v.303/5664, 2004); W. S. Hwang, et al., "Patient-Specific Embryonic Stem Cells Derived from Human SCNT Blastocysts," *Science* (v.308/5729, 2005).

Bill Kte'pi
Independent Scholar

# Kriegstein, Arnold

**PROFESSOR ARNOLD R. KRIEGSTEIN** is the director of the Institute for Regeneration Medicine at the University of California, San Francisco. He gained his bachelor's degree in biology from Yale University in 1971 and then proceeded to New York University, where he gained his master's of science degree in physiology in 1974. He then worked on his doctoral thesis on physiology and completed his medical degree at New York University, graduating with both in 1977.

His doctoral thesis was "Development of Sea Hare, *Aplysia californica*," a 68-page work in which Kriegstein managed to study in detail the development of the nervous system of the *A. californica*, which led to an article, "Development of the Nervous System of *Aplysia californica*," published in the *Proceedings of the National Academy of Sciences* in 1977. This in turn led to Kriegstein's interest in the human nervous system and the problems that arose when it was damaged. From his work then to his work now, Kriegstein has been involved in regeneration medicine, in which stem cells and other areas have been investigated to help regenerate damaged and injured tissue and organs.

From 1978 until 1981, Kriegstein was a neurology resident in the Harvard Longwood Area Program at the Peter Bent Brigham Hospital, the Beth Israel Hospital, and the Boston Children's Hospital in Boston, Massachusetts. He then moved to Stanford University as the assistant professor of neurology at Stanford's Department of Neurology from 1981 until 1988. During that time, from 1982 until 1984, he was a Mellon scholar, and in 1986 he was the Stanford University William M. Hume Faculty Scholar.

In 1987 he was appointed by the Italian Ministry of Public Education as the visiting professor of neurology and lecturer in clinical neuroscience at the University of Bari in the southeast of Italy. This position lasted until 1989, and in 1991 Kriegstein won the Wellcome Research Travel Award to Britain and was appointed clinical associate professor at the Department of Neurology at Yale University, New Haven, Connecticut. He remained there until 1993 and was also an associate research scientist at the Department of Neurobiology at Yale.

In 1994 Kriegstein was appointed associate professor of neurology at the College of Physicians and Surgeons of Columbia University, New York, and was also jointly appointed in the departments of neurology and pathology and at the Center for Neurobiology and Behavior in New York. In 1999 Kriegstein was promoted to professor of neurology at the College of Physicians and Surgeons of Columbia University, receiving the Javits Neuroscience Investigator Award in the same year, and remained there as professor of neurology until 2001, when he was further promoted to become the John and Elisabeth Harris Professor of Neurology (in pathology and in the Center for Neurobiology and Behavior) at the College of Physicians and Surgeons of Columbia University. In 2004, Kriegstein was appointed professor of neurology at the University of California, San Francisco, and also director of the Institute for Regeneration Medicine at the same university.

Throughout his distinguished medical career, Kriegstein has written extensively for many scientific and medical journals; his first major work was as a coauthor, with J. J. Lo Turco, of "Clusters of Coupled Neuroblasts in Embryonic Neocortex," which was published in *Science* in 1991. His first paper for which he was lead author was written with B. A. Armitage and P. Y. Kim, being "Heroin Inhalation and Progressive Spongiform Leukoencephalopathy," published in the *New England Journal of Medicine* in 1997. Other journals to which he has contributed include the *Journal of Cell Biology*, *Neuron*, *Clia*, *Cerebral Cortex*, *Journal of Neuroscience*, and *Stem Cells*. One of his papers, cowritten with S. C. Noctor, A. C. Flint, T. A. Weissman, and R. S. Dammerman, "Neurons Derived from Radial Glial Cells Establish Radial Units in Neocortex," was published in *Nature* in 2001, receiving much acclaim.

Since starting his in-depth research into stem cells and related fields in 1984, he has been involved in many projects. Three that he has completed involved research on glycine receptors and the disorders of corticogenesis, conducted with the support of the National Institutes of Health; another project for the Citizens United for Research in Epilepsy on the pathogenesis of cortical lesions in a model of tuberous sclerosis; and the third, for the Lieber Foundation, was on exploring the role of the neurodevelopmental mechanisms that may underlie schizophrenia. There are also four major ongoing projects. The first was about intercellular signaling in neocortical development, which involved a large number of experiments designed to illuminate how epigenetic signals, including those from amino acid neurotransmitters and their receptors, are involved in the influencing of critical events in early corticogenesis, as well as the mechanisms that were involved in the regulating of symmetrical and asymmetrical cell divisions.

Another ongoing project, starting in 1997, covered the physiology of radial units in corticogenesis. This involved trying to address new questions that had emerged and that concerned the clonal relationship of neural progenitor cells and their daughter neurons. It involved a particular focus on the role of gap junctions in cortical development.

The third ongoing project undertaken by Kriegstein was about microcephaly in regards to brain formation and behavior. In this project, Kriegstein and his team have been examining the dynamics of proliferation in the embryonic telencephalon in normal and also in mutant mice to gain further insights into the mechanisms that the mice use to regulate neurogenesis in health and disease. His last major ongoing research project, with the U.S. Army Medical Research and Materiel Command, was on the role of tuberin and hamartin in cortical neuron migration.

**SEE ALSO:** Columbia University; New York.

**BIBLIOGRAPHY.** "In Heated Heroin, a Dangerous Dragon," *New York Times* (November 16, 1999); "Kriegstein, Arnold R. Biographical Sketch," www.stanford.edu (cited February 2008); Nicholas Wade, "Some Scientists See Shift in Stem Cell Hope," *New York Times* (August 14, 2006).

Justin Corfield
Geelong Grammar School

# Kyoto University

**KYOTO UNIVERSITY IS** located in Kyoto, Japan; it is the second oldest Japanese University. The mission of the university is "to sustain and develop its historical commitment to academic freedom and to pursue harmonious coexistence within human and ecological community on this planet." It is known for focusing on basic science research, then generating industry from this research, and finally sharing the knowledge gained with the community in educational endeavors. There are three campuses—two are in Kyoto while the third campus is technically in Uji; nevertheless, the campuses are within close proximity and can be said to all be in Kyoto.

Kyoto University has a long and eventful history. Notable events include the founding in 1897 as Kyoto Imperial University, with a college of science and engineering (currently these units are two separate colleges). Two years later, the College of Law and Medicine, as well as the university hospital and university library were built. In 1947 the name was changed to Kyoto University, and the Center for Molecular Biology and Genetics was established in 1988.

One of the many institutes at the university is the Institute for Frontier Medical Sciences. The institute was established in April 1998 to promote research and science in regenerative medicine with a mission to carry out basic science investigations as well as to foster regenerative medicine. An adjunct facility within the institute is the Stem Cell Research Center. The Center was founded in April 2002 "to advance basic research and medical application in the field of the regenerative medicine using stem cells such as human embryonic stem cells." It is composed of the five Laboratories of Cell Processing, Embryonic Stem Cell Research, Reprogramming Research, Stem Cell Differentiation, and Stem Cell Engineering.

The Laboratory of Cell Processing collaborates with the Laboratory of Embryonic Stem Cell Research. It began in 2005 to develop the production and maintenance of lines of stem cells for research and clinical purposes. The laboratory aspires to be a stem cell bank for future scientists. The Laboratory of Embryonic Stem Cell Research uses self-renewable human embryonic stem cell lines from three consenting donors to conduct investigations into the molecular mechanisms of this self-renewing property. The Laboratory of Stem Cell Differentiation studies the stem cells of the cardiovascular system, specifically in the functioning, angiogenesis, and repair of this system. The Laboratory of Stem Cell Engineering focuses on nuclear reprogramming events that determine the switch from the state of being one type of cell such as a stem cell into another cell type. The knowledge gained may one day be used to cause the reverse; that is, to induce pluripotent stem cell identity in a somatic (adult, differentiated) cell.

The university is overseen by a president, with four vice-presidents and two auditors. Additionally, a board of seven executive directors manages the university.

**SEE ALSO:** Differentiation, In Vitro and In Vivo; International Laws; Japan.

**BIBLIOGRAPHY.** Japan Human Cell Society, "The Japan Human Cell Society," jhcs.umin.jp (cited November 2007); Kyoto University, "Institute for Frontier Medical Sciences, Kyoto University," www.frontier.kyoto-u.ac.jp (cited November 2007); University Hospital Information Network, "The Japan Human Cell Society," center.umin.ac.jp (cited November 2007).

Claudia Winograd
University of Illinois, Urbana-Champaign

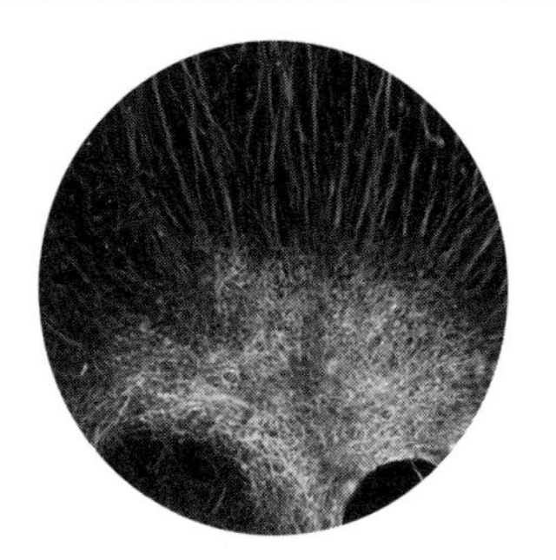

# L

## Lanza, Robert

**ROBERT P. LANZA** is currently the Chief Scientific Officer of Advanced Cell Technology in Worcester, Massachusetts, and an adjunct professor at the Institute for Regenerative Medicine of Wake Forest University School of Medicine. His work is focused on using stem cells, tissue engineering, and cloning to provide therapies for incapacitating diseases and conditions like diabetes and Parkinson's disease. He is known for cloning an endangered gaur named Noah and the first human embryo; however, Lanza is most famous for establishing a new technique for stem cell isolation from human embryos, similar to preimplantation genetic diagnosis.

Lanza grew up in Stoughton, Massachusetts, where he displayed an early aptitude for science. He received B.A. and M.D. degrees from the University of Pennsylvania where he was both a University Scholar and Benjamin Franklin Scholar. Later, he studied with two Nobel laureates, Gerald Edelman at Rockefeller University and Rodney Porter at Oxford University. Lanza has also worked with well-known scientists like Jonas Salk, who developed the polio vaccine, and Christiann Barnard, who performed the first heart transplant.

He has authored many books and manuals including the *Handbook of Stem Cells*, *Essentials of Stem Cell Biology*, and *Principles of Tissue Engineering*, which is the most seminal text in the field. He is the recipient of the 2005 Rave Award for Medicine by *WIRED Magazine* and the 2006 All Star Award for Biotechnology.

### ANIMAL CLONING

At Advanced Cell Technology, Lanza's scientific team was the first group to clone an endangered species. Noah the gaur, an oxlike animal found in Southeast Asia, was cloned using an unconventional somatic cell nuclear transfer technique. Born in January 2000, Noah died within 48 hours because of a bacterial infection unrelated to cloning. The results of this study were published in the journal *Cloning*.

The researchers used 692 enucleated cow eggs and combined them with the nucleus of a male gaur's skin cells, creating nearly 81 blastocysts, or embryos containing roughly 100 cells. They then implanted 42 of the 81 blastocysts into 32 surrogate cows; only eight became pregnant. Fetuses were removed from two cows for scientific analysis, four cows had spontaneous abortions at the second month of pregnancy, the seventh cow had a late-term abortion, and only Noah survived until birth.

This technique differs from the process used by Ian Wilmut to clone Dolly the sheep in 1997, where another phylogenetically similar species was used to host the embryo. This may explain the low rate of success, but even when scientists attempt to clone a cow without the embryonic transfer technique, only one or two births can be achieved when starting with 100 cow eggs. Nevertheless, this discovery has launched the possibility of rescuing endangered species like gaurs, of which roughly 36,000 remain. Yet, some scientists argue that cloning does not rescue the genetic diversity within a species.

Other interspecies embryo transfers of endangered organisms, such as those of an Indian desert cat into a domestic cat and a bongo antelope into a more common African antelope, have yielded success in live births. With these recent achievements, Lanza's team plans to use black bears to clone pandas, an endangered species that only has 1,000 remaining animals in southwest China. Yet, the Chinese government has some reservations on the technique due to its low rate of success and arguable benefits.

## HUMAN EMBRYONIC CLONING

The introduction of human embryonic cloning, or therapeutic cloning, to the world was inspired by the union of three personalities at Advanced Cell Technology: Jose B. Cibelli, Michael D. West, and Robert P. Lanza. After 20 years of engineering tissues that fail to engraft in human patients due to immune rejection, Lanza set out to clone a human embryo and derive stem cells from it to generate an ideal immunocompatible therapy.

Human embryonic cloning is achieved by somatic cell nuclear transfer using an enucleated human egg and a nucleus from a somatic cell. Lanza is a proponent for therapeutic cloning but states that cloning for the purpose of implantation, or reproductive cloning, places too much risk on the mother and potential child. Advanced Cell Technology began by appointing Ronald Green of the Ethics Institute of Dartmouth to head the bioethics committee as well as Harvard's Ann Kiessling-Cooper to aid in the collection of eggs. They accepted eggs from women 24 to 32 years of age who had at least one child. Skin cells were collected from patients who may gain therapeutic benefit from the derived stem cells, such as those suffering from diabetes. Out of 71 eggs from seven volunteers, two divided into four-cell embryos and one divided into six on October 31, 2001, where they hoped for a blastocyst. Not only did the cells stop dividing, but they were unable to derive stem cells from the clones.

Despite these shortcomings, they were able to parthenogenetically, or asexually, drive an egg cell into a blastocyst without fertilization. This may prove to be less ethically controversial, but will only work for women. The egg cell was triggered to divide during diploidy and prior to haploidy. Their work, however, did not yield a blastocyst containing an inner cell mass useful for generating stem cell lines. Both the therapeutic cloning and parthenogenesis studies were reported online in *The Journal of Regenerative Medicine* on November 25, 2001.

In a separate parthenogenesis study by Advanced Cell Technology published in *Science* on November 30, 2001, thirty cattle were cloned, but six died after birth, with the remainder showing no abnormalities. Interestingly, the telomeres of the clones' calves were identical to control calves. This suggests that cloning actually resets the biological clock and may serve as a source of "youthful" tissue for an aging population.

## ALTERNATIVE SOURCES

In an attempt to evade legislation and reduce ethical controversy, Lanza and his group established an embryonic stem cell line without destroying an embryo, as described in *Nature* on August 23, 2006. He believes that this is the last step to sidestep the controversy on embryonic stem cell research. Yet, objectors argue that his new technique puts the embryo at risk.

The technique was performed on a two-day-old embryo, where the fertilized egg has divided into eight cells or blastomeres. These cells are used in fertility clinics during in vitro fertilization to screen for Down syndrome and other genetic abnormalities. Typically, one cell is obtained from the mass, leaving seven cells to be implanted into the recipient after the screening is complete. Known as preimplantation genetic diagnosis, Lanza's group derived an embryonic stem cell line from a blastomere. Conventionally, stem cell lines are obtained from blastocysts, yet harvesting these cells destroys the embryo. Stem cells from a blastomere are nearly identical to those derived from a blastocyst. Still, this new technique did not satisfy President Bush's objections, and he vetoed legislation on the embryonic stem cell research in July 2006.

Proponents for embryonic stem cell research cite that over 2,000 babies have been born from preimplantation genetic diagnosis with no sign of increased risk for disease. Others maintain that more data need to be collected. Brian Hart, a spokesman for Senator Sam Brownback, Republican of Kansas, says that this new technique simply creates a twin, and the twin is then killed when the cell line is created. Lanza argues, however, that twinning occurs at a later stage of embryonic development, and there is no evidence that a single blastomere can form a person.

**SEE ALSO:** Cloning; Human Embryonic Stem Cells; Nuclear Transfer, Somatic; Tissue Culture.

**BIBLIOGRAPHY.** Jose B. Cibelli, Robert P. Lanza, Michael D. West, and Carol Ezzell, "The First Human Cloned Embryo," *Scientific American* (November 24, 2001); Joannie Fischer, "The First Clone," *U.S. News & World Report* (November 25, 2001); Robert P. Lanza, Betsy L. Dresser, and Philip Damiani, "Cloning Noah's Ark," *Scientific American* (November 2000); Nicholas Wade, "In New Method for Stem Cells, Viable Embryos," *The New York Times* (August 24, 2006).

John S. Kuo
University of Wisconsin

## Lasker Foundation

**THE LASKER FOUNDATION** was started by Mary and Albert Lasker in 1942 to promote scientific understanding of biomechanical processes and of the means for treating diseases. To meet this goal, the Lasker Foundation focused on securing increased federal funding for biomedical research within the United States. The foundation chose to provide seed money for research as well as advocate for increased federal funding.

The Lasker Foundation Award Program began in 1945 to recognize new discoveries by scientists, physicians, and people in public service leading to advances in fundamental knowledge, treatment, and prevention of human illness and disease. The foundation has presented over 300 awards, and 75 of these recipients have also been awarded the Nobel Prize. The original awards were for basic medical research, clinical medical research, and public service, and in 1996, the Albert Lasker Award for special achievement in medical science was added.

The basic medical research award is awarded to scientists for performing fundamental research contributing to knowledge, concepts, or techniques leading to a reduction in disability, morbidity, and mortality from human disease. The clinical medical research award is awarded to investigators for clinical application of innovative therapies for treating patients.

The public service award, originally named for Albert Lasker and renamed for Mary Lasker in 2000, is awarded to those who have promoted funding for medical research through federal legislation or the creation of public health programs. The award honors Mary Lasker for her efforts over decades of advocating to alleviate human disease. She focused on cancer initially and became a driving force in the National Cancer Act of 1971 by approaching legislators and rallying public support. Her advocacy efforts led to increased funding from the National Institutes of Health and to the expansion of programs. She also joined the efforts of other advocacy groups and research organizations for women's health, mental health, cardiovascular health, and other causes.

The Lasker Awards Society was founded in 1997 to ensure that the awards program is able to continue. The planned giving program allows individuals and corporations to donate money to the program through bequests and other gifts. Fairness of the award is maintained by having award recipients chosen by a panel of international experts, so making a donation does not ensure the donor a say in who should receive the Lasker Awards.

In 2005 Ernest A. McCulloch and James E. Till received the basic medical research award for their stem cell research experiments, which allowed for the identification of the stem cell and set in motion all areas of current stem cell research on both adult and embryonic stem cells.

The Lasker Foundation maintains a Web site with research papers, including reports on stem cell research, history, future implications, profiled scientists, and leading opinions and quotes from leading scientists and experts, as well as answers to frequently asked questions.

The research center at the Audubon Center at Columbia University is located in the Audubon Biomedical Science and Technology Park, which opened in 1995 and is dedicated to biomedical research. The Mary Woodard Lasker Biomedical Research Building houses start-up biotechnology and biomedically related companies to ensure that scientific innovation is turned into clinical applications to treat disease.

### REGENERATIVE MEDICINE MEETING

The Lasker Foundation hosted a meeting at Stanford University in 2007 on regenerative medicine. The term *regenerative medicine* refers to the use of stem cells to repair, replace, or regenerate tissues and organs. The meeting allowed scientists and specialists from a variety of related scientific fields, including cell biology, nanotechnology, applied physics, bioengineering, biocomputation, chemical biology, and tissue engineering, to meet, network, and discuss ways of advancing regenerative technology by using stem cells to repair diseased or damaged tissues and organs. The collaborative was chaired by Irving L. Weissman, M.D., from the Department of Pathology at the Stanford University School of Medicine.

**SEE ALSO:** Columbia University; New York; Stanford University.

**BIBLIOGRAPHY.** Lasker Foundation, "Lasker Awards," www.laskerfoundation.org (cited November 2007).

Lyn Michaud
Independent Scholar

# Lineages

**STEM CELLS ARE** immature, undifferentiated cells that can divide and multiply for an extended period of time, differentiating into specific types of cells and tissues. Autogenous stem cells are derived from the patient being treated, while allogenous stem cells are derived from other individuals. Stem cells available commercially are currently mainly allogenous (donor derived).

While it is believed that allogenous stem cells will not produce an immune response, this is not known with certainty. Autogenous stem cells, on the other hand, reduce the risk of rejection and, provided they are handled correctly, remove the risk of cross-infection from allogenous transplanted tissue. In addition, autologous stem cell transplant recipients will not require immunosuppressive drugs to combat rejection.

Stem cells may be totipotent, multipotent or unipotent. This means that they are able to differentiate into any tissue, several types of tissue or one type of tissue, respectively. The process by which stem cells are derived from one type of tissue and differentiate into other types of tissue is referred to as plasticity or transdifferentiation. Multipotent stem cells consist of three major types of tissue: ectodermal (skin and nerves), mesodermal or mesenchymal (bone, cartilage, muscle and adipose), and endodermal (intestines and other). The two main categories of stem cells are embryonic stem cells and adult stem cells, defined by their source.

Embryonic stem cells (ESCs) are derived from the cells of the inner cell mass of the blastocyst during embryonic development. ESCs have the capacity to differentiate into any cell type and the ability to self-replicate for numerous generations. A potential disadvantage of ESCs is their ability to differentiate into any cell lineage and to proliferate endlessly unless controlled. The clinically observed teratoma is a tumor that is an example of ESCs growing into a "different and undesired tissue." ESC scan be obtained only from embryos, and therefore are associated with ethical issues.

## ADULT STEM CELLS

Adult stem cells, an alternative source for stem cells, can be collected from umbilical cord, amniotic fluid, bone marrow, adipose tissue, brain and teeth. Adult stem cells are not subject to the ethical controversy that is associated with embryonic stem cells; they can also be autologous and isolated from the patient being treated, whereas embryonic stem cells cannot.

The newly discovered induced pluripotent stem cells (iPS) cells are adult or somatic stem cells that have been coaxed to behave like embryonic stem cells. iPS cells have the capacity to generate a large quantity of stem cells as an autologous source that can be used to regenerate patient-specific tissues. However, even the authors of these recent reports have cautioned that any carcinogenic potential of iPS cells should be fully investigated before any commercialization can be realized.

Amniotic fluid-derived stem cells (AFSCs) can be isolated from aspirates of amniocentesis during genetic screening. An increasing number of studies have demonstrated that AFSCs have the capacity for remarkable proliferation and differentiation into multiple lineages such as chondrocytes (for cartilage), adipocytes (for fat), osteoblasts (for bone), myocytes (for muscle), endothelial cells, neuron-like cells and live cells. The potential therapeutic value of AFSCs remains to be discovered.

Umbilical cord blood stem cells (UCBSCs) are derived from the blood of the umbilical cord. There is a growing interest in their capacity for self-replication and multilineage differentiation, and UCBSCs have been differentiated into several cell types that resemble cells of the liver, skeletal muscle, neural tissue, pancreatic cells, immune cells and mesenchymal stem cells. Several studies have shown the differentiation potential of human UCBSCs in treating cardiac and diabetic diseases in mice. The greatest disadvantage of UCBSCs is that there is only one opportunity to harvest them from the umbilical cord at the time of birth. Similarly, amniotic stem cells can be sourced only from amniotic fluid and are therefore subject to time constraints.

Bone marrow-derived stem cells (BMSCs) consist of both hematopoietic stem cells that generate all types of blood cells and stromal cells (mesenchymal stem cells) that generate bone, cartilage, other connective tissues and fat. BMSCs are currently the most common commercially available stem cell. They can be isolated from bone marrow aspiration or from the collection of peripheral blood-derived stem cells following chemical stimulation of the bone marrow, by means of subcutaneous injection, to release stem cells.

Adipose-derived stem cells (ASCs) are typically isolated from lipectomy or liposuction aspirates. They have been differentiated into adipocytes, chondrocytes, myocytes, and neuronal and osteoblast lineages, and may provide hematopoietic support. ASCs express some, but certainly not all, of the cell markers that bone marrow MSCs express. While ASCs have an advantage in that adipose tissue is plentiful in many individuals, accessible and replenishable, the ability to reconstitute tissues and organs using ASCs versus other adult stem cells has yet to be comprehensively compared and documented.

Dental stem cells (DSCs) can be obtained from the pulp of the primary and permanent teeth, from the periodontal ligament, and from other tooth structure. Periodontal ligament-derived stem cells are able to generate periodontal ligament and cementum. Extracted third molars; exfoliating/extracted deciduous teeth; and teeth extracted for orthodontic treatment, trauma or periodontal disease are all sources of dental stem cells from the dental pulp. The dental pulp offers a source of stem cells postnatally that is readily available, with a minimally invasive process that results in minimal trauma. Exfoliating or extracted deciduous teeth offer extra advantages over other teeth as a source of stem cells. Stem cells from deciduous teeth have been found to grow more rapidly than those from other sources, and it is believed that this is because they may be less mature than other stem cells found in the body. Additional advantages of sourcing stem cells from exfoliating deciduous teeth are that the cells are readily available, provided they are stored until they may be needed later in life; the process does not require a patient to sacrifice a tooth to source the stem cells; and there is little or no trauma.

The structures of interest to the dental profession are the enamel; dentin; dental pulp; cementum; periodontal ligament; craniofacial bones; temporomandibular joint, including bone, fibrocartilage and ligaments; skeletal muscles and tendons; skin and subcutaneous soft tissue; salivary glands; and so forth. Without exception, neural crest-derived and/or mesenchymal cells form all these dental, oral and craniofacial structures during native development. Several populations of adult stem cells have been explored for the regeneration of dental, oral and craniofacial structures, including BMSCs, ASCs, and DSCs, which, despite important differences between them, are likely the subfamily of mesenchymal stem cells (MSCs).

MSCs in general have several important properties: adherence to cell culture polystyrene, self-replication to multiple passages and differentiation into multiple cell lineages. Mesenchymal cells natively form connective tissue, including bone, cartilage, adipose tissue, tendon and muscle, and participate in the formation of many craniofacial structures. MSCs can differentiate into multiple cell lineages, including but not limited to chondrocytes, osteoblasts, myoblasts, and adipocytes.

**SEE ALSO:** Cells, Adult; Cells, Embryonic; Cells, Sources of.

**BIBLIOGRAPHY.** *Cell Stem Cell*, www.cellstemcell.com (cited April 2008); Science Daily, www.sciencedaily.com (cited April 2008); StemCells.net, www.stemcells.net (cited April 2008).

Fernando Herrera
University of California, San Diego

# Liver

**THE LIVER IS** a critical organ for clearing the body of toxins, as well as for regulating blood sugar levels. It also is a chief organ for mobilization of fat stores in the body. Damage to the liver can consequently affect the physiology of the entire body. Although in a healthy person the liver can regenerate damaged cells and thus maintain a healthy state, in some people this regenerative capability is compromised. Research into stem cell therapy for liver damage may lead to therapeutic breakthroughs for the benefit of patients with liver damage. Liver damage can occur as a result of various insults. For example, ingesting toxins such as poisons or alcohol harms the liver. Liver inflammation can also result in liver damage, such as during a viral infection or auto-immune disorder. There are several viruses, such as all types of Hepatitis viruses, which can compromise the liver.

In general, the liver is an organ that has a remarkable ability to regenerate itself. After minor damage, the liver can often recuperate its healthy state through regeneration. Yet sometimes the liver cannot keep up its regeneration with the pace of its damage, such as during a severe viral infection, a chronic auto-immune disorder, or with chronic alcohol intake. In these cases, fibrous tissue is laid down in damaged areas, causing a scar. The clinical term is *cirrhosis* of the liver. This regeneration may be supported by a population of hepatic stem cells. Research indicates that this stem cell population is actually the hepatocytes, or liver cells, themselves. Cultured hepatocytes can undergo clonal expansion, which is regenerative cellular division. There are a number of circulating factors that are known to stimulate the division of hepatocytes, including (i) hepatocyte growth factor (scatter factor) whose levels increase soon after partial hepatectomy (ii) TNF-alpha, (iii) Interleukin-6 and epidermal growth factor. How these factors control stem cell division and thus liver regeneration is the focus of many studies.

Liver cirrhosis makes a person much more susceptible to liver cancer, or hepatic carcinoma. The

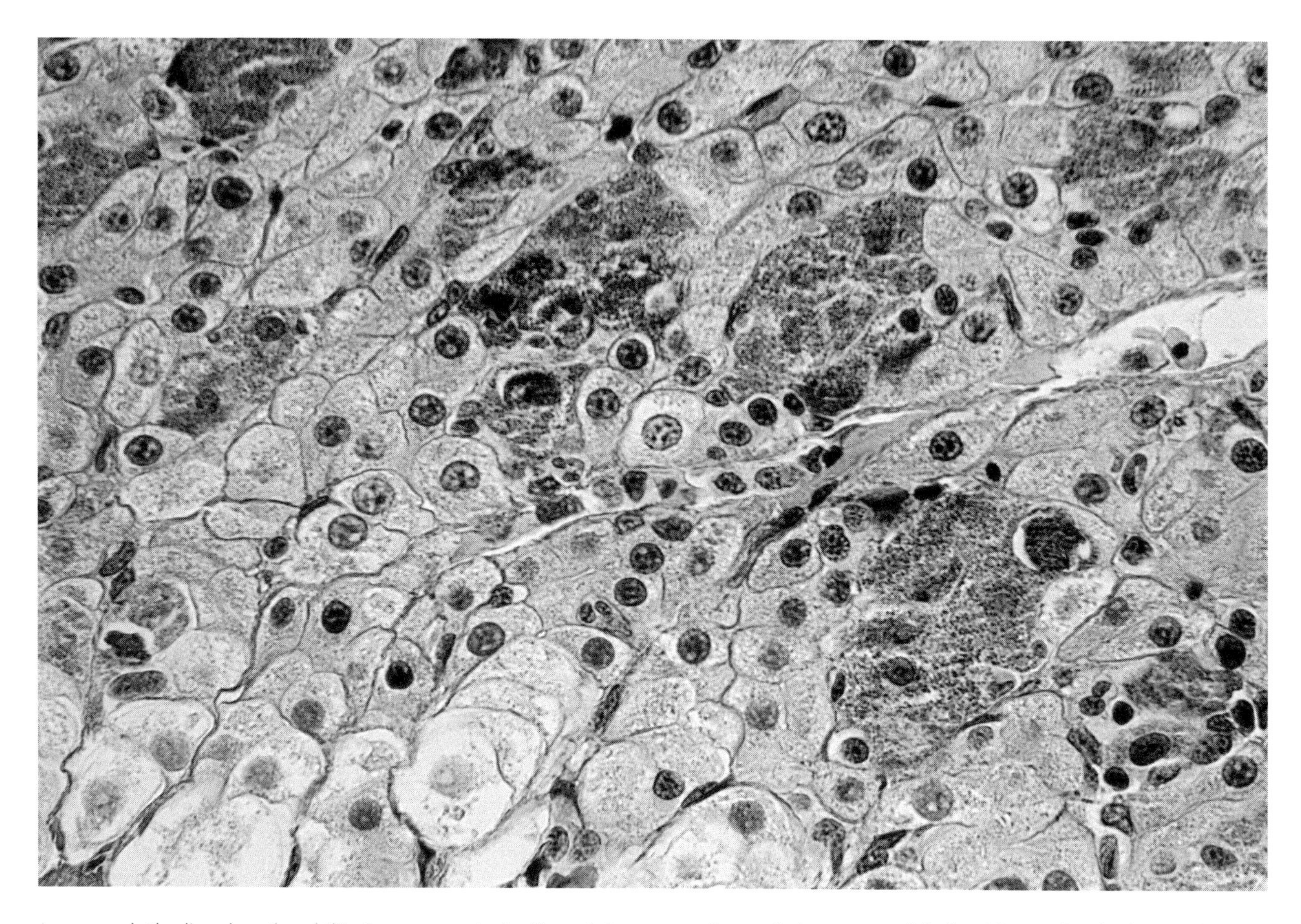

*In general, the liver has the ability to regenerate itself, and the stem cell population responsible for this may be the liver cells themselves, such as those shown above.*

damaged liver is continuously trying to regenerate cells to replace the damaged tissue, and any cell population that undergoes constant division and differentiation, and therefore has repeatedly replicating nucleic acid, is more vulnerable to genetic mutations. Therefore, in a person with cirrhosis, the liver DNA is more susceptible to mutations in important regulatory genes for cell growth and differentiation than in a healthy person without as much hepatocyte proliferation. If in addition to having cirrhosis, the person is ingesting toxins such as alcohol, or any one of the harmless substances that become metabolized in the liver into toxins, that person now has a "double hit" effect and is even more susceptible to liver cancer.

Scientists are working toward a better understanding of the population of hepatic stem cells that are constantly dividing and differentiating. Determining the factors that stimulate proliferation and differentiation can lead to a better understanding of risk factors for liver cancer, and potentially to therapies. It may also be possible to generate hepatocyes from human embryonic stem cells, although the spontaneous regeneration of adult liver makes this less important in many cases.

**SEE ALSO:** Cancer; Differentiation, In Vitro and In Vivo; Gut Stem Cells; Pancreas; Self-Renewal, Stem Cell; Tissue Culture.

**BIBLIOGRAPHY.** M. R. Alison, R. Poulsom, S. J. Forbes, "Update on Hepatic Stem Cells," *Liver* (December 2001); A. D. Burt, B. C. Portmann, and L. D. Ferrell, *MacSween's Pathology of the Liver* (Churchill Livingstone, 2006); M. Kojiro, *Pathology of Hepatocellular Carcinoma* (Wiley-Blackwell, 2006); K. Okita, *Stem Cell and Liver Regeneration (Frontiers in Hepatology)* (Springer, 2004).

Claudia Winograd
University of Illinois, Urbana-Champaign

# Losordo, Douglas

**DOUGLAS W. LOSORDO** is the director of the Feinberg Cardiovascular Research Institute; professor of medicine and associate professor of medicine at Tufts University School of Medicine, having been appointed to that role in 2004; and director of the Cardiac Catheterization Laboratory, St. Elizabeth's Medical Center, Northwestern University Feinberg School of Medicine, Evanston, Illinois. He graduated with a bachelor's of science degree from the University of Vermont, Burlington, in 1979 and remained at the university for the next four years, completing his medical degree, before taking up his residency at St. Elizabeth's Medical Center, Boston, and then proceeding to a fellowship in molecular biology, interventional cardiology, and cardiology at St. Elizabeth's Medical Center. He is now board certified in internal medicine, cardiovascular disease, and interventional cardiology and is a fellow of the American College of Cardiology, as well as the American Heart Association, the American Association for the Advancement of Science, the American College of Physicians, the American College of Chest Physicians, and the Society for Cardiac Interventions and Angiography.

Losordo joined the faculty at Tufts University School of Medicine in Boston, Massachusetts, in 1983 and remained there for the next 23 years, being promoted to professor of medicine in 2004. In 2001 he was appointed chief of cardiovascular research at St. Elizabeth's, and in 2003, he was promoted to acting chief of cardiology. He joined Northwestern University's Feinberg School of Medicine in late 2006 as the director of the Cardiovascular Research Institute.

Throughout his medical career, Losordo has been heavily involved in many professional organizations. He has been a member of the committee of the National Institutes of Health's (NIH's) Ad Hoc Study Section in Molecular Medicine and Atherosclerosis, the NIH Special Emphasis Panel in Tissue Engineering and the Atherogenic Microenvironment, and also the NIH National Heart, Lung, and Blood Institute Special Emphasis Panel. From 2006 until 2007, he was also the chair of the American Society of Gene Therapy's Cardiovascular Gene Therapy Committee. In addition, he is a member of the American Association for the Advancement of Science.

Losordo has served on the editorial boards of *Cardiovascular Radiation Medicine Including Molecular Interventions, Circulation, Circulation Research, Journal of the American College of Cardiology, Stem Cells,* and *Vascular Medicine.* He is currently the associate editor of *Cardiovascular Revascularization Medicine* and *Circulation Research.* He has written about 130 articles for many scientific and medical journals, including the *American Journal of Pathology, Circulation, Endocrinology, Journal of Applied Physiology, Journal of the American Society of Nephrology, Journal of Molecular and Cellular Cardiology, Microvascular Research, Radiology,* and *Trends in Cardiovascular Medicine.*

At present, Losordo is the national principal investigator of a study taking place at 15 centers around the United States that are involved in the testing of the use of adult stem cells in patients who are suffering from severe angina. He has also been active with a study funded by NIH that involves the study of adult stem cells to help improve the ability of patients who are suffering from blocked arteries to walk.

**SEE ALSO:** Cells, Adult; Clinical Trials Within U.S.: Heart Disease; Heart; Heart Attack.

**BIBLIOGRAPHY.** Gina Kolata, "Lack of On-the-Spot Revival May Doom Cardiac Victims," *New York Times* (November 14, 1991); "Douglas W. Losordo," www .fcvri.northwestern.edu (cited February 2008); M. Ii and D. W. Losordo, "Statins and the Endothelium," *Vascular Pharmacology* (v.46/1, 2007); "Stem Cells to Heal Hearts," www.cbsnews.com, May 27, 2004 (cited November 2007); F. G. Welt and D. W. Losordo, "Cell Therapy for Acute Myocardial Infarction: Curb Your Enthusiasm?" *Circulation* (v.113/10, 2006).

Justin Corfield
Geelong Grammar School

# Louisiana

**THE STATE OF** Louisiana encourages the biotechnology industry, including adult stem cell research for economic development and scientific innovation. Growth in biotechnology and biomedicine for translating basic research into medical therapies is possible through appropriate legislation and funding, as well as strong collaborative networks for scientific research for industrial, academic, and clinical institutions throughout the state.

The Louisiana Alliance for Biotechnology provides networking opportunities between academic and commercial researchers to encourage economic growth and the transfer of basic research into commercially viable products. The Biomedical Research Foundation of Northwest Louisiana promotes regional scientific growth and development in coordination with Louisiana State University Medical Center in Shreveport.

The foundation operates the Biomedical Research Institute and a Positron Emission Tomography Imaging Center for diagnosis and research in various fields, including immunology, neurological and cardiovascular cellular communication, signal transduction, and neurosciences. The foundation's clinical application is performed by the Center for Biotechnology Innovation with a focus on research in energy, photonics, biogenetics, orthopedics, and medical informatics. The foundation is also developing a research and technology park called the International Technology Center to focus on biomedical healthcare delivery and biotechnology. This effort brings together nine of the academic institutions in north Louisiana.

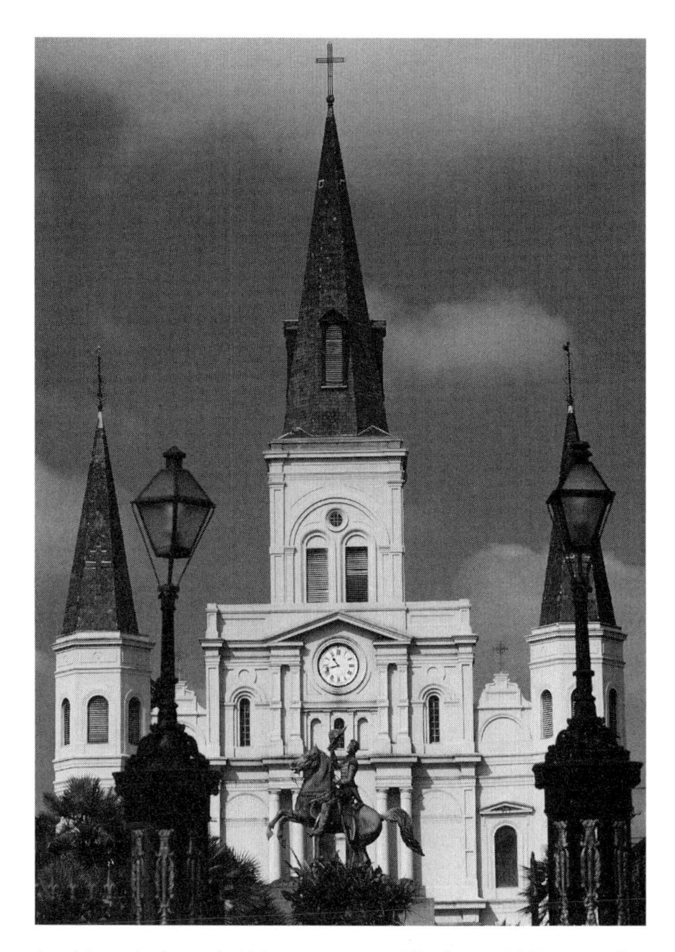

*Louisiana is the only U.S. state to specifically prohibit research on human embryos.*

The Louisiana Gene Therapy Research Consortium was established in 2000 with funds given by the state of Louisiana for enhancing economic growth and innovation by attracting researchers, building research laboratories, and producing gene and cell therapies to be used in human clinical trials.

## LAWS, REGULATION, AND FUNDING

At present, no federal legislation in the United States is in place to regulate stem cell research (except by executive order to not allow federal funding for generation of new embryonic stem cell lines and limiting research on embryonic stem cell lines); this leaves each state responsible for determining policy and funding for stem cell research. Louisiana is the only state to specifically prohibit research on human embryos and restricts human embryonic stem cell research.

For expansion of the biotech industry in Louisiana, the division of economic development has set up three centers within the state, in Baton Rouge, New Orleans, and Davenport, to provide financial assistance with a small business investment company fund, business development services, and wet laboratory incubator space. Their financial support has allowed the creation of a Good Manufacturing Practice Laboratory for stem cell research and funding for the Louisiana Cancer Research Centers of New Orleans and for the Gene Therapy Research Consortium. They also work with start-up companies to bring to the marketplace the application of research from Louisiana universities.

## STEM CELL RESEARCH

Pennington Biomedical Research Center at Louisiana State University in Baton Rouge provides research laboratories and inpatient and outpatient medical clinics. The center opened in 1988 with funds provided by a philanthropic gift from C. B. "Doc" Pennington in 1980. The center is home to eight basic research laboratories, three clinical research units, 19 core service laboratories, and conference space.

The center's researchers specialize in a variety of disciplines including molecular biology, genomics and proteomics, and biochemistry. Though dedicated to nutrition and its related health issues, the center's research foci include tissue and organ regeneration postinjury/damage, characterization and biological mechanisms including formation of adult stem cells and adipose tissue, and the epigenetic basis for human diseases of obesity, hypertension, and adult-onset diabetes.

Tulane University, in addition to providing education, is also a research university with active studies in biotechnology including vaccine and drug development, pain-control therapies, and gene therapy. Basic research is translated into clinical therapy and commercial products by the Office of Technology Development. In 2000 the university formed the Tulane Center for Gene Therapy with the goal of developing therapeutic treatment for a variety of human diseases, using adult stem cells through autologous donation and then turning them into therapy for osteoporosis, osteoarthritis, Parkinson's disease, spinal cord injury, stroke, and Alzheimer's disease. The center also provides career development and community education, encouraging dialogue on social, legal, and ethical issues related to gene therapy. Funding for the center is provided through grant funding from national, state, and private sources, including the National Institutes of Health, the Louisiana Gene Therapy Research Consortium, Tulane University Health Sciences Center, Healthcare Company, and private foundations.

In addition to research, the center is a stem cell provider of human adult stem cells, rat stem cells, and mouse stem cells for researchers internationally, with a signed Tulane University Materials Transfer Agreement and handling fee. The center isolates, expands, and characterizes the stem cells in the laboratory and provides protocols for expansion as well as information on the cells.

The Louisiana State University is a public institution of higher learning, with majors in the physical sciences and with schools of medicine in New Orleans and Shreveport. The main campus of the university system is located in Baton Rouge, with campuses throughout the state. Research on stem cells includes survival of stem cells after freezing and their capability to proliferate and differentiate, developing technology in engineering stem cells in sheets or three-dimensional structures for transplant, and working with the Pennington Center to develop protocols for the cryopreservation of human adipose adult stem cells. Clinical research through the Gene Therapy Program at the Health Sciences Center at the School of Medicine in New Orleans includes translating the basic science of genetic involvement in disease into clinical therapy to prevent or treat some cancers or to restore function to diseased tissues or organs.

**SEE ALSO:** *Individual U.S. State Articles*; Biotechnology, History of; Clinical Trials Within U.S.: Batten Disease; Clinical Trials Within U.S.: Blind Process; Clinical Trials Within U.S.: Cancer; Clinical Trials Within U.S.: Heart Disease; Clinical Trials Within U.S.: Peripheral Vascular Disease; Clinical Trials Within U.S.: Skin Transplants (Burns); Clinical Trials Within U.S.: Spinal Cord Injury; Clinical Trials Within U.S.: Traumatic Brain Injury; Ethics; Federal Government Policies; Moral Status of Embryo; Special Interest/Lobby Groups; United States.

**BIBLIOGRAPHY.** Louisiana Alliance for Biotechnology, "About Us," www.labiotech.org (cited November 2007); Louisiana Gene Therapy Research Consortium, "Overview," www.lagenetherapy.org (cited November 2007); Pennington Biomedical Research Center, "About Us," www.pbrc.edu (cited November 2007); Tulane Center for Gene Therapy, www.som.tulane.edu (cited November 2007).

Lyn Michaud
Independent Scholar

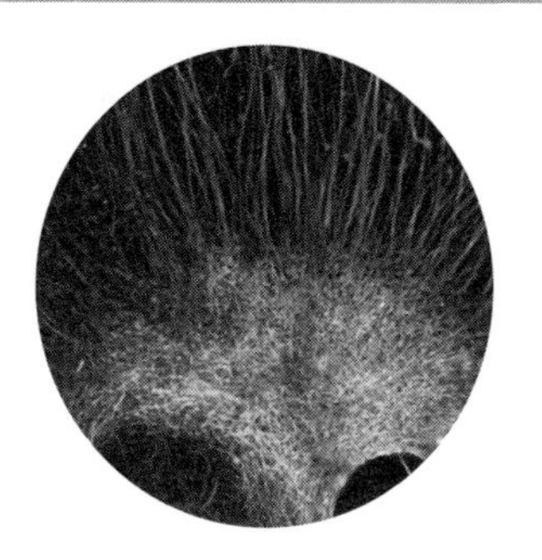

# M

## Macklis, Jeffrey

**DR. JEFFREY MACKLIS** is the director of the Massachusetts General Hospital–Harvard Medical School Center for Nervous System Repair, and is the program head of neuroscience/nervous system diseases at the Harvard Stem Cell Institute at Harvard University. His laboratory at the Division of Medical Sciences at Harvard University has the long-term goal of working on ways of helping with brain and spinal cord repair. Specifically, this involves cellular repair of injured or degenerated complex cerebral cortex and also cortical output circuitry. By its very nature, this involves dealing with motor neuron problems and diseases, working out ways of dealing with amyotrophic lateral sclerosis and multiple sclerosis, as well as spinal cord injury.

Before moving to Harvard, Macklis attended the Massachusetts Institute of Technology (MIT), completing his bachelor's of science thesis at the Department of Electrical Engineering and Computer Science in 1979, before going to the graduate school at MIT, studying within the Harvard-MIT Division of Health Sciences and Technology. Macklis gained his medical degree with honors from Harvard University Medical School in 1983; his thesis was on noninvasive laser lesioning of dye-targeted mammalian neurons. Subsequently, he was a postdoctoral student in developmental neuroscience with Richard Sidman at Harvard Medical School. In 1986, he was living at Phoenixville, Pennsylvania

Macklis has an interest in both medicine and science. He trained clinically in internal medicine at Brigham and Women's Hospital, Boston, and in adult neurology in the Harvard-Longwood Neurological Training Program. He was also working in the Basic Science Division of Neuroscience at Children's Hospital Boston until 2003, when he moved to Massachusetts General Hospital to establish the Massachusetts General Hospital–Harvard Medical School Center for Nervous System Repair. He has been director of this center since then.

Altogether, Macklis has been the author or coauthor of 60 papers, including eight as the lead author, and has been sole author of two papers. These two papers were: "Transplanted Neocortical Neurons Migrate Selectively into Regions of Neuronal Degeneration Produced by Chromophore-Targeted Laser Photolysis," published in the *Journal of Neuroscience* in September 1993, and "Neurobiology: New Memories from New Neurons," published in *Nature* on March 15, 2001.

Macklis's laboratory continues to study precursor biology and the molecular development of the key cortical neuron lineages, including the corticospinal motor neurons. Initial results have been promising, with experiments indicating that signals directing neuronal migration and specific differentiation of immature neurons and from cortical stem cells can be reexpressed in adult mammals. Macklis is always very realistic about translating these exciting findings to the clinic, but his work may one day open up the possibility of finding treatments for a number of degenerative diseases of the brain.

**SEE ALSO:** Amyotrophic Lateral Sclerosis; Multiple Sclerosis; Spinal Cord Injury.

**BIBLIOGRAPHY.** J. Chen, S. S. P. Magavi, and J. D. Macklis, "Neurogenesis of Corticospinal Motor Neurons Extending Spinal Projections in Adult Mice," *Proceedings of the National Academy of Sciences* (v.101/46, 2004); Harvard Stem Cell Institute, www.hsci.harvard.edu (cited February 2008); R. M. Macklis and J. D. Macklis, "Historical and Phrenologic Reflections on the Nonmotor Functions of the Cerebellum: Love under the Tent?" *Neurology* (v.42, 1992); S. S. Magavi, B. R. Leavitt, and J. D. Macklis, "Induction of Neurogenesis in the Neocortex of Adult Mice," *Nature* (v.405, 2000).

Justin Corfield
Geelong Grammar School

# Maine

**THE STATE OF MAINE** in the United States has no specific laws regarding stem cell research, though the state has a long history in progressive biomedical research dating back to the founding of Jackson Laboratory on Mt. Desert Island in 1929. The state has made a commitment to monetary investment in research and development for their modest biomedicine industry to support innovation while creating jobs and improving the economy.

In March 2007 a bill (LD 1402 An Act to Authorize a General Fund Bond Issue to Enhance Funding for Stem Cell Research in Maine) was introduced into the Maine legislature. The bill would have directed bond revenue to fund stem cell research and establish an umbilical cord bank in the state. Along with the bill, the sponsor offered an amendment to limit the funding to adult stem cells to avoid the embryonic stem cell controversy. However, the bill did not progress and appears to be dead due to legislative rules.

With no federal funding available for stem cell research, Maine researchers must rely on grant money and state support. In 2006 the governor made funding of stem cell research a priority and set a goal of achieving $1 billion annual expenditure on biomedical research in Maine by the year 2010. Investment by the State of Maine on building infrastructure (labs and equipment) is expected to result in a return on investment through grant funding from outside sources, including a recent National Institutes of Health grant and opportunities for increased biotech business development in commercially viable products and therapies.

Jackson Laboratory in Bar Harbor was started in 1929 by Clarence Cook Little as a cancer research facility. The mission of Jackson Laboratory is to perform primary genetic research and provide resources and education to support other researchers in treating human disease. To meet this goal, the laboratory breeds mice, inducing over 800 varieties of targeted genetic traits and diseases. These mice as well as frozen embryos and DNA samples are available for shipment to investigators worldwide.

In addition to the breeding program, researchers at Jackson Laboratory are studying cancers, immunology, neurobiology, metabolic diseases, developmental and reproductive biology and computational biology (genes). In 1956 a research team at Jackson Lab transplanted blood forming cells from the living into anemic mice. The majority of the anemic mice were cured within 60 days, providing the first evidence of stem cell transplant ability to cure disease.

Current stem cell research in animal models includes the use of adult stem cells as possible treatment for genetic disorders like lysosomal storage disease, minimizing the effect of graft-versus-host disease after stem cell transplant and the direct implantation of neuronal stem cells into the brain to solve the problem of minimal stem cell entry into the central nervous system.

The Maine Medical Center Research Institute (MMCRI) in Scarborough opened in 1996. With both laboratory and clinical research spaces, the institute maintains academic ties with the University of Maine at Orono, University of Vermont Medical School, Dartmouth Medical School, the Jackson Laboratory, and the University of New England College of Osteopathic Medicine. The center grew from the previous success in research with funding from the National Institutes of Health dating back to the 1950s. At MMCRI, a research team identified signaling pathways and the genes controlling stem cell renewal and differentiation as well as discovering the possibility of using adult stem cells in developing a wide range of tissue cells. The institute focuses on research, education, and patient care.

The University of Maine at Orono opened in 1868 and over time developed a reputation as a nationally recognized research school. In collaboration with the Maine Medical Center Research Institute and the Jackson Laboratory, the university now offers a Ph.D. program in functional genomics, which includes laboratory rotations at each partner's institution and encourages having more than one mentor to enhance understanding of the biological mechanisms as well as the technology. Current stem cell research at the university is focused on the analysis of cell surface proteins for signaling and response as well as the dynamic processes involved.

The Mount Desert Island Biological Laboratory located in Salisbury Cove was founded in 1898 as the Tufts Summer School of Biology. The mission of the laboratory is the study of marine life for advancing knowledge of developmental and life mechanisms with correlations to human health, especially in the areas of cardiovascular, pulmonary, and renal disease. The laboratory has the special distinction of being one of only four NIEHS Marine and Freshwater Biomedical Science Centers.

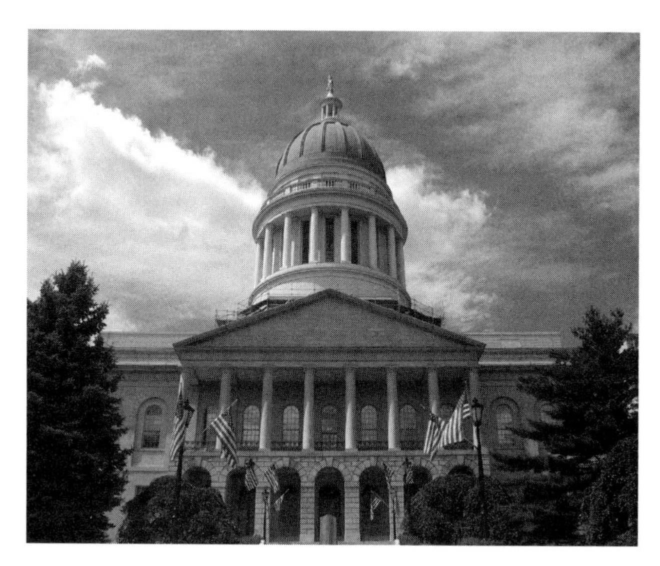

*The governor of Maine made stem cell research a priority in 2006 and set a goal of $1 billion in annual research by 2010.*

The Mount Desert Island Stem Cell Symposium held on August 10–11, 2007, was jointly hosted by the Jackson Laboratory and the Mount Desert Island Biological Laboratory. The conference focused on the molecular genetics of embryonic and adult stem cells and their role in the development of potential therapies for human disease. Speakers from leading academic research institutions and biomedical companies presented research and opportunities.

**SEE ALSO:** Cells, Adult; Mouse ES Cell Isolation; United States.

**BIBLIOGRAPHY.** Jackson Laboratory, "Facts about the Jackson Laboratory," www.jax.org (cited November 2007); MDI Biological Laboratory, www.mdibl.org (cited November 2007); Ann B. Parson, *The Proteus Effect: Stem Cells and their Promise for Medicine* (Joseph Henry Press, 2004); State of Maine Press Release, "Governor Announces Commitment to Increase Funding for Biomedical and Stem Cell Research" (September 20, 2006).

Lyn Michaud
Independent Scholar

# Mammary Stem Cells

**THE MAMMARY GLAND** is a dynamic organ, capable of extensive growth, regeneration, and remodeling. The growth demands placed on the mammary gland during embryonic development and throughout adulthood, suggests a function for mammary stem/progenitor cells. Indeed, functional testing of mammary stem cell activity in rodent models has revealed the presence of subpopulations of cells with the ability to recapitulate adult mammary gland development. As yet, there are no markers known that are specifically expressed only by stem cells that can reveal their activation or distribution. Although the contribution of mammary stem cells to breast cancer has yet to be determined, it has been proposed that these cells may play a significant role in mammary tumorigenesis.

Mammary glands are secretory organs derived from the epidermis, which are unique to all members of the class *Mammalia*. Mammary glands exist in both female and male mammal species, although in males the mammary glands are rudimentary and nonfunctional. In females, the mammary gland consists of a branching network of ducts embedded in a fat pad, which coalesce at the nipple and respond to local and humoral factors to produce milk in response to suckling.

## GROWTH DEMANDS FOR MAMMARY EPITHELIAL CELLS

There are four processes that demand cell growth and may be mediated by embryonic or adult mammary stem cells: (1) Specification and invagination of the embryonic mammary placode. Embryonic specification of mammary placodes starts along two epithelial ridges, known as milk lines, that are formed in the epidermis. Mammary rudiments are formed by further invagination of the ectoderm to form simple ductal structures, which are present at birth. (2) Expansion of the ductal tree during colonization of the mammary fat pads in juveniles. Ductal outgrowth occurs in response to the female endocrine environment, and is led by specialized, proliferative centers called terminal end buds. The mitotic index is very high in the terminal end buds, and it is likely that the ductal stem cells are concentrated in these structures. In the adult these growth centers regress. Ducts comprise heterogeneous cells, broadly divided into a basal layer of myoepithelial cells that produce and adhere to the basement membrane, and a single layer of suprabasal luminal cells, that face the ductal lumen. Luminal cells can have multiple layers in actively dividing juvenile tissues and preneoplastic conditions. (3) Cycle-associated proliferation. The hormonal cycles typical of mammalian females can generate mitotic indices in mammary epithelia that are typical of pregnancy, but only briefly (hours long), and the proliferative phase is followed by regression and cell apoptosis. (4) Expansion and differentiation during pregnancy, to produce the lactation-competent mammary gland.

During pregnancy, postcoitus, proliferative humoral signals (from pituitary, ovary, and placenta) induce the extensive proliferation of the lobuloalveoar lineage, which branch off from the permanent adult ductal structure. Postpartum, the luminal epithelial cells terminally differentiate to produce milk (by apocrine secretion) and the myoepithelial cells contract in response to oxytocin (to express milk). During weaning, the majority of lobuloalveolar cells involute. During pregnancy, the mitotic index rises to almost 30 percent continuously.

## MAMMARY STEM CELL ASSAY

To date (November 2007), there is no known marker specifically expressed by mammary stem cells, and so they have not been directly visualized during growth, differentiation or neoplasia. There is, however, a functional assay for rodent mammary stem cell activity, which is the transfer of whole populations (using limiting dilutions) or purified subpopulations, into cleared fat pads (the isotopic growth site) of juvenile (or adult) rodents.

Using immunoincompetent hosts and stromal support, human breast stem cells can also be assessed this way. Results obtained from fat pad assays suggest that stem cell activity does not change with age or parity of the female gland, but that it is reduced after serial regeneration of ductal trees. Using flow cytometry, some investigators have purified cell populations enriched for their stem cell activity. In fact, they claim that just one cell can seed the growth of a completely new ductal tree, and this new tree includes a normal component of both mammary lineages.

This fits the operating definition of a stem cell. From limiting dilution assays, the frequency of stem cells can be inferred, and that is found to remain constant at approximately 1:1,400. Since this frequency is also typical of glands after serial transplantation, it is inferred that mammary stem cells can divide symmetrically, and that their proportion in the final population is maintained and constant.

### MAMMARY STEM CELLS AND BREAST CANCER

As for other tumors, it is very attractive to propose that somatic stem cells are a fast track precursor cell for mutation. To date, there is no clear evidence for recruitment of normal somatic cells, though it may be true that breast tumors have cancer stem cell subpopulations.

If these cells have properties in common with other cancer stem cells, their growth, response to damage (for example, genotoxins), and death may be regulated by different means than the tumor majority, and their successful elimination will need a separate treatment protocol.

**SEE ALSO:** Cells, Adult; Cells, Developing; Cells, Mouse (Embryonic); Developmental Biology.

**BIBLIOGRAPHY.** S. Liu, G. Dontu, and M. S. Wicha, "Mammary Stem Cells, Self-Renewal Pathways, and Carcinogenesis," *Breast Cancer Research* (v.7/3, 2005); W. A. Woodward, M. S. Chen, F. Behbod, and J. M. Rosen, "On Mammary Stem Cells," *Journal of Cell Science* (v.118, 2005).

Nisha A. McConnell
Caroline M. Alexander
University of Wisconsin, Madison

## Markers of Stemness

**STEM CELLS ARE** unspecialized cells that possess properties such as self-renewal, high potential for proliferation, and the ability to become a variety of cell types in the body. Self-renewal is the process of generating more stem cells. Differentiation is the process of becoming different cell types. Embryonic stem cells are isolated from very early stage embryos that possess the ability to develop into all different cell types in an individual. Adult stem cells, in contrast, are isolated from specific tissues that can only differentiate into cell types in that specific tissue under normal conditions. However, in rare occasions, the adult stem cells can become cell types of other tissues—a phenomenon known as transdifferentiation.

Markers of stemness are special properties and molecular signatures that distinguish stem cells from other differentiated cell types in the body. This special molecular signature can be a unique gene expression pattern or posttranslational modifications that determine unique function of stem cells. The expression of these genes controls the establishment, survival, and maintenance of stem cells in undifferentiated states. Many growth factors and signaling molecules in the body regulate the specific gene expression pattern. The molecular signature of stem cells is commonly identified by the gene microarray method to globally assess the gene expression pattern of stem cells and differentiated cells at different stages. By comparing the expression of genes in embryonic and adult stem cells, the common molecular signatures in adult and embryonic stem cells can be defined.

### EXAMPLES

OCT-4, SSEAs, CD133, ABCG2, and Nestin are several commonly used stemness markers. OCT-4 is one of the most commonly used markers for identifying embryonic stem cells. OCT-4 is required for embryonic stem cell self-renewal, to generate more stem cells, and for multiple lineage differentiation, to generate different cells in the body. Several other genes are also related to this property, such as Sox2 and Naong. Stage-specific embryonic antigens (SSEAs) are molecules that regulate cell–cell communication and interaction with intracellular structures. There are several SSEA proteins expressed in different tissue at various stages of development in embryonic stem cells and adult stem cells. CD133 is a sugar-attached protein that is expressed on the surface of blood stem cells and several tissue-specific stem cells such as neuron, breast, prostate, and colon stem cells. Recent studies suggest that CD133 is also expressed in cancer stem cells. ABCG2 (ATP-binding cassette superfamily G member 2) is a membrane transporter that is responsible for Hoechst-exclusion side-population stem cells by transporting Hoechst dye out of the stem cell membrane. Nestin is expressed predominantly in neuron stem cells, but its expression is absent in mature neuron.

## IDENTIFICATION AND APPLICATION

Stem cell markers are gene expression products that are uniquely related to stem cells. They are typically proteins or carbohydrates that are specifically expressed in stem cells. These markers are relatively specific and are usually expressed at a low level or are not expressed at all in terminal differentiated cells. However, most of the stem cell markers are not expressed exclusively in stem cells: Some of the stem cell markers are also expressed on many other differentiated cells in various tissues, and in tumor stem cells at different levels.

So far, more than 100 stem cell markers have been identified in different tissues or at different stages of development, but the functional roles of most stem cell markers are not clear. Stem cell markers play a very important role in scientific research. Antibodies to stem cell markers are the most commonly used tools for the initial identification of stem cells in the tissue. Antibodies to stem cells are generated by immunizing animals with proteins associated with stem cell markers. Fluorescence-labeled antibodies to stem cell markers are used to identify stem cells or localize the stem cell niche—an area enriched for stem cells. Several antibodies to stem cell markers can be used in combination to define different types of stem cells based on differential expression of these markers.

## STEM CELL MARKERS AND STEM CELL FUNCTION

The criteria used to define the stem cell markers and the functional roles of the identified stem cell markers are heavily debated issues in stem cell research. The stem cell functional assay is a more reliable method for testing whether or not isolated cells are stem cells. Stem cell functional assays include in vitro cell proliferation and differentiation assays, as well as an in vivo assay to test whether or not isolated stem cells can generate the same types of tissues when transplanted to animals.

However, the stem cell functional assay is time consuming and is difficult to perform in most cases. Thus, antibodies against stem cell markers become very important tools for the initial identification of stem cells. When defining stem cells, the expression of stem cell markers can only be used as an initial screening method and guideline to help identify and isolate stem cells for further characterization. It is not sufficient to determine stem cells based solely on the surface markers in the absence of other supporting properties of stem cells.

## IDENTIFYING STEM CELLS IN A MIXED POPULATION OF CELLS

Stem cells only make up a small proportion of the cells in any given tissue, and the expression of stem cell markers is tissue and developmental stage dependent. Analysis and interpretation of stem cell marker expression results is limited by purity, and small numbers of stem cells can be isolated from a large population of differentiated cell types in the tissue. When stem cells are induced to differentiate to other cell types, the differentiated cells then cease to express stem cell markers and express differentiation markers. Stem cell markers are not exclusively expressed in stem cells; some differentiated cells also express stem cell markers at different levels. Most of the cells that express only one stem marker are usually not authentic stem cells. Multiple stem cell markers should be used in combination to define true stem cells in the tissue. Different tissues may express different types of stem cell markers. At present, there are no stem cell markers that can be used to identify all types of stem cells. In contrast, some stem cell markers can indicate stem cells in one tissue but have no predictive value in stem cells in other tissues. For example, stem cell antigen 1 is useful for the identification of mouse blood and prostate stem cells, but it is not consistently expressed in mouse breast ductal stem cells. To make things even more complicated, stem cell marker expression is highly dependent on the microenvironment for stem cell survival.

The microenvironment for stem cells is called the stem cell niche. It is often difficult to compare stem cell marker expression without having the information on its microenvironment. Isolated stem cells will exit quiescent status and start to differentiate to different cell types under different microenvironments. Thus, appropriate control is often needed when using stem cell markers from one system to interpret results in another system. Use of molecular genetics to manipulate these "stemness" genes may help to clearly decipher the functional role of stem cell markers in the establishment and maintenance of stem cells.

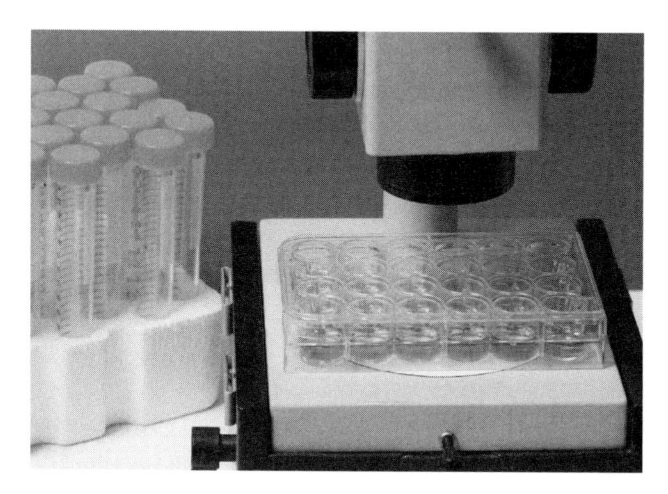

*Markers of stemness distinguish stem cells from other differentiated cell types in the body.*

## APPLICATION OF OTHER STEM CELL PROPERTIES

In addition to using an antibody to stain for stem cell markers, several other assays based on stem cell properties have also been used to identify stem cells. Stem cells are more quiescent and divide more slowly in comparison with differentiated cells in tissue. Therefore, stem cells can preserve labeled DNA for a longer period of time. Taking advantage of this property, DNA is labeled with molecular markers, and "slow cycling" cells are determined. The fact that stem cells can exclude dye in living cells has also been applied to the isolation of stem cells. The molecular mechanism of dye exclusion in stem cell is the specific expression of an ion channel that exports dye and other foreign reagents to the outside of cells. This property is related to cancer stem cells resistant to chemotherapeutic therapy. However, the dye exclusion property is not universally found in all stem cells; in some tissues, the dye exclusion cells are not stem cells. For example, mammary gland dye exclusion cells are not stem cells. This method is valuable only when used in combination with other methods. DNA labeling retention, dye exclusion, and antibody staining can be used in combination to identify and isolate stem cells in the tissue. In addition, several signaling pathways, including TGF-beta, Wnt/beta-catenin, Bmi-1, Shh, and Notch, have been shown to be activated in stem cells or in the area where the stem cells are located. This property can also be used in stem cell identification and characterization.

To accurately define stem cells in tissue is an important goal in stem cell research. The identification of stem cell markers unique to specific tissues and the determination of their relationship with functional stemness genes will have a significant effect on tissue stem cell research and potential clinical applications.

**SEE ALSO:** Cells, Adult; Cells, Embryonic.

**BIBLIOGRAPHY.** National Academy of Science, "Stem Cells at the National Academies," dels.nas.edu (cited November 2007); National Institutes of Health, "Stem Cell Basics," stemcells.nih.gov (cited November 2007); *Scientific American*, "The Stem Cell Challenge," www.sciam.com (cited November 2007); Tell Me about Stem

Cells, "Basic Information about Stem Cells," www.tellmeaboutstemcells.org (cited November 2007).

Daniel Xudong Shi
University of Wisconsin, Madison

# Maryland

**THE STATE OF** Maryland excels in biomedical education at Johns Hopkins University and the University of Maryland, as well as with numerous commercial researchers. Stem cell research is made possible through appropriate legislation, public support, and a combination of public and private funding sources, though with limited availability and instant competition for such sources, increased state funding and leveraged private investment are necessary to retain and attract top stem cell researchers and to encourage commercial growth.

As no federal legislation in the United States regulates stem cell research (except by an executive order to not allow federal funding to be used for embryonic stem cell research except on human embryonic stem cell lines created before August 9, 2001, each state is responsible for determining policy and funding for stem cell research. Maryland law encourages stem cell research, though it prohibits state-funded stem cell researchers from engaging in human reproductive cloning. The Maryland Stem Cell Research Act of 2006 allowed unused material from assisted reproduction and oocytes to be donated for use in research and also created the Maryland Stem Cell Research Fund, as well as appointing a commission to review proposals and administer funds to provide grants for adult and embryonic stem cell research.

Funding for research is available through the National Institutes of Health, state funding, and private foundations and research grants. The Howard Hughes Medical Institute, founded in 1953 by Howard Hughes, is a philanthropic organization located in Chevy Chase. The organization provides $700 million a year for research, made available to researchers around the country, with projects chosen through national competition, as well as $80 million in grants for science education. In addition to funding, the Howard Hughes Medical Institute also performs cross-discipline research at its campus in Virginia.

## UNIVERSITIES

Johns Hopkins University opened in 1876 and is located in Baltimore. It has achieved global acclaim for both education and research, with additional campuses in Rockville; Nanjing, China; and Bologna and Florence, Italy. The university has nine academic divisions, including the school of medicine, which shares a campus with Johns Hopkins Hospital, where patients from around the world are treated and participate in clinical trials. The school of medicine has received the most grants of any medical school from the National Institutes of Health.

The Stem Cell Resources Center at the Institute of Cell Engineering centralizes the cross-disciplinary research being performed at Johns Hopkins. The center was established in 2001 to support research on cell fate and basic stem cell science with the goal of translating this research into medical therapies to treat a wide range of human diseases including musculoskeletal and cardiovascular diseases and diabetes. The center's research facilities were completed in 2004 and include two floors with laboratories, offices, and resources to attract faculty and perform research.

The University of Maryland performs basic research and administers clinical therapy based on stem cell research. A Biosciences Research Building supports the research of the College of Chemical and Life Sciences with laboratory space and sophisticated core instrumentation facilities, as well as two Biosafety Level-3 (BSL- 3) containment facilities with space for seminars and conferences.

At the University of Maryland, the Marlene and Stewart Greenebaum Cancer Center has an active program, using autologous and allogeneic bone marrow and stem cell transplantation in treating many different types of cancer including Hodgkin's lymphoma, non-Hodgkin's lymphoma, multiple myeloma, testicular cancer, leukemia (acute and chronic) and aplastic anemia.

**OTHER ORGANIZATIONS**

Osiris Therapeutics, located in Baltimore, is a commercial company developing products from adult bone marrow cells for clinical trials testing products to use in treating autoimmune disorders, heart attacks, and arthritis. Their current clinical trials include two biologic products: Prochymal is being tested for the treatment of steroid-refractory acute graft-versus-host disease in patients post–bone marrow transplant and to treat patients with Crohn's disease. The other clinical trial is on Chondrogen, used to regenerate the meniscus of the knee and prevent osteoarthritis. The company's product Osteocel is the first biological product to induce bone growth. The University of Miami Miller School of Medicine is using mesenchymal stem cells provided by Osiris in treating heart attack patients with the hope of decreasing damage to the heart muscle.

Maryland Families for Stem Cell Research, based in Annapolis, is an organization to educate the public on the benefits of stem cell research and the potential for clinical application, as well as to advocate for public policy and funding for this research. The organization depends on networking by members with academic, clinical, and biotech commercial professionals to educate the public and lawmakers on biomedical research and regenerative medicine.

**SEE ALSO:** Johns Hopkins University; Osiris Therapeutics, Inc.; University of Miami.

**BIBLIOGRAPHY.** Howard Hughes Medical Institute, www.hhmi.org (cited November 2007); Maryland Families for Stem Cell Research, www.marylandcures.org (cited November 2007); Osiris Therapeutics, Inc., www.osiris.com (cited November 2007); Ann B. Parson, *The Proteus Effect: Stem Cells and their Promise for Medicine* (Joseph Henry Press, 2004); Stem Cell Resources Center, www.hopkins-ices.org (cited November 2007).

Lyn Michaud
Independent Scholar

# Massachusetts

**MASSACHUSETTS EXCELS IN** the biomedical field. The commonwealth has strong, internationally recognized academic research institutions and clinical centers, as well as a growing biomedical industry, with stem cell and regenerative medicine companies. The legislation is supportive of stem cell research, and the state is setting aside funds for embryonic stem cell research. Past successes have included performing the first skin graft grown from human stem cells in 1983.

The only federal legislation regulation of stem cell research is an executive order prohibiting federal funds from being used for embryonic stem cell research, except those using embryonic stem cell lines created before August 9, 2001. Each state is therefore responsible for determining its policy and funding for stem cell research.

Stem cell research in Massachusetts falls under the 2005 act enhancing regenerative medicine, which permits and encourages stem cell research on adult, placental, umbilical cord blood, and human embryonic stem cells. The law permits the creation of embryos for research by therapeutic cloning, using somatic cell nuclear transfer. Cloning for human reproductive purposes is prohibited, and the law includes penalties for violating regulations.

To clarify the regulations for creating embryos for research, an act on biotechnology regulation also was enacted in 2006. This act makes it clear that creating embryos for research may be done only by somatic cell nuclear transfer, parthenogenesis, or other asexual means. Though embryos may not be created for research through in vitro fertilization procedures, excess embryos from assisted reproduction may be donated for research with the informed consent of the donors. Regulations prohibit payment for embryos, human gametes, or cadaveric tissue.

The legislature also overrode a governor's veto to create an institute for stem cell research and regenerative medicine at the University of Massachusetts and established an investment fund to create a life science center for regenerative medicine and biotechnology in 2006. With a planned investment of $1 billion over 10 years, the Massachusetts Life Sciences Initiative will provide investment to public and private institutions, growing life sciences research, development, and commercialization, as well as building ties between sectors of the Massachusetts life sciences community. In addition to funding, this strategy of focusing on medicine and science research will provide funds to researchers for work before NIH grant funding, build an infrastructure for research, and support the translation of Massachusetts research innovation into clinical applications with tax incentives and other assistance.

The Massachusetts Biotechnology Research Park was created in 1985 in Worcester for biotechnology research and production. The park is across the street from the University of Massachusetts Medical Center and is home to over a dozen biotechnology companies, not-for-profits, and academic institutions. The facilities include wet laboratory space and locations for buildings designed for the business. CenTech Park–Emerging Technology Research and Manufacturing located in Grafton is near the Tufts University School of Veterinary Medicine. The park is intended for emerging technology companies.

## ACADEMIC STEM CELL RESEARCHERS

The Harvard Stem Cell Institute, founded in 2004, supports the collaborative work of the university, medical school, teaching hospitals, and researchers to bring together basic science innovation with clinical expertise to translate innovations into clinical applications. The institute supports research into all aspects of stem cell biology, including both embryonic and adult stem cells. Their primary emphasis is on the search for new therapies for serious diseases, including, among others, diabetes, neurological diseases, cardiovascular diseases, blood diseases, and cancer. The institute receives private donation support and National Institutes of Health grant funds.

The University of Massachusetts is a public research university system with campuses statewide and a medical school and a teaching hospital in Worcester. The University of Massachusetts Memorial Healthcare is home to the commonwealth's public cord blood bank, as well as researchers in cell biology, stem cell research for use in bone disease and blood disorders, and clinical research with the goal of translation of their findings to clinical application in cardiovascular and blood disease, cancer, and diabetes.

The Massachusetts legislature set aside funding for an institute for stem cell research and regenerative medicine at the university, which will integrate the system-wide strengths in human and animal stem cell research as well as biological material and cell/tissue engineering. The hope is to build core lab facilities, enhance the academic programs, and use the strength of the Massachusetts Biologic laboratories in translating basic science innovations into clinical applications.

Massachusetts Biologic Laboratories became part of the University of Massachusetts in 1997. The laboratory manufactures vaccines and other biologic products at locations in Jamaica Plain and Mattapan. The laboratory is licensed by the U.S. Food and Drug Administration for vaccine manufacturing.

The Whitehead Institute for Biomedical Research, established in 1982, is affiliated with the Massachusetts Institute of Technology, though it is an independent not-for-profit. The institute was started by businessman and philanthropist Edwin C. "Jack" Whitehead to establish a research institute dedicated to biomedical science and the translation of this science to clinical therapy. Research at the institute related to stem cell research includes mapping stem cell circuitry. Their successes have included developing the first transgenic mouse model of a severe human genetic disease, the first mouse clone carrying an inserted gene, therapeutic cloning for the correction of immune deficiency in mice, and restoring neurological function in animal models with Parkinson's symptoms.

Worcester Polytechnic Institute was founded in 1865 as an engineering and technology university. In 2006 the institute formed a joint research agreement between the Biology and Biotechnology Department, the Bioengineering Institute, and CellThera Inc., a Worcester-based biotechnology company, to develop regenerative techniques for limbs and digits damaged by injury. Researchers at Worcester Polytechnic in multiple disciples will be involved in the project, including those with expertise in tissue engineering, wound healing, and stem cells.

## CLINICAL STEM CELL RESEARCHERS

Children's Hospital of Boston was established in 1869 and provides both patient care and innovative research. Researchers in the Stem Cell/Developmental Biology Program investigate stem cells in human development and in the disease process, with the goal of creating novel treatments for diabetes, heart disease, spinal cord injury, and other human illnesses. The Stem Cell Program at Children's Hospital is affiliated with the Harvard Stem Cell Institute.

Massachusetts General Hospital, in Boston, has a Center for Regenerative Medicine that opened in 2005 and focuses on stem cell research to bring together innovations in basic science with clinical expertise to create innovative therapies for treating leukemia, lymphoma, various cancers, diabetes, and other illnesses with tissue damage. The core laboratories in the center are funded by and associated with the Harvard Stem Cell Institute and include cell sorting.

## PRIVATE BIOTECHNOLOGY BUSINESSES

Viacord Cord Blood Banking Service, located in Boston, is a private company that provides Cord Blood Banking Services for customers to preserve cells so they will be available for transplant if needed. This service means that the cord blood will be available for the family's use, unlike a public banking service, where the umbilical cord may be donated for use by any patient. Viacord also is focused on stem cell research for treating cancer and cardiac disease.

Advanced Cell Tech is headquartered in California but has a laboratory facility in Worcester. The company's research in stem cell differentiation is focused on regenerative medicine, with the goal of using the cells for transplant by developing many different cell types including skin, neuronal, lung, heart, liver, and pancreatic beta cells.

**SEE ALSO:** Children's Hospital, Boston; Harvard University; Massachusetts General Hospital; Massachusetts Institute of Technology; Whitehead Institute.

**BIBLIOGRAPHY.** Advanced Cell Technology, "Research," www.advancedcell.com (cited November 2007); Children's Hospital of Boston, "Research," www.childrens-hospital.org (cited November 2007); Harvard Stem Cell Institute, www.hsci.harvard.edu (cited November 2007); Massachusetts Biologic Laboratories, www.ummbl.org (cited November 2007); Massachusetts Life Sciences Center, "Mission," www.masslifesciences.com (cited November 2007); Massachusetts General Hospital, "Regenerative Medicine," www.massgeneral.org (cited November 2007); University of Massachusetts Stem Cell Research and Development Working Group, "A Strategy for Advancing Stem Cell Research and Regenerative Medicine at the University of Massachusetts" (Report to Board of Trustees, February 2, 2007); Viacord, "Research," www.viacord.com (cited November 2007); Whitehead Institute, "History," www.wi.mit.edu (cited November 2007); Worcester Polytechnic Institute, www.wpi.edu (cited November 2007).

Lyn Michaud
Independent Scholar

# Massachusetts General Hospital

**MASSACHUSETTS GENERAL HOSPITAL** is a teaching hospital (of Harvard Medical School) and biomedical research facility in Boston, Massachusetts. It is owned and operated by Partners HealthCare (which also owns Brigham and Women's Hospital and North Shore Medical Center). In addition, it is part of the consortium of hospitals that operates Boston MedFlight and is a member of the Dana-Farber/Harvard Cancer Center. Founded in 1811, the original hospital was designed by the famous American architect Charles Bulfinch. It is the third oldest general hospital in the United States and the oldest and largest in New England. John Warren, professor of anatomy and surgery at Harvard

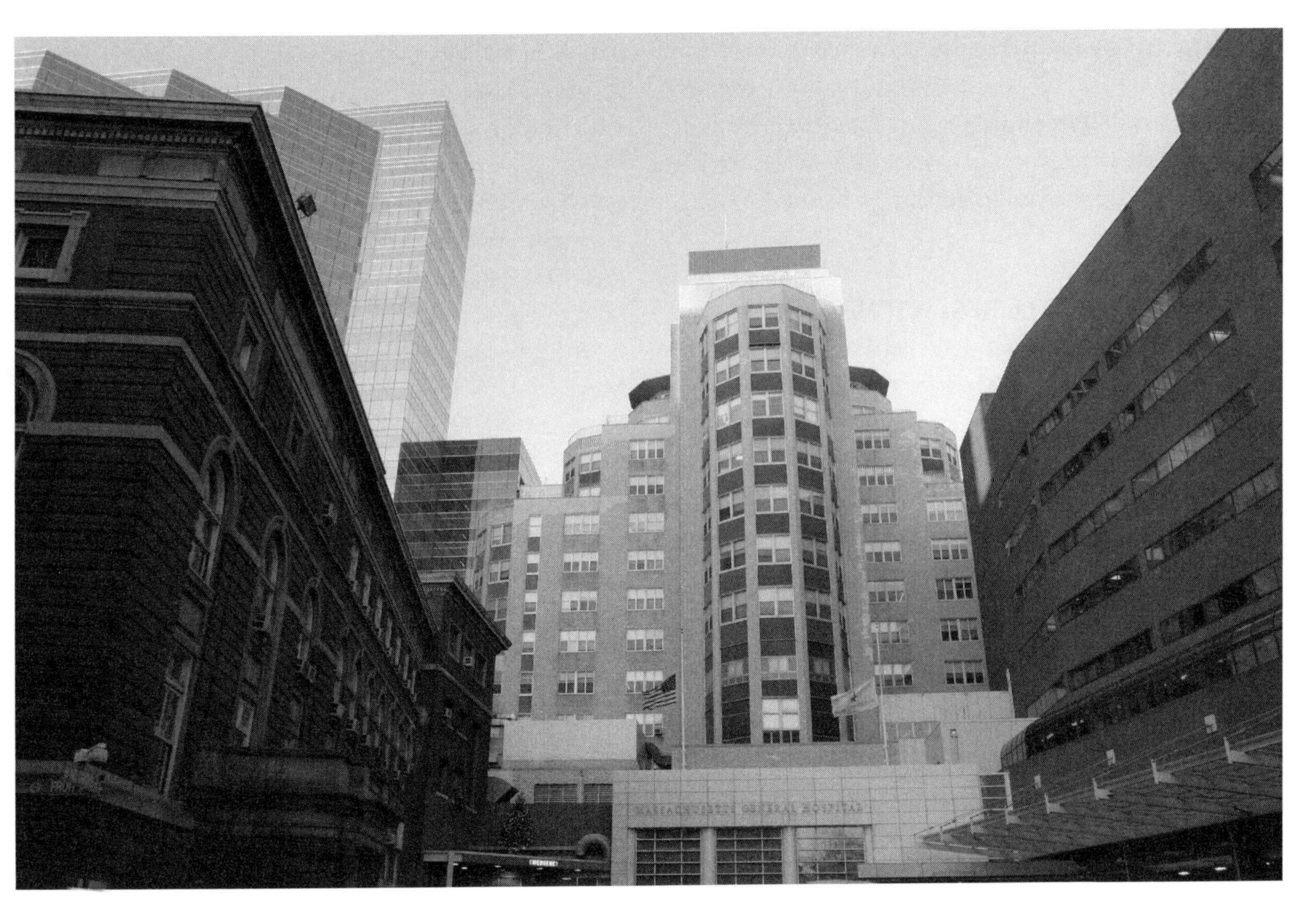

*The Center for Regenerative Medicine at Massachusetts General Hospital prioritizes research with practical potential for patient benefit and supports work in the field of tissue repair and regeneration.*

Medical School, which was located in Cambridge at the time, spearheaded the move of the medical school to Boston. Warren's son, John Collins Warren, along with James Jackson, led the efforts to start the Massachusetts General Hospital. Because all those who had sufficient money were cared for at home, Massachusetts General Hospital, as was the case with most hospitals that were founded in the 19th century, was intended to care for the poor. During the mid- to late 1800s, Harvard Medical School was located adjacent to Massachusetts General Hospital.

## CENTER FOR REGENERATIVE MEDICINE

The Center for Regenerative Medicine is dedicated to understanding how tissues are formed and how they may be repaired in case of injury. Its primary goal is to develop novel therapies to regenerate damaged tissues and thereby overcome debilitating chronic disease. The success of this effort requires a cohesive team of scientists and clinicians with diverse areas of expertise, but with a shared mission and dedication to the larger goal of curing chronic diseases. Central to the center's overall design and mission is the provision of technological services to tissue regeneration and stem cell research throughout the Harvard-wide community. Although these facilities support the center's research activities, they will also be made available to other stem cell researchers within the Harvard Stem Cell Institute (HSCI)'s region, further enhancing collaboration and also eventually providing an additional revenue source supporting the center.

In addition, the center is committed to creating and sustaining collaborative relationships throughout Massachusetts General Hospital, the Harvard-affiliated hospitals, and with national and international researchers. The center's unparalleled focus on stem cell and tissue regeneration research is evident within the center and in the collaborations it forms. One aspect of this is the development of tools (such as the facilities) and biomedical capabilities of key principal investigator labs (such as tissue engineering and somatic cell nuclear transfer) that will support many potential future stem cell–based therapies. Another aspect is the focus on its own collaborations and its role with HSCI that offers significant opportunities for both success and impact. The areas of focus include the blood and immune system, cancer, neurological diseases, cardiac diseases, and diabetes.

The center is using stem cell biology to inform novel strategies for tissue repair in three lines: replacement parts along the model of current stem cell transplant techniques, but extended in disease application and to novel tissue constructs; as a tool to develop drug therapies to enhance endogenous tissue repair; and as a model for understanding mechanisms of degenerative disease and cancer that may change drug development schemas.

The center is pursuing each of these three parallel paths either directly through its membership or indirectly through collaboration. The center emphasizes fundamental biology but prioritizes areas with practical potential for patient benefit and that will provide core resources to assist a broad investigative community. In the longer term, it also supports active development in the field of tissue engineering, with the goal of integrating stem cell science into the creation of biocompatible and genetically compatible laboratory-grown organs.

HSCI is currently focused on basic research and clinical translation in five principal disease areas: cancer, diabetes, nervous system diseases (such as amyotrophic lateral sclerosis and Parkinson's), blood diseases (including AIDS), and cardiovascular disease. These diseases are among the early priorities for HSCI, but its mission is broader and encompasses basic research on all aspects of stem cell biology, with special emphasis on areas in which there is a potential opportunity to improve human health.

## EDUCATION

HSCI faculty members are involved in teaching more than 18 separate undergraduate and graduate level courses, including a new undergraduate course titled "Ethics, Biotechnology, and the Future of Human Nature," taught by Doug Melton, scientific codirector of HSCI, and Michael Sandel, HSCI's ethics and public policy program leader. Professors Melton and Sandel also led a faculty seminar, with well-known outside speakers, titled "Between Two Cultures," to get both humanists and scientists to talk about the ethical and policy issues of stem cell science. Graduate and medical school courses range from basic biology and clinical applications to workshops and informal lunchtime seminars on medical ethics.

With support from the Sternlicht Director's Fund, HSCI has announced the creation of the Sternlicht Awards for Graduate Students in Diabetes. Awards are made to students in the Harvard University Graduate School of Arts and Sciences who are working in the field of diabetes-related stem cell research.

The HSCI Undergraduate Summer Research Internship Program was established to provide students with an opportunity to gain hands-on experience in stem cell research by working in the labs of HSCI faculty members. In 2005, 26 Harvard undergraduates were selected to participate in the program. Through a grant from the Howard Hughes Medical Institute, HSCI was later able to expand the program to include nine non-Harvard students, in addition to 25 Harvard undergraduates. The program included a weekly seminar series of lectures and discussion, which was also open to the broader HSCI community. The students concluded their summer work with scientific posters and presentations of their work. To support the training of clinician scientists with expertise in stem cells, HSCI funds a Medical Scientist Training Fellowship for M.D.-Ph.D. students whose thesis projects or long-term research goals involve stem cells.

**SEE ALSO:** Harvard University; Massachusetts.

**BIBLIOGRAPHY.** Harvard Stem Cell Institute, www.hsci.harvard.edu (cited November 2007); Harvard University, www.harvard.edu (cited November 2007); Massachusetts General Hospital, Center for Regenerative Medicine, www.massgeneral.org/regenmed (cited November 2007).

Fernando Herrera
University of California, San Diego

# Massachusetts Institute of Technology

**THE MASSACHUSETTS INSTITUTE** of Technology (MIT) is one of the most prestigious and influential institutions of higher education in the United States, with an international reputation for outstanding research and education programs. As MIT has developed into a world-class research university, it has developed a number of unique partnerships with other research institutions in the United States and throughout the world that have augmented and contributed significantly to the field of stem cell research.

MIT was started as a result of the commitment and vision of William Barton Rogers and others, who sought to create a university that emphasized technology and science. These were particularly important concerns during the early 1860s, when MIT was launched, during the incipient Industrial Revolution.

Rogers' idea focused on three pillars of education, known later as the "Rogers Plan." Rogers called for the creation of a university that stressed the value of "learning by doing," the value of useful and applicable knowledge, and the value of blending together both liberal arts and professional education curriculums. In 1861 the Commonwealth of Massachusetts, recognizing the value of such an institution, granted a charter establishing MIT.

However, with the onset of the American Civil War, the development of MIT was somewhat curtailed. During MIT's early years of existence, neighboring Harvard University proposed a merger between the two schools that was ultimately rejected by MIT.

In 1909 MIT moved to its current campus, located on a mile-long section along the Charles River in Cambridge, Massachusetts. The move facilitated the growth of MIT and also enhanced its reputation within the collegiate realm. In the 1930s, MIT began to develop a stronger basic research focus, which has continued to flourish to this day, focusing more exclusively on the sciences such as biology, physics, and chemistry, rather than focusing on the more vocational aspects of the sciences or of engineering, such as drafting.

As World War II loomed, MIT became a major center for scientific research in the United States, particularly for research devoted to defense purposes. The war led to significant expansions in MIT's research role in the nation, as well as the growth of labs on and near the MIT campus. Following the conclusion of World War II, the United States faced the enormous challenge of the Cold War period. Because of the perceived technological race between the United States and the Soviet Union, research and research cooperation between the U.S. government and MIT took on renewed vigor during this period, contributing to another period of massive growth at MIT. Because of the university's growth and expansion of its research programs, MIT is recognized as one of the most prestigious and important research institutions in the United States and performs a scientific leadership role that it continues into the modern era.

## RESEARCH AT MIT

MIT has been recognized as contributing to advances in many different scientific fields. Historically, MIT researchers helped lay the groundwork for a wide variety of scientific fields with broad practical applications. MIT researchers developed some of the earliest and most advanced electronic circuitry design and helped develop technologies such as radar, the internet, and the synthesis of penicillin, many of which have revolutionized modern life. In recent years, MIT scientists contributed significantly to the genetic analysis of diseases such as Lou Gehrig's disease and Huntington's disease and also took the lead in completing the Human Genome Project.

MIT fosters research collaboration among MIT faculty, graduate students, and undergraduates, as well as with other institutions. MIT currently works closely with other universities across the United States and the world in many areas of research. Research institutes such as the Whitehead Institute represent efforts by MIT to expand collaborative focus with recognition that greater collaboration frequently leads to superior research having a positive and beneficial effect on society.

MIT programs such as the Undergraduate Research Opportunities Program enable undergraduates to participate broadly in advanced research on campus. This program frequently involves a majority of the MIT undergraduate population and provides them with the opportunity to become involved in research very early in their college experience.

## STEM CELL RESEARCH

As the role of MIT has expanded beyond defense-related research, it has played an important role in advancing molecular and cellular biology, and specifically stem cell research. Much of the groundbreaking stem cell research that occurs at MIT is conducted at the Whitehead Institute, an institute that MIT helped to develop as a fiscally independent entity. All Whitehead Institute members are jointly appointed in MIT's Biology Department, and their labs are staffed by MIT postdoctoral fellows and both graduate and undergraduate students.

The role of the Whitehead Institute and of the larger MIT research community in stem cell research has continued to expand in recent years, with a number of recent scientific advances that may transform the stem cell research field.

In December 2007, MIT-Whitehead researchers including Rudolf Jaenisch and others announced that sickle cell anemia had been successfully treated in mice, using stem cells derived from mouse fibroblasts (skin cells), without the traditional use of an oocyte or an embryo. The discovery came on the heels of other announcements from researchers at MIT and other institutions that it was possible to develop viable embryonic-like stem cells without destroying an embryo or oocyte. These advances could represent a watershed change in the field of stem cell research, helping to avoid some of the more difficult moral questions that have long plagued this field of research.

Frequent objections to stem cell research result from the harvesting of embryonic stem cells from embryos and from the use of human oocytes in the creating these cells. The new technique offers a potential method of avoiding this ethical dilemma and improving future stem cell therapeutics by creating stem cells specific to each individual patient. The announcement that embryonic-like stem cells derived from mouse fibroblasts had been used to successfully combat sickle cell anemia in mice adds credibility to the hope that this technique might be used therapeutically in the future.

Others within the Whitehead Institute and MIT are working to advance stem cell research in a number of different ways. Dr. Harvey Lodish of the Whitehead Institute has worked extensively with hematopoietic stem cells to develop new culturing techniques and practical methods of using adult hematopoietic stem cells in treating hematological disease.

Significant research has also taken place at MIT with the goal of understanding and regulating stem cell differentiation. For stem cells to become useful therapies, it is of great importance that we direct the final fates of stem cells. The principle of stem cell differentiation is a cornerstone underlying much of the current research, which aims to use stem cells for practical and therapeutic ends.

It is hoped that the growth of new collaborations and partnerships between MIT institutions and other research institutions will build further on this research and aid in the development of new research with broad implications for biology, medicine, and a wide array of scientific fields.

**SEE ALSO:** Cells, Adult; Cells, Sources of; Harvard University; Massachusetts; Whitehead Institute.

**BIBLIOGRAPHY.** Massachusetts Institute of Technology, www.mit.edu (cited November 2007); Whitehead Institute, www.wi.mit.edu (cited November 2007).

JOHN S. KUO
UNIVERSITY OF WISCONSIN

# Mayo Clinic

**IN ACCORDANCE WITH** its long history of cutting-edge medical care, the Mayo Clinic is now a leader in clinical research trials using stem cells for the treatment of human illness. The combination of patient care, medical education, and research ensures translation of basic research into patient therapies. Throughout its history, the Mayo Clinic has attracted medical professionals who have focused on improving medical practice and treatment. Some innovations initiated at the clinic have become global standards of practice, including medical charting and intramural communications. Medical research at the clinic began in 1907 with the establishment of research and diagnostic laboratories.

The Mayo Clinic is located in Rochester, Minnesota, with centers in Jacksonville, Florida, and Scottsdale, Arizona. All the centers provide identical clinical services and coordinated research. The founding clinic in Rochester grew from the medical practices of D. William W. Mayo and his two sons William J. Mayo and Charles Mayo. Recognizing the need for a hospital in Rochester after the devastating tornado of 1883, they, along with the Sisters of St. Francis, opened St. Mary's hospital in 1889; this hospital became part of the Mayo Clinic in 1986.

In 1919, a partnership of physicians, including the Mayos, created a not-for-profit association called the Mayo Properties Association, and the Mayos donated the clinic properties and equipment to this association. The Mayo Clinic provided $2 million for the founding of a medical school at the University of Minnesota in 1917. Physicians at the Mayo Clinic also taught at the medical school until the Mayo Clinic opened its own medical school in 1972.

In 1983, the Mayo Clinic began publishing health information targeted at consumers/patients through newsletters, books, and Internet content. The revenue from their publishing endeavors is used to support Mayo Clinic programs including medical education and research.

## EDUCATION

The Mayo Medical School is an independent, degree-granting institution focusing on small class size in relation to faculty size for promoting enhanced patient care, and on clinical research, as well as graduate medical education and residencies in a variety of specialties, and accredited Continuing Medical Education to help physicians and other health professionals to keep current on skills and knowledge.

The Mayo School of Health Sciences focuses on educating allied health professionals. The school offers training to nurses and in a wide range of clinical support services, including laboratory, imaging, therapy, research, and pharmacy services. The Mayo Graduate School focuses on education and research opportunities in the biomedical sciences including virology, immunology, molecular biology, pharmacology, and related academic disciplines focused on improving the understanding and treatment of human disease.

## STEM CELL TREATMENT

Stem cell transplants at the Mayo Clinic are performed by the blood and marrow transplant team, who have specialties in oncology and hematology as well as diverse other specialties. The transplant may be autologous (stem cells are collected from the patient for storage and reinfusion) or allogenic (cells are obtained from a relative or unrelated compatible donor) and are available to adult and children for a variety of diseases.

The Mayo Clinic offers stem cell treatment to adults for amyloidosis, aplastic anemia, genetic-kinked cancers (leukemias, lymphoma, multiple myeloma, and myelodysplastic syndrome), and solid tumors (ovarian, testicular, and brain). The treatment is also offered for children and adolescents for adrenoleukodystrophy, anemias (aplastic, Fanconi's, and sickle cell), leukemias, lymphomas, and some brain tumors, as well as solid tumors and some genetic-linked diseases.

The stem cell transplant is used after chemotherapeutic conditioning to kill cancer cells. The stem cells create new bone marrow and stem cells. The procedure can cure some diseases and put others into remission. Some complications may include graft-versus-host disease, stem cell failure, organ damage, blood vessel damage, cataracts, and secondary cancers. Clinical research at the Mayo Clinic focuses on alleviating these complications.

## RESEARCH

Focused on the understanding and treatment of human disease, the Mayo Clinic focuses on both basic and clinical research. Funding for this research comes from a variety of sources including monies raised from Mayo Clinic programs, National Institutes of Health grants, and other federal and private grants and donations, as well as from the biomedical industry.

The stem cell research laboratory at the Mayo Clinic is directed by Dr. Stanimir Vuk-Pavlovic and focuses on stem cells as a research tool and possible treatment for human disease. The focus of the lab is basic science, using hematopoietic (blood) stem and progenitor cells and the translation of new knowledge into clinical practices for transplantation and cellular immunotherapy. The stem cell lab also investigates cell development and its role in cancer and other diseases.

One problem with using stem cells in clinical application is the possibility of tumor development if the stem cells grow out of control. The researchers have discovered a method to suppress cancer genes. In a mouse model, and using embryonic stem cells in which they suppressed the cancer genes, the researchers differentiated the stem cell into cells that would differentiate into cardiomyocytes to repair damaged heart tissue. The result showed repair of the heart muscle without the development of tumors. The researchers intend to continue this research in the hope of applying a similar technique to human stem cells for use in regenerative medicine.

Researchers at the Mayo Clinic are continuously participating in stem cell research clinical trials, whether they are reviewing protocols, administering and evaluating medical applications, or retroactively studying medical records. When they are accepting/recruiting patients for studies, they have a searchable database set up on their Web site based on medical condition, organ system, or location (Rochester, Scottsdale, or Jacksonville). The information is also available at clinicaltrials.mayo.edu and on the government's Web site clinicaltrials.gov, with searches by keyword.

The Mayo Clinic is currently chairing active studies related to stem cell transplant treatment following conditioning treatment in patients with Ewing's sarcoma, acute myeloid leukemia, multiple myeloma, neuroblastoma, scleredema, and lymphoma. They are also investigating related conditions associated with having stem cell transplants, including treating graft-versus-host disease, the development of idiopathic pneumonia, and treatment and use of cytomegalovirus vaccine in donors and recipients of allogenic hematopoietic stem cell treatment.

## OTHER ACTIVITIES

The faculty, staff, and researchers at the Mayo Clinic are active in organizations to promote biomedical education, stem cell research, and collaboration on a national and international level. The researchers at the Mayo Clinic also widely publish their research findings in scientific and clinical journals. The listing of recent published articles can be found on their Web site. Samplings of some of their stem cell articles from 2007 include findings from using hematopoietic stem cell transplantation and assessing patients for adverse effects and outcomes; basic knowledge on programming, deriving, and differentiating stem cells; and treatments for diseases.

The Mayo Clinic is active in Minnesota government as it relates to healthcare, education, and research. Representatives from the Mayo Clinic have testified in hearings and served on committees including the governor's Bio-Science Council regarding finance bills (S.F. 2456 and S.F. 2757) to encourage the development of Minnesota's bioscience industry and a finance bill (S.F. 2754) to provide operating expenses for a research partnership between the Mayo Clinic and the University of Minnesota.

**SEE ALSO:** Bone Marrow Transplants; Clinical Trials (Adult Cells); Minnesota.

**BIBLIOGRAPHY.** Clinical Trials, www.clinicaltrials.gov (cited November 2007); Mayo School of Health Sciences, www.mayo.edu (cited November 2007); Minnesota Legislature, "Finance and Higher Education," www.senate.leg.state.mn.us (cited November 2007); "Researchers Safely Regenerate Failing Mouse Hearts with Programed Embryonic Stem Cells," www.newscitech.com/mayo-clinic (cited November 2007); Vuk-Pavlovic Stem Cell Lab, "Research," mayoresearch.mayo.edu (cited November 2007).

Lyn Michaud
Independent Scholar

# McKay, Ronald D. G.

**RONALD D. G. MCKAY** is the senior investigator at the Laboratory of Molecular Biology within the National Institute of Neurological Disorders and Stroke at the National Institutes of Health. A native of Scotland, McKay was awarded his doctorate from the University of Edinburgh in 1974 and came to the United States to join the Cold Spring Harbor Laboratory in 1978. He joined the faculty of the Massachusetts Institute of Technology in 1984 before coming to the National Institutes of Health in 1993.

McKay has an impressive history, working in some of the top molecular biology labs including that of Dr. Southern, famous for the "Southern Blot" technique. His research gradually shifted toward stem cell biology. In 1988 McKay proved that neuronal precursors from many regions of the brain could be identified and grown in the culture dish. These findings helped open up new possibilities for researchers interested in stem cell biology and the development of stem cell–based therapies in the repair of degenerative disorders of the brain. McKay was also a pioneer in using mouse embryonic stem cells to generate neurons. Oliver Brustle (now a leading stem cell scientist in Germany) worked on these techniques while a postdoc with Dr. McKay.

In more recent studies, McKay and his team generated dopamine neurons from mouse embryonic stem cells. The cells were, in turn, injected into the brains of rats that were experimentally induced with Parkinson's disease. The rats showed a marked decrease in symptoms. Because human embryonic stem cells can also be turned into dopamine-producing cells, it is believed this might be the basis for a new therapy for Parkinson's patients in the future, although many hurdles still remain. Dr. McKay's paper was a "proof of principle" that this idea may work. McKay's lab now focuses on uncovering many aspects of basic stem cell biology, particularly how cells are able to self renew and differentiate.

Dr. McKay has played a leading role in stem cell research at the NIH and continues to be a world leader in neural stem cell biology.

**SEE ALSO:** Cells, Adult; Cells, Embryonic.

**BIBLIOGRAPHY.** O. Brustle, et al., "Embryonic Stem Cell-Derived Glial Precursors: A Source of Myelinating Transplants," *Science* (v.285, 1999); H. A. Cameron and R. D. G. McKay, "Adult Neurogenesis Produces a Large Pool of New Granule Cells in the Dentate Gyrus," *Journal of Comparative Neurology* (v.435, 2001); S.-H. Lee, N. Lumelsky, L. Studer, J. Auerbach, and R. D. G. McKay, "Efficient Generation of Midbrain and Hindbrain Neurons from Embryonic Stem Cells," *Nature Biotechnology* (v.18, 2000); N. Lumelsky, et al., "Differentiation of Embryonic Stem Cells to Insulin-Secreting Structures Similar to Pancreatic Islets," *Science* (v.292, 2001); L. Studer, V. Tabar, and R. D. G. McKay, "Transplantation of Expanded Mesencephalic Precursors Leads to Behavioral Recovery in Hemiparkinsonian Rats," *Nature Neuroscience* (v.1, 1998); C. Vicario-Abejon, C. Collin, and R. D. G. McKay, "Hippocampal Stem Cells Differentiate into Excitatory and

Inhibitory Neurons," *European Journal of Neuroscience* (v.12, 2000); C. Vicario-Abejon, C. Collin, R. D. G. McKay, and M. Segal, "Neurotrophins Induce Formation of Functional Excitatory and Inhibitory Synapses between Cultured Hippocampal Neurons," *Journal of Neuroscience* (v.18, 1998).

Heather K. Michon
Independent Scholar

# McMaster University

**MCMASTER UNIVERSITY IS** a highly regarded medium-sized research-intensive university located in Hamilton, Ontario, Canada, with an enrollment of 18,238 full-time and 3,836 part-time students (as of 2006). McMaster, or "Mac," as it is known, comprises six faculties: science, health sciences, engineering, humanities, social sciences, and business. The campus is located in the residential neighborhood of Westdale, adjacent to Hamilton's Royal Botanical Gardens.

McMaster has a large number of well-known comedian graduates including Martin Short, John Candy, Eugene Levy, and Ivan Reitman. McMaster has been particularly renowned for its academic strengths, most notably in the fields of health sciences and engineering. The university has been named Canada's most innovative medical-doctoral university eight times in the past 11 years by *Maclean's* in its annual ranking of Canadian universities. McMaster earned the designation of Research University of the Year in 2004 on the basis of its ability to attract and capitalize on its research income.

McMaster's research activities exceed those of universities twice its size, and no Canadian university receives a higher proportion of research funding relative to its operating budget than McMaster. McMaster launched Canada's first school of computational engineering and science in 2005, dedicated to developing expertise in the third wave of scientific research involving stimulation, modeling, and optimization. The new school brings together over 50 faculty members from engineering, science, business, and health science to collaboratively conduct research and advance education.

The university's health sciences reputation started with the foundation of its medical school in the 1960s with nontraditional small-group problem-based learning tutorials, which have since been adopted by other programs. However, it quickly grew, adding programs in occupational therapy, physical therapy, midwifery, and other allied fields. A portion of Albert Einstein's brain is preserved and held for medical research at the McMaster brain bank. Researchers there have identified differences in his brain that may relate to his genius for spatial and mathematical thinking.

## STEM CELL AND CANCER RESEARCH INSTITUTE

Established in 2006, the McMaster Stem Cell and Cancer Research Institute (SCC-RI) is a unique research facility in Canada. The institute's vision and mandate is to explore the underlying cellular and molecular origins that initiate human cancer by employing human stem cells as a model system. The institute houses impressive shared facilities designed to help mitigate the high cost of human stem cell research that has made entry into the field almost prohibitive for investigators in Canada.

The institute has grown rapidly and is home to a team of four leading-edge stem cell investigators and their research programs, with another 32 postgraduate students, postdoctoral fellows, laboratory assistants, and staff. With its particular focus on human embryonic stem cell (ESC) research, the SCC-RI provides interested graduate students and postdoctoral fellows an exciting opportunity to pursue this specialized training in Canada. The institute provides an open forum to educate the public about this important research and work, with sectors developing ethical guidelines and policy for therapeutic applications to ensure that Canadians will receive the best healthcare possible.

Dr. Bhatia, senior scientist and director of the SCC-RI, has made several important advancements in human stem cell research, particularly related to blood forming stem cells. Although he believes stem cells can serve as sources for cellular and organ replacement in tissue damaged by trauma or genetic influences, and for disease intervention, he focuses on human cancer and on using human stem cells to understand how cancer begins and how treatment may be revolutionized, based on this new knowledge. Dr. Bhatia's research program sets out to understand the molecular mechanisms that orchestrate somatic and embryonic human stem cell development. His laboratory can be subdivided into three themes of interest, and although each is unique in its own way, they all possess complementary overlap to allow for an enhanced understanding of the overall nature of novel human stem cell populations, the basis of human cell fate decisions and cellular programming, and how these may relate to rare cancer-initiating cells in the human.

Dr. Doble's expertise in the area of cell signaling and ESC biology further consolidates the institute's strengths and its focus on human stem cell biology, as it is applied to our understanding of human cancers. Dr. Doble's research program aims to unravel critical regulatory nodes in the minimal network of the signal transduction pathways required for the maintenance of pluripotent ESCs. Specifically, he will examine the role of GSK-3 in human ESC self-renewal and create novel "knock-in" models to understand Wnt and Notch signaling in human ESC biology on the basis of a prototype double-knockout mouse ESC model system that he has successfully developed. The ultimate goal of Dr. Doble's work is to understand the signaling pathways that govern the growth and maintenance of human ESCs in a fully defined medium. This will permit the optimization of conditions required for differentiation of human ESCs into cell types compatible with therapeutic interventions for the treatment of tissue injury and disease in humans.

Dr. Sheila Singh joined the McMaster Stem Cell and Cancer Research Institute in July 2007. Before her arrival at McMaster, Singh completed a doctoral degree at the Hospital for Sick Children. She obtained her degree within the Surgeon Scientist Training Program at the University of Toronto, where she completed her residency training, specializing in pediatric neurosurgery. Dr. Singh's research program is centered on the study of cancer stem cells. She recently identified an abnormal stem cell that may drive the formation of brain tumors. Using the cell surface protein CD133, Dr. Singh has characterized a rare subpopulation of brain tumor cells that exclusively generate a replica of the patient's tumor and exhibit self-renewal ability in vivo through serial retransplantation. Her research program focuses on further molecular and genetic characterization of the brain tumor–initiating cell and the molecular signaling pathways that are dysregulated in this cell, allowing brain tumorigenesis.

Dr. Christopher Wynder joined SCC-RI in June 2006 with an appointment as assistant professor in the Department of Biochemistry and Biomedical Sciences. Dr. Wynder's research program aims to understand epigenetic regulation of pluripotency in ESCs and targeting of histone-modifying enzymes to regulate differentiation and transformation in human ESCs.

The McMaster Stem Cell and Cancer Research Institute was launched by the generous support of Canadian philanthropist and businessman Michael G. DeGroote, as well as by recent support from philanthropist David Braley, who donated $15 million to McMaster University that was specifically designated for creating an ESC library.

**SEE ALSO:** Canadian Stem Cell Network; National Institutes of Health.

**BIBLIOGRAPHY.** Life Site News.com, www.lifesite.net (cited November 2007); McMaster University, www.mcmaster.ca (cited November 2007); McMaster University, Faculty of Health Sciences, www.fhs.mcmaster.ca (cited November 2007).

Fernando Herrera
University of California, San Diego

# Medical Research Council

**THE MEDICAL RESEARCH COUNCIL** (MRC) is a publicly funded organization in the United Kingdom (UK) that supports research in the medical sciences within the UK and Africa. Although the MRC receives annual grant-in-aid funding from Parliament through the Office of Science and Innovation, its choices about what research to fund are made independently of the government. The MRC supports medical research through research grants and career awards to scientists, by funding research centers at universities, and through MRC research facilities. Research is organized into five areas (2006–07 research funding in parenthesis): Physiological Systems and Clinical Sciences (£97.3 million), Health Services and Public Health (£89.8 million), Neurosciences and Mental Health (£108.7 million), Infections and Immunity (£85.8 million), and Molecular and Cellular Medicine (£192.1 million).

The MRC is governed by the MRC Council, led by (in 2008) chairman Sir John Chisholm and Deputy Chairman Sir Leszek Borysiewicz. The Executive Board is responsible for day-to-day management of the organization, while five Research Boards allocate MRC funds to support scientific research, and the Training and Development Board. MRC Technology is an affiliated company which works with industry to translate scientific findings into practical applications: in 2006-2007 MRC income from technology transfer licensing was £47 million. The Medical Research Foundation is an independently managed charity associated with the MRC that receives donations from the public to support medical research.

The MRC currently funds over 130 stem cell research projects, fellowships, and studentships and supports major stem cell programs in three MRC institutes and two MRC centers, the Centre for Stem Cell Biology and Medicine in Cambridge, and the Centre for Stem Cell Research in Edinburgh. The MRC is also the chief contributor to the UK Stem Cell Bank, which stores stem cells derived from adult, fetal, and embryonic tissues and may be used by approved scientists from around the world. The UK Stem Cell Bank was founded in 2004, jointly funded by the MRC and the Biotechnology and Biological Sciences Research Council, and was the first such institution in the world. The

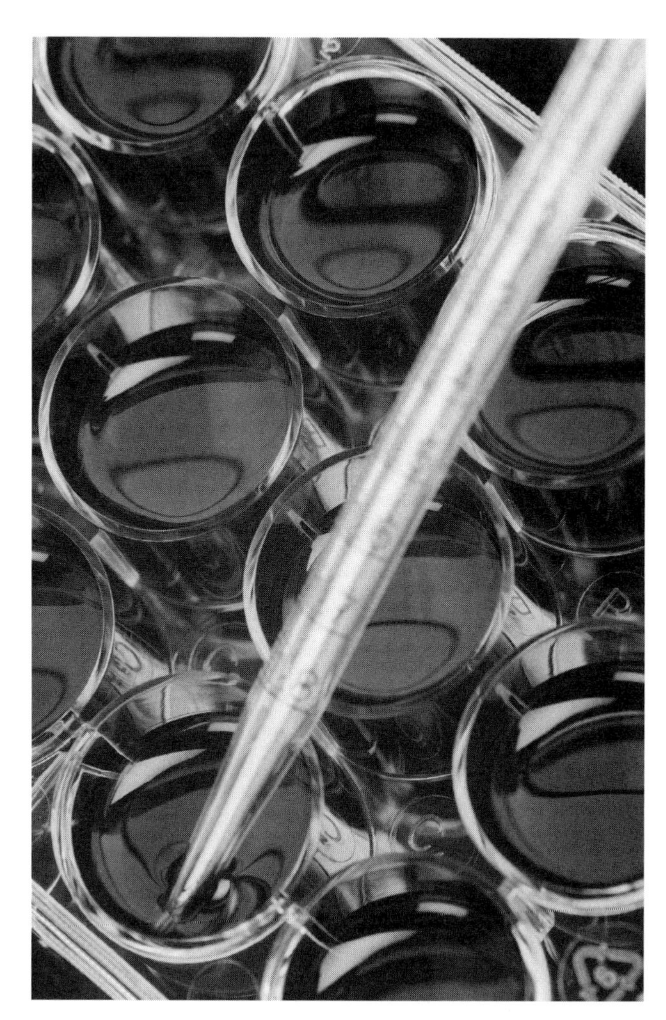

*The MRC is the chief contributor to the UK Stem Cell Bank, which was the first such institution in the world.*

first two hESC lines in the UK were approved for deposit in May 2004, and as of November 2007 63 human embryonic stem cell (hESC) lines had been approved for banking.

The MRC launched the International Stem Cell Forum (ISCF) in 2003 along with eight other international funding agencies, in order to create standardized global criteria for creating, storing and maintaining stem cell lines. The ISCF, which today has 21 member organizations in 19 countries, has three major projects: The International Stem Cell Initiative (ISCI), which aims to characterize the properties of a range of hESC lines and establish a registry; the International Stem Cell Banking Initiative, which aims to establish best practices and guides for banking and development of hESC lines; and carrying out a global review of ethical issues and regulations and intellectual property issues related to cell research.

**SEE ALSO:** UK National Stem Cell Network; United Kingdom.

**BIBLIOGRAPHY.** Medical Research Council, www.mrc.ac.uk (cited April 2008).

Sarah Boslaugh
BJC HealthCare

# Medical Tourism and Stem Cells

**MEDICAL TOURISM REFERS** to traveling, usually outside one's home country, in order to obtain medical treatments or care. Although people have traveled in search of medical care for hundreds, if not thousands, of years, for instance to towns where springs were reputed to have healing powers, the term *medical tourism* usually refers to travel in order to undergo medical or dental procedures that may be unavailable or very expensive in the traveler's home country, or which may only be available after a long wait.

Although no official statistics are kept on how many individuals seek healthcare abroad every year, for the United States in 2006 estimates range from 150,000 to 400,000. These numbers are expected to increase as more of the public becomes familiar with the concept, and as more companies specializing in medical tourism enter the market. Such companies serve as a combination travel agent and medical services coordinator, arranging everything from airplane flights and accommodations to medical and surgical procedures and posttreatment care.

In addition, the Joint Commission International, the international arm of the accrediting organization for U.S. hospitals (JCAHO, the Joint Commission on Accreditation of Healthcare Organization) has begun granting accreditation to overseas hospitals, which will aid medical tourists in selecting hospitals that meet the standards of care available in their home countries.

Economic factors are the main driving force behind medical tourism. Most medical tourists come from industrialized countries such as the United States, Canada, Japan, Israel, and from the countries of Europe and the Middle East. The medical services are usually offered in countries such as Costa Rica, India, and Thailand, which have a cadre of well-trained doctors and nurses and modern medical facilities, but where the costs of medical care are much lower than in the traveler's home country.

Reasons for seeking medical care abroad vary. One reason is that often the desired procedure is not covered by insurance (for instance, plastic surgery, LASIK eye surgery, or dental implants) and the need to pay out-of-pocket motivates the search for the lowest price for care of reasonable quality. Some countries have become centers for particular types of surgery not usually covered by health insurance plans; for instance, Thailand is a leading center for sex reassignment surgery.

Another motivating force is the need to pay out-of-pocket for medical care because of a lack of health insurance. This reason applies in particular to the United States, where about 45 million people were uninsured in 2005. As with procedures not covered with medical insurance, having to pay out-of-pocket for medical procedures encourages the patient to seek out the best price.

A third motivating factor is the long waiting period for elective surgical procedures in some countries; for instance, citizens of Great Britain and Canada may have to wait a year or longer for hip replacement surgery. Organ transplants are another type of surgery that often motivates medical tourism, since in most industrialized countries there is a long waiting list for available organs. The supply may be greater in poor countries, in particular for organs such as kidneys that can be transplanted from a live donor, although it raises issues of medical imperialism as well as the complications that may ensue from a complex medical procedure undertaken away from the patient's home country.

Finally, some procedures may not be available in the patient's home country. Procedures based on stem cells are a good example of this. Because of restrictive laws and lack of funding in the United States, other countries have taken the lead in stem cell research, and some therapies based on stem cells not available in the United States are offered in Singapore and Thailand. For instance, as of August 2007, five hospitals in Thailand and Singapore offered stem cell therapy for end-stage heart disease. The treatment procedure involves harvesting blood from the patient, isolating and expanding angiogenic precursor cells (a procedure that is performed in Israel), then injecting the cells into the heart muscle or reinfusing them via an angiographically directed catheter. Stem cells are a relatively new area of medical research, and it is likely that more such procedures will be developed in the future, and if they remain unavailable in the United States, more Americans will become medical tourists in order to seek them out.

The lower costs of surgery abroad have motivated some U.S. insurance companies to pay for overseas surgery that previously would have been conducted in an American hospital. The commercial Web site medicaltourism.com estimates that a heart bypass conducted in the United States costs about $130,000, versus $11,000 in Thailand or $10,000 in India. The same Web site estimates the cost of hip replacement at $43,000 in the United States versus $12,000 in Thailand or Singapore, and costs for a hysterectomy to be $20,000 in the United States versus $3,000 in India. Among the insurance companies that now offer reimbursement for medical care abroad are Health Net of California, which will pay for healthcare services delivered in Mexico, and Blue Cross/Blue Shield and BlueChoice HealthPlan, both of South Carolina, which include Thailand's Bumrungrad International Hospital among the hospitals for which they will reimburse care.

While some medical tourism is clearly professional there is also a dark side. People with terminal diseases will seek treatments within clinics offering "stem cell treatment"—often costing $40,000 or more. Great caution should be applied until these treatments are validated in well controlled studies.

**SEE ALSO:** China; Ethics; India; Singapore; Thailand.

**BIBLIOGRAPHY.** Forbes.com, "Medical Tourism Takes Flight," July 6, 2007, www.forbes.com (cited April 2008); Medical Tourism, medicaltourism.com (cited April 2008); Neil Osterweil, "Americans Gamble on Bargain Surgery Abroad," *MedPage Today*, August 13, 2007, www.medpagetoday.com (cited April 2008); Josef Woodman, *Patients Beyond Borders: Everybody's Guide to World-Class Medical Tourism* (Healthy Travel Media, 2007).

Sarah Boslaugh
BJC HealthCare

# Melton, Doug

**DOUGLAS MELTON IS** currently a leading embryonic stem cell researcher and the Thomas Dudley Cabot Professor in the Natural Sciences at Harvard University. In addition, Doug Melton is the codirector of the Harvard Stem Cell Institute, chair of the Life Sciences Council at Harvard's Faculty of Arts and Sciences, and since 1994, a Howard Hughes Medical Institute Investigator. He received his bachelor's of science degree in biology, Phi Beta Kappa, from the University of Illinois, Urbana, in 1975 and a bachelor's of arts from Cambridge University in history and the philosophy of science as a Marshall Scholar. He also received his doctoral degree from Cambridge University, at Trinity College, under the supervision of J. B. Gurdon and while working in the Medical Research Council Laboratory of Molecular Biology. He is also a member of the National Academy of Sciences (since 1995), the Institute of Medicine (2001), and the American Academy of Arts and Sciences (1995).

Melton's research aims to understand how human stem cells become different types of tissues, particularly the pancreas and its insulin-producing beta cells. Melton began as a scientific researcher studying development, RNA processing, and translation in frog (*Xenopus laevis*) oocytes. However, in 1993, when his infant son was diagnosed with type 1 diabetes mellitus, a disease in which the insulin-producing cells of the pancreas are destroyed, Melton changed his research's direction to address the development of vertebrate organs from stem cells. His son and daughter are now in their teens, and both are affected by this disease; as diabetics, they are at risk of future blindness, organ failure, and heart disease. Melton has been quoted in an interview in the *New York Times* saying, "Like any parent, I asked myself, 'What can I do?' . . . I wanted my children to know I was doing everything I could for them." An ultimate goal of his work is to make transplantable pancreatic tissue for diabetic patients by understanding how the pancreas develops and how to instruct embryonic stem cells to make pancreatic tissue.

## BREAKTHROUGHS

Melton's laboratory's recent work has had a variety of major breakthroughs. In 2004 an article from his laboratory in *Nature* reported that preexisting beta cells of the pancreas primarily duplicate to replenish their numbers, rather than resulting from pluripotent stem cells differentiating. One year later, Melton's group showed that embryonic stem cells could fuse with and reprogram the transcriptional state of a somatic cell. In early 2007 another article in *Nature* from Melton's laboratory demonstrated that the number of cells in the pancreas progenitor cell pool limits mice pancreas size.

Using funding from the Howard Hughes Medical Institute, the Juvenile Diabetes Association, and alumni of Harvard University, Melton helped continue his stem cell research independent of federal funding after August 9, 2001, and provided a number of human embryonic stem cell lines for free to other researchers.

## HONORS

Melton has received many awards and honors. As a undergraduate, he was an Edmund J. James Scholar from 1975 to 1978. In 1981 he won the Max Perutz Prize and the Camille and Henry Dreyfus Award. Between 1983 and 1986, Melton was a Searle Scholar. In 1991 Melton received the George Ledlie Prize, a Harvard award given in recognition of the individual who "since the last awarding of said prize has by research, discovery or otherwise made the most valuable contribution to science, or in any way for the benefit of mankind." That same year, he was received an American Society of Biochemistry and Molecular Biology Young Investigator Award. In 1995 he received the Richard Lounsbery Award from the National Academy of Sciences and became an honorary member of the Japanese Biochemical Society in 1996. In 2002 Melton was awarded the Eliot P. Joslin Medal.

Melton rose quickly through the ranks of academia. From 1981 to 1984, he was assistant professor, and from 1984 to 1987, he was associate professor at the Department of Biochemistry and Molecular Biology at Harvard University. From 1987 to 1988, Melton was named the John L. Loeb Associate Professor of the Natural Sciences at Harvard, and since 1988, he has been a professor of molecular and cellular biology at Harvard. He concurrently holds additional positions as a biologist (medicine) at the Massachusetts General Hospital in Boston (since 1993), an associate member of Children's Hospital Boston (1994), a Howard Hughes Medical Investigator (1994), and the Thomas Dudley Cabot Professor in the Natural Sciences (1999).

Melton has also had editorial positions with a variety of publications. In addition, he is a member of the National Institutes of Health/National Institute of Diabetes and Digestive and Kidney Diseases Ad Hoc Strategy Planning Group (2000) and is the treasurer of the International Society on Stem Cell Research (2002). He is also a member of the Beta Cell Biology Consortium, along with Joshua LaBaer and Lori Sussel. His most well-known editorial positions include being the review board editor of *Science*, from 1997 to 2001; being U.S. editor of *Development*, 2003; and being on the editorial board of *Proceedings of the National Academy of Sciences* from 2003 to 2004. In 2003, he was also an editor of *Neurobiology* and *Cytokine & Growth Factor Reviews*. From 2003 to 2004, he was both on the advisory board for *Genome Biology* and an editor of the e-journal *Regenerative Medicine*.

Although information regarding his nonacademic work has not been updated recently, Melton serves on the boards of at least two scientific companies. Melton was a director and the scientific founder of Ontogeny Inc., which later merged with other biotechnology companies to form Curis, a drug development company hoping to use cell-signaling pathway technology and functional genomics to transform medicine in cancer and neurological and cardiovascular diseases. Melton is also on the scientific board of Scatterbrain, a scientific consultancy firm that seeks to provide appraisals of the originality, quality, and feasibility of experimental approaches.

**SEE ALSO:** Diabetes; Harvard University; Macklis, Jeffrey; Massachusetts General Hospital.

**BIBLIOGRAPHY.** Harvard Stem Cell Institute, www.hsci.harvard.edu (cited November 2007); Harvard University, www.harvard.edu (cited November 2007).

JOHN BYUN
INDEPENDENT SCHOLAR

# Methods of Growing Cells

**THERE ARE MANY** different types of stem cells, and a variety of methods can be used to culture them. This discussion will focus on embryonic stem (ES) cells and the subsequent derivation of neural stem cells (NSCs). ES cells are a source of pluripotent stem cells, which means that they have the potential to give rise to all the cell types of an individual (over 200). In contrast, NSCs are an example of multipotent stem cells, which can generate a limited number of cell types—in this case, cells of the central nervous system, consisting of neurones, astrocytes, and oligodendrocytes.

There are three key requirements for ES cell culture: Cells should remain undifferentiated and retain a normal karyotype (the number of chromosomes) and the ability to generate all three germ cell layers (pluripotency). To this end, inter alia, it is important to provide stable culture conditions that do not create selection pressure. In general, growing ES cells is technically demanding and labor intensive. For example, the cells require a complete change of media every 24 hours (feeding), both to remove harmful products but also to replenish growth factors and nutrients. In addition, fresh medium should be prepared every seven days because it becomes alkaline with time—a point applicable to most cell culture media.

## MOUSE ES CELLS

Mouse ES (mES) cells are generated from the inner cell mass of preimplantation blastocysts and are grown on tissue culture plates in an incubator. Typically, mES cells will double in number approximately every 20 hours, requiring at around three to four days the ES cell plate to be passaged (split), usually in a ratio of 1:3. The process of passaging or reseeding can be continued indefinitely, allowing the generation of potentially unlimited numbers of mES cells.

MES and human ES (hES) cells are usually grown on feeders, but they can also be cultured in feeder-free conditions (although this is more technically challenging). The majority of embryonic stem cell culture systems rely on mitotically inactivated mouse feeder cells, mouse embryonic fibroblasts (MEFs), to provide factors critical for the growth and maintenance of pluripotency of ES cells. MEFs are derived from 12.5-day-old mouse embryos that are mechanically and enzymatically dissociated before culture in feeder medium. No growth factors are necessary. These fibroblast cells can be rendered incapable of further cell division through gamma-irradiation or the use of antimitotics such as mitomycin C, which is necessary to prevent the feeders from growing uncontrollably at the expense of the ES cells. Both MEFs and ES cells can be cryopreserved and stored in freezing medium for some years. To avoid freeze-induced fracturing, transfer of cells for long-term storage into liquid nitrogen is done gradually.

Feeder-free culture of mES cells involves the addition of high concentrations of LIF (leukemia

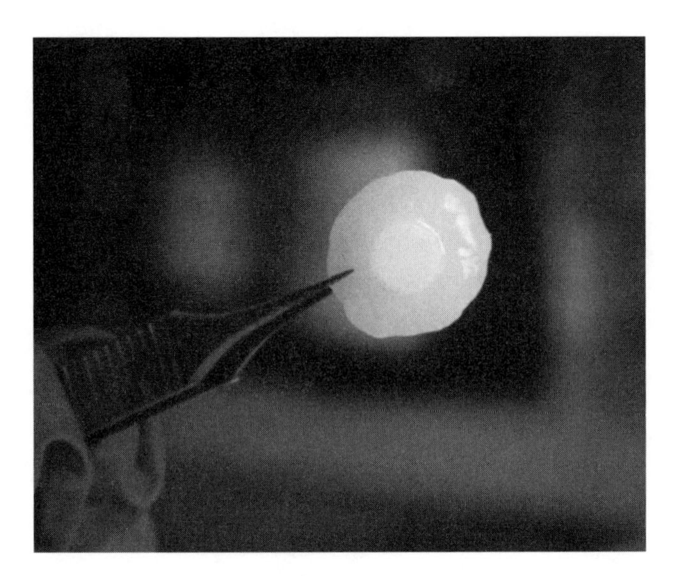

*Growing ES cells is technically demanding and labor intensive, and they require a complete change of media every 24 hours.*

inhibitory factor). However, mES cells are more generally grown on a feeder layer of MEFs supplemented with LIF in the culture medium (though the LIF is not strictly necessary). On reaching approximately 80 percent confluence (by area), mES cells are enzymatically passaged with trypsin. It is important to gently rinse the plates with sterile saline first, which removes any residual traces of serum from the culture medium, because serum inactivates the enzyme. Typically, the ES colonies will detach within approximately two to three minutes following the addition of trypsin.

Serum-containing media is then added to neutralize trypsin and is followed by centrifugation. The resulting cell pellet is resuspended in standard ES culture medium and gently mechanically triturated (mixed) to avoid clumping or formation of aggregates before seeding onto new culture plates. Seeding density matters; the cells must not be plated too sparsely or allowed to grow too densely, as this can select an abnormal population of fast-growing cells with a limited differentiation capability.

Indeed, quality control of ES cell cultures is essential, and it is well-recognized that ES cells can acquire karyotypic abnormalities (loss, or acquisition, of one or more chromosomes) after periods in culture. Thus, it is a requirement of ES culture systems to periodically karyotype the cells. On a smaller scale, there may also be a problem with individual colonies differentiating (no longer pluripotent) on a culture plate, which can be detrimental to the rest of the culture. These colonies have a different appearance, which means that they can be removed mechanically—a process termed *pruning*.

## HUMAN ES CELLS

In contrast to mES cells, which are comparatively robust and straightforward to culture, hES cells are less easily grown. HES cells were first isolated in 1998, 17 years after the isolation of mES cells. Broadly, culture of human ES cells follows the same principles as mES cells, but significant methodological interspecies differences exist (e.g., a requirement for LIF in mES cell culture that is not required for hES culture).

HES cells were initially derived by James Thomson in 1998 from embryos donated during in vitro fertilization treatment, with full consent and ethical approval. This opens up the possibilities of using such cells to study early human development, including maintenance of pluripotency and lineage commitment, drug discovery, and potentially, in the longer term, as a source of cells for transplantation.

At present, the most common method of growing human ES cells again involves the use of feeders, most typically MEFs. This, however, is not ideal, as research moves toward the goal of generating good manufacturing practice clinical grade hES cell cultures; the aim of such systems is to completely remove animal products from the culture process, thereby generating clinically compatible cells. Encouraging recent evidence has shown that this is a feasible goal with the successful propagation of hES cells on Matrigel-coated plates supplemented with a variety of growth factors. However, Matrigel is a proprietary formulation derived from mouse sarcoma lines, so it remains an animal product, and its components are undefined. Thus, some important challenges remain in the culture of hES cells, which includes learning how to grow scaleable numbers of cells under defined, animal-free, and controlled conditions.

Culture requirements of various hES cell lines are basically similar with some (generally minor) modifications contingent on the specific line. The culture medium is supplemented with basic fibroblast growth factor (FGF-2) at different concentrations depending on the hES cell line. hES cells are seeded onto MEFs at densities ranging from 200,000 to 1 million per 60-mm culture dish, which is another variable that changes according to the cell line. Feeding consists of complete exchange of the media every 24 hours, and passaging is required every 48 hours to one week, once the plates reach confluence or the individual colonies are large, depending on the characteristics of the cells being cultured. Some lines are passaged with collagenase; others with trypsin.

It is now established practice to be able to culture both mES and hES cell lines. This opens up the possibility of generating defined cell types from these ES cells, of which NSCs are an example.

## HUMAN ES CELL–DERIVED NSCS

It is the ability of human ES cells to generate unlimited numbers of specialized cells that makes them so attractive to the field of regenerative medicine. ES cells, unlike many other stem cells, can be patterned, allowing the imposition of a region-specific identity. Thus, one type of neurone can have different characteristics and functions, depending on the area in which it is located. An example of this would be dopaminergic neurones, which can be found in more than one area of the central nervous system; however, it is only those with the identity of midbrain dopaminergic neurones that have the potential to reverse the disability seen in Parkinson's disease.

Neurological medicine is an example of a discipline in which insights that will lead to treatments for many currently untreatable disorders are most needed. Such disorders include stroke, Alzheimer's disease, Parkinson's disease, motor neurone disease, and multiple sclerosis. Considerable excitement exists around the experimental opportunities afforded by hES cell–derived NSCs as a disease modeling and drug discovery and testing resource. In addition, the ability to generate specific types of neurones appropriate to individual disease, such as midbrain dopaminergic neurones for Parkinson's disease, could have direct clinical application.

To meet these requirements, the first step is to direct the differentiation of ES cells toward an NSC platform. It is now possible to generate highly enriched populations of NSCs. The most widely applied ES cell neuralizing systems employ spontaneous differentiation (embryoid bodies) with mechanical and growth-factor-mediated expansion, together with the addition of retinoic acid to ES cell aggregates, or coculture with stromal cells and conditioned media. More recently, defined systems have been developed that take advantage of the default pathway of ES cells, which is to differentiate into neural stem cells, using a chemically defined medium (CDM). The ES cell colonies can be detached from the culture plate by incubation with collagenase and are then transferred into CDM, where they round off to become spheres over a day or so. Without further growth factor or morphogen manipulation, on differentiation (see later) on cover slips, these NSC spheres will generate anterior forebrain neurones, mirroring normal human development. However, it is also possible to caudalize these NSCs through exposure to the morphogen retinoic acid, resulting in a spinal cord positional identity.

Using any of these methods to generate NSCs from ES cells, over the course of a few days (4–8 days in the mouse system; 8–16 days in the human system) the spheres stop expressing pluripotency markers such as OCT-4, instead upregulating neural stem cell markers such as Musashi and Nestin. They can continue to be propagated in substrate-free conditions (as spheres) or grow as an adherent monolayer, in both cases with the addition of the neuroepithelial mitogens EGF and FGF-2.

Spheres need to be fed every three days, which involves transferring the medium containing the spheres into a conical tube and allowing the NSCs to settle by gravity, removing most of the medium, resuspending the cells in fresh medium, and transferring them back to the culture dish. Passaging is required every 10–14 days, once the spheres are approximately 1 mm in diameter (i.e., visible to the naked eye and the size of a pinhead). Passaging can be mechanical, with a tissue chopper that cuts the spheres into small sections, or with enzymes such as accutase. Similar to ES cells, NSCs can be cryopreserved at any point in their freezing medium and thawed out for experiments at a later date.

To initiate differentiation, the spheres are plated on poly-L-ornithine and laminin-coated cover slips in plating medium. Feeding involves exchanging half of the medium on alternate days. Early spheres—before day 45—generate predominately neurones after one to two weeks on the cover slips, and these neurones stain for both glutamine and GABA.

Later spheres give rise to a smaller proportion of neurones but also generate astrocytes and 1–2 percent oligodendrocytes. The proportion of neurones from these later spheres can be increased by adding neurotrophic factors, such as BDNF and GDNF, to the plating medium.

Culture of ES cells is not easy, but the system is now well established. The ability to grow ES cells is extremely attractive to the field of regenerative medicine, because of their ability to respond to cues and thus generate defined cell types. One area where such advances are particularly eagerly awaited is neurology, and it is to be hoped that with the generation of neural stem cells, it will be possible to offer treatments for currently untreatable disorders.

**SEE ALSO:** Cells, Embryonic; Feeder/Feeder-Free Culture; Human Embryonic Stem Cells; Mouse ES Cell Isolation; Neurosphere Cultures; Self-Renewal, Stem Cell.

**BIBLIOGRAPHY.** L. M. Hoffman and M. K. Carpenter, "Characterization and Culture of Human Embryonic Stem Cells," *Nature Biotechnology* (v.23/6, 2005).

Sybil R. L. Stacpoole
Siddharthan Chandran
University of Cambridge

# Michael J. Fox Foundation

**THE MICHAEL J. FOX** Foundation, which was founded in 2000, is named after the actor, who won fame in the 1980s for his role on the hit U.S. television show *Family Ties*, in which he played Alex Keaton, a boy genius. The foundation itself was founded by the actor after he was diagnosed with Parkinson's disease. Fox's fame evolved as he moved to the big screen in the mid-1980s with his role in the *Back to the Future* series, running from 1985 to 1990. Fox did several films in the 1990s before returning to the television screen in the hit series *Spin City* (1996–2001). It was during the filming of *Spin City*, in 1998, that it was revealed that Fox was suffering from Parkinson's disease. Before revealing his illness, Fox had first undergone an experimental brain surgery after being diagnosed with the illness in 1991. He first showed symptoms in 1990 during the filming of *Doc Hollywood* but was incorrectly diagnosed.

Fox married Tracey Pollan, his former costar on "Family Ties," in 1988. The couple has four children. Three of them were born after he was diagnosed with Parkinson's disease. Fox was born in Canada but now has dual U.S.-Canadian citizenship. Although he continues to make occasional guest appearances on television, his main focus has shifted to political advocacy.

Through his own illness, Fox learned firsthand of the struggles associated with the degenerative disease. During the third season of *Spin City*, Fox decided to retire from show business to focus on being an advocate for Parkinson's research. Fox then started the Michael J. Fox Foundation, a foundation with a strong drive to support Parkinson's disease research. Fox testified on Capitol Hill in 1998 before the Senate Appropriations Committee in an effort to increase governmental spending in stem cell research. Before testifying in front of the senate subcommittee, Fox decided to discontinue his Parkinson's medication so that committee members could both see and hear the true symptoms and life changes that are associated with Parkinson's disease. Similar to many Parkinson suffers, Fox has developed dyskinesia and adverse effects directly related to his medication. These adverse effects include difficulty speaking, cluttering of speech, difficulty sitting still, and swaying from side to side. In 2002 Fox released a book about his life titled *A Lucky Man*, with all proceeds going to his foundation.

Fox is a strong supporter of stem cell research. There have been promising advances in stem cell research related to Parkinson's disease; however, experts in the field reiterate that the disease is complex and that the proper research is possibly years away. Fox supported Republican Arlen Specter's 2004 Senate campaign because of the candidate's strong support of advancing stem cell research. In 2006 Fox voiced strong support for the Stem Cell Research Enhancement Act of 2005, which was vetoed by President George W. Bush. In 2006 Fox endorsed several politicians who showed a strong commitment to expanding and funding embryonic stem cell research. These candidates included Jim Doyle, Ben Cardin, and Claire McCaskill, all of whom went on to win their respective elections. Fox has said that failure to fund stem cell research within the United States will lead to foreign researchers "having more say" in the direction in which the research will progress.

## PARKINSON'S DISEASE

The foundation's mission is to aggressively fund research related to Parkinson's disease. Parkinson's disease is a progressive movement disorder that is chronic, with symptoms worsening over time. It is estimated that 40,000 Americans are diagnosed with Parkinson's disease annually. Many more suffer from the disease but are not diagnosed. The incidence of the disease increases with age; however, 15 percent of patients with Parkinson's disease are younger than 50 years. The most common symptoms of Parkinson's disease include hand, arm, leg, or jaw tremors; stiffness in the limbs or trunk; slowed movements; and balance difficulties. Fox's initial symptom was twitching in a single finger. The etiology of Parkinson's disease is unknown, although genetic and environmental causes are currently being studied. There is some evidence that there may be a hereditary component, although most cases are not genetically related. The disease is commonly treated with medications, although there is no cure. Surgery is rarely performed but is sometimes done in rare cases.

Parkinson's disease is progressive in that patients typically suffer a decline in functioning and may become unable to perform the activities of daily living, such as bathing, driving, or walking. Individuals affected with the disease often have a reduced quality of life and can become quite debilitated. The economic costs of the disease average more than $25 billion annually in the United States. Medication costs average $2,500 per person, and surgical intervention can exceed $100,000 per procedure.

The foundation has funded research since its inception in 2000. Fox has voiced a desire to determine a genetic marker for Parkinson's disease because 80 percent of dopamine-producing cells are dead by the time most people are diagnosed with the disease. He is hopeful that if the disease could be identified earlier, aggressive treatments could help prevent the severe symptoms and debilitation that are the common progression of the disease. Fox has high hopes that stem cell research can be the key for Parkinson's and is dedicated to ensuring the continuation of funding from his own organization, along with strong political advocacy for government funding.

## RESEARCH PLANS

To date, the Michael J. Fox Foundation has provided funding in excess of $104 million to Parkinson's research. The foundation's mission is divided into four distinct steps. The first step is to develop the course. The foundation has brought together 350 scientists from throughout the world who specialize in Parkinson's disease research. The aim is to support the most promising research and to concentrate the foundation's efforts in that area, build collaborations, and plan future endeavors.

The second step is to identify research that can be directly translated into practice and that can aid Parkinson's patients. Experts from the research community are chosen as advisers to review proposals from researchers. Proposals are scored on the basis of how readily the research can be translated into new treatments, along with the potential to reach the foundations' final goals, namely, higher-quality treatments and eventually a cure for Parkinson's disease.

The third step is speed and accountability. Although some government research institutions can take up to 9–12 months to proceed through the application, review, and start-up phase, the Michael J. Fox Foundation has most projects up and running within two months. The foundation works collaboratively with the researchers to set short-term goals throughout the project to ensure that essential milestones are being met. Foundation staff members are actively involved in the evaluation of outcomes and progress. They also serve to problem solve if unexpected barriers arise and work hand in hand with the researchers to set future goals and directions as needed.

The final step is moving forward. Once research and project outcomes are provided, the foundation moves quickly to either implement the findings or find a collaborating partner to pick up the next needed step. Research as a process in itself can yield both positive and negative findings. The foundation considers both sets of findings beneficial in learning what can and cannot work in helping patients living with Parkinson's disease. Negative findings can also help the advisers to determine research priorities and guide future research awards.

The foundation is a 501(c) 3 nonprofit organization recognized by the United States Internal Revenue Service. The organization makes a very public distinction between their mission and Michael J. Fox as a celebrity. They emphasize that the foundation is dedicated to Parkinson's research and that they are not a mechanism to contact the celebrity. They are unable to provide signed autographs, portraits, or other fan-related services and ask that such requests not be made because they divert staff members from their organizational duties. They also note that Michael J. Fox, as a Parkinson's patient, prefers to keep his own medical progress private.

**SEE ALSO:** Christopher Reeve Foundation; Federal Government Policies; Parkinson's Disease.

**BIBLIOGRAPHY.** Michael J. Fox Foundation, www.michaeljfox.org (cited November 2007).

Michele R. Davidson
George Mason University

# Michigan

**A LOT OF** work has been done in the state of Michigan on stem cells. The University of Michigan and prestigious hospitals such as the Henry Ford Hospital and many others have been working on human stromal cells and stem cells, finding out ways in which they can be used as potential lifesaving cures and treatments. Much work has been carried out to improve the outcome after stroke, traumatic brain injury, and cancer.

The laws in the state of Michigan with regard to stem cell research are different from those in other states. Michigan law bans any research that destroys embryos for nontherapeutic purposes. Michigan law also bans the use of the somatic cell nuclear transfer procedure. Many of the states that have enacted legislation prohibiting human cloning have distinguished between reproductive and therapeutic cloning, but Michigan does not. Michigan, like South Dakota, forbids therapeutic cloning.

Michigan Citizens for Stem Cell Research and Cures is a nonprofit organization formed to educate the citizens of the state of Michigan, including public officials and policy makers, about the complex science, the biomedical potential, and the current policies affecting stem cell research in Michigan to promote informed decision making on this important issue.

In 2000 the researchers at the Henry Ford Health Sciences Center Department of Neurology tested a hypothesis and found that intracerebral grafting of a combination of bone marrow (BM) with brain-derived neurotrophic factor enhances differentiation of BM cells and significantly improves motor recovery. Because most of the active studies involve rats, before involving human beings, fresh BM was harvested from adult rats. It was anticipated that this may provide a powerful autoplastic therapy for human neurological injury and degenerative disorders.

## BRAIN INJURIES AND STROKE

In 2001 a significant step was taken by the Department of Neurosurgery at the Henry Ford Health Sciences Center. Rats were subjected to traumatic brain injury (TBI), and marrow stromal cells (MSCs) were injected into the tail vein 24 hours after TBI.

The rats were killed 15 days later. It was found that MSCs injected intravenously significantly reduced motor and neurological deficits. On the basis of this data, the researchers suggested that the intravenous administration of marrow stromal cells may be a promising therapeutic strategy that may be useful in treating TBI and that warrants further investigation.

The same year, researchers tested the hypothesis that intravenous infusion of bone marrow–derived MSCs enter the brain and reduce neurological functional deficits after stroke in rats. Significant recovery of somatosensory behavior was found. To test the efficacy of various delivery routes of stem cells, the researchers injected MSCs into the internal carotid artery of the adult rat after TBI. They came up with the suggestion that intra-arterial transplantation of MSCs along with intravenous and intracerebral transplantation is also a viable route for the administration of MSCs for the treatment of TBI, as MSCs infused intra-arterially after TBI survive and migrate into the brain.

As human umbilical cord blood cells (HUCBC) are rich in stem and progenitor cells, a team of researchers went ahead and tested whether intravenously infused HUCBC could enter the brain, survive, differentiate, and improve neurological functional recovery after stroke in rats. In addition, it was also tested whether ischemic brain tissue extract selectively induces chemotaxis of HUCBC in vitro. Treatment with HUCBC significantly improved functional recovery, and significant HUCBC migration activity also was present. Therefore, HUCBC transplantation may provide a cell source to treat stroke.

The specific mechanisms by which introduced MSCs provide benefit remain to be elucidated. Various growth factors have been shown to mediate the repair and replacement of damaged tissue. Vascular endothelial growth factor (VEGF) is a growth factor responsible for growth of new vessels. It was confirmed that intravenous infusion of human bone marrow stromal cells promotes VEGF secretion, VEGF receptor 2 expression, and angiogenesis in the ischemic boundary zone of the host brain after stroke.

More recently, Dr. Asim Mahmood and his team of doctors at the Henry Ford Hospital Department of Neurosurgery investigated the effects of a combination therapy of marrow stromal cells and statins (atorvastatin) after TBI in rats in 2007. It was found that when administered in combination with MSCs, atorvastatin increases MSC access or survival within the injured brain and enhances functional recovery compared with monotherapy with MSCs or atorvastatin alone.

TBI causes extensive loss of cerebral parenchyma; however, no strategy for reconstruction has been clinically effective. Human marrow stromal cells (hMSCs) were used to treat rats subjected to TBI, and no significant changes in the lesion volume were found, although functional outcome was improved significantly. To identify new ways of delivering hMSCs into the injured brain and to maximize the therapeutic benefits of hMSC treatment, the team of doctors at the Henry Ford Hospital transplanted collagen scaffolds into the lesion cavity of the injured cortex after TBI. After an array of function tests and histopathology analysis, it was found that collagen scaffolds populated by hMSCs improve sensorimotor function, reduce the lesion volume, and foster the migration of hMSCs into the lesion boundary zone after TBI in rats and may be a new way to reconstruct the injured brain and improve neurological function after TBI.

## CANCER

According to the scientists at the University of Michigan, only a small minority of all the neoplastic cells in human breast cancers are capable of forming new malignant tumors. These tumor-inducing cells have many of the properties of stem cells. They make copies of themselves by a process called self-renewal and produce all the other kinds of cells in the original tumor. The scientists isolated cells from primary or metastatic breast cancers that were removed from nine women treated for cancer at the University of Michigan's Cancer Center. University of Michigan scientists suggested that this might explain why current treatments for metastatic breast cancer often fail. According to them, the wrong cells were being targeted with the wrong treatments. Instead, drugs targeted at the tumor's stem cells need to be developed. To have any real cures in advanced breast cancer, it is absolutely necessary to eliminate these cells.

Cancer has its own rejuvenating stem cells. The progression of some cancers, including leukemia, appears to be driven by cancer stem cells—rare cancer cells that have a greater ability to proliferate than other cancer cells and are therefore the most malignant. A research team from the University of Michigan has found a way to distinguish these bad cells from the normal stem cells that they closely resemble and to kill the cancer stem cells without harming the normal stem cells in the same tissue.

The study, carried out by Sean J. Morrison, Ph.D., director of the University of Michigan's Center for Stem Cell Biology, proves that it is possible to identify differences in the mechanisms that maintain normal stem cells and cancer stem cells, and to therapeutically exploit these differences to kill the cancer stem cells without harming normal stem cells at the same tissue. Morrison is also a Howard Hughes Medical Institute investigator and was part of a University of Michigan team that made the breakthrough discovery that breast cancer has its own stem cells.

**SEE ALSO:** Cancer; Cells, Embryonic; Cells, Umbilical; Clinical Trials Within U.S.: Traumatic Brain Injury; Morrison, Sean; Stroke; University of Michigan.

**BIBLIOGRAPHY.** Xiaoguang Chen, et al., "Human Bone Marrow Stromal Cell Cultures Conditioned by Traumatic Brain Tissue Extracts: Growth Factor Production," *Journal of Neuroscience Research* (v.69/5, 2002); Dunyue Lu, et al., "Collagen Scaffolds Populated with Human Marrow Stromal Cells Reduce Lesion Volume and Improve Functional Outcome after Traumatic Brain Injury," *Neurosurgery* (v.61/3, 2007); Asim Mahmood, Dunyue Lu, Changsheng Qu, Anton Goussev, and Michael Chopp, "Treatment of Traumatic Brain Injury with a Combination Therapy of Marrow Stromal Cells and Atorvastatin in Rats," *Neurosurgery* (v.60/3, 2007); "U-M Scientists Find 'Stem Cells' in Human Breast Cancer," www.cancer.med.umich.edu (cited November 2007).

S. Qader Quadri
Dow University of Health Sciences

# Microenvironment and Immune Issues

**THE MOLECULES FOUND** within a microenvironment—such as an area of injury—may be found in the form of peptides or proteins or may be bound to other cells. An understanding of microenvironmental influence on stem cells requires an interdisciplinary approach among engineering, science, and different areas of biology. Such an understanding is needed as part of the mechanism leading to successful stem cell therapy.

Proposed therapies with stem cells require several experimental considerations. A major issue relates to the rejection of implanted stem cells when they are taken from one donor and then given to another recipient. This type of stem cell transfer is referred as allogeneic transplantation. The major cause of rejection is the polymorphism found within major histocompatibility class 2 (MHC-2). This indicates that it would be difficult to find an individual that closely matches the MHC-2 of another person. To circumvent the problem of rejection, it is proposed that stem cells from the same individual be used to treat the disease, referred to as autologous stem cell treatment. However, this might not be always possible because the disease could be caused by genetic alterations, and the transfer of stem cells from one organ to another organ where the disease is expressed could result in the continued expression of the dysfunctional gene.

## TISSUE INJURY AND INFLAMMATION IN STEM CELL THERAPY

In addition to the issues regarding allogeneic versus autologous stem cell delivery, a key point to consider in stem cell therapy is the interaction between the implanted stem cells and molecules within the area of tissue injury. The maintenance of stem cells involves several genes, and in particular those that are linked to cancer biology. During tissue injury, such as in traumatic brain injury, spinal cord injury, or myocardial infarction (heart attack), the immune system will migrate toward the regions of insult. Once in the area, the immune cells will produce several soluble mediators, such as cytokines and chemokines. These two families of mediators are small molecules that act locally and can bind to specific receptors on stem cells.

Once the cytokines are bound to stem cells, biological responses are triggered. The resulting functions depend on the signal elicited by the soluble mediators. The functions could be beneficial and assist in the repair process, or they can be deleterious. Deleterious functions could occur if the reaction attracts additional immune cells to exacerbate the inflammation; activates genes in the stem cells that can cause tumor formation; or activates genes in the stem cells to prematurely produce factors, which would be produced by specialized cells. For example, a cytokine with proinflammatory properties can induce the production of neurotransmitters in stem cells even before the stem cell has matured to form neurons. Although this premature function does not appear to be a normal physiological response, the current science cannot prove or disprove the benefit or hindrance to such an outcome.

The goal in stem cell therapy is for an effective outcome in stem cell repair. The following are relevant questions to be kept in mind when considering stem cell delivery within the context of varying microenvironments. First, should one type of stem cell serve as effective therapy for a particular type of tissue injury over another type? This question refers to the possibility of bone marrow stem cells being effective for spinal cord injury and gut stem cell for cardiac repair. Second, should the particular type of stem cell depend on the extent of tissue injury? For example, brain stem cells might be better for repair in a situation of acute tissue injury, whereas embryonic stem cells might be more effective in cases of chronic tissue injuries. Third, would microenvironmental influence determine the developmental stage at which stem cells are delivered to an area of tissue injury? This latter question is important because an inflammatory mediator might cause a deleterious effect on a stem cell, but less so on a partly differentiated stem cell.

One hypothesis is to take advantage of inflammatory mediators that are released by tissue injury, as would occur by infarcted heart, which would attract endogenous stem cells, or would aid in the delivery of stem cells directly or close to the area of injury. The basic premise of this approach is that some of the inflammatory mediators will exhibit chemoattractant properties for stem cells. Another approach is to determine whether it would be efficient to deliver the stem cells locally at the site of injury. However, the question is whether the stem cells should be delivered through an engineered material. The advantage is that the stem cells would be contained within a local region rather than escaping to another region, where they could encounter a different microenvironment. For example, stem cells delivered to a region of spinal cord injury, if it reaches the intestinal area, could take cues from the region and form any type of tissue. A new tissue such as bone would be harmful in the area.

The delivery of an engineered product, such as biomaterials, brings up another problem of long-term sustenance in the body. The material might become harmful in long-term implantation and in this case would need to be degraded at a specific time. The time needed for dissolving the material will require flexibility. In injuries with severe inflammation, the response could be different than responses in cases of minimal inflammation. Thus, it might be necessary to deliver multiple implantations.

**SEE ALSO:** Cancer; Cells, Embryonic; Spinal Cord Injury; Self-Renewal, Stem Cell; Transdifferentiation.

**BIBLIOGRAPHY.** S. J. Greco and P. Rameshwar, "Enhancing Effect of IL-1α on Neurogenesis from Adult Human Mesenchymal Stem Cells: Implication for Inflammatory Mediators in Regenerative Medicine," *Journal of Immunology* (v.179, 2007); N. Rosenthal, "Prometheus's Vulture and the Stem-Cell Promise," *New England Journal of Medicine* (v.349, 2003).

Pranela Rameshwar
University of Medicine and Dentistry of New Jersey

# Microscope

**A MICROSCOPE IS** an instrument used to observe structures that are too small to be seen by the naked eye. It usually does so by using different lenses that can refract waves, and when focused, these waves can give an image that is much larger then the object itself. This instrument, which is of vital importance, especially to the field of health sciences, has a very interesting history.

When early man saw natural glass for the first time in the volcanic rocks, little did he know of the uses it was to have. Even the person standing in front of the first coated glass, appreciating the perfect reflection it had to offer—so unlike the wavering reflections given by flowing streams and stagnant pools—must have known little of the real beauty hiding within that light-reflecting piece of art. How amused early man would have been when the reading stone was used in 1000 C.E. or when Salvino D'Armate created the first wearable spectacles in 1284. D'Armate, in turn, did not know that the very glass that he was using to strengthen weakening eyesight would soon give us sight into a world where a naked human eye was nothing but blind.

Though lenses (named after the seeds of lentil they resembled) existed even before the birth of Christ, it was not until 1590 that any kind of proper microscope was invented. Zaccharias Janssen and his son Hans, two Dutch spectacle makers, while experimenting with a few lenses in a tube, realized that nearby objects appeared greatly enlarged. Little did they imagine, though, that the simple instrument they had just made would be the predecessor of a scientific apparatus that would form the basis of histology, microbiology, embryology, and numerous other fields.

In 1609, Galileo, who knew about the older experiments with lenses, made the first microscope with a focusing device. However, Galileo's main interest was in space and the heavenly bodies, for which he needed a telescope. The person who actually worked on the microscope and earned the title of "father of microscopy" was Anton van Leeuwenhoek.

The microscope's further journey was not as slow paced as its original invention, and the microscope soon was being modified to offer better and bigger images. Many scientists worked on it and improved the basic design by adding to it. The compound microscope, invented in 1509, became the basis for all the light microscopes used afterwards. This basic design was improved radically, and additions and subtractions were made in the design according to the individual user.

However, it was not until 1665 that the microscope helped make a discovery that was to change the basis of biology—and thus every field that is related to the study of life—forever. In 1665 Robert Hook used a microscope to examine a piece of dead log and found it to be made of "empty honeycomb-like boxes." He called them *cells*. This generated a wave of excitement among scientists, who now had a basic idea of the basic unit of life. Later, it was again the microscope that led to the discovery of the structures within the cell and thus gave birth to many fields that today are of vital importance.

Taking the study of microscopic life further, Anton van Leeuwenhoek made a simple microscope (with one lens) and studied blood, yeast, insects, and many other things in 1674. However, his simple microscope was not a solution to all problems—things much smaller than a cell existed, and in vast numbers, and this microscope only showed a two-dimensional structure. Therefore, different scientists worked to overcome this difficulty, with each overcoming a different set of problems, yet none answering all of them.

The greatest discovery in this regard was of the electron microscope, which uses electrons as the source of illumination, rather than light, and allowed scientists to see structures much smaller than the wavelength of visible light, broadening the horizons of our understanding of life. This discovery, made by Ernst Ruska, won Ruska a Nobel Prize in 1986. However, the electron microscope does not allow us to see living material, as the light microscope does. This is why all sorts of microscopes are still in use, because no individual machine is perfect.

## TYPES OF MICROSCOPES

The different kinds of microscopes include compound microscopes, ultramicroscopes, phase contrast microscopes, dissecting microscopes, electron microscopes, and scanning tunneling microscopes, among others. Compound microscopes are the simplest of all microscopes and are still the most widely used worldwide. They use a visible light source to illuminate the object to be seen. The light source might be sunlight or a bulb. The microscope offers a range of magnifications that can be adjusted by using lenses of different powers, but unfortunately, the best resolution it can give is 200 nm, or 2,000 Armstrong units. This limitation is the result of its use of visible light, which has a specific range of wavelengths. If objects smaller than that are to be observed, then other kinds of microscopes must be used. Another disadvantage to the compound microscope is that it can only provide a two-dimensional image.

The problem of the resolution was to some extent solved when Richard Zsigmondy invented the ultramicroscope in 1903, which allowed scientists to view objects much smaller in size than the wavelength of light. The objects are held in liquid or gaseous suspension in an enclosure with an intensely black background and illuminated with a convergent pencil of very bright light entering from one side and coming to focus in the field of view.

The phase contrast microscope was invented by Frits Zernike in 1932. It is used to view transparent or colorless biological material. This discovery won its inventor a Nobel Prize in 1953. The phase contrast technique employs an optical mechanism to translate minute variations in phase into corresponding changes in amplitude, which can be visualized as differences in image contrast. One of the major advantages of phase contrast microscopy is that living cells can be examined in their natural state without having been killed, fixed, and stained.

The difficulty with microscopes only showing two-dimensional images was solved by the invention of the dissecting microscope, which shows three-dimensional images, but its magnification is very low, and hence structures such as cells cannot be viewed separately.

All these microscopes use light as the source of illumination, but to study the microworld in more detail, a microscope was needed that uses a source with much smaller wavelength than visible light. The electron microscope, invented in 1931, uses electrons as the source of illumination and has a resolution 1,000 times stronger than that of the light microscope. However, this was not the last step in the progressive field of microscopy. In 1981 Gerd Binnig and Heinrich Rohrer invented the scanning tunneling microscope, which allows scientists to observe three-dimensional images of substances as small as atoms. This microscope remains to date the most accurate image-providing microscope. Gerg Binnig and Heinrich Rohrer received a Nobel Prize in 1986.

Many other types of microscopes are in use today, and new additions and advancements are constantly being made in the important and ever-growing field of microscopy. To this day, the microscope remains of the utmost necessity to numerous fields of study.

**SEE ALSO:** Cells, Adult; Cells, Human; In Vitro Fertilization.

**BIBLIOGRAPHY.** Sally Morgan, *From Microscopes to Stem Cell Research: Discovering Regenerative Medicine* (Heinemann, 2007); Jutta Schickore, *The Microscope and the Eye: A History of Reflections, 1740–1870* (University of Chicago Press, 2007).

Tahawur Abbas Khaleeq
National University of Science and Technology

# Minnesota

**MINNESOTA IS A** state in the central northern part of the continental United States. It is bordered to the east by the Canadian states of Ontario and Manitoba, by Lake Superior and Wisconsin to the east, Iowa to the south and South and North Dakota to the west. It became the 32nd state of the union in 1858 and its name is derived from a word used by the Sioux people who previously owned the land. The state has a land area slightly in excess of 87,000 square miles and a population of just under 5 million.

Since its settling by Europeans, the state has been dominated by immigrants from Germany and the Scandinavian countries, who have brought a certain cultural and religious sensibility with them and who have more or less flourished in the farming, timber, and resource-extraction industries that have covered the prairies, woodlands, and lakes of Minnesota. However, in recent years, a higher level of ethnic diversity has been witnessed, particular in the twin cities of St. Paul and Minneapolis, in which more than half of the state's population live, and which house the bulk of its commerce, government, cultural, and social institutions.

Partly as a result of liberal voter registration rules and a good standard of education, Minnesota has acquired a reputation for high levels of engagement with the political process and with general support for progressive and liberal policies. Senator Paul Wellstone, for example, was before his untimely death in a plane crash a leading and articulate exponent of the potential benefits of stem cell research. However, it would be wrong to characterize the situation as purely partisan, as leading figures of all shades of opinion in Minnesota have supported the research, while others have been opposed to it for one reason or another. Although generalizations are often invidious, it appears that most Minnesotans are quite prepared for stem cell research to take place within their state and are prepared to debate the appropriate checks and balances that would help guide researchers most appropriately. Controversy within the state on this issue is not prominent compared to certain other parts of the country.

One of the principal institutions supporting stem cell research in the state is the Stem Cell Institute at the University of Minnesota, which has a mission statement saying: "Our mission is to further our understanding of the potential of stem cells to improve human and animal life." The institute has received some $15 million in capital investments from the university since its inception in 1999 and a total of funding in excess of $43 million. More than 500 people are involved in the research, which has yielded 15 current U.S. patents relating to stem cells and targets diseases in seven primary areas: cancer, neurology, cardiology, liver, diabetes, vessel, and genetic.

Seventeen university departments and schools work together in this institute, which, thereby, acts as a focal point for joint research and development. One early success at the institute was the demonstration of how adult human bone marrow cells can differentiate in vitro to become hepatocytes—effective liver cells that can do the principal functions of original liver cells. Other work shows similar ability to differentiate into other functional cells related to target areas.

**SEE ALSO:** *Individual U.S. State Articles*; Biotechnology, History of; Clinical Trials Within U.S.: Batten Disease; Clinical Trials Within U.S.: Blind Process; Clinical Trials Within U.S.: Cancer; Clinical Trials Within U.S.: Heart Disease; Clinical Trials Within U.S.: Peripheral Vascular Disease; Clinical Trials Within U.S.: Skin Transplants (Burns); Clinical Trials Within U.S.: Spinal Cord Injury; Clinical Trials Within U.S.: Traumatic Brain Injury; Ethics; Federal Government Policies; Moral Status of Embryo;.

**BIBLIOGRAPHY.** "Adult Bone Marrow Stem Cells Can Become Liver Cells, Minnesota Researchers Report," *Science Daily* (May 15, 2002), www.sciencedaily.com (cited February 2008); Annette Atkins, *Creating Minnesota: A History from the Inside Out* (Minnesota Historical Society Press, 2007); William E. Lass, *Minnesota: A History*, 2nd ed. (Norton, 2000); The Stem Cell Institute at the University of Minnesota, www.stemcell.umn.edu (cited February 2008).

John Walsh
Shinawatra University

# Mississippi

**IN EARLY FEBRUARY** 2006, the Mississippi House of Representatives passed a bill that forbids stem cell research using embryonic stem cells or even somatic cell nuclear transfer (SCNT), a form of therapeutic cloning. SCNT involves injecting an adult stem cell into an unfertilized egg, effectively cloning the adult cells. Opponents to this process argue that it could rapidly lead to human cloning. Supporters of SCNT argue that scientists are not trying to clone humans but, rather, to clone customized organs or tissues that could be used to restore the health of the original donor of the adult stem cell. These customized tissues would not present the risks of traditional organ transplants because the recipient's immune system would recognize the new organ as its own and thereby not reject it.

On July 18, 2006, the U.S. Senate convened to vote on a proposed bill (H.R.810) that would amend the Public Health Service Act and provide federal funding for research on human embryonic stem cells. This bill was passed by the Senate but was later vetoed by President George W. Bush. In the vote, the two Mississippi senators voted in favor of the bill, despite February's indication of where the state of Mississippi stood on stem cell research. These senators were Thad Cochran and Trent Lott, both Republicans.

Despite the political standstill on stem cell research, scientists in Mississippi are continuing to seek education in the field of stem cells. In early 2002, the University of Mississippi (UM) held the Symposium on the Scientific, Ethical, Legal, and Societal Impact of Stem Cell Research, sponsored in part by the Trent Lott Leadership Institute at UM. The goal of this symposium was to bring together experts from the four title fields as well as graduate students, senior researchers, and members of the public, to discuss openly all sides of the stem cell issue and raise awareness of the challenges and potential benefits involved in stem cell research.

In 2006 the Office of Research and Sponsored Programs at UM announced a call for research proposals to investigate the role of stem cells with developmental biology of the brain as well as brain tumors. This research would be funded by the Goldhirsch Foundation Brain Tumor Research Awards Program, out of Branford, Connecticut. The money would therefore be supplied by a state that supports stem cell research. Although a project out of this program would not necessarily be supported by the state of Mississippi, a Mississippi scientist could still conduct the research. This disparity is resolved by the fact that the bill passed by the Mississippi House of Representatives allows Mississippians to seek stem cell research opportunities outside of the state.

**SEE ALSO:** *Individual U.S. State Articles*; Biotechnology, History of; Clinical Trials Within U.S.: Batten Disease; Clinical Trials Within U.S.: Blind Process; Clinical Trials Within U.S.: Cancer; Clinical Trials Within U.S.: Heart Disease; Clinical Trials Within U.S.: Peripheral Vascular Disease; Clinical Trials Within U.S.: Skin Transplants (Burns); Clinical Trials Within U.S.: Spinal Cord Injury; Clinical Trials Within U.S.: Traumatic Brain Injury; Ethics; Federal Government Policies; Moral Status of Embryo; Special Interest/Lobby Groups; United States.

**BIBLIOGRAPHY.** M. Bellomo, *The Stem Cell Divide: The Facts, the Fiction, and the Fear Driving the Greatest Scientific, Political and Religious Debate of Our Time* (American Management Association, 2006); C. B. Cohen, *Renewing the Stuff of Life: Stem Cells, Ethics, and Public Policy* (Oxford University Press, 2007); C. Fox, *Cell of Cells: The Global Race to Capture and Control the Stem Cell* (Norton, 2007); B. Harrison, "Stem Cell Ban Passes House," *Daily Journal* (February 9, 2006); K. R. Monroe, R. Miller, and J. Tobis, eds., *Fundamentals of the Stem Cell Debate: The Scientific, Religious, Ethical, and Political Issues* (University of California Press, 2007); M. Ruse and C. A. Pynes, eds., *The Stem Cell Controversy: Debating the Issues (Contemporary Issues)* (Prometheus, 2006); C. Vestal, "States Take Sides on Stem Cell Research," www.stateline.org (cited January 2008).

Claudia Winograd
University of Illinois, Urbana-Champaign

# Missouri

**THE DEBATE ON** stem cell research rages on in the state of Missouri. Many states have successfully enacted some legislation that addresses the specific uses and means of harvesting human embryonic stem cells, and Missouri has followed suit. Missouri law currently forbids the use of state funds for cloning for reproductive purposes but does permit cloning for research. It does not specifically prohibit research on the human fetus/embryo but does not allow research on a fetus that was alive before abortion, thereby eliminating the so-called abortion-for-research practice. The law also prohibits the sale of human tissue for research and cloning purposes.

Missouri is one of three states (including Iowa and Massachusetts) that affirm the legality of human embryonic stem cell research but that do not provide state funding for this scientific endeavor. Many organizations, such as the Missouri Coalition for Lifesaving Cures and the Missouri Right to Life, are active in the state on both sides of this important ethical and legislative issue. This was widely considered to be the key issue that decided Missouri's U.S. Senate seat race in 2006. Also in 2006, the legislature passed the Stem Cell Research and Cures Initiative, a constitutional amendment that gives constitutional backing to the right to conduct stem cell research and for patients to receive the therapies developed through it. There are many stem cell research programs active in Missouri today under these legislative provisions.

The battle did not end there, however. The constitutional language allowing stem cell research is still rather vague. Recently, a group called Cures Without Cloning has proposed an amendment to the existing Missouri law that would outlaw somatic cell nuclear transfer, a form of cloning in which the nucleus of a human cell is injected into an unfertilized human egg, which is then stimulated to grow. Anticloning groups contend that a cloned human exists after an embryo is made with this technique. Many other groups are still reviewing this new proposal and the current language of the law. It is not likely that the matters related to embryonic stem cell research will be completely settled for a long time.

One of the largest privately funded research organizations in Missouri and a primary financial supporter of the stem cell research–related ballot initiative is the Stowers Institute for Medical Research in Kansas City. This organization was founded in 1994 and established in Kansas City, Missouri, by James and Virginia Stowers, who were both cancer survivors and independently wealthy after founding American Century Investments Corporation. In 2007 the Stowers Institute housed 24 independent research programs and employed over 420 scientists, research associates, and technicians. The mission of the Stowers Institute is to seek more effective means of preventing and curing disease through basic research on genes and proteins that control fundamental processes of cellular life. The $30 million campaign for the stem cell research ballot initiative was funded in large part by the Stowers family.

At the University of Missouri in Columbia, many scientists are currently performing research using embryonic stem cell lines in animals. The

Transgenic Animal Core, directed by Dr. Elizabeth Critser, assists scientists from many different labs in preparing transgenic animals for various research projects. This facility has been involved in the creation of well over 100 transgenic animals. Research here also targets the development of cell lines from sources other than the embryo or fetus. Dr. Elmer Price was able to isolate adult stem cells from the blood of swine that have been able to grow into neurons and blood vessel cells. Still, these adult stem cells have not been as easy to differentiate and develop into different tissues as embryonic stem cells.

At Washington University in St. Louis, Dr. Jeffrey Gordon and Dr. Michael Lovett have collaborated to join the Stem Cell Genome Anatomy Project and to focus their research on gastric and intestinal stem cells. This research is part of a much larger consortium funded by the National Institutes of Health that seeks to study and characterize tissue-specific progenitor cells and to use these in bioinformatics and bioengineering techniques. Many other researchers at Washington University have focused on the development of pluripotent stem cells into fully developed adult cells such as neurons and other tissues. This has been a rather hot field, as stem cells must not only survive after implantation but must also grow into the developed tissues of interest to be useful.

Not only are many scientists at St. Louis University working on the scientific aspects of stem cell research but the ethics department is also on the forefront of the stem cell ethics debate. Dr. Gerard Magill is the director of the Center for Care Ethics and chairman of the program for healthcare ethics at St. Louis University. He is one of the prominent ethicists specializing in the more difficult ethical aspects of stem cell research and human cloning and has written several books and many scholarly papers on the topic.

Sigma-Aldrich is the largest for-profit company engaging in stem cell research in Missouri. With its headquarters in St. Louis, Sigma-Aldrich is a leading life science and high-technology company. It provides many products and reagents used in genomics and stem cell research around the world. Although the company does not directly perform stem cell research, it is integral in supporting the expansion of this scientific research field for others.

Overall, Missouri is very active in every aspect of stem cell research. The Missouri legislature has been a battleground for this issue for the past several years, which has had far-reaching consequences in other states across the country. Missouri researchers are integral in key stem cell breakthroughs and nationally funded projects. The battle will no doubt continue within Missouri and the rest of the country, while the shape of the stem-cell environment is influenced and different groups continue to battle over this controversial topic.

**SEE ALSO:** *Individual U.S. State Articles*; Biotechnology, History of; Clinical Trials Within U.S.: Batten Disease; Clinical Trials Within U.S.: Blind Process; Clinical Trials Within U.S.: Cancer; Clinical Trials Within U.S.: Heart Disease; Clinical Trials Within U.S.: Peripheral Vascular Disease; Clinical Trials Within U.S.: Skin Transplants (Burns); Clinical Trials Within U.S.: Spinal Cord Injury; Clinical Trials Within U.S.: Traumatic Brain Injury; Ethics; Federal Government Policies; Moral Status of Embryo; Special Interest/Lobby Groups; United States.

**BIBLIOGRAPHY.** National Conference of State Legislatures, "State Embryonic and Fetal Research Laws," www.ncsl.org (cited November 2007); State of Missouri, www.missouri.edu (cited November 2007); Christine Vestal, "Embryonic Stem Cell Research Divides States," www.stateline.org (cited November 2007).

John S. Kuo
University of Wisconsin

# Montana

**IN FEBRUARY 2005,** the Montana State Legislature passed a bill that urged U.S. President George W. Bush and the U.S. Congress to support stem cell research. The bill was titled Senate Joint Resolution No. 18 and was a combined resolution of the Montana Senate and House of Representatives. The bill stressed that the contemporary lines of stem cells were contaminated and could therefore not be used therapeutically; it also cited the states of California, Illinois, New Jersey, New York, and Wisconsin for either having already established stem cell research centers or for establishing groundwork to do so and noted that polls showed that the majority of American citizens favored stem cell research.

On July 18, 2006, the U.S. Senate convened to vote on a proposed bill (H.R.810) that would amend the Public Health Service Act and provide federal funding for research on human embryonic stem cells.

This bill was passed by the Senate but was later vetoed by President George W. Bush. In the vote, the two Montana senators voted against each other—Democrat Max Baucus was in favor of the bill and Republican Conrad Burns opposed it.

On April 20, 2007, Dr. Irving Weissman, a Montana native and premier stem cell scientist, gave a free public lecture at Montana State University (MSU). His lecture was titled "Stem Cell Research and the Future." Weissman received his bachelor's degree from Montana State College in 1961; Montana State College became Montana State University in 1965, and Weissman was subsequently recognized with an honorary MSU degree in 1992. He also served as a high school intern at the McLaughlin Research Institute (MRI), an independent nonprofit research center located in Great Falls, Montana, and affiliated with MSU.

MRI Director Dr. George A. Carlson conducts research on neurological disorders. One facet of his lab is investigating the development and differentiation of central nervous system stem cells (CNS-SC). CNS-SC can be isolated and studied in the laboratory, outside of the brain, to determine what causes them to develop into neurons or glial cells, the support cells of the brain. Carlson studies CNS-SC in his lab with the hope of developing a future therapy for Alzheimer's disease in which critical neurons either die or lose their proper function. Potentially, CNS-SC could be programmed to differentiate into healthy neurons that could replace the effete cells and treat or cure Alzheimer's disease.

In 2004, Carlson, in collaboration with California-based company StemCells, Inc., was awarded a prestigious grant from the National Institutes of Health. The total sum awarded amounted to $465,000 and was to be put toward Carlson's research on CNS-SC.

**SEE ALSO:** *Individual U.S. State Articles*; Biotechnology, History of; Clinical Trials Within U.S.: Batten Disease; Clinical Trials Within U.S.: Blind Process; Clinical Trials Within U.S.: Cancer; Clinical Trials Within U.S.: Heart Disease; Clinical Trials Within U.S.: Peripheral Vascular Disease; Clinical Trials Within U.S.: Skin Transplants (Burns); Clinical Trials Within U.S.: Spinal Cord Injury; Clinical Trials Within U.S.: Traumatic Brain Injury; Ethics; Federal Government Policies; Moral Status of Embryo; Special Interest/Lobby Groups; United States.

**BIBLIOGRAPHY.** M. Bellomo, *The Stem Cell Divide: The Facts, the Fiction, and the Fear Driving the Greatest Scientific, Political and Religious Debate of Our Time* (American Management Association, 2006); C. B. Cohen, *Renewing the Stuff of Life: Stem Cells, Ethics, and Public Policy* (Oxford University Press, 2007); R. Ecke, "McLaughlin Grant to Aid Stem Cell Research," *Great Falls Tribune* (October 9, 2004); C. Fox, *Cell of Cells: The Global Race to Capture and Control the Stem Cell* (Norton, 2007); K. R. Monroe, R. Miller, and J. Tobis, eds., *Fundamentals of the Stem Cell Debate: The Scientific, Religious, Ethical, and Political Issues* (University of California Press, 2007); Montana Legislature, "Senate Joint Resolution No. 18," data.opi.state.mt.us (cited January 2008); M. Ruse and C. A. Pynes, eds., *The Stem Cell Controversy: Debating the Issues (Contemporary Issues)* (Prometheus, 2006); C. Vestal, "States Take Sides on Stem Cell Research," www.stateline.org (cited January 2008).

Claudia Winograd
University of Illinois, Urbana-Champaign

# Moral Status of Embryo

**DETERMINING THE MORAL** status of a human embryo means that a moral principle is applied to biological facts by human reasoning at some point in a biological process. The point in the process chosen unites natural facts as understood by humans with ideas of ought, or right, or moral principle(s). The evaluative reasoning used to make a moral judgment about the moral status of an embryo has numerous consequences. The consequences significantly affect the embryo, individuals related to the embryo, and society as well.

The moral status of a fetus that is the product of natural reproduction is a matter that has been generally settled around the world from millennia of human experience. The developments of modern medicine making abortion very safe have reopened the issue of the moral status of a fetus in a natural pregnancy. In an example of the fact that law and morals are not always in agreement, the issue of abortion has been settled in Anglo-American law with the decision that an embryo as it develops into a fetus is not given full legal rights until after birth.

The politics of the abortion controversy have affected the moral debate about the status of embryos that are the product of advancing reproductive technology. Many of those who claim a moral status for an embryo in all cases of natural pregnancy extend this claim to both in vivo and in vitro fertilization.

It is generally understood that an embryo begins its existence when a sperm fertilizes an egg. In normal reproduction, this cycle ends with birth of the being the embryo was destined to become at fertilization. Actually, the early development of an embryo is not quite so simple nor so determined because the biological development of a fertilized egg is a much more complicated process than it was understood to be by previous generations. The process involves a variety of possibilities that affect the future of the embryo, and therefore its possible moral status. As a consequence, the moral status of an embryo as a human being at conception is a matter of serious debate for a number of reasons. Some reasons are religious, and others are secular.

In general, most controversy about the moral status of an embryo in regard to stem cell research is about the life of the embryo between fertilization and its development to about the 14th day of in vitro fertilization. Broadly, the stages in reproduction can be called the prefertilization stage, the early development stage, and the later development stage. Only the early development stage arouses moral controversy. The prefertilization stage usually does not raise moral controversy, and the later developmental stage is not controversial because the embryo was successfully implanted, with the pregnancy then proceeding normally.

There is a problem, however, that arises in using the term *stages*, in that it seems to imply that the stages are *events*. This is really an older way of looking at the reproductive process, which rendered the act of fertilization of an egg an event, which seems to suggest that it is fixed. Contemporary science has shown that reproduction, whether natural or technologically assisted, is a fluid process in which a number of things can occur that can produce several possible futures for the embryo in its earliest stages of development. This understanding makes it more difficult to mark some point in the process as a definitive biological development.

The prefertilization stage involves both spermatozoa and ova (eggs). Before fertilization, these are called gametes. Sperm and eggs are each produced by the process of gametogenesis. In the gametocyte phase, the gametes divide by meiosis into gametes in organs that are called gonads in animals. To date, there have been very few—if any—moralists argue that there is a moral status to the unfertilized eggs or to sperms. They are not generally viewed as having a moral status.

Strictly speaking, if spermatozoa and ova, before fertilization, were given moral status, there would be a duty to protect them, so that every egg ovulated must be somehow fertilized and all sperm must be used for this purpose. In reality, most sperm are not used to fertilize ova because, even when implanted during sexual intercourse, the woman is not ovulating, or a contraceptive may be used that is a spermicidal agent, or the sperm is lost in nighttime wet dreams or in masturbation. In contrast, most ova are never fertilized because women are not married, or if married, their husband is absent for some reason, or contraception is being practiced for some other reason.

It does not seem to be the plan of nature or (in Thomas Jefferson's words) the plan of nature's God that all eggs and sperms ever produced should accomplish their biological purpose, assuming that there is teleology inherent in nature. It has indeed seemed to some observers that nature is somewhat wasteful or overabundant in guaranteeing the reproduction of the species. Nor is it likely that prefertilization gametes have ever been given moral status. The situation changes, however, when fertilization occurs.

The second stage of reproduction, early development, includes fertilization and the first 8- to 12-cell divisions. Fertilization occurs when a spermatozoon unites with an ovum to form a zygote. The fertilization occurs either by nature through sexual intercourse or by artificial means. In the case of a normal pregnancy, there is a long tradition of moral evaluation of the developing embryo. However, in both the case of natural fertilization and that of reproductive technology that permits in vitro fertilization, the process is rather more complicated and fluid than was previously understood. This fluidity in the number of things that can happen during the earliest divisions of the zygote presents problems to claims that a human being is created at the moment of conception, whether naturally or in vitro.

## IN VITRO FERTILIZATION

The issue of stem cell research and the moral status of an embryo is a product of modern medical technology. Thanks to advances in reproductive technology, it has become possible for childless couples to have children from their own genetic materials though in vitro fertilization. From this great modern medical wonder have come blessed bundles of joy to numerous couples. However, the process of in vitro fertilization has also created new conditions that have evoked moral controversy.

Before the development of cryogenic freezing for preserving indefinitely in vitro fertilized embryos, the problem of what to do with the surplus embryos was answered by nature. The fertilized embryos lost their viability in less than a week. Within six or seven days, a preimplantation embryo disintegrates inside of the cell.

Unless all embryos were to be implanted, there would, of necessity, be a loss of fertilized embryos. The reason for the loss is that in harvesting eggs from a woman's ovaries, the drugs used to stimulate ovulation need to be strong enough to produce several times the number of eggs actually needed. This is because implantation, a demanding physical experience, was not guaranteed, so at least two embryos are implanted. The issue of what to do with the surplus embryos was not an issue until after the development of cryogenic freezing, which led to the embryos being able to be kept indefinitely.

The growing number of frozen embryos in existence raised the issue of what to do with them if they were not to be used by the couple from who they were produced. The reasons for not using them were several, including the fact if all the frozen embryos were used, it might mean bearing far more children than the coupled wanted. So what ought to be done with preimplantation zygotes? Were they to be simply flushed? Were they to be donated unwillingly or unwillingly, knowingly or unknowingly, to sterile couples who could not produce their own in vitro embryos? Or should couples be made to pay rent in a liquid nitrogen bank indefinitely? What was to be done with them by the embryo bank after they had been there for years and contact had been lost with the couples to whom they belonged?

The moral status of the preimplantation embryo is a matter of controversy for Roman Catholics, Evangelicals, some conservative Christians, and others. In their view, at the moment of conception, the new zygote acquires a moral status. For many others, such as most Jews, Muslims, secularists, liberal Christians, and others, the fertilized egg does not acquire moral status until it is part of a successful pregnancy that has developed to the point of quickening.

## STEM CELL RESEARCH

Debates on the moral status of the preimplantation embryos have developed after decades of legal and moral debates on abortion. The battles waged since the American *Roe v. Wade* (1973) legal case have contributed to the debate on preimplantation views on the status of frozen embryos. Also contributing to the debate has been the development of stem cell research. Neither in vitro fertilization nor stem cell research existed as fields of research when the abortion controversy began.

Many researchers and those who could benefit from their research are eager to use the surplus preimplantation embryos. The researcher seeks to learn about the nature of stem cells in their earliest stages because it is hoped that cures of a great number of diseases will be discovered from this research. However, embryonic research destroys the embryo. The question of moral status then involves the question of whether or not a preimplantation embryo has a moral status. If so, is it permissible to conduct experiments? If not, then how are the embryos to be handled?

## RELIGIOUS ETHICS

The grounds for deciding the moral status of preimplantation embryos are either religious or secular. The religious grounds arise from the belief that a human being is created at conception. The belief that preimplantation embryos have a moral status is grounded in a general regard for the sanctity of life. This position is sometimes called the biological humanity view. However, this is a stance that rests on the development of religious ethics from biblical passages, none of which are specifically referring to preimplantation embryos. Prohibitions against abortions by Christians have used the passages in the Bible on accidental miscarriage and other principles to prohibit abortion virtually since the beginning of Christianity.

Applying the principles of abortion debates to the preimplantation zygotes has resulted in the moral judgment that the use of embryonic stem cells is morally offensive. The appropriate response to the unwanted frozen embryos is to either persuade the couples to whom they belong to give them to infertile couples who do not have even the option of in vitro fertilization or to allow the embryos to die and to give them proper burial.

In response, the use of unwanted preimplantation embryos is urged as morally proper by many Christians on the grounds that relieving the suffering of the sick is a religious duty. The ministry of healing is held in high regard by Christians because they look to the God and to numerous healing works of the apostles including Saint Luke (the Physician) and others. Some arguments that have been made are that all healing must be in response to prayer and faith. Among most Christians, the use of "means of grace," which includes medicines or medical research, is theologically very acceptable.

Other principles that have been offered by Christians include looking at the consequences of the research versus the consequences of not performing the research. The development of reproductive technology involved the destruction of embryos because losses were incurred in the creation of the technology. However, the net effect of the technology has been a great increase in human happiness. Babies have been and will continue to be born to what would otherwise be childless couples. The loss to humanity is viewed by those making these kinds of arguments as small because the preimplantation embryos would never have been born anyway. Counterarguments that the wrongs that create benefits are not morally acceptable are not likely to be persuasive to families who have children gained via reproductive technology.

Looking at the consequences of acts is a type of ethics. It is in opposition to the duty ethics that are advocated by those who claim that it is a moral fact that at conception all of the moral and legal rights of a full adult ought to be conferred on the preimplantation embryo. The response could be that the claim is a form of legalism or, more precisely, the practices of casuistry, or that the claim that it is a moral fact is actually a moral judgment that has attached a moral claim to a biological fact in a manner that may not be justifiable. The fact is, all moral decisions have consequences, including costs and benefits, to both the individuals involved and the moral community as well.

The moral debates often use analogous reasoning. One analogy that has been used is to compare the beginning-of-life issues surrounding the preimplantation embryo with an end-of-life situation. It is now technologically possible to preserve a person in a vegetative state long after their brain has ceased to emit waves indicating that it is functioning. This technologically produced situation would not have existed if nature were permitted to handle the future of the individual. However, with technology and at mounting cost, the individual could be kept "alive." The analogy is that the same could be done to preserve preimplantation embryos. The call for heroic efforts for the artificially alive is not one that many moralists would find acceptable because the costs to society would be tremendous and would be borne by many as yet unborn.

## THE "CONCEPTIONIST" POSITION

If the claim that a human being exists at conception is made, then the claim rests on viewing the naturally fertilized embryo the same as an in vitro embryo. However, the rejection of the moral claim of full humanity for preimplantation embryos is made by many Christians on the grounds that the analogy of natural fertilization and in vitro fertilization is a false analogy. Natural reproduction for bearing children and using reproductive technology for producing children are technically different.

Those who believe that conception is the event that defines a human being argue that it is the time of ensoulment. Therefore, to abort a fetus or to destroy a preimplantation embryo is to damage a being made in the image of God. Some holding this position have argued that the whole process of in vitro fertilization is immoral and therefore results in murder because it involves the death of embryos. However, if instead of fertilizing the eggs harvested for the in vitro process the ova gametes were simply frozen and only one used at a time, then the process would not result in the loss of embryos. The cost of this approach would be high for each attempted implantation, however, with most couples finding it unaffordable.

Another argument that is made against the claim of full humanity for preimplantation embryos is that to simply flush them is to not accord them human dignity. General agreement on this point has not been found to answer the question of what ought to be done with the growing surplus of "unwanted" preimplantation embryos. Many of those who wish to accord full humanity to preimplantation embryos urge their respectful burial. Conducting a funeral for the embryos would sanctify them for the religious but would be viewed by others as simply a religiously sanctioned form of dumping the embryos down the drain.

In opposition to the view that proper burial is the morally appropriate way to dispose of surplus preimplantation embryos is the moral claim that there are great benefits to be gained by using the embryos that will not waste them. The medical advances are potentially great and the relief of human suffering also enormous. The embryos would—even if accepted as fully human—be analogous to soldiers that fall in battle. Their sacrifice would be for the good of the whole moral community.

The "conceptionist" position entails a moral issue that may arise from successful developments in future stem cell research. If a cure for some disease(s) were developed through the use of preimplantation embryonic research, it would be morally offensive to use it because it would be the product of "murders." How many people enduring the suffering of a family member(s) with diseases such as Parkinson's would deny treatments and allow the suffering to continue to maintain moral purity? Although the question is currently hypothetical, it is a logical consequence of rigorously following the "conceptionist" position.

The problem with moral reasoning by some in the Christian faith is that their attempts to be morally pure seem to be denials of salvation by grace. Moreover, the human condition is one of existence in a fallen world in which ethical action is morally imperfect or ambiguous.

## OTHER VIEWPOINTS

Secular grounds for determining the moral status of preimplantation embryos are several. The sentient being view operates from the observation that an embryo, until about the 14th day of development, is not a sentient being. It can neither feel pain nor communicate. On the grounds that to be a human being is to be a being that communicates, some secular moralists have denied a moral status to zygotes in early development. Another view is that of the genetic humanity. This position claims that human embryos are humans entitled to all rights. Of course, this means that all preimplantation embryos have a right to implantation and that there are wombs that have a duty to receive them.

The species argument claims a special status for embryos as members of a special species. Some have argued that this is a form of "speciesism," which can be viewed as a form of racism. The assertion is somewhat circular, claiming that a species is valuable because is a member of a species.

Another moral view point that is derived from natural reason is the one that asks what kind of beings can have rights. The goal then is to develop a doctrine of rights that protects interests. Something can be viewed as having a moral status it if matters. A preimplantation embryo that is surplus and scheduled for disposal at a future time is one without real interests or with only those interests that are imputed to it by human adults.

The moral claim that embryos have a moral status is based on the "person view." This position claims that because humans have psychological attributes called personality they therefore have a moral status. This position, as critics have noted, has not explained why sentience creates moral rights. In general the fact that humans exist does not prove that they have rights. Having a biological life is not the same as having a biographical life. The claim to a moral status is simply a moral claim advanced as an interpretation of the facts of nature. The moral status of embryos in the case of preimplantation embryos is supported by some and denied by others. If a solution to this dispute is available, it may emerge with a better understanding of human nature from reason or revelation.

**SEE ALSO:** Advocacy; Cells, Embryonic; Ethics; In Vitro Fertilization; Religion, Buddhist; Religion, Catholic; Religion, Christian; Religion, Hindu; Religion, Jewish; Religion, Muslim; Religion, Protestant; Stem Cells, Bush Ruling.

**BIBLIOGRAPHY.** Janet T. Arnes, *Stem Cell Research: Issues and Bibliography* (Novinka, 2006); Michael Bellomo, *The Stem Cell Divide: The Facts, the Fiction, and the Fear Driving the Greatest Scientific, Political and Religious Debate of Our Time* (AMACOM, 2006); Robert P. George and Christopher Tollefsen, *Embryo: A Defense of Human Life* (Doubleday, 2008); Ronald M. Green, *The Human Embryo Research Debates: Bioethics in the Vortex of Controversy* (Oxford University Press, 2001); David Guinn, ed., *Handbook of Bioethics and Religion* (Oxford University Press, 2006); Eve Herold, *Stem Wars: Inside Stories from the Frontlines* (Macmillan, 2006); Suzanne Holland, Karen Lebacqz, and Laurie Zoloth, eds., *The Human Embryonic Stem Cell Debate: Science, Ethics, and Public Policy* (MIT Press, 2001); David Albert Jones, *Soul of the Embryo: Christianity and the Human Embryo* (Continuum International, 2004); Helga Kuhse and Peter Singer, eds., *Unsanctifying Human Life* (Wiley, 2002); Glenn McGee and Arthur L. Caplan, *The Human Cloning Debate* (Berkeley Hills, 2004); John F. Peppin. Mark J. Cherry, and Ana Iltis. *Religious Perspectives in Bioethics* (Taylor & Francis, 2004); Michael Ruse and Christopher A. Pynes, eds., *The Stem Cell Controversy: Debating the Issues*, 2nd ed. (Prometheus, 2006); Francoise Shenfield, *Ethical Dilemmas in Reproduction* (CRC Press, 2002); Nancy E. Snow, ed., *Stem Cell Research: New Frontiers in Science and Ethics* (University of Notre Dame Press, 2003); Bonnie Steinbock, *Life before Birth: The Moral and Legal Status of Embryos and Fetuses* (Oxford University Press, 1996); Brad Stetson, ed., *The Silent Subject: Reflections on the Unborn in American Culture* (Praeger, 1996); John A. Tichell and Scott B. Rae, "The Moral Status of Fetuses and Embryos," in *The Silent Subject: Reflections on the Unborn in American Culture* (Praeger, 1996).

Andrew J. Waskey
Dalton State College

# Morrison, Sean

**SEAN MORRISON, PH.D.,** is a researcher at the University of Michigan who examines different properties of stem cells from different tissues, namely the precursors of hematopoietic (blood and immune) cells and cells of the peripheral nervous system. Stem cells are cells that are at the top of the differentiation line; developing from these primitive cells are all types of cells in that certain tissue. Morrison and his lab investigate the intrinsic regulatory mechanisms of these stem cells, focusing specifically on cell self-renewal and cell aging. They are looking to see whether critical mechanisms are conserved between different stem cell lines, that is, do cells from the hematopoietic precursors and nervous cell precursors have similar cellular processes? A general answer the researchers have come up with is that yes, they do.

With regard to stem cell aging, the accepted theory is that stem cells wear out as the person ages. However, Morrison's laboratory has figured out that aged stem cells do not wear out; instead, they have a gene, *Ink4a*, that shuts them down in a programmed manner. Through understanding how age-specific functions in stem cells work, new treatments can be developed for health problems such as degenerative diseases. Overall, stem cells drive growth and regeneration in most tissues, so a theory is that age-related morbidity can be determined by aging stem cells.

Morrison has discovered that stem cells (in the hematopoietic and nervous systems) have conserved cellular changes as they age. The researchers are looking into how conserved gene expression changes lead to these conserved cellular changes. Through an appreciation of how stem cells proliferate and how the genes that protect them from aging, the aging process is better realized. It is also thought that some cancers come from the transformation of stem cells; by understanding how stem cells turn themselves off, new methods of cancer treatments can be uncovered.

Morrison's laboratory also examines the role of stem cells in organogenesis, which is organ development of the fetus. By understanding how stem cells facilitate organogenesis, it becomes feasible to see how disease is linked to stem cells—diseases such as congenital issues that are rooted in stem cell malfunction. Hirschsprung's disease is one such case. This is where defects in development and migration of neural crest stem cells in developing intestines lead to the infant's intestines having no neural stimulation to move food and feces along the gut. It can lead to chronic constipation and stretching of the intestines. Morrison has discovered there are two pathways that are defective. Without these pathways providing the proper signals, proper regulation of neural crest cell migration does not occur, and neurons do not get into gut tissues. The importance of this is that possible therapy with stem cells may be able to essentially bypass the effects of these inappropriate pathways.

Morrison's laboratory also discovered that hematopoietic stem cells differ from neural crest stem cells in how they create their specific organ systems. The hematopoietic stem cells do not specialize regionally. This is apparent because blood stem cells are in different places of the body throughout fetal and adult life, yet they all come out the same; thus, these stem cells have intrinsically identical organogenesis mechanisms. In contrast, the peripheral nervous system is very dependent on spatial location of the stem cell. Where the stem cells are located very directly dictates what sort of cell it will become. Morrison's laboratory is looking at how these differences are encoded in the genes of the stem cells.

Finally, Morrison and his researchers also look at and compare stem cell renewal regulatory mechanisms and cancer cell proliferation mechanisms. They have discovered that the gene *Bmi-1* is required for self-renewal (but not for differentiation) of all adult stem cells. It works by repressing p16 Ink4a (a cyclin-dependent kinase inhibitor) and p19 Arf (a p53 agonist). This shows that stem cells need ways to prevent premature senescence so that they can self-renew throughout person's life. An interesting point is that *Bmi-1* is conserved between stem cell lines and distinguishes stem cells cell cycle regulation from regulation of other, more restricted, progenitors. Because certain cancers, such as childhood leukemias, have their own stem cells, through being able to tell the difference between the cancerous cells and normal stem cells, treatment protocols can be developed. Leukemias are cancers composed of mutated blood-forming cells; the mutation essentially turns otherwise normal stem cell self-renewal mechanisms permanently on.

The laboratory has also discovered that stem cells in the embryo and adult are different from those in the developing fetus, citing that fetal blood cells in umbilical blood act differently than adult blood stem cells. They have found a gene called *Sox17*, which regulates hematopoietic cells in fetal mice but not adults, which can help regenerate blood systems when transferred from fetuses to adults. Without this gene, a blood system cannot develop. The next question to be answered is, Is this gene inappropriately activated in these childhood leukemias? Treatment involving Sox17 expression can also help stimulate blood-forming cells after bone marrow transplantation.

Morrison attended college at Dalhousie University in Halifax, Nova Scotia, Canada, receiving a bachelor's of science. He then attained his doctoral degree from Stanford University in immunology, where he identified key markers that are unique to blood cells. It was through this discovery that it was discovered that stem cells are present in adults. Before this, it was thought that adults did not have stem cells in their bodies. As a postdoctorate fellow in the Caltech lab of David Anderson, he was the first to isolate uncultured neural crest stem cells—cells that develop into the nerves and support cells of the peripheral nervous system.

Morrison is a Henry Sewall Professor in Medicine at the University of Michigan Medical School, research associate professor at the University of Michigan Life Sciences Institute, and director of the University of Michigan Center for Stem Cell Biology. He is also a Howard Hughes Medical Institute Investigator. Awards Morrison has won include the Seale Scholar Award, Mental Illness Research Association Milestone Award, *Technology Review* magazine's 100 young innovators (2002), and the Presidential Early Career Award for Scientists and Engineers.

When asked about the inspiration for his work, Morrison says:

> The greatest opportunities to change medicine arise from fundamental scientific discoveries, and I believe those opportunities exist in stem cell biology. Stem cell biology is so central to a variety of important scientific and clinical questions that it commands a lot of attention from researchers in diverse fields. That attracted me, because if I invest years of my life answering a question, I really want people to care what the answer is.

**SEE ALSO:** Cells, Adult; Michigan; University of Michigan.

**BIBLIOGRAPHY.** "LSI Team Identifies Gene that Regulates Blood-Forming Fetal Stem Cells," lsi.umich.edu/newsevents/discoveries/2007-07-26 (cited October 2007); "Mechanisms that Regulate Stem Cell Function in Diverse Tissues," www.hhmi.org/research/investigators/morrison.html (cited October 2007); "The Morrison Laboratory," www.umich.edu/~stemcell (cited October 2007); "Sean J. Morrison, Ph.D.," www.hhmi.org (cited October 2007); "Research," lsi.umich.edu/facultyresearch/labs/morrison/ (cited October 2007).

Caroline M. Sebley
Kansas City University of Medicine and Biosciences

# Mount Sinai School of Medicine

**MOUNT SINAI SCHOOL** of Medicine (MSSM) is a medical school located in the borough of Manhattan in New York City. The official name is Mount Sinai School of Medicine of New York University because of its academic affiliation with New York University (NYU). However, MSSM is independent of NYU; that is, MSSM has its own facilities, board of trustees, administration, student body, faculty, admissions offices, tuition fees, and endowment. MSSM also raises its own funds. MSSM and the Mount Sinai Hospital occupy a four-block area adjacent to Central Park in the community of Carnegie Hill. MSSM and Mount Sinai Hospital make up the Mount Sinai Medical Center. Mount Sinai Hospital was established in 1852 as the Jews' Hospital in the City of New York, but another century would pass before a school of medicine was created. Over the years, Mount Sinai Hospital built a well-earned reputation for the excellence of its patient care and clinical research programs. The laboratories and wards of Mount Sinai Hospital became a mecca for trainees interested in pathophysiology and basic science research.

In the late 1950s, Mount Sinai Hospital was ranked number 27 in the United States among institutions receiving National Institute of Health funds, an exceptional achievement for a hospital with little academic affiliation. Schools and colleges of medicine from Columbia University to NYU to Cornell University have sought the opportunity to use Mount Sinai Hospital as one of their primary teaching sites. For Mount Sinai Hospital to maintain its leadership position in the areas of clinical medicine and basic science research, it was decided that it would create the first, solely hospital-based medical school in the United States.

MSSM was chartered in 1963; in 1968, Mount Sinai School of Medicine of the City University of New York (CUNY) commenced its first class of future physicians. MSSM quickly became one of the leading medical schools in the United States, with Mount Sinai Hospital gaining international recognition for advances in patient care and the discovery of disease. After an extensive search and analysis, and after some setbacks, on January 1, 1998, NYU's hospital facilities were initially spun off as a separate, nonprofit organization and subsequently were joined with Mount Sinai Hospital to form Mount Sinai–NYU Health, an umbrella organization that joined the two hospitals. Throughout this process, the New York University School of Medicine continued to be a part of NYU; in 1999, with the approval of the board of regents of the University of the State of New York, MSSM, itself a separate nonprofit organization, changed its academic affiliation from CUNY to NYU. The merger between the NYU Medical Center and the Mount Sinai Medical Center and their facilities has since been dissolved, though MSSM's academic affiliation with NYU remains.

According to *U.S. News & World Report*, among medical schools, MSSM is currently ranked number 27 in the United States in medical research and number two in the United States in geriatrics. MSSM is also ranked number 20 in the United States among medical schools receiving National Institutes of Health grants.

MSSM's four missions of quality education, patient care, research, and community service follow the "commitment of serving science." The majority of students take part in some aspect of community service before graduating from MSSM. Notably, this participation includes the East Harlem Health Outreach Partnership, which was developed by the students of MSSM to create a health partnership between the East Harlem community and the MSSM, providing quality healthcare, regardless of ability to pay, to uninsured residents of East Harlem.

## THE BLACK FAMILY STEM CELL INSTITUTE

In 2005, financier Leon D. Black donated $10 million to MSSM to establish the Black Family Stem Cell Institute. The institute is currently directed by Gordon Keller, Ph.D., professor of gene and cell medicine. The Black Family Stem Cell Institute was established at MSSM to create a comprehensive research program that fosters the study of stem cell biology. The institute is an interdepartmental center that provides an outstanding interactive environment for the development of highly competitive research programs in both embryonic and adult stem cell biology within the MSSM.

The MSSM has state-of-the-art core facilities, including microarray, mouse genetics, microscopy, microsurgery, flow cytometry, and a newly established training facility for human embryonic stem (ES) cell research. Research in stem cell biology holds great promise for developing new treatments for many diseases through replacement of nonfunctional or malignant cell populations. Stem cells could potentially provide the basis for replacement therapies in diseases such as type 1 diabetes, Parkinson's disease, cardiovascular disease, and liver disease, as well as in cancers. Realization of these goals will require an understanding of the mechanisms responsible for the establishment of different organ systems in the embryo and for the maintenance of their function in the adult.

The community of stem cell biologists at Mount Sinai is committed to translating the great promise of stem cell biology into clinical advances at the bedside in a timely and safe manner. Both ES and tissue-restricted adult stem cells will be investigated in an environment in which interdisciplinary collaborations are encouraged and facilitated. The ultimate goal of scientists at the Black Family Stem Cell Institute is to improve their understanding of the behavior of stem cell to manipulate their fate for the treatment of human diseases.

The Black Family Stem Cell Institute will include research on ES and adult stem cells. Given that ES cells are of early embryonic origin and have the potential to generate any cell type in the body, scientists at the Black Family Stem Cell Institute are committed to understanding the mechanisms that govern lineage induction, tissue specification, and development in the normal embryo, with the goal of duplicating these processes in the ES cell system.

Adult stem cells are essential for the replacement of cells with a finite life span and for the maintenance of tissues. Although the best of characterized adult stem cells are those of the hematopoietic system, studies in recent years have provided strong evidence for the existence of stem cells in many other tissues, including the liver, skeletal muscle, brain, and skin. By integrating the biology of ES cells, embryonic development, and adult stem cells, scientists can focus on building or expanding expertise in a number of different areas, including the hematopoietic, cardiac, skeletal muscle, hepatocyte, and pancreas systems. Existing strengths in the biological research of several stem cell systems, as well as expertise in bone marrow, liver, and kidney transplantation in the clinic, place Mount Sinai in a strong position to develop a broad stem cell program.

## DEPARTMENT OF GENE AND CELL MEDICINE

The Department of Gene and Cell Medicine was established in 1996 at MSSM to promote and accelerate the science and technology on the development of gene and cellular therapeutics. Initially, the department focused on various aspects of gene therapy research, such as understanding basic virology, efficient gene delivery into cells, and incorporation of these genes into the genome. Ideally, a viral vector is delivered to target cells such as the patient's liver or lung cells. The vector then unloads its genetic material containing the therapeutic human gene into the target cell. The therapeutic gene is incorporated into the cell's genome and produces a functional protein product, which restores the target cell to a normal state and potentially cures the disease.

The department has since broadened its scope to integrate gene therapy and stem cell biology. In addition to targeting diseased tissues directly, such as the liver, the department is also studying how to deliver genes to stem cells, specifically, hematopoietic stem cells (developmentally immature cells that form blood). This approach produces functioning gene product in all the cells of a specific tissue, such as all blood cells.

**SEE ALSO:** Developmental Biology; Keller, Gordon; New York.

**BIBLIOGRAPHY.** Black Family Stem Cell Institute, www.blackfamilystemcell.org (cited November 2007); Mount Sinai Department of Gene and Cell Medicine, www.mssm.edu/gene_cell (cited November 2007); Mount Sinai School of Medicine, www.mssm.edu (cited November 2007).

Fernando Herrera
University of California, San Diego

# Mouse ES Cell Isolation

**MOUSE EMBRYONIC STEM** (ES) cells are pluripotent and have the ability to divide into any cell types that form an organism. They are derived from early embryos before they implant into the uterus (blastocysts). Blastocysts are made of an outer layer (trophectoderm) that aids implantation and eventually forms the placenta, and an inner cell mass that will give rise to the germ layers and the organism. ES cells are produced by removing the inner cell mass of a blastocyst. After isolation, the blastocyst is no longer able to complete implantation and thus is destroyed.

## CHARACTERISTICS

Researchers have come up with a list of criteria that ES cells must fulfill. ES cells must have normal chromosomes, meaning that they have the number and length of chromosomes of its organism counterpart. ES cells also express a high level of telomerase activity. Telomerase activity is associated with immortality of cells; the high level of expression indicates ES cells' relatively long replicative life span. In addition, ES cells are characterized by unique cell markers not observed in other early cell types. These highly expressed cell markers include stage-specific embryonic antigens (SSEA), human cell surface keratan sulphaterated antigens (TRA), a stem cell unique transcription factor, Oct-4 and alkaline phosphatase activity. Finally, ES cells have the developmental potential to form any components of the three embryonic germ layers, ectoderm, endoderm and mesoderm. This is generally proven by transplanting the ES cells back into immune compromised mice and looking for teratoma formation where all three germ layers are present.

## METHODS

The methods used to isolate ES cells are generally conserved from organism to organism, although there are also important differences. Early isolation faced difficulty in establishing a suitable stage for isolation, developing a suitable media that will maintain isolated ES cells in an undifferentiated state, and culturing ES cells in an in vitro environment.

In the 1980s, Dr. Evans was the first to describe how mouse ES cells can be isolated and was awarded the Nobel prize in physiology or medicine for this work in 2007. His group showed that mouse ES could be derived from the blastocyst. The isolation of mouse ES cells begins with fertilizing the embryo through copulation between a superovulated female and normal male mouse. Seventy-six hours after detecting a copulation plug, early blastocysts are flushed out of the mouse uterus. These fertilized embryos (zygotes) are cultured overnight in DME solution supplemented by 10 percent fetal calf serum until the late blastocyst stage. The inner cell mass is then separated from the trophectoderm via immunosurgery with rabbit antiserum. The separated inner cell mass is cultured on irradiated mouse embryonic fibroblasts to imitate the in vivo environment of the uterus. These fibroblasts are inactivated to prevent further cell growth and division of the fibroblasts. More recently Dr. Austin Smith established that the mouse feeder layers could be removed as long as leukemia inhibitor factor (LIF) was added to the medium.

Early isolation faced problems of cross-contamination by embryonal carcinoma cells because of the inability to differentiate these cells morphologically. Genetic analysis of specific genes like glucosephosphate isomerase were reported as assays to confirm the identity of derived mouse ES cells.

After two to three weeks of growth, the isolated mouse ES cells grow into colonies. These individual ES cell colonies have to be selected and dissociated for further expansion into cell lines. A sample of cells from each selected colony will be taken for karyotype analysis in the early passages. Cell marker expression, morphology analysis will also be carried out to ensure the integrity of isolated ES cells. Mouse ES cells expressed only levels of SSEA-1, but not SSEA-4 or SSEA-3. Variations between mice and humans in the embryonic genome expression, structure and function of uterine components, and structure of inner cell mass suggest basic species differences between early mouse and human development. These various differences have motivated researchers to find an animal model closer to human embryo development.

A decade passed before successful isolation of ES cells in a primate (the rhesus monkey) was accomplished. In November 1998, shortly after the successful derivation of non-human primate ES cells, the same researcher, Dr. James Thomson, achieved the feat of isolating human ES cells.

In recent years, following the success of human ES cell isolation, other papers have been published on the isolation of canine, bovine, and other animal ES cells. The successful isolation of human ES cells is a recognized breakthrough in scientific technology, but is also a key to a Pandora's box of bioethics and politics.

**SEE ALSO:** Cells, Embryonic; Cells, Mouse (Embryonic); Experimental Models; Feeder/Feeder-Free Culture; Homologous Recombination; Non-Human Primate Embryonic Stem Cells; Self-Renewal, Stem Cell.

**BIBLIOGRAPHY.** M. J. Evans and M. H. Kaufman, "Establishment in Culture of Pluripotential Cells from Mouse Embryos," *Nature* (v.292, 1981); Gail R. Martin, "Isolation of a Pluripotent Cell Line from Early Mouse Embryos Cultured in Medium Conditioned by Teratocarcinoma Stem Cells," *Proceedings of the National Academy of Sciences of the United States of America* (v.78/12, 1981).

Ka Yi Ling
University of Wisconsin

# MRI Tracking

**MAGNETIC RESONANCE IMAGING** (MRI) is traditionally used in the clinical setting to generate an image of the inner body and the organization of its tissues. An MRI scan can be used diagnostically to detect abnormalities such as hemorrhages

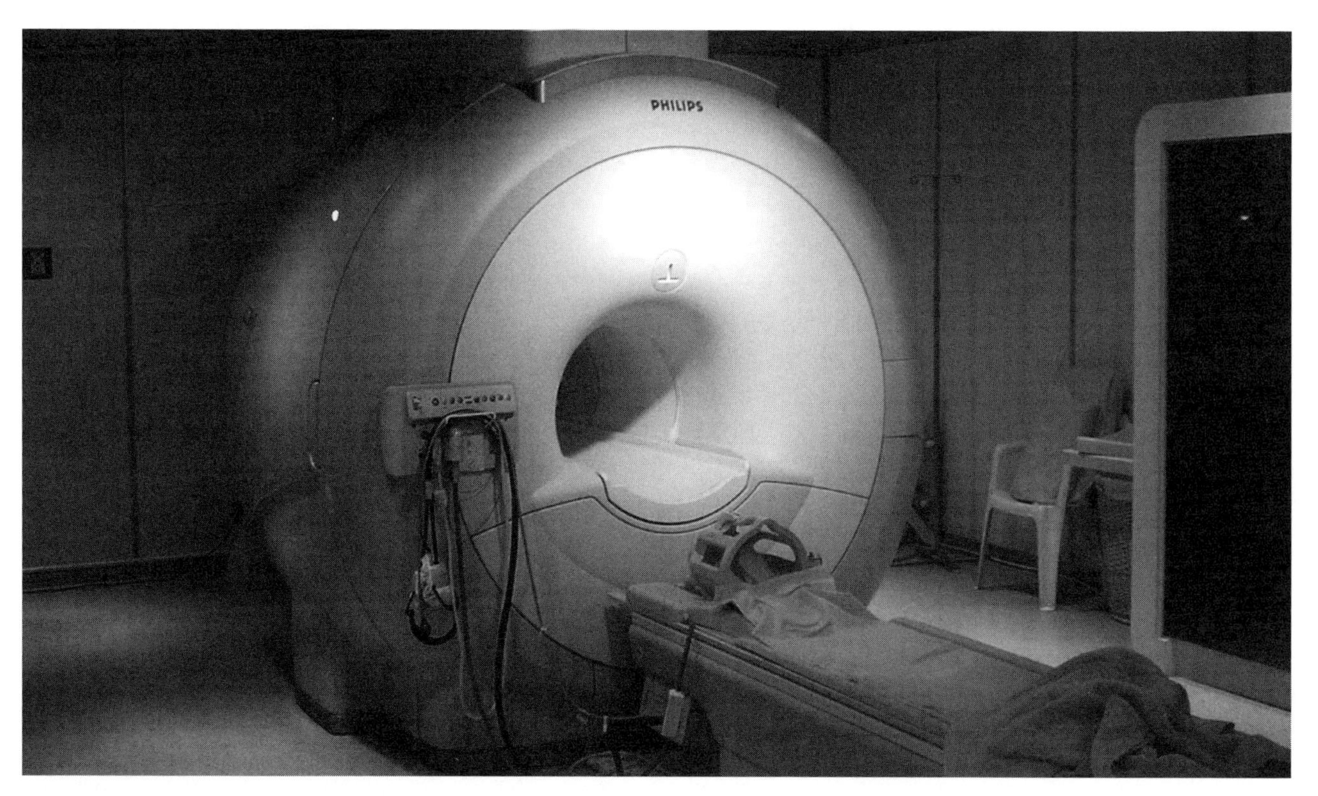


*MRI can be exploited by scientists and clinicians alike; stem cell researchers are using MRI tracking to confirm whether stem cells injected in humans localize to damaged tissue.*

or other internal bleeds, musculoskeletal lesions, and tumors. The mechanisms behind MRI involve using a high-power magnet to align all the hydrogen atoms in a given tissue area. These atoms are then manipulated in such a way as to record their locations, and a computer can process this information and generate a two-dimensional, black-and-white image of one plane of the tissue examined. These planes can be viewed sequentially, allowing the clinician to visualize the abnormality noninvasively. The principles of MRI can be exploited by scientists and clinicians alike; one example of using MRI technology is MRI tracking.

If stem cells are to be used as a therapeutic mechanism to stimulate repair of damaged tissue, it must first be determined that injected stem cells do in fact localize to the damaged tissue. In animal models, it is relatively easy to inject stem cells labeled with some sort of marker and then kill the animal to observe where the stem cells went. This process is not feasible in humans. An option for tracking stem cells that have been injected into a human could be a biopsy of the damaged site and analysis for presence of labeled stem cells, as well as observation regarding extent of tissue repair. Yet biopsy is an invasive procedure, often involving surgery and resulting in patient discomfort, and it may introduce infection because of the opening of the body cavity. To circumvent the need to biopsy, yet still locate the injected stem cells, MRI tracking was developed.

MRI tracking is carried out by labeling the unit to be tracked (such as stem cells) with the supermagnetic molecule iron oxide. Iron oxide leaves a signal void, which stands out against the black-and-white MRI image. Thus it is possible to monitor the location and infiltration of labeled injected stem cells by conducting MRI scans and observing the localization of the iron oxide particles. MRI tracing is noninvasive and therefore does not have a risk of ensuing infection.

MRI tracking has been carried out successfully in research labs. Scientists at the University of Oxford in the United Kingdom showed that MRI tracking could be used to trace blood monocytes, labeled with iron oxide, as they migrated to damaged heart tissue and differentiated into macrophages. Some scientists from this laboratory also work with stem cells, and in collaboration with researchers at Imperial College in London, they used MRI tracking to follow bone marrow stem cells and their potential recruitment to the site of damage in heart tissue following a myocardial infarct. The model organism for these studies is the rat.

Investigators at Johns Hopkins University School of Medicine used MRI tracking to monitor the recruitment and function of mesenchymal stem cells, also labeled with iron oxide, to damaged heart tissue in dogs that had undergone surgery to simulate myocardial damage from a heart attack. It is important to note that although MRI tracking may be used in humans in the future, the technological aspects are still being worked out in animal models.

**SEE ALSO:** BrdU/Thymidine; Johns Hopkins University; Lineages.

**BIBLIOGRAPHY.** C. A. Carr, et al., "MRI Tracking of Systemically Administered Bone Marrow Stem Cells," *Journal of Molecular and Cellular Cardiology* (v.42/6, 2007).

Claudia Winograd
University of Illinois, Urbana-Champaign

# Multiple Sclerosis

**MULTIPLE SCLEROSIS (MS)** is an inflammatory, demyelinating, autoimmune disease of the central nervous system, with permanent lesion formation leading to disability in the young and old, and in men as well as women. This disease is notorious for making a patient totally bedbound, not only resulting in bed sores but also inviting all kinds of infections to the disabled, depressed patient. Although intensive therapy has a key role in managing this complex disease, even in this era of advancement, the slowing accumulation of neurological damage in MS has remained mostly irreversible. Along with

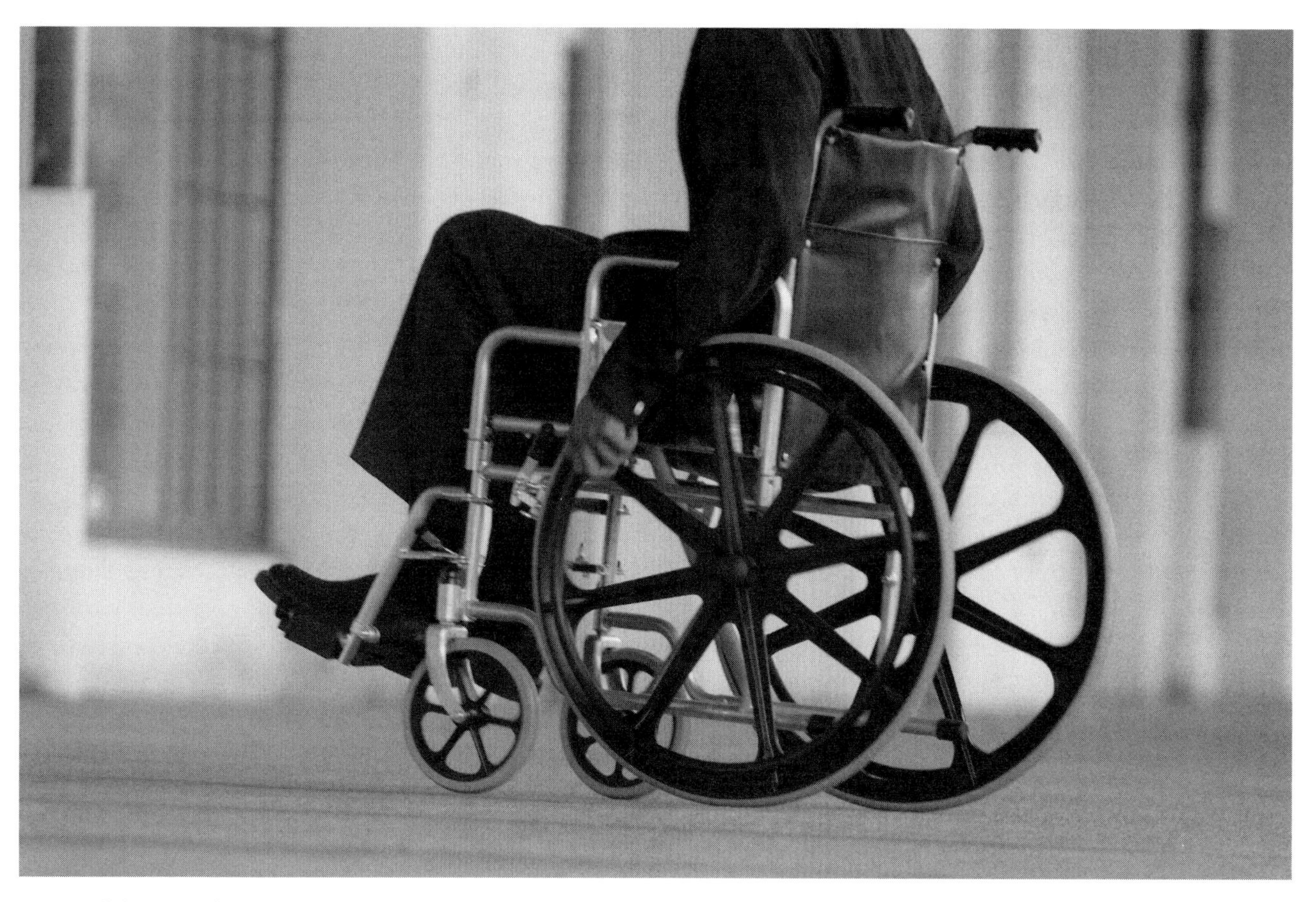

*Stem cell therapies for the debilitating disease of multiple sclerosis are showing promise, and studies are now in progress on procedures that use a patient's own bone marrow cells instead of embryo-derived cells.*

therapies that improve blood circulation, mitochondrial energy production, and antiinflammatory, antimicrobial, and antioxidant factors, there is increased optimism among scientists about slowing and perhaps reversing the disease with a comprehensive program that includes stem cell therapies.

There are different forms of MS, including relapsing remitting (attacks are followed by improvement), primary progressive (the disease progresses without remission), secondary progressive (initial remission followed by progressive disability), and relapsing progressive (disability occurs and accumulates between and during attacks). Although the cause of MS has not yet been found, neuroresearchers agree that whatever the cause, inflammation destroys the myelin sheath of the brain and spinal cord. The myelin sheath is an insulating structure around the nerves, which are responsible for the quick traveling of impulses. Once this myelin is affected, signal transmission is slowed down considerably, giving rise to the signs and symptoms of MS. In the brain and spinal cord, special glial cells, called oligodendrocytes, are responsible for the manufacture and maintenance of this myelin sheath. This is where the role of stem cells is being evaluated. When stem cells were injected into the demyelinated area of the brain and spinal cord, regrowth of the affected neurons is observed. Stem cells, both embryonic and adult, can potentially be used to deliver molecules that repair or help in the reformation of damaged tissue of the central nervous system.

The disease is more common in females than males, but the disability is more pronounced when it affects males. A variety of signs and symptoms have been highlighted, including memory problems, decline in reasoning function of the brain, loss of coordination of body parts, paralysis, body weakness, urinary retention, urinary incontinence, sexual problems, visual problems, facial weakness, depression, pain symptoms, emotional disturbances, and a few other presentations have been observed and evaluated by the neurologists.

## STEM CELL RESEARCH

Because most of the active study involves mice, before human beings are involved, the first task for scientists was to find a lesion similar to MS in mice. Experimental autoimmune encephalomyelitis (EAE) was developed and found to be characteristically identical to MS in humans. The researchers then labeled neural stem cells of adult mice with iron particles and injected these labeled stem cells into the tail vein of mice with EAE. Labeling the neural stem cells with iron particles is of significance because iron particles interfere with magnetic fields and can be detected on magnetic resonance imaging (MRI). To the great satisfaction of the researchers, the injected neural stem cells started reaching the EAE—the damaged area—within the first 24 hours. Gradual improvement in symptoms appeared as the myelin sheath started to be repaired by the newly arrived stem cells.

Many of the researchers used the embryonic stem cells in their hunt for a successful treatment recipe for patients with MS. One such study used embryonic stem cell suspensions containing stem cells obtained from active growing cells of four-to-eight-week-old cadaver embryos. After administration of these embryonic stem cell suspensions into MS patients, they were patiently observed. This treatment resulted in an improved range and quality of motions in the extremities, normalized muscle tone, decreased fatigue and general weakness, and improved quality of life. Most of the patients involved in the study showed no further progression of disability.

A purified, multipotent stem cell has now been isolated from bone marrow and umbilical cord blood; these stem cells have been named CD 34 (+). The CD 34 (+) cell is capable of migrating to an injured or damaged area and proliferating into the specific cells required for the repair of that tissue. These cells basically transform into the neuroprotective glial cells, predominantly the oligodendrocytes and their progenitors. Histopathologically, these cells are capable of balancing the immune system (it is this imbalance in the immune system that targets the body's own myelin sheath). This potency of CD 34 (+) cells is now being applied for treating MS. Similar multipotent cells, called mesenchymal stem cells, which are found in the bone marrow and umbilical cord blood, have been extracted. These cells specialize into adipocytes, osteocytes, chondrocytes, or glial cells depending on the specific growth factors influencing them.

Recently, a new procedure involving a patient's own bone marrow cells being injected, instead of embryo-derived cells, has been developed. This trial involves bone marrow stem cells of the same patient extracted from his or her bones, preferably the pelvic bones, and then being processed in the lab. The marrow stem cells are then effectively injected into the veins of the same MS patient. An MRI scan done before is then compared with the postinjection stage, for structural changes. These studies are in their initial stages, and a proven outcome in human beings is expected in the coming few years.

Many researchers have been studying and applying the concepts of remyelination, which involves extraction of the stem cells and then culturing them in the laboratory. In this way, bone stem cells have been induced to differentiate into oligodendrocyte-like cells. This demonstration is of real hope for MS patients. The newly cultured oligodendrocyte like-cells are now being tested on animal models, and a positive outcome there will lead to trials on human beings. When efforts to know more were intensified, it was discovered that the phenomenon of remyelination involves myelin repair by oligodendrocyte progenitor cells. When these oligodendrocyte progenitor cells are implanted near the defective area, the outcome is striking. Many substances stimulate the production of these cells, including platelet-derived growth factor A, brain-derived neurotrophic factor, and neurotrophin 3.

Researchers have also found a factor termed *Fyn tyrosine kinase*, which can increase the production of myelin base protein. When observed closely, this myelin base protein plays an essential role in the remyelination of axons. The gene that codes for Fyn tyrosine kinase has also been isolated and termed the *fyn* gene. Studying stem cells closely has led to the coding and successful isolation of the previously unknown *fyn* gene. Another angle of focus is to first analyze and diagnose the deficient factor or gene in the respective MS patient. Once the defect is identified, a number of combinations can be tried, depending on the deficiency. For instance, for an individual who has a deficiency of *fyn*, incorporating umbilical cord stem cells containing the *fyn* gene will be of great benefit. All these studies have mostly been carried out on animal models, so the exact reaction of human beings is not perfectly understood.

Moreover, efforts are also underway to use stem cells to help in the discovery of new genes and molecules that can cease the progression or help repair the damaged zone. These stem cells can also be of help in manufacturing new drugs that can treat MS. Places like the Netherlands and Mexico were initially the only hope for people suffering from MS, but gradually all the countries of the world, including the United States and the United Kingdom, intensified their efforts to find a cure for this debilitating disease. The use of embryonic and fetal stem cells for research purposes has been a cause of protest from different circles. Therefore, not all countries have been able to contribute to their full potential. The alternatives, including using stems cells from cadaver embryos, stem cells from umbilical cord blood, and recently, stem cells from the patient's own bone marrow, have opened new avenues for scientists and researchers.

Many of the patients suffering from MS are now optimistic and are willing to participate in the dozens of trials underway; the results have been very good. Some of the participants have found themselves improving and living an independent life because of this stem cell revolution. However, the work is still in its initial stages; with the hopeful outcome seen in mice models, the incorporation of the whole process into the all-important human patient is yet to happen. The future of stem cell therapy in treating patients of MS looks bright.

**SEE ALSO:** Amyotrophic Lateral Sclerosis; Moral Status of Embryo; Mouse ES Cell Isolation; Stem-Like Cells, Human Brain; Spinal Cord Injury; Stroke; Tissue Culture.

**BIBLIOGRAPHY.** National Multiple Sclerosis Society, www.nationalmssociety.org (cited October 2007); "Stem Cells to Treat Multiple Sclerosis," www.unmc.edu (cited October 2007); "Stem Cell Treatment Improves the Quality of Life in Patients with Multiple Sclerosis," www.stemcelltherapies.org (cited October 2007).

Atif Zafar
Dow University of Health Sciences

# Mummery, Christine

**CHRISTINE MUMMERY IS** a professor of developmental biology at Universiteit Utrecht in the Netherlands and the group leader of the Mummery Group, part of the Netherlands Institute for Developmental Biology. She earned her doctoral degree in biophysics from Guy's Hospital Medical School in London and did her postdoctoral work at Hubrecht laboratory at the Netherlands Institute. Much of her research has focused on the use of stem cells in the treatment of cardiovascular disease.

The Mummery Group is dedicated to the research of both stem cells and adult cells in cardiovascular pathology. Their three main goals are to study the genetic and molecular development of the cardiovascular system, to develop models of the human cardiovascular system in culture to better study both normal development and the effect of disease, and to produce cells suitable for cardiovascular cell repair therapies. They have already made advances in improving the methodology for producing cardiomyocytes, or heart cells, from embryonic stem cells.

Mummery and her lab have taken a novel approach to the use of stem cells in the treatment of heart disease. Rather than inject stem cells into a damaged heart tissue, as had been tried in previous studies, they used stem cells to grow cardiomyocytes. They induced heart attacks in mice and then injected these mature cardiomyocytes into the heart muscle. The results were initially promising, but the effect faded within about a month. Careful study of the process showed that the introduced cardiomyocytes were not lining up correctly with existing cells, reducing their efficiency.

Mummery accepted a fellowship to Radcliffe in 2007–08 to continue her studies in the structure of cardiomyocytes. She is developing a new approach to her study that would involve creating heart tissue from stem cells and grafting the new tissue onto a damaged heart muscle.

**SEE ALSO:** Cells, Adult; Clinical Trials Within U.S.: Heart Disease.

**BIBLIOGRAPHY.** A. Beqqali, et al., "Genome-Wide Transcriptional Profiling of Human Embryonic Stem Cells Differentiating to Cardiomyocytes," *Stem Cells* (v.24, 2006); R. Carvalho, et al., "Defective Paracrine Signaling by TGF b in Yolk Sac Vasculature of Endoglin Mutant Mice: A Paradigm for Hereditary Haemorrhagic Telangiectasia," *Development* (v.131, 2004); L. van Laake, et al., "Endoglin Has a Crucial Role in Blood Cell-Mediated Vascular Repair," *Circulation* (v.114, 2006); S. Chuva de Sousa Lopes, et al., "BMP Signaling Mediated by ALK2 in the Visceral Endoderm Is Necessary for the Generation of Primordial Germ Cells in the Mouse Embryo," *Genes and Development* (v.18, 2004); R. Passier, et al., "Increased Cardiomyocyte Differentiation from Human Embryonic Stem Cells in Serum-Free Cultures," *Stem Cells* (v.23, 2005); D. van Hoof, et al., "A Quest for Human and Mouse Embryonic Stem Cell-Specific Proteins," *Molecular and Cellular Proteomics* (v.5, 2006).

Heather K. Michon
Independent Scholar

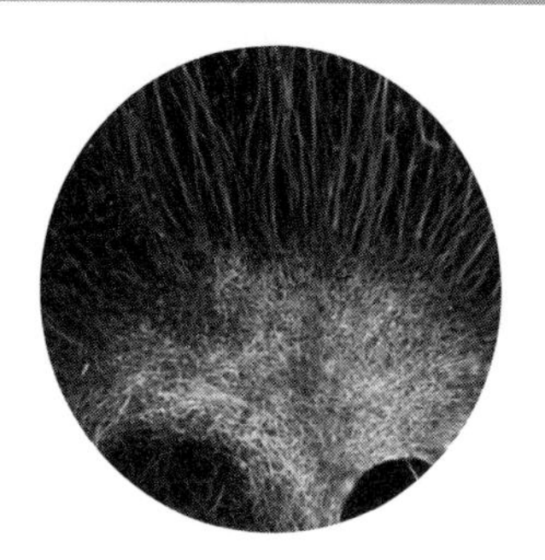

# N

## National Academy of Sciences

**THE NATIONAL ACADEMY** of Sciences (NAS) is the leading scientific community in the United States. It is composed of invited citizen members and foreign associates who represent the most prominent and highly regarded scientific researchers in engineering as well as life sciences, who use their research for the improvement of general welfare. It is one of the National Academies; other Academies are the National Academy of Engineering, the Institute of Medicine, and the National Research Council.

President Abraham Lincoln created the NAS on March 3, 1863. It was to serve the government to "investigate, examine, experiment, and report upon any subject of science or art," according to its Act of Incorporation. Its role is thus to provide scientific advice that will shape public policy. Over time, the NAS expanded into the four National Academies, of which the current NAS is one member Academy. The NAS headquarters are in Washington, D.C. The NAS is led by a council composed of 12 councilors and 5 officers. These leaders are elected annually by the Academy.

As the national scientific advisor, the Academy has been asked to address stem cell research. On December 8, 2003, then Academy President Bruce Alberts issued a statement against the proposed United Nations global law banning somatic cell nuclear transfer. In this statement, the Academy position was defined as explicitly opposed to cloning of human beings, yet in favor of scientific research that would lead to therapeutic regenerative medicine.

To explain its stance on stem cell research for medicine versus human cloning, the Academy has published two major studies: *Stem Cells and the Future of Regenerative Medicine* (2001) and *Scientific and Medical Aspects of Human Reproductive Cloning* (2002). The first publication was authored by the Committee on the Biological and Biomedical Applications of Stem Cell Research, the Board on Life Sciences National Research Council, and the Board on Neuroscience and Behavioral Health Institute of Medicine. It addresses adult and embryonic stem cells, and includes a chapter titled "Opportunities for and Barriers to Progress in Stem Cell Research for Regenerative Medicine." Importantly, as its first finding, the study concludes that while research in mouse and other species stem cells is important, it is not a sufficient substitute for human study, and it therefore recommends that "studies with *human* stem cells are essential to make progress in the development of treatment for *human* disease, and this research should continue."

The second publication was authored by the Committee on Science, Engineering, and Public Policy, Policy and Global Affairs Division; the Board on Life Sciences, Division on Earth and Life Studies; and the other three Academies within the National Academies. It addresses cloning—animal, human, and in the context of assisted reproduction. As a major finding, the study proposes to ban human reproductive cloning. This type of cloning is defined as the cloning of an individual human. This opposition being outlined and defended, the study then continues to support somatic cell nuclear transfer as a method for research of stem cells for therapeutic purposes. Major disease populations cited by the study as potentially benefiting from this research include Alzheimer's disease, amyotrophic lateral sclerosis, and Parkinson's disease, as well as spinal cord injury patients.

**SEE ALSO:** Cloning; International Laws; Nuclear Transfer, Somatic.

**BIBLIOGRAPHY.** NAS, *Scientific and Medical Aspects of Human Reproductive Cloning* (National Academy Press, 2002); NAS, *Stem Cells and the Future of Regenerative Medicine* (National Academy Press, 2001).

Claudia Winograd
University of Illinois, Urbana-Champaign

# National Institutes of Health

**THE NATIONAL INSTITUTES** of Health (NIH) is an agency that is part of the U.S. Department of Health and Human Services; the NIH is the primary agency in the government of the United States that is responsible for biomedical research. The NIH is also one of the leading institutions for research in the world.

The NIH Web site stemcells.nih.gov has a wealth of information available to all regarding stem cell research; the site provides a great deal of information regarding basic stem cell background, the potential of stem cell research, federal funding opportunities, policy, and training. NIH publications that provide a comprehensive review of the progression of stem cell research are provided on the Web site, along with stem cell basics for those who would like a general overview of stem cells and their potential uses, as well as frequently asked questions regarding healthcare, research and policy, cell line availability, and funding, along with research regarding stem cells and disease and an extensive glossary of technical and scientific terms. The NIH site also provides links to current research, the stem cell registry, upcoming events regarding stem cell research, funding for research, training programs, and scientific literature. Databases are available for searching primary abstracts on stem cell literature; primary scientific literature about embryonic stem cell research and stem cell experimentation with regard to the treatment of disease is also provided on PubMED.

## BIOLOGY OF STEM CELLS

Stem cells have a remarkable capability to develop into many different cell types. Stem cells can divide infinitely to develop into other cells in the body. When stem cells divide into *daughter* cells, the daughter cell has the ability to either remain a stem cell or become a cell with more specialized cell functions, such as being a red blood cell or a brain cell. Three classes of stem cells exist: totipotent, multipotent, and pluripotent.

A fertilized egg can be considered totipotent; the potential of the mass is total and it can give rise to a multitude of cells within the body. Totipotency is the ability of a cell to divide and produce all of the undifferentiated cells within an organism. The growth and development of a living being is said to begin when a sperm fertilizes an egg and creates a single totipotent cell, the zygote. After fertilization, the cell begins to divide and produce other totipotent cells; these totipotent cells begin to specialize within a few days after fertilization. The totipotent cells specialize into pluripotent cells, which they develop into the tissues of the developing body. Pluripotent cells can further divide and specialize into multipotent cells, which produce cells of a particular function.

Multipotent cells, in contrast, can only give rise to a small number of cell types. For example, a hematopoietic cell, or a blood stem cell, can develop into several types of blood cells but cannot develop into liver cells or other types of cells; the differentiation of the cell is limited in scope. A multipotent blood cell can produce red and white blood cells, for example. At the end of cellular divisions during differentiation, the cells are terminally differentiated, meaning that they are considered to be devoted to that specific cellular function.

Pluripotent stem cells can give rise to any type of cell in the body except those needed to develop a fetus or adult because they lack the potential to support the extraembryonic tissue (e.g., the placenta). Pluripotent stem cells have the capability to differentiate into any of the three germ layers: the endoderm, the mesoderm, or the ectoderm. The endoderm consists of tissues and organs such as the lungs, the gastrointestinal tract and the stomach lining; the mesoderm consists of the blood, bone, and muscle; and the ectoderm consists of the nervous system and epidermal tissues. Pluripotent stem cells are isolated from embryos that are only several days old; cells from these stem cell lines can be cultured in the lab and grown without limit.

Stem cell lines can be grown in the laboratory and frozen for storage or for distribution to other researchers; these lines can provide an infinite amount of stem cells. A researcher can use the stem cell line indefinitely instead of having to isolate the stem cells again; this is other advantage of having a stem cell line. In the future, scientists hope to replace damaged genes with new ones by using stem cells to treat disease; scientists will also be able to use therapies to overcome the problems that are involved with immune rejection.

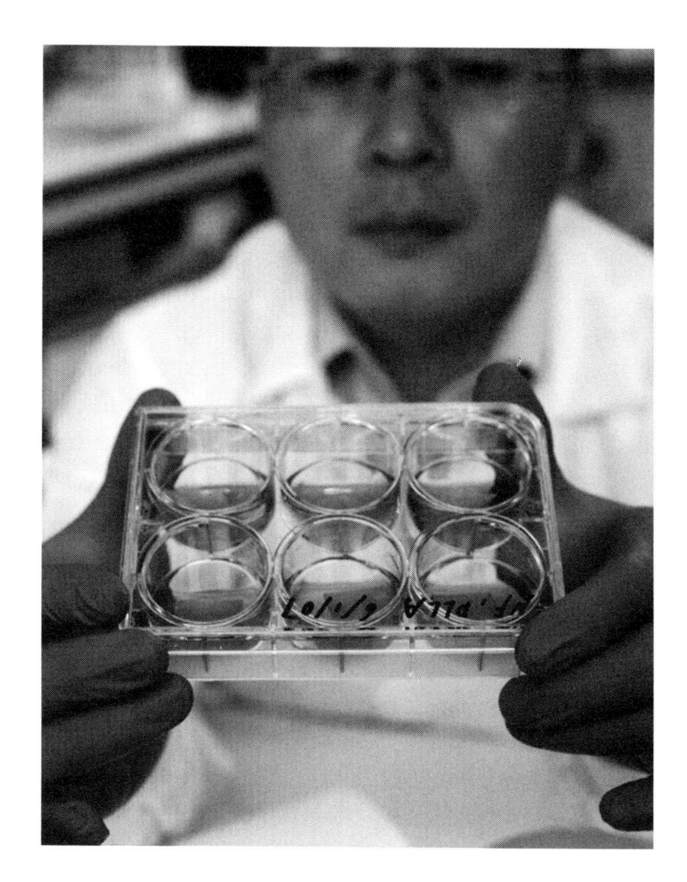

*In 2007 the NIH made a major advancement by using heart cells derived from hESCs to help restore rat heart function.*

## ETHICS

There are many ethical issues surrounding the use of both embryonic and adult stem cells; embryonic stem cells are controversial because the pro-life movement believes that human life becomes a human person at or shortly after conception. This mind-set contributes to the thought that the removal of stem cells from an embryo, which effectively kills the embryo, is technically equivalent to murdering a 70-year-old man or a 10-year-old girl. Regardless of the supposed health benefits, this position holds that even saving the lives of millions of people does not justify the killing of millions of other "humans." The use of adult stem cells is generally much less disputed because the cells exist in humans and may be obtained without causing injury or death. Recently, they have been discovered in more locations in the human body and are becoming increasingly useful, but embryonic stem cells are far more differentiable and more plastic. The use of adult cells, however, does help to avoid the ethical issue because they are previously existing cells.

Ethical issues regarding stem cell research consider the moral results of using stem cell technology. Legal issues require a unique fusion of researchers, scientists, policy makers, and the public to decide how government will be involved in the scientific arena: funding, technology regulation, and so forth. Social issues entail the effect of technology on society and public issues.

## FEDERAL POLICY

Stem cell research is inextricably linked to public policy; this fundamental bond will continue to grow, and so it is important to make the public and legislators more aware of research developments and clinical applications of stem cells.

On August 9, 2001, President George W. Bush announced that federal funds could be awarded for researching using human embryonic stem cells (hESCs) only if certain strict criteria were met. The law stated that the derivation process of destroying the embryo had to initiate before August 9, 2001; furthermore, the stem cells had to be derived from an embryo that was created solely for reproductive purposes and was no longer needed; then, informed consent had to be obtained for the donation of the embryo, and the donation could not involve any financial stimulus.

According to the NIH Stem Cell Registry, the NIH has consulted with the investigators who have derived the cells from federally funded hESCs. States may pass laws to permit hESC research using state funds only; Congress has not to date passed a law that bans states this right, and so a state may pay for hESC research that is not eligible for federal funding.

President Bush signed a law on August 9, 2001, banning the use of federal funding for research done on any new embryonic stem cell lines and restricting the funding to what he claimed were "60 preexisting genetically diverse stem cell lines." Dissenters immediately began to call him out on this figure. The director of the National Institutes of Health informed Congress that only 11 such stem cell lines are readily available for research fitting Bush's restrictions, and that all of these lines are potentially contaminated by viruses from mouse feeder cells. As a result of these funding restrictions, new research is being thwarted and essentially choked. Although researchers at Johns Hopkins have since discovered a method of developing cell lines using human feeder cells, they cannot proceed with federal funding because the method still does not qualify under Bush's policy. The policy has stalled the progress of stem cell research throughout the United States.

HESCs are believed to have a much greater developmental potential than adult stem cells; hESCs are pluripotent, meaning that they have the ability to give rise to cells found in nearly all tissues of the developing embryo. Conversely, adult stem cells are thought to be multipotent, meaning that their development is restricted to specific types of cells. Adult stem cells are less controversial and are much easier to acquire, but much more potential lies within the functionality of the hESCs.

## CURRENT STEM CELL RESEARCH

Several advancements and experiments in stem cell research have been made at the NIH, specifically with relation to medicine and techniques. In 2007 heart cells derived from hESCs helped to restore rat heart function, a major advancement in cardiovascular research. Scientists hope to repair and replace damaged heart muscle cells with stem cells in the future. In the laboratory of C. E. Murry, NIH-funded investigators developed a novel technique to create a large number of heart muscle cells from hESCs. Improved heart function was examined in rat hearts, which offers great promise for the effective treatment of human heart disease.

Other advancements in stem cell research have been equally exciting; for example, researchers were able to isolate adult stem cells for the first time in tendons, procedures were developed to differentiate between stem cells lines and the development of hESCs for different types of neurons, tissue-matched human stem cells were created without cloning, olfactory stem cells were identified in mammals, hair follicles were regenerated in mice, hESCs developed into lung tissue, adult stem cells were able to develop into skeletal muscle, nonembryonic human stem cells were matured in the rat spinal cord, stem cells responsible for pancreatic cancer were identified, and stem cells were generated in amniotic fluid.

### FUTURE OF STEM CELL RESEARCH

Many people question the effectiveness of hESCs; scientists have only been performing experiments with hESC since about 1998. When federal funds that supported hESC research were limited with President Bush's decision on federal funding in 2001, academic researchers suffered: Almost all researchers depend on federal funding to support their laboratory experiments. Because of the federal fund restrictions, however, scientists have only recently begun to develop stem cells and conduct experimentation. Although hESCs are believed to have great potential for the advancement of medicine, extensive research is still necessary to offer therapies for disease and therapy. Hematopoietic stem cells (HSCs) are blood-forming stem cells in bone marrow. At present, these stem cells are the only type of stem cell that is conventionally used to treat human disease; for example, doctors have been using the HSCs of bone marrow for bone marrow transplants for over 40 years.

Although the potential of adult stem cells has been tested and observed in the treatment of other types of human disease (such as kidney cancer), the studies have only involved a limited number of subjects (patients), and not enough experimentation has been conducted to extensively use stem cells for treating human disease. Nonetheless, the unique properties of hESCs offer great potential in the understanding of embryonic development, disease, cancer, and biomedical engineering.

**SEE ALSO:** Clinical Trials Within U.S.: Blind Process; Federal Government Policies; Regulations Overview; Stem Cells, Bush Ruling; United States.

**BIBLIOGRAPHY.** T. Lougheed, "New US Guidelines for Research on Human Embryos," *Canadian Medical Association Journal* (v.172/13, 2005); National Institutes of Health, "NIH Stem Cell Information Home Page," stemcells.nih.gov (cited October 2007); Gene Outka, "The Ethics of Stem Cell Research," The President's Council on Bioethics (April 2002); "Save Embryonic Stem Cell Research," *Scientific American* (v.284, 2001).

Krishna Subhash Vyas
University of Kentucky

# National Right to Life Committee

**THE NATIONAL RIGHT TO LIFE** Committee is the most powerful pro-life organization in the United States, working through education and legislation mainly against abortion, human cloning, healthcare reform, euthanasia, and related issues.

The association was created in 1973 in response to a U.S. Supreme Court decision released on January 22 of that year, legalizing the practice of human abortion in all the federal states through the entire nine months of pregnancy. Before that Supreme Court case—*Roe v. Wade*—the abortion debate had been confined to the legislatures of the states, 17 of which had legalized abortion under certain circumstances and 33 of which had voted to continue to protect human life from conception onward.

A pregnant single woman (Roe) brought a class action lawsuit challenging the constitutionality of the Texas criminal abortion laws, which proscribed procuring or attempting an abortion except on medical advice for the purpose of saving the mother's life. A licensed physician (Hallford), who had two state abortion prosecutions pending against him, was allowed to arbitrate. A childless married couple (the Does) separately attacked the laws, basing their alleged injury on the future possibilities of contraceptive failure pregnancy, unpreparedness for parenthood, and impairment of the wife's health. A three-judge District Court, which consolidated the action, held that Roe and Hallford and the members of their classes had standing to sue and presented justiciable controversy.

The court declared the abortion statutes void as being vague and overbroadly infringing individuals' Ninth and Fourteenth Amendment rights. The court ruled the Does' complaint not justiciable. Appellants directly appealed to the court on the injunctive rulings, and the appellee cross-appealed from the District Court's grant of declaratory relief to Roe and Hallford.

*Roe v. Wade* is one of the most controversial and important cases in U.S. Supreme Court history. The focal holding of this case was that abortion is allowed for any reason up until the point at which the fetus is able to live outside the mother's body, even if with artificial aid. This condition (called fetus viability) is usually fixed between 24 and 28 weeks of pregnancy, and the court held that abortion after viability must still be accessible when required to ensure a woman's health.

## HISTORY

The *Roe v. Wade* decision elicited national disputation that survives to this day. When the Supreme Court legalized abortion on demand in all 50 states, various state right-to-life groups saw the need to combine their efforts and coordinate a national response. By May 1973, 30 state pro-life groups had elected representatives to serve on a board of directors, and the National Right to Life Committee was formally incorporated on May 14 of the same year.

In June 1973, this group of pro-life leaders met in Detroit for the first convention of a new organization that was to be nondogmatic, nonpartisan, and have its board consist of an elected representative from each of the 50 states. These first board members included experts in the field of science, medicine, philosophy, ethics, constitutional law, and religion. During the summer of 1973, the organization's first national office was opened in Washington, D.C., with six full-time employees.

In the early years, different programs helped the pro-life movement to grow and expand. One particularly successful campaign, the "Mission Possible" Minnesota project, provided other freshman state groups with leadership training and financial assistance. From 1985 to 1994, the group joined other important pro-life organizations, for example, supporting a boycott of the Upjohn Company for its research on drugs to induce abortion. Since its official beginning, the National Right to Life Committee has grown to represent over 3,000 chapters in all 50 states. The board of directors now consists of a director from each state, elected by the state group, as well as an internal elected nine-member executive committee, a fully staffed national office, and millions of supporters.

Today, the National Right to Life Committee has the staff and experience to get its pro-life message heard and influence critical legislation affecting the lives of the unborn, the aged, and the medically dependent and disabled. The *NRL News* is the movement's newspaper of record, providing a monthly report and discussing upcoming educational, legislative and political events.

The National Right to Life Committee has a number of departments but three primary functions: education, legislation, and political action. The NRL Educational Trust Fund sponsors educational advertising and distributes brochures and booklets detailing fetal development and abortion's effect and works with churches, students, and minority groups to facilitate their involvement with the pro-life cause.

## STEM CELL RESEARCH

Recent scientific advancements in human stem cell research have brought the status of human embryos into focus. Pro-life organizations as well as the National Right to Life Committee are against killing embryos and human cloning because they believe that each human being begins as an embryo. Stem cells can be obtained from umbilical cord blood and from a large number of adult (nonembryonic) tissues, as well as from human embryos.

Although the potential of embryonic stem cells remains untested, adult stem cell treatments have been used for many years to successfully treat leukemia and related bone/blood cancers through bone marrow transplants. Human embryonic stem cell research is particularly controversial because starting a stem cell line requires the destruction of human embryos or therapeutic cloning.

Human cloning is human asexual reproduction. It may be accomplished by introducing the nuclear material from one or more human somatic cells into a fertilized or unfertilized egg cell, the nuclear material of which has been removed or inactivated to produce a human embryo that is virtually genetically identical to an existing or previously existing human being. This particular method is called somatic cell nuclear transfer.

Parthenogenesis is another asexual form of reproduction typical of some species in which growth and development of an embryo in females occurs without fertilization by males. This method of cloning is begun using an electrical or chemical stimulus to artificially produce the beginning of an embryo. Research on human parthenogenesis is focused on the production of embryonic stem cells for use in the medical treatment of degenerative diseases.

Regardless of whether the embryo is subsequently implanted into a woman and reaches the point of live birth or is destroyed for research or experimentation, human cloning has occurred. The National Right to Life Committee promotes a global ban on human cloning for any purpose. The committee believes that human cloning must be banned because it represents the modification and possible commercialization of human life. It would create a class of human beings who exist not as ends in themselves but as the means to achieve the ends of others. It would be a gateway technology for further genetic manipulation and control of human beings.

The National Right to Life Committee believes strongly that a ban on cloning as a means of producing live human beings will prove to be unenforceable unless it also bans cloning for any other purpose—including the use of cloning to produce human embryos as sources of stem cells or for other experimentation. In addition, the committee views referring to this latter use of cloning as "therapeutic cloning" as prejudicial and misleading, as it has not yet been proved that cloning is necessary for or useful in the production of medical therapies.

The position of the National Right to Life Committee is in opposition to that of many important researchers, who believe that stem cells have virtually unlimited application in the treatment and cure of many human diseases and disorders including Alzheimer's disease, diabetes, cancer, and so on. President Bush's position is very close to that of the National Right to Life Committee; during his first week in office, he reinstated the Mexico City Policy, which prevents tax funds from being given to organizations that perform and promote abortion overseas. He also threatened to veto an appropriation bill unless a provision overturning the policy was removed. He declared that federal funds will not be used for stem cell research that requires the destruction of human embryos.

**SEE ALSO:** Advocacy; Federal Government Policies; Moral Status of Embryo; *Roe v. Wade*; Stem Cells, Bush Ruling.

**BIBLIOGRAPHY.** National Institutes of Health, "Report of the Human Embryo Research Panel" (November 1994); "National Right to Life Committee," www.nrlc .org (cited October 2007).

Anna Maria Destro
Eastern Piedmont University
School of Medicine

# National Stem Cell Bank

**OVER THE PAST** few years, stem cells have played a major role in our approach toward medical issues. The availability of different stem cell lines encourages modern and state-of-the-art therapeutics for the future. This promises to save many lives and lead to great advancements in medical treatment.

The National Stem Cell Bank (NSCB) stores different human embryonic stem cell lines (hESCs). Located near the University of Wisconsin campus in Madison, this bank contains the stem cell lines that are listed on the National Institutes of Health (NIH) Stem Cell Registry. These stem cell

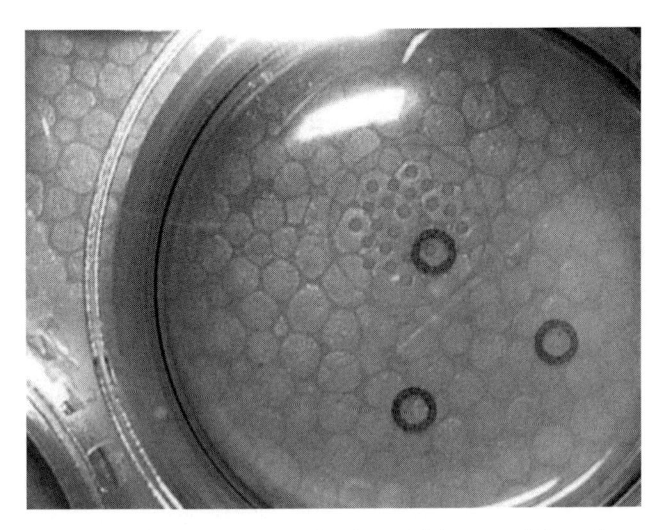

*The National Stem Cell Bank holds 13 of the 21 cell lines that are on the National Institutes of Health registry.*

lines are the only ones for which federal funding is allowed for research.

Led by Derek Hei and James Thomson, the NSCB was launched in October 2005 after President George W. Bush announced its federal support. There were some restrictions. Funded research conducted on the cells derived from extra embryos is allowed only on those embryos created as a product of in vitro fertilization, after having the consent of the owner of the stem cells.

The WiCell (University of Wisconsin, Madison, cell bank) laid down the foundation and created the infrastructure for the growth and distribution of cells. The only thing remaining to be focused on was the development of a quality system and standard operating procedures for investigating and recording all aspects of cell production and the testing methods used. Another main task of the bank was to manage the business and other legal issues with the cell line providers.

As stated by Derek Hei, current president of the NSCB, the main objectives of the bank are to produce, characterize, and distribute the NIH Registry Cell Lines (including 21 hESC lines). The bank also aims at introducing techniques for culturing and characterizing hESCs. The bank is willing to share these techniques with the research community worldwide (i.e., to provide technical support to all those researchers who experiment using the cells at academic and nonprofit institutions).

The cell lines with which the NSCB is currently working have a great importance in the United States because only these lines are allowed to be used for NIH-funded research. Research in other cell lines requires private funding. During the first two years of its existence, the bank has succeeded in launching its own Web site, which proved to be of great benefit, as it allows people from the world over to order and get detailed information about the cell lines in which they are interested.

The University of Wisconsin was chosen to be the birthplace for the NSCB because the university has staff members who have experience when it comes to working with embryonic stem cells, and the bank has benefited from the university's accumulation of knowledge and history of that research.

The university's College of Agriculture and Life Sciences (which consists of 21 academic departments) has conducted more than 600 distinct lines of research. The National Research Council ranks this department among the top 10 in the country. The whole faculty of the university, including researchers from different departments, provides a beneficial and productive council of experts, who can surely extend their expertise and collaborate with the WiCell.

## RESEARCH

The University of Wisconsin, Madison, also provides a multidisciplinary research center, which aims at researching human development, developmental disorders, and disabilities related to the brain. This clinical research center provides materials for synthesizing and testing services for the range of different pharmaceutical compounds. The cell lines for research and other biological materials of use can be brought to the clinic, further enhancing the bank's resources for research.

Derek Hei's intellect and experience increased the success of this project fourfold. He is the lead investigator at the NSCB and a director of the Waisman Clinical Biomanufacturing Facility. With a postgraduate degree from the University of California, Berkeley, in biochemical engineering and an undergraduate degree in chemical engineering from the University of Wisconsin, Madison, his many years spent in the biotechnology industry contribute positively to his role in the NSCB.

Hei considers the strength of the university itself the reason behind WiCell getting the NIH contract. Other reasons include that the university provides its own research facilities for the stem cell lines and at the same time offers outreach education to the community of researchers across the world. In addition to the bank's goal of advanced characterization of the stem cells, another important task is to enable the distribution of these stem cells at a lower cost. This will help the researchers associated with nonprofit institutions to extend the scope of their research.

Another renowned personality involved in the NSCB is Dr. James Thomson, who, along with Derek Hei, leads the NSCB. Thomson is a professor at the University of Wisconsin, Madison, who received his doctorate in molecular biology from the University of Pennsylvania. Thomson is especially well known for his innovative work in the isolation and culture of nonhuman primate cells and hESCs. Thomson has the honor of leading a group that was known to be the first to report the isolation of embryonic stem cell lines from a nonhuman primate. This work led to the successful isolation of hESC lines. At present, Thomson and his group are focused on understanding how embryonic stem cells choose between self-renewal and the decision to differentiate. Thus, Thomson, along with the other people at the NSCB, benefits the bank with his research and wealth of knowledge.

## PROCEDURES

The basic reason behind the creation of the NSCB is the formation of master cell banks. These are gatherings of those cells that have differentiated again and again and have undergone many testing procedures, so that the cells are free from any virus, pathogen, or any other infecting agent. Such types of cells can be used for clinical trials without the danger of being infected. The researchers can perform clinical procedures on these pathogen-free cells.

The first thing that is taken into account when depositing stem cell lines in the NSCB is whether the cells to be deposited are present on the NIH registry. Basically, two types of cells are taken: those that are to be distributed immediately and those that are to be developed in the master cell banks.

After accepting the cells from different donors, the next step involves rigorous testing of these cells. The cells undergo different procedures that actually test for them to be sure that they are free from any abnormalities. Once all the tests prove that the cells are free of disease and other infectious agents, a certificate is issued to the researchers, who are free to further study these stem cells. This certificate provides a guarantee to researchers that the cells have no abnormalities. The procedure used in the bank is quite foolproof and ensures the perfection of the stem cells stored there.

The bank has taken certain measures to promote the first of the two master cell banks. The bank has the honor of establishing and creating research plans for differentiation and characterization methods. An example of this includes a method of estimating the condition of the cells with the help of the markers that express on the surface of these cells, called cytometry.

The University of California, San Francisco, has also deposited some cells with the NSCB in September 2006. With this addition, the NSCB will now have a deposit of 13 of the 21 cell lines that are on the NIH registry.

The NSCB has an advisory board, which guides the policies and decisions of the bank. The NSCB Scientific Advisory Board is led by Dr. Ron McKay of NIH. Mr. Jack Harding works as the NSCB scientific officer. The position of vice chair is held by Dr. Sue O'Shea of the University of Michigan. This board represents all those providers who have deposited their cell lines in the NSCB.

Derivation of the embryonic stem cell lines will always be there, along with differing views on the moral and ethical status of cell lines. Morally, the procedure to use stem cell lines as a source of treatment is not considered appropriate, and in many countries, like France and Italy, this practice is not allowed. It is still thought that other treatments should be introduced, rather than using the one involving different stem cell lines. It is also thought that procedures should be created through which stem cells can be obtained by other means, as from the bloodstream of an adult person or from tissue culture.

Another concern of the NSCB is the likelihood of finding a match for the stem cells. Because of the donation patterns, a match cannot always be found. It has been determined that Caucasians find a match 88 percent of the time, but only 58 percent of the time is a match found for other racial groups. Donation of stem cells by people of nonwhite racial groups is now being encouraged.

According to Derek Hei, the development of nonhuman primate cells may or may not address these controversial issues. Research work has to be done to comprehend the differences between hESCs and nonhuman primate cells.

Demonstrating pluripotency also has been a topic of discussion. Teratoma estimates have been done on each of the cell lines, but researchers are thinking of repeating these testing procedures on the new master cell banks that are produced for each of the different stem cell lines. In addition, they will perform directed differentiation studies for different lineages such as cardiac, hematopoietic, neural, pancreatic, and endoderm lineages.

It is difficult to predict the future, especially because of the recent advances in nonhuman primate cells. Several more banks also will soon be developed around the world that will deposit and develop groups of cell lines, such as HLA-diverse lines for transplantation procedures.

It is believed that the NSCB will eventually attract groups of scientists and individuals with other expertise from all across the world to come together and work as a group. The bank will serve as a place for the collaboration of people from around the world, and this will be beneficial for the progress and development of science. As a result of this increased international interaction, donors will be encouraged to deposit their cell lines. This will further help in developing better relations among different research groups. Thus, in short, the whole science community will benefit from international collaboration on stem cell research.

Stem cell lines from the NSCB can be ordered for research being performed anywhere in the world. For stem cells to reach underdeveloped countries like Cambodia, Sudan, Ethiopia, and so forth requires different companies to develop therapeutics in a way that will address the regulatory requirements of each country. Here, the only role of the NSCB will be to provide these companies with well-characterized and vigorously tested super-clean cells that will, in turn, be used as a starting point for the development of therapeutics in these underdeveloped countries.

There are a number of groups that have been able to grow up to $10^9$ total cells, as stated by Derek Hei. This is a large number of cells and is sufficient to produce cells for limited clinical applications. It is believed that if work on the different stem cell lines continues at the same rate it is now, in the coming two to five years, it will result in the production of two to three logs more cells per batch. This increase in the production of stem cells will be a great advantage.

A place where the stem cell lines can be saved and used for further research and treatment methods is definitely needed at this time. As projects similar to these continue to begin all over the world, more people will benefit. What should be done now is to create awareness among people worldwide of the importance of these stem cell lines in the treatment of many blood and immune system–related genetic diseases, cancers, and other blood disorders.

**SEE ALSO:** Cells, Embryonic; International Laws; National Institutes of Health; Thomson, James; University of Wisconsin, Madison; WiCell.

**BIBLIOGRAPHY.** National Stem Cell Bank, www.wicell.org (cited May 2008).

Madiha Anwar Baig
National University of Science and Technology

# Nebraska

**NEBRASKA'S HISTORY OF** biomedical research in the academic and medical fields has brought the state national recognition for work such as that of researchers at the University of Nebraska Medical Center, who in 1997 injected liver cells into diseased tissue, resulting in improved function and in the patient no longer needing a liver transplant. However, developments in the legislative area resulting from ethical and social debate may hinder both future innovation and the attracting of top researchers in stem cell research if a research ban and penalty for such research is approved.

As no federal legislation in the United States regulates stem cell research (except by an executive order to not allow federal funding to be used for embryonic stem cell research except on human embryonic stem cell lines created before August 9, 2001), each state is responsible for determining policy and funding for stem cell research. Nebraska law also limits the use of state funds from the tobacco settlement to the state healthcare cash fund from being used for human embryonic stem cell research.

A bill was introduced in 2007 and carried over into 2008 that would ban both human reproductive and therapeutic cloning using somatic cell nuclear transfer. In addition to the ban, the bill seeks to classify this type of research activity as a felony with harsh penalties. Funding for research is available through the National Institutes of Health, state funding, and private foundations and research grants.

## UNIVERSITY OF NEBRASKA

Research in the department of virology at the University of Nebraska includes the interaction between the neurological and immune systems and the laboratory's discovery that T cells mount a spontaneous response to protect injured neurons. Their research also includes central nervous system regeneration of damaged retina in a mouse model using rodent embryonic progenitor cells. The long-term goals include returning vision in cells that do not naturally regenerate.

The stem cell and bone marrow transplantation team at the University of Nebraska Medical Center is involved in over 400 research protocols and clinical trials for cancer, heart diseases, diabetes, musculoskeletal disease, and other illnesses. In addition to treatment, the center's research is conducted to improve post-transplant quality of life by reducing transplant-related complications. One such study follows peripheral stem cell transplant patients for sleep disturbances, fatigue, and pain and compares the biological indicators of sleep quality and cycles, as well as determining the effect on caregivers' sleep quality and cycles.

After the success in 1997 of injecting liver cells, researchers have turned to studying the possibility of using human embryonic stem cells to create liver cells. The scientists at the University of Nebraska Medical Center are working with National Institutes of Health–approved stem cell lines in mouse models. As with all research, preliminary testing is necessary before federal grant money can be requested, as federal money is limited to research that has been shown to be viable, and even then, funding is very competitive.

The Nebraska Center for Cellular Signaling, established in 2003 through National Institute of Health funding, created a center of biomedical research in Nebraska. The center is the result of collaboration between the University of Nebraska–Lincoln, Creighton Medical School, and the University of Nebraska Medical Center. The center's mission is to improve oral and dental health. To meet this goal, researchers focus on cellular biology (adhesion and motility and cancer biology), with projects on oral and colon cancer, DNA damage, ubiquitin ligases, and signaling.

## NEBRASKANS FOR RESEARCH

Nebraskans for Research was formed in 2000 as an advocacy and public education group to support medical research within the state, including stem cell research. The organization's goals are to gain increased funding for biomedical research for economic growth and improved medical treatments for human disease and illnesses, as well as attracting top researchers to the state. To meet this goal, the organization promotes the successes of Nebraska researchers to the public through online content, media coverage, and conferences or lectures showcasing a variety of topics from ethics, to basic research, to accomplishments. With a goal of training future scientists, the group also develops programs for science teachers to use in their classes.

**SEE ALSO:** *Individual U.S. State Articles*; Biotechnology, History of; Clinical Trials Within U.S.: Batten Disease; Clinical Trials Within U.S.: Blind Process; Clinical Trials Within U.S.: Cancer; Clinical Trials Within U.S.: Heart Disease; Clinical Trials Within U.S.: Peripheral Vascular Disease; Clinical Trials Within U.S.: Skin Transplants (Burns); Clinical Trials Within U.S.: Spinal Cord Injury; Clinical Trials Within U.S.: Traumatic Brain Injury; Ethics; Federal Government Policies; Moral Status of Embryo; Special Interest/Lobby Groups; United States.

**BIBLIOGRAPHY.** University of Nebraska Medical Center, "Two UNMC Research Teams to Begin Projects Using Bush-Approved Embryonic Stem Cell Lines," www.unmc.edu (cited February 2005); University of Nebraska–Omaha, www.unomaha.edu (cited November 2007); Nebraskans for Research, "Overview of LB 700," www.nebraskansforresearch.org (cited November 2007).

Lyn Michaud
Independent Scholar

# Netherlands

**THE NETHERLANDS HAS** a long history of work in developmental biology, from the collection of embryonic material from a variety of species by Ambrosius Hubrecht, dating from the late 1800s, to the study of embryos by Peter Nieuwkoop and continuing with Christine Mummery's work in the 1980s of using mouse embryonic stem cells to study control of growth and differentiation in early development, and moving into human embryonic stem cells. Current stem cell research is able to progress because of government support, with appropriate legislation and funding, strong scientific research foundation, public support of biomedical research, and international cooperative relationships and partnerships.

The September 1, 2002, Embryo Act allows for research on fertilized eggs and provides rules for the creation and treatment of embryos related to assisted reproduction. The Organ Donation Act, which has been in force since 1998, allows anyone 12 years of age and older in the Netherlands to register their organ and tissue donation preference in a central donor register. Spare embryos that were unused for in vitro fertilization may be donated with the consent of the persons who donated the gametes. For embryos to be used for research, the law mirrors that for the Dutch Medical Research Act covering protection of human test subjects. The research is subject to ethical review and consent from the parents (for whom the embryos were created) or the donors, as appropriate. The law allows researchers to derive human embryonic stem cells from excess embryos. When the law was enacted, a five-year ban on embryo creation was included and would be reviewed at the end of the five years to determine the status of the ban. The act prohibits human reproductive or therapeutic cloning, the creation of human–animal hybrids and gender determination.

Funding is provided through government sources, the European Science Foundation, the Netherlands Organization for Scientific Research, project grants from Dutch and international sources, and from the biomedical and pharmaceutical industries.

## ORGANIZATIONS

Stem Cells in Development and Diseases was established in 2004 through government funding as a consortium to understand the genetics and regulation of human disease to advance technology and clinical/therapeutic application. The consortium brings together researchers in stem cell, developmental, and molecular biology with biotechnology industry researchers. Their common goal is determining the control-cell identity in stem cells and tissues. Research being done by this consortium is focused on three areas: signaling, regulation, and stem cells and differentiation.

The Dutch Program for Tissue Engineering was also established in 2004 through government funding. It encourages collaborative cross-discipline research by academic and clinical and industry professionals to translate tissue engineering technology into clinical applications. Stem cell technology is one of the three areas of focus with the research objectives of isolating, growing, and differentiating stem cells for tissue repair for musculoskeletal and cardiovascular and skin tissues.

The Dutch Forum for Regenerative Medicine also intends to use stem cell research and tissue engineering. Regenerative medicine relies on controlling cell development to grow healthy tissues, using cell-based therapy to improve organ function in diseased or injured organs and tissues instead of drugs or devices.

The Netherlands Organization for Health Research and Development distributes funding for scientific research by open applications or restricted programs, with research performed on topics chosen by the organization. They fund programs where the researcher directs the program and managed research, where the researchers work toward specific goals. In the spirit of international collaboration, the organization cohosted a Therapeutic Cloning Conference to bring together British and Dutch policy makers and scientists for a debate on how best to translate the fundamental science of cloning into clinical application. The Netherlands maintains international collaborations and networks in the area of stem cell research including the International Stem Cell Forum and the EuroStemCell Project.

## RESEARCH UNIVERSITIES

Erasmus University Rotterdam was founded in 1913 as a business school and has incorporated a broad range of academic disciplines throughout the years, including a merger with the Medical College in 1973. The Erasmus Medical Center integrates teaching, research, and medical care with their research in biomedical sciences. The biomedical cluster plays a leading role in the field of genomics (analysis of genes and proteins) and bioinformatics. Stem cell research is accomplished through collaborative networks, and one Erasmus professor is the project leader for determining the mechanism for blood stem cell renewal.

The Hubrecht Institute is a research institute located in Utrecht. It was established in 1916 and has roots dating back to Professor Ambrosuis Hubrecht, who taught zoology at Utrecht University. He was a contemporary of and correspondent with Charles Darwin. Dr. Hubrecht collected embryonic material from many species. The first Hubrecht laboratory was housed in his residence and has moved and expanded since then. The Hubrecht Institute is known for its pioneering work in developmental biology.

Current research at the institute covers a range of areas of study in biology, including gene activation/inactivation, organ development (heart, intestine, brain), cancer biology, regenerative medicine, and embryonic stem cells. Funding for Hubrecht's research comes from the Royal Netherlands Academy of Arts and Sciences and from public and private grants from the national and international pharmaceutical industry. The institute's stem cell projects include stem cells used in development, disease, validation, and implementation of the Embryonic Stem Cell Test to be used for developmental toxicity testing, as approved for animal testing.

Utrecht University is located in Utrecht with proximity to other renowned institutes for networking. The university offers a wide range of academic education in the biomedical field, up to doctoral coursework. Research and education in biomedical and life sciences is offered within the Academic Biomedical Center for collaboration across disciplines and includes the University Medical Centre Utrecht, Pharmaceutical Sciences (containing the departments of Medicine, Veterinary Medicine, Science, Biology, and Chemistry), and Hubrecht Institute for Developing Biology and Stem Cell Resources. The center also ensures the translation of innovations to medical application by supporting entrepreneurial activity. Research related to stem cells includes the discovery of signaling pathways on digestive tract stem cells, cardiovascular research, drug innovation, growth and differentiation of stem cells, synthesis and characterization, and imaging.

### KNOWLEDGE PROJECT IN DEVELOPMENTAL BIOLOGY

A comprehensive working group of prominent and successful developmental, stem cell, and molecular scientists within the Netherlands collaborates on fundamental processes in developmental biology and includes stem cell research to create cellular therapies for the treatment of human diseases. Under the auspices of this network, research collaborations are possible on the developmental processes of human disease. However, through the realization of the innovative Knowledge Research Project in biomedical technology, a larger, highly advantageous and more integrated/interactive program is achieved. Previously, this has not been possible because of the lack of an appropriate subsidy scheme. Although the European Community offers subsidy opportunities for integrated research programs between many European laboratories, funding through this program allows for structured research within the Netherlands.

**SEE ALSO:** European Consortium for Stem Cell Research—EuroStemCell; International Society for Stem Cell Research; International Stem Cell Forum; Mummery, Christine.

**BIBLIOGRAPHY.** Dutch Program for Tissue Engineering, "Abstract," www.dpte.org (cited November 2007); Ministry of Health, Welfare, and Sport, "Embryo Act," www.minvws.nl (cited November 2007); Stem Cells in Development and Disease, "About," www.stemcells.nl (cited November 2007); Academic Biomedical Center, www.abc.uu.nl (cited November 2007); Erasmus University Rotterdam, www.eur.nl (cited November 2007); Hubrecht Institute, "Information," nlob.know.nl (cited November 2007).

Lyn Michaud
Independent Scholar

# Neuralstem

**NEURALSTEM IS A** biotherapeutics company with corporate headquarters in Rockville, Maryland. The corporate mission of Neuralstem is to apply stem cell research to the treatment of diseases of the central nervous system (CNS) including ischemic paraplegia, traumatic spinal cord injury, amyotrophic lateral sclerosis (ALS, aka Lou Gehrig's disease), and Parkinson's disease. Treatment is promoted with Neuralstem's patented human neural stem cell technology.

Neuralstem's stock is publicly traded on the American Stock Exchange (AmexR) under the ticker symbol CUR; previously, Neuralstem was traded over the counter under the symbol NLRS. Karl Johe (Ph.D.), Richard Garr (J.D.), and Merrill Solomon founded the company in 1996. Dr. Johe is the scientific founder and current chairman of the board of directors of the company. Prior to creating the company, he worked for the National Institute for Neural Disorders and Stroke, which is one of two dozen institutes that comprise the National Institutes of Health. Richard Garr is the current president and chief executive officer of Neuralstem. The company was strengthened in 2007 by the appointment of Scott V. Ogilvie and William C. Oldaker as independent members of the board of directors. It also appointed John Conron as its chief financial officer.

Through stem cell research, Neuralstem has been able to produce mature commercial quantities of neural stem cells. These kinds of stem cells have the ability to differentiate into different kinds of cells that can become physiologically relevant human neurons and glia. The technology used by Neuralstem has the power to direct the differentiation of mature adult stem cells into specific neural cells. The cells can then be injected into the human body to be used as therapies.

Approval of the Food and Drug Administration (FDA) is needed before any stem cell therapies can be used in the treatment of otherwise incurable diseases. Neuralstem has developed a patent-protected technology that it calls Human Neural Stem Cell technology. Neuralstem holds a number of stem cell patents. Its patents are "Isolation, Propagation, and Directed Differentiation of Stem Cell from Embryonic and Adult Central Nervous Systems of Mammals" (US patent 5,753,5060); "In Vitro Generation of Differentiated Neurons from Cultures of Mammalian Multi-potential CNS Stem Cell" (US patent 6,040,180); "Method for Generating Dopaminergic Cells Derived from Neural Precursors" (US patent 6,284,539); "Stable Neural Stem Cell Lines" (Australian patent 755849).

The technology invented by Neuralstem allows it to isolate stem cells from central nervous system tissue. It then puts the isolated stem cells into in vitro material, which allows the cells to grow by division (up to 60 doublings) into cells numbering into the multiple billions. Its process controls differentiation of the cells. They grow into mature cells, which can be used in therapies in the nerve tissue of the spinal cord of humans or into human brain tissue.

The Neuralstem process can use undifferentiated stem cells from humans to make a variety of specific types of nervous system cells. In May 2007 the journal *Neuroscience* contained a report by researchers at the University of California at San Diego that they had successfully returned function to experimental animals that had been treated with neural stem cells produced by Neuralstem. The stem cells used were a modal of Ischemic Spastic Paraplegia (ISP). In humans, ISP disease can result from surgery that seeks to repair aortic aneurysms. In December 2007 Neuralstem signed a Clinical Trial Research Agreement with the University of Pennsylvania's Department of Anesthesiology and Critical Care. Clinical trials will be conducted at the University of Pennsylvania Hospital using Neuralstem stem cell technology on patients with ISP.

**SEE ALSO:** Cells, Adult; Cells, Neural; Clinical Trials (Adult Cells); Stem Cell Companies.

**BIBLIOGRAPHY.** Neuralstem, Inc., www.neuralstem.com (cited April 2008); Seeking Alpha, "Neuralstem: Wall Street Analyst Forum Presentation Transcript," May 22, 2007, seekingalpha.com/article/36284-neuralstem-wall-street-analyst-forum-presentation-transcript (cited April 2008).

Andrew J. Waskey
Dalton State College

# Neurosphere Cultures

**THE ADULT CENTRAL** nervous system has long been viewed as comprising tissue that is incapable of cell neogenesis and, particularly, lacking the ability to support production of new neuronal cells. Yet, discoveries made over the last two decades have radically altered this perspective. In fact, the discovery that some regions of the mature brain are the site of intense neurogenesis throughout life has changed our understanding of how the brain maintains its cytoarchitecture and functional integrity while, at the same time, possessing an inherent degree of plasticity and significant regeneration capacity.

The biological entity at the root of this neurogenetic process is the neural stem cell. Although bearing somewhat distinct functional properties depending on their age and location, neural stem cells are involved in the production of new mature brain cells throughout life, including embryonic and fetal development. The in vitro approach that is most widely used to isolate and quantify these neural stem cells from the vast majority of the central nervous system tissues across species, higher primates and humans included, is the neurosphere technique that is described here. It is worth emphasizing how the neurosphere method also allows for the expansion of the neural stem cell population pool ex vivo while, at the same time, making it possible to measure critical stem cell features in the candidate neural cells, such as self-renewal, fate potential, and differentiation properties.

## THE NEUROSPHERE METHOD

The neurosphere system can be applied to many different tissues, be they of adult, fetal, or embryonic origin, from virtually all mammalian species, including humans. In its most common applica-

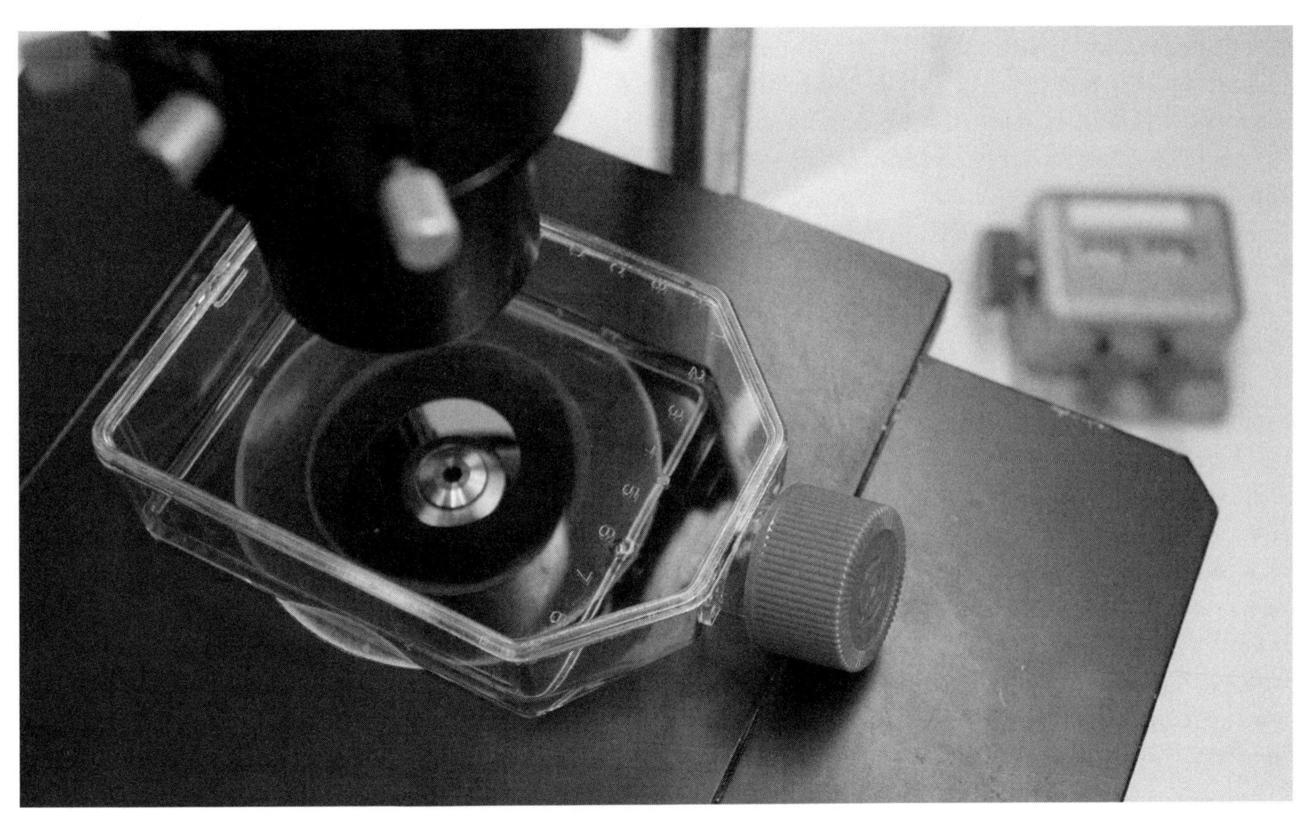

*The discovery that some regions of the mature brain are the site of intense neurogenesis throughout life has changed some of our understanding of the brain. The biological entity at the root of this process is the neural stem cell.*

tion, donor tissue is predigested enzimatically and then mechanically dissociated to yield a single-cell suspension, which is then plated under quite stringent growth conditions. This procedure establishes a selective culture system in which most of the primary differentiated/differentiating central nervous system cells found in the primary tissue die out soon after plating, whereas the undifferentiated stem cells enter into a state of active proliferation.

Four main conditions must absolutely be satisfied for the neural stem cells to become the prevalent cell type in these cultures: there must be low cell density ($<5 \times 10^4$ cells/cm$^2$), there must be an absence of serum, and there must be the addition of the appropriate growth factors (i.e., EGF or FGF2), and there must be a plating substrate warranting loose cell adhesion (poly-L-lysine or polyornithine may be used). Under these conditions, cells from a freshly dissociated brain attach loosely to the substrate, with the majority (99 percent) rapidly dying out. At the same time, a tiny fraction of undifferentiated neural precursors, mostly neural stem cells, become hypertrophic, round up, and engage into active proliferation while adhering loosely to the culture vessel. The progeny of these proliferating precursors preferentially adhere to each other while dividing and, eventually, form spherical clusters that, because of their increasing mass, eventually lift off the substrate and float in suspension. These have been named *neurospheres*, from which comes the name of the technique.

## SUBCULTURING

In giving rise to neurospheres, neural stem cells undergo symmetric cell cycles in which the two daughter cells are identical to their mother. This occurs in concomitance with additional asymmetric and symmetric divisions in which one or both cell progeny are more differentiated/mature cells. There are two important consequences of this phenomenon. First, in the neurosphere assay, the number of stem cells expands over time and, second, each neurosphere turns out to be a cluster of both neural stem cells and more mature precursors. Depending on the species, age, and area of origin within the brain, anywhere between 10 and 50 percent of the total cells generated in a neurosphere are neural stem cells. This is the reason why neurospheres are routinely subcultured by harvesting, followed by mechanical dissociation, and by replating under the initial growth conditions—as in the primary culture, the more mature cells rapidly die out, whereas the newly generated neural stem cells continue to proliferate, giving rise to secondary spheres that can then be further subcultured. If single, primary, or serially passaged neurospheres are dissociated and plated under clonal conditions, the number of new neurospheres provides an estimate of the number of neural stem cells in the original sphere. This is particularly true if the appropriate neurosphere size cutoff is applied to exclude from counting those small spheres generated by cells that are capable of transient proliferation, such as transient amplifying cells.

The subculturing procedure can be repeated nearly indefinitely in a sequential fashion. Thus, as each stem cell gives rise to many stem cells during the formation of a neurosphere, the result will be the progressive and exponential increase in the number of stem cells in the neurosphere cultures over serial subculturing. If properly carried out, this procedure will produce a linear cell growth curve when plotted onto a semilogarithmic graph.

One of the most important features of this system is that, as at each subculturing steps all but the neural stem cells are selected away, the overall expansion of the total cell number is, in fact, resulting from the division and amplification of the neural stem cells. Hence, there will be a direct correlation between the slope of the growth curve and the proliferation/expansion of the size of the neural stem cell pool. The latter is inherently linked to the relative ratios between the overall number of symmetric cell cycles generating two stem cells and the other kinds of divisions occurring within the stem cell pool as a whole. Hence, by analyzing the kinetic of expansion in a neurosphere culture, one is able to gain information as to the expansion of the neural stem cell pool size and the mode of division occurring within the neural stem cell population, which can eventually be confirmed by the neurosphere formation clonal assay.

A direct consequence of the property above is that any deviation from a linear growth kinetic in a neurosphere culture turns out to be an indication of the alteration of the expected growth stability of the neural stem cells when grown by this system. In particular, a downward deviation of the curve will point to loss of capacity for amplification/self-maintenance and may be an indication of altered or poor growth conditions, senescence, toxicity, or the fact that the cells that have been isolated are most likely transit-amplifying precursors rather than true stem cells.

## MULTIPOTENCY

Neural stem cells are multipotent (i.e., generate neurons, astrocytes, and oligodendrocytes), and this property ought to be stably reproduced in neurosphere culture, particularly at the clonal level when they are induced to differentiate. The latter is routinely obtained by plating neursopheres onto a good adhesive substrate, such as lamnin or matrigel, followed by growth factor removal. Variations on this basic theme include addition of various trophic factors, cytokines, and serums to support the generation, survival, or maturation of the desired mature central nervous system cell types. Not only ought neurospheres retain the ability to generate all three major neural cell types over long-term subculturing but the relative ratios of the different cell types being generated at each time must not vary.

In conclusion, the neurosphere assay allows researchers to isolate candidate neural stem cells from the brain and to validate and study their stemness and functional properties in vitro under chemically defined conditions. These cells are also easily manipulated to test the effect of candidate molecules on the neural stem cell physiology, as well as their effect on neural stem cell growth, survival, fate potential and choice, differentiation, and maturation. At the same time, it allows for the steady and prolonged expansion of cultured neural stem cells, thus providing a plentiful and renewable, standardized source of multipotent neural precursors. These precursors can be not only used for basic research but also to generate safe and reproducible preparations of various types of mature neural cells for preclinical and clinical studies for the cure of neurodegenerative disorders while allowing for the control of critical graft parameters such as cell maturation and enrichment.

**SEE ALSO:** Cells, Adult; Cells, Embryonic; Cells, Neural; Neuralstem.

**BIBLIOGRAPHY.** Norman Doidge, *The Brain that Changes Itself: Stories of Personal Triumph from the Frontiers of Brain Science* (Viking Adult, 2007); R. Ian Freshney, Glyn N. Stacey, and Jonathan M. Auerbach, *Culture of Human Stem Cells* (Wiley-Liss, 2007); Fred H. Gage, Gerd Kempermann, and Hongjun Song, *Adult Neurogenesis* (Cold Spring Harbor Laboratory Press, 2007).

Angelo L. Vescovi
University of Milan Bicocca

# Nevada

**IN APRIL 2005,** a Nevada university, along with one in Pennsylvania, began discussing the opening of a new medical center in Las Vegas that would incorporate stem cell biology with organ transplants. The University of Pittsburgh Medical Center (UPMC) and the University of Nevada School of Medicine (UNSM) proposed to establish the joint academic medical center in downtown Las Vegas at Union Park. Faculty would come from both universities; however, although the UNSM would profit both financially and intellectually from the new medical center, most of the financial backing would come from UPMC.

On July 18, 2006, the U.S. Senate convened to vote on a proposed bill (H.R.810) that would amend the Public Health Service Act and provide federal funding for research on human embryonic stem cells. This bill was passed by the Senate but was later vetoed by President George W. Bush. In the vote, the two Nevada senators voted against each other: Republican John Ensign was opposed to the bill, and Democrat Harry Reid supported it. Senator Reid helped to introduce another Stem Cell Research Enhancement Act for 2007. It was passed by the U.S. Senate on April 11, 2007, and the House passed it two months later, but President George W. Bush vetoed it later that month.

A doctor in Nevada named Alfred Sapse claims he can cure a wide range of diseases by implanting stem cells from dried placentas under the skin of his patients. He claims to have had astonishingly positive results with test studies in Odessa, Ukraine; however, although Sapse says the results were published, the papers have not been found. Nevertheless, Sapse has established StemCell Pharma Inc., where he acts as president and founder, to conduct his procedures. Sapse has not explained how his technique circumvents the requirement for donated cells to match the HLA, or human leukocyte antigen, haplotype of the recipient; the chance of HLA haplotypes matching between two unrelated individuals is rare.

At the University of Nevada at Reno, scientists are developing the ability to grow human organs in sheep from human stem cells injected into sheep embryos still inside the pregnant ewe. These organs would be used for transplants back into the initial stem cell donor, who would be given bone marrow stem cells. The procedure is still in development as the researchers determine how to ensure that the new organs will be 100 percent human. In addition, the researchers must prove that the carrying animal, here the sheep, does not harbor any diseases that could be transplanted along with the organ. This research is led by Dr. Esmail Zanjani. Also working on stem cell biology at the University of Nevada at Reno are Dr. Graca Almeida-Porada, who is focusing on human stem cell biology, tissue engineering, and stem cell expansion and modulation, and Dr. Christopher Porada, who is working with in utero gene therapy and stem cell transplantation.

**SEE ALSO:** *Individual U.S. State Articles*; Biotechnology, History of; Clinical Trials Within U.S.: Batten Disease; Clinical Trials Within U.S.: Blind Process; Clinical Trials Within U.S.: Cancer; Clinical Trials Within U.S.: Heart Disease; Clinical Trials Within U.S.: Peripheral Vascular Disease; Clinical Trials Within U.S.: Skin Transplants (Burns); Clinical Trials Within U.S.: Spinal Cord Injury; Clinical Trials Within U.S.: Traumatic Brain Injury; Ethics; Federal Government Policies; Moral Status of Embryo; Special Interest/Lobby Groups; United States.

**BIBLIOGRAPHY.** M. Bellomo, *The Stem Cell Divide: The Facts, the Fiction, and the Fear Driving the Greatest Scientific, Political and Religious Debate of Our Time* (American Management Association, 2006); C. B. Cohen, *Renewing the Stuff of Life: Stem Cells, Ethics, and Public Policy* (Oxford University Press, 2007); C. Fox, *Cell of Cells: The Global Race to Capture and Control the Stem Cell* (Norton, 2007); K. R. Monroe, R. Miller, and J. Tobis, eds., *Fundamentals of the Stem Cell Debate: The Scientific, Religious, Ethical, and Political Issues* (University of California Press, 2007); *Pittsburgh Business Times*, "UPMC Sees Stem-Cell Research in Vegas Plans," pittsburgh.bizjournals.com (cited January 2008); M. Ruse and C. A. Pynes, eds., *The Stem Cell Controversy: Debating the Issues (Contemporary Issues)* (Prometheus, 2006); StemCell Pharma Inc., www.stemcellpharmainc.com (cited January 2008); C. Vestal, "States Take Sides on Stem Cell Research," www.stateline.org (cited January 2008).

Claudia Winograd
University of Illinois, Urbana-Champaign

# New Hampshire

**FAMOUS FOR ITS** "first in the nation" presidential primary, New Hampshire has traditionally been a conservative enclave compared with its more liberal neighbors of Vermont and especially Massachusetts. Its all-American reputation is underscored by its inspiration for the settings for Thornton Wilder's *Our Town*, Grace Metalious's *Peyton Place*, John Knowles's *A Separate Peace*, and the *Archie* comic's Riverdale High School. Its "Live Free or Die" motto and lack of broad-based taxes have attracted a variety of summer and permanent residents, from the bikers who converge on the Lakes Region for Bike Week to the libertarian Free State Initiative, which plans to have 20,000 members move to the state with the intent of influencing local politics in their favor. Since the Cold War, southern New Hampshire has been home to many giants of the technology and defense industries, many of whom relocated their plants to the state to take advantage of its proximity to Boston and the local tax benefits.

Since the start of the Republican Party, only five non-Republican presidential candidates have won New Hampshire's support: John Kerry, Bill Clinton, Lyndon Johnson, Franklin Roosevelt, and Woodrow Wilson. The inclusion of Kerry and Clinton on that list may be an indication of the state's slow softening and liberalizing as a school funding crisis forces a reexamination of the state tax structure that has been so key to New Hampshire's identity. As of the 2006 midterm elections, for the first time since 1915, all of the representatives from New Hampshire are Democrats. As of 2008, the state has legalized same-sex civil unions, though whether that is a sign of liberalism or old-fashioned libertarianism is debatable—traditionally hands-off, the state is the only one with no seatbelt law and also lacks motorcycle helmet laws, mandatory automobile insurance, sales tax, and personal income tax.

The senior senator from New Hampshire Republican Judd Gregg has voted solidly pro-life and against fetal tissue research, a stance he has upheld since his days as a congressman and the state's governor. However, in April 2007, he was one of the few Republicans to support the Stem Cell Research Enhancement Act, having also supported the 2005 Stem Cell Research Enhancement Act. Each act sought to broaden the number of embryonic stem cell lines available for federally funded research to include stem cells derived from embryos created for fertility treatments and then discarded, while continuing to forbid such funding for embryos created specifically for research. Both acts passed the House and Senate but were vetoed by President Bush. The chairman of the Senate Health, Education, Labor, and Pensions Committee when former president Ronald Reagan died after a decade-long struggle with Alzheimer's, Gregg's views on stem cell research may have been affected by the conservative icon's illness; he had come of political age in Reagan's America, was elected to the House of Representatives for his first term on the same day Reagan was elected to the presidency, and was elected as governor in 1988 while endorsing Vice President George Bush as Reagan's successor. When Reagan's widow Nancy made a plea on behalf of embryonic stem cell research, Gregg acknowledged to the press that her support would undoubtedly influence the debate.

Junior Senator John E. Sununu (son of George H. W. Bush's chief of staff John H. Sununu) is more conservative than Gregg in science and technology issues and was among the hardline Republicans opposing the various stem cell bills drafted after the August 9, 2001, executive order.

Though New Hampshire has no legislation on stem cell research, its laws on surrogate parenthood are relevant. By New Hampshire law, the preembryo—that is, the cell mass resulting from a fertilized ovum, before being implanted—must not be kept ex utero (unimplanted) for more than 14 days after being fertilized without being cryogenically preserved, and no preembryo that has been donated for use in research can then be used for in vitro fertilization.

New Hampshire has no legislation on cloning. A 2004 Research America survey found that 79 percent of New Hampshire respondents opposed the use of cloning for reproduction (16 percent supported it), whereas 74 percent supported therapeutic cloning (20 percent were opposed). A poll conducted for Boston television station WBZ in advance of the 2008 New Hampshire primary found that, when asked about specific issues, most New Hampshire respondents opposed stem cell research (presumably embryonic stem cell research) by a small margin. The exceptions were supporters of Barack Obama, Rudolph Giuliani, and John McCain, who supported stem cell research by an equally small margin.

**SEE ALSO:** Federal Government Policies; Stem Cells, Bush Ruling.

**BIBLIOGRAPHY.** Robert B. Harmon, *Government & Politics in New Hampshire* (Vance Bibliographies, 1990); Dante J. Scala, *Stormy Weather: The New Hampshire Primary and Presidential Politics* (Palgrave Macmillan, 2003).

Bill Kte'pi
Independent Scholar

# New Jersey

**NEW JERSEY,** the Garden State, is one of the 13 original colonies of the United States and has become a densely populated region with an intensively used transportation system mostly used to take people and goods out of the state. The state has, perhaps a little unfairly, come to symbolize the rundown industrial northeast of the country and to be associated with corrupt politics and organized crime. New Jersey residents might resent these imputations but have, nevertheless, found it difficult to create much of a sense of distinctive identity.

The state is bounded by the Atlantic Ocean, New York State, Delaware, and Pennsylvania. It has a total land area of just over 8,700 square miles, making it the fifth smallest in the country, but has a population estimated at being just over 8,500,000, which is the country's 11th largest. Its capital city is Trenton, and other large urban areas include Newark, which is a larger city than the capital. The state has one of the most ethnically and religiously diverse populations of any in the country, which has become associated, since the 1980s at least, with progressive politics, resulting in the regular election of Democratic candidates.

The general sentiment toward ethical issues is in line with this political loyalty, and hence there appear to be majorities that are in favor of same-sex unions and are pro-choice in the case of abortions. In this environment, the state administration has forged ahead with stem cell research. The State of New Jersey Commission on Science and Technology offers funding for stem cell research, a free source of stem cells for research, and the nurturing of a supportive environment for such research, including funding and support for the necessary infrastructure. The commission has set out its main commitments as being

> to advance New Jersey's position as a leader in scientific research and bring the benefits of stem cell research to New Jersey residents; to encourage and enable the state's renowned research and life sciences communities to develop quality, innovative treatments for patients; to support ground-breaking research that contributes to the understanding of stem cells and their potential and the translation of such research to patient treatment; and to generate economic opportunity and job growth in New Jersey by accelerating commercialization of new therapies and new technologies related to stem cell research.

State administrators have shown a dedication to preserving state laws and resisting the imposition of unwanted values or policies from elsewhere.

## STEM CELL RESEARCH FUNDING

The Stem Cell Research Grant Program offered $10 million in funds to a range of academic, not-for-profit, and for-profit organizations that have been able to provide appropriate proposals for achievable research projects. The program recognizes the importance of such research contributing to the economy as a whole and the fact that organizations creating relationships working together may provide better results than they can working alone. The provision of business incubators in the state has demonstrated the ways in which these forms of synergy can produce productive results from a commercial perspective. Existing projects have already sought to find stem cell–related treatments aimed at tackling Alzheimer's and Parkinson's diseases, spinal cord injuries, stroke, and brain trauma. Facilities funded in the state include the Stem Cell Institute of New Jersey in New Brunswick, the New Jersey Institute of Technology in Newark, the Elie Katz Umbilical Cord Blood Program, and the Garden State Cancer Center, among others.

However, the state's progress toward a scientific utopia for stem cell and other forms of research has not always been a smooth one. In late 2007, Governor Jon Corzine proposed on a statewide ballot that a $270 million bond be created to fund the various initiatives promoting stem cell science. This measure, together with another concerning sales tax reallocation, was rejected by the voters, which is being taken to mean that the electorate prefers these state priorities, if they are to be priorities, to be funded directly rather than by the state taking on debt. However, other interpretations have also been proposed. Even so, it seems that state administrators intend to push forward with plans to make the Garden State the country's leading location for life sciences. Corzine has, for example, reportedly invested his own money in developing the research infrastructure, and given the nature of state politics, it seems unlikely that opponents of stem cell research on ethical grounds will be elected to high office over the short or medium terms.

Private sector interests are also likely to be powerful motivating forces in continuing the initiative. Corzine, in October 2007, for example, opened the Christopher Reeve Pavilion as part of the New Jersey Institute of Stem Cell Research. The late Mr. Reeve was an internationally famous actor who suffered spinal damage that eventually led to his death as the result of a horse-riding accident. A native New Jerseyan, Reeve was a passionate campaigner on behalf of stem cell research, which, it is anticipated, will eventually provide a cure for his own condition as well as for so many others.

**SEE ALSO:** *Individual U.S. State Articles*; Biotechnology, History of; Clinical Trials Within U.S.: Batten Disease; Clinical Trials Within U.S.: Blind Process; Clinical Trials Within U.S.: Cancer; Clinical Trials Within U.S.: Heart Disease; Clinical Trials Within U.S.: Peripheral Vascular Disease; Clinical Trials Within U.S.:

Skin Transplants (Burns); Clinical Trials Within U.S.: Spinal Cord Injury; Clinical Trials Within U.S.: Traumatic Brain Injury; Ethics; Federal Government Policies; Moral Status of Embryo; Special Interest/Lobby Groups; United States.

**BIBLIOGRAPHY.** Scott Goldstein, "What Next for Stem-Cell Research?" *NJBIZ* (v.20/47, 2007); Alan J. Karcher, *New Jersey's Multiple Municipal Madness* (Rutgers University Press, 1999); Michael Siegel, Maxine N. Lurie, and Marc Mappen, eds., *Encyclopedia of New Jersey* (Rutgers University Press, 2004); State of New Jersey Commission on Science and Technology, www.nj.gov/scitech (cited November 2007); "Stem Cell Institute of New Jersey Breaks Ground," *Constructioneer* (v.62/24, 2007).

John Walsh
Shinawatra University

# New Mexico

**ON JULY 18, 2006,** the U.S. Senate convened to vote on a proposed bill (H.R. 810) that would amend the Public Health Service Act and provide federal funding for research on human embryonic stem cells. This bill was passed by the Senate but was later vetoed by President George W. Bush. In the vote, the two New Mexico Senators voted against each other: Democrat Jeff Bingaman was in favor of the bill and Republican Pete Domenici opposed it.

Also in 2006, New Mexico Governor Bill Richardson proposed a budget of $10 million of state funds to be dedicated to supporting stem cell research. The money would build a new research center at the Health Sciences Center of the University of New Mexico campus at Albuquerque (with an allocated $4 million), as well as hire research faculty (using another $4 million) and train graduate students for future careers in stem cell research (with the remaining $2 million). The purpose of using state funds to build the research center as well as to support faculty and students is to circumvent the federal law prohibiting stem cell research with federal funds. States, however, are free to choose their own stances on stem cell research. Governor Richardson was approached by New Mexico's Roman Catholic Bishops, who urged him to reconsider his proposal to use embryonic stem cells.

In January 2008, the U.S. Senate again passed a bill in favor of allowing federal funds to support stem cell research while forbidding human cloning. This bill, 2008 Senate Bill 23, or the Biomedical Research Act, was sponsored by New Mexico Senator John C. Ryan and was supported by Governor Bill Richardson.

At present, within the University of New Mexico Health Sciences Center (UNM HSC), there is a graduate training program in development and stem cell biology. Stem cell–related research focuses on embryonic stem cells in terms of their cell cycle and its regulation and how these regulatory schemes are related to those schemes of cancer cells, as well as neural stem cells and the harnessing of such cells to treat disorders such as Parkinson's disease, Alzheimer's disease, and numerous other degenerative disorders. In addition, neural stem cells could be used to treat spinal cord injury patients, and further understanding of these stem cells could shed light on the molecular biology of brain tumors.

Another focus of the research at UNM HSC is on adult human renal stem cells. These cells can be harvested from the adult kidney and studied. Such investigations might lead to customized treatment of chronic kidney failure or other renal diseases. Scientists at UNM HSC also study human blood and bone marrow stem cells.

Another university in New Mexico, the New Mexico State University (NMSU), also recognizes the importance of stem cell research. Although little research that is directly related to stem cells is carried out at NMSU, scientists there are encouraged to stay abreast of the biological science regarding stem cells. In fact, the main Web page of the office of the vice president for research highlights stem cell research breakthroughs in its Global Research News Section. Smaller universities such as the Eastern University of New Mexico and the Western

University of New Mexico do not have the facilities to conduct stem cell research, yet they keep their students and faculty informed through classes and seminars that address stem cell biology.

**SEE ALSO:** *Individual U.S. State Articles*; Biotechnology, History of; Clinical Trials Within U.S.: Batten Disease; Clinical Trials Within U.S.: Blind Process; Clinical Trials Within U.S.: Cancer; Clinical Trials Within U.S.: Heart Disease; Clinical Trials Within U.S.: Peripheral Vascular Disease; Clinical Trials Within U.S.: Skin Transplants (Burns); Clinical Trials Within U.S.: Spinal Cord Injury; Clinical Trials Within U.S.: Traumatic Brain Injury; Ethics; Federal Government Policies; Moral Status of Embryo; Special Interest/Lobby Groups; United States.

**BIBLIOGRAPHY.** M. Bellomo, *The Stem Cell Divide: The Facts, the Fiction, and the Fear Driving the Greatest Scientific, Political and Religious Debate of Our Time* (American Management Association, 2006); C. B. Cohen, *Renewing the Stuff of Life: Stem Cells, Ethics, and Public Policy* (Oxford University Press, 2007); C. Fox, *Cell of Cells: The Global Race to Capture and Control the Stem Cell* (Norton, 2007); K. R. Monroe, R. Miller, and J. Tobis, eds., *Fundamentals of the Stem Cell Debate: The Scientific, Religious, Ethical, and Political Issues* (University of California Press, 2007); Office of the Vice President for Research at NMSU, research.nmsu.edu (cited January 2008); M. Ruse and C. A. Pynes, eds., *The Stem Cell Controversy: Debating the Issues (Contemporary Issues)* (Prometheus, 2006); C. Vestal, "States Take Sides on Stem Cell Research," www.stateline.org (cited January 2008); S. Vorenberg, "Guv Proposes Stem Cell Program at UNM," www.abqtrib.com (cited January 2008).

Claudia Winograd
University of Illinois, Urbana-Champaign

# New York

**NEW YORK IS** located in the northeastern part of the continental portion of the United States and is one of the 13 original colonies. It is bounded by three smaller states to the east—Vermont, Massachusetts, and Connecticut; by the Atlantic Ocean, New Jersey, and Pennsylvania to the south; and on the north and west by two of the great lakes, Lake Ontario and Lake Erie, and two Canadian provinces, Quebec and Ontario. The land area of the state is in excess of 54,000 square miles, and its population is approaching 19 million people.

Although the capital is Albany, the state is dominated by the city of New York, which is one of the world's leading cities in terms of financial trading, business activity, tourism, cultural production, and integration of migrants to the country and its culture. The iconic Statue of Liberty is in the state, as is Ellis Island, which was once a principal port of entry for immigrants, including political and economic refugees. The city of New York and, to a lesser extent, the state as a whole contain a wide diversity of people of different ethnic groups and represent a serious attempt by urban and state-level administrations to create a workable, livable urban area in which multiculturalism, in the sense of people living together harmoniously while maintaining separate ideologies, thrives.

Long-term demographic changes mean that California now exceeds New York according to many of the indices by which states and cities are ranked, although the latter retains its size and vitality. The harsh winter climate in New York, which does not benefit from the Gulf Stream that has made Western Europe so much more conducive to economic and cultural development, is perhaps influential in the migration of development westward as, after all, New York represents a staging post for migrants seeking a better life for themselves and their children. However, the domination of the city over the state has tended to mean that people outside the city often feel that their interests are overshadowed by those of urban residents. Other states in the United States, such as Washington and Arizona, have also found that preponderant urban areas often dominate rural and provincial areas to an extent that may be resented by members of the latter.

Because the state is full of such a wide variety of people who are fueled by so many different political, religious, and ethical ideologies, it is not surprising that it has witnessed numerous debates about the possible use of stem cells in medical research. The preponderance of political discourse in the state in recent decades has tended to favor a generally liberal consensus, with many Democratic Party representatives being elected to public office not only in New York City but also in other urban areas, including Albany, Buffalo, and Syracuse.

Various organizations exist within the state to promote stem cell research. For example, the New York Stem Cell Foundation is a well-resourced organization that provides support for research and for various outreach activities. Through grants and publications, it works to promote a positive attitude toward the benefit of stem cell research. It is true that many interests within the state recognize the potential importance of stem cell research for economic development and, indeed, profit making. More than 300 degree-awarding tertiary-level educational institutes are established in the state, and many of these have faculty members who are ready and willing to work on relevant research if they are permitted to do so.

State officials have been attempting to pass legislation not just to permit stem cell research on a broad range of areas but also to donate state funds to support it. The proposed budget ranges between half and one and a half billion dollars. The State Assembly has, for some years, been broadly in support of such an initiative, but it has been unable to secure an agreement that would pass the approval of the governor, the Assembly and the Senate. To increase the chances of success, proposed bills have used imprecise language to avoid specific issues, but this has also provoked further debate. The plans are considered quite urgent because there is evidence of a brain drain of leading researchers that has already begun to affect the state.

**SEE ALSO:** *Individual U.S. State Articles*; Biotechnology, History of; Clinical Trials Within U.S.: Batten Disease; Clinical Trials Within U.S.: Blind Process; Clinical Trials Within U.S.: Cancer; Clinical Trials Within U.S.: Heart Disease; Clinical Trials Within U.S.: Peripheral Vascular Disease; Clinical Trials Within U.S.: Skin Transplants (Burns); Clinical Trials Within U.S.: Spinal Cord Injury; Clinical Trials Within U.S.: Traumatic Brain Injury; Ethics; Federal Government Policies; Moral Status of Embryo; Special Interest/Lobby Groups; United States.

**BIBLIOGRAPHY.** Jill Gardiner, "New York Could Face Stem Cell Brain Drain," *New York Sun* (October 9, 2006); Andrea Gawrylewski, "Stem Cell Funding in the NY Pipeline," *Scientist* (March 26, 2007); Kenneth T. Jackson and David S. Dunbar, eds., *Empire City: New York through the Centuries* (Columbia University Press, 2005); Milton M. Klein, *The Empire State: A History of New York* (Cornell University Press, 2005); New York Stem Cell Foundation, www.nyscf.org (cited November 2007).

John Walsh
Shinawatra University

# Niche Self-Renewal

**WITHIN THE BODY,** normal stem cells appear to be able to divide for the lifetime of the organism because they exist in a microenvironment called a niche. These niches provide tissue support (adult stem cells are often on the basement membrane, surrounded by specific cell types called stromal cells) and signaling (between niche and stem cells, hormonal, neural, and metabolic pathways) that control the action of stem cells in a dynamic that sustains the tissue. With few exceptions, stem cells always remain in the niche and may be attached by adhesion molecules.

Researchers at the Howard Hughes Medical Institute identified the types of cells that make up the niche in *Drosophila* by altering/marking individual stem cells. They learned that stem cells could migrate to a new spot and function as a stem cell and that regulatory signaling could be performed by cap cells because of their abundance and constant ratio with stem cells, and they also suggested that the cap cells may act as an adhesion molecule.

The niche provides an environment in which to regulate and maintain the cells in an undifferentiated state and to signal when new cells are needed. This strict genetic regulation ensures that stem cells do not grow out of control. Stem cell niches have been identified in blood, brain, breast, prostate, large and small intestines, and skin. Loss of this control results from mutations in the stem cells caused by exposure to chemicals or radiation or by improper copying before cell division.

## SIGNALING PATHWAYS

Signals to regulate cell behaviors include genes, and the cascade of events triggered by gene activity dictate stem cell fate and function. Among these signaling pathways are the *BMI-1*, *Notch*, *Sonic Hedgehog*, and *Wnt* genes. The Wnt signaling pathway may directly promote stem cell self-renewal, as has been shown in mice, and may influence stem cell function indirectly through the niche.

The BMI-1 (from the Polycomb group of transcription repressors) signaling pathway has been identified in hematopoietic and neuronal stem cells and is likely to regulate the self-renewal of other types of somatic stem cells. Sonic hedgehog signaling controls many aspects of growth, and studies have shown that it controls stem cell–like cells in mouse embryonic neocortex and cell proliferation in the adult ventral forebrain and in the hippocampus and that it is required for cell proliferation in the mouse forebrain's stem cell niche.

The Notch pathway plays an important role in many stem cell niches, including the hematopoietic system, gut, mammary gland, and muscles. On activation, the ligand interacts with the Notch receptor in the neighboring cell and activates it to induce and maintain stem cell division.

## STEM CELL DIFFERENTIATION

Adult stem cells replenish the cells lost by normal tissue turnover. When signaled to divide, the division may be asymmetric (of the two daughter cells, one remains in the niche as a stem cell and the other becomes a progenitor cell and leaves the niche to develop into a specialized cell) or symmetric (both daughter cells are stem cells that remain in the niche). The niche must provide signals telling the cells to remain undifferentiated, or they will quickly begin proliferating and differentiating, as that is the default programmed behavior and only the niche signal holds it in check. Progenitor cells move away from the niche under escort by guardian cells. Stem cells remain undifferentiated because of their unique capacity for self-renewal; with increasing specialization, they lose their proliferative ability and stop dividing.

In *Drosophila*, the placement of the mitotic spindle (perpendicular or parallel) to the cell interface results in asymmetric or symmetric division. Pluripotent mouse embryonic stem cells multiply symmetrically in culture and are suspected to be asymmetrical in the body.

If cell differentiation happened more frequently than self-renewal, the stem cell population within a niche would decrease, and if self-renewal continued unchecked, the result would be tumor development. The niche provides the necessary balance. The niche environment is responsible for the induction or inhibition of stem cell differentiation, based on the size of the niche and the composition. Signals emanating from the surrounding tissue and the supporting extracellular matrix sustain the cell identity and direct its behavior.

All functional cells arising from stem cells develop into an intermediate-differentiated progenitor cell that, through further division and differentiation through several stages, becomes a mature cell that has lost the ability to proliferate or alter its own destiny and is considered terminally generated.

In all the body systems with stem cell niches, the regenerative cells may not divide with high frequency, but the capacity for proliferation is high. By using fluorescent labeling to mark skin stem cells, researchers have shown that in response to stimulation, cells can divide rapidly within the stem cell niche.

Stem cells have the potential for regenerative medicine in repairing injured or diseased tissue and because of their purported role in tumor initiation. The niche may also play a role in cancer stem cells, making it a possible target for clinical therapy to destroy cancer as an adjunct to using chemotherapy or irradiation to destroy the proliferating tumor cells. Stem cells in the mammary gland are under the control of reproductive hormones as well as the niche to produce new tissues to create a more complex mechanism of stem cell renewal and differentiation, as well as the possibility for tumor development. A similar case is seen in the prostate, where the stem cell niche is in the basal cell layer within the region of the gland that is proximal to the urethra, which has been identified as the prostate stem cell niche.

**SEE ALSO:** Cells, Embryonic; Developmental Biology; Differentiation, In Vitro and In Vivo; Division Types (Symmetrical and Asymmetrical); Self-Renewal, Stem Cell.

**BIBLIOGRAPHY.** Michael F. Clarke and Michael W. Becker, "Stem Cells: The Real Culprits in Cancer?" *Scientific American* (July 2006); "Defining a Niche that Regulates Stem Cells," *Science Daily* (October 16, 2000); Howard Hughes Medical Institute, "Defining a Niche that Regulates Stem Cells," www.hhmi.org (cited January 2008); Devon A. Lawson, et al., "Isolation and Functional Characterization of Murine Prostate Stem Cells," *Proceedings of the National Academy of Sciences* (v.104/1, 2007); "Niche Control of Stem Cell Function," *Science Daily* (January 10, 2008); Verónica Palma, et al., "Sonic Hedgehog Controls Stem Cell Behavior in the Postnatal and Adult Brain," *Development* (v.132, 2005); In-Kyung Park, Sean J. Morrison, and Michael F. Clarke, "Bmi1, Stem Cells, and Senescence Regulation," *Journal of Clinical Investigation* (v.113/2, 2004); Chris Pierret, et al., "Elements of a Neural Stem Cell Niche Derived from Embryonic Stem Cells," *Stem Cells and Development* (v.16/6, 2007); Ellen J. Ward, et al., "Stem Cells Signal to the Niche through the Notch Pathway in the *Drosophila* Ovary," *Current Biology* (v.16/23, 2006).

Lyn Michaud
Independent Scholar

# Non-Human Primate Embryonic Stem Cells

**STEM CELL RESEARCH** is a controversial topic. Some people argue that stem cell research is the beginning of a slippery slope to reproductive cloning, whereas proponents, including medical researchers, state that stem cell research is essential and has the potential for significant medical benefit. In light of this controversy, on August 9, 2001, U.S. President George W. Bush announced that federal taxpayer funding for human embryonic stem cell research would be limited to research using stem cells lines that are currently in existence.

Research has been ongoing for many years to circumvent the ethical issues surrounding research on human embryonic stem cells. Researchers have been developing techniques of isolating stem cells that are as universal and potent as human embryonic stem cells but that do not involve human embryos. The potential benefit of using embryonic stem cells holds great promise for the field of medicine, including potential therapies or even cures for Parkinson's disease, multiple sclerosis, cardiac disease, and spinal cord injuries.

One way to circumvent the ethical dilemma of using human embryos is to use stem cells from nonhuman primates. There are some unique advantages and disadvantages of using cells from nonhuman primates, such as rhesus and cynomolgus monkeys. One potential advantage of these primates is that they have a very close genetic relationship to human beings, which allows more clinically relevant research to be conducted. Researchers have estimated the genetic similarity between some nonhuman primates and humans to be greater than 98.5 percent. This is particularly important in neural degenerative disease applications. In these applications, the mouse is inadequate as a transplantation or disease model because of the genetic variability between humans and mice.

In addition, National Institutes of Health funding can currently be obtained to make unlimited stem cell lines from nonhuman primates, as opposed to using human embryonic stem cells.

Also, because these primates have been studied extensively over the years, many disease models of these primates exist. Experimentation with nonhuman primates' embryonic stem cells is an important prerequisite to beginning to use human embryonic cells, especially because of ethical and moral considerations. The major disadvantage is that these cells ultimately are not human and are therefore unlikely to be used in clinical transplant programs.

## CLONING

The majority of cloning studies published to date have been in mice, using a technique called somatic cell nuclear transfer. This involves transplanting the nucleus containing an individual's DNA to an egg cell that has had its genetic material removed. This technique of somatic cell nuclear transfer has worked fairly well in mice but has not historically produced satisfactory results in primates.

However, researchers at the Health & Science University in Portland, Oregon, in November 2007 were able to isolate nonhuman primate embryonic stem cells and clone them. Being able to isolate embryonic stem cells and successfully clone them is an important milestone for two important reasons. First, embryonic stem cells harvested from in vitro fertilization (IVF) are not genetically identical to the host, whereas embryonic stem cells isolated and cloned from a particular host are genetically identical, which is a benefit when infusing them back into the same host. Any infusion of the IVF-obtained stem cells back to a host would undoubtedly result in rejection without continuous application of an immunosuppressive drug, which in and of itself is fraught with adverse effects. Second, being able to isolate embryonic stem cells from primates circumvents the ethical issues regarding the use of human embryonic stem cells.

Researchers led by Dr. Shoukhrat Mitalipov took nuclei from skin cells of an adult monkey and implanted them into cells of an egg from a fertile monkey after the nucleus had been removed. They then stimulated the cells into forming a round and hollow formation of cells—a type of immature embryo called a blastocyst. Extracting the innermost cells, the researchers were able to create two embryonic stem cell lines identical to the host.

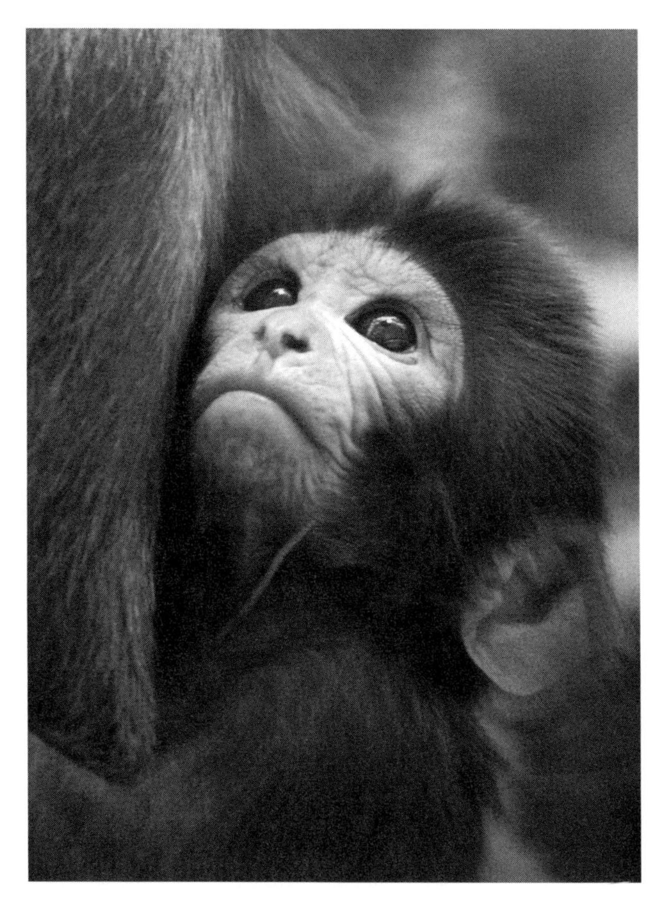

*The genetic similarity between some nonhuman primates and humans may be greater than 98.5 percent.*

## THERAPEUTIC CLONING VERSUS REPRODUCTIVE CLONING

This type of work is known as therapeutic cloning. Therapeutic cloning should be distinguished from reproductive cloning. As opposed to reproductive cloning, therapeutic cloning involves extracting stem cells to fuse with an egg, and after maturation, the blastocyst can be induced to form a tissue that is desired by the researcher. If therapeutic cloning is continued and induced, then it can potentially involve reproductive cloning, which has been performed on sheep, but not yet on monkeys. Although theoretically it is possible to use somatic cell nuclear transfer to clone—so-called reproductive cloning—the process is extremely difficult. In fact, Dolly the sheep, the first cloned animal, was born via reproductive cloning only after experimenting with 277 eggs.

### LIMITATIONS AND UPCOMING ADVANCES

It is important to note that there are many limitations to overcome when working with nonhuman primate embryonic stem cells. The primate cell lines used for research are more cumbersome with regard to their requirements for growth. They require considerably more technical expertise and attention when compared with the mouse growth requirement. Another limitation with primate embryonic stem cells is that they can sometimes spontaneously differentiate. This causes the cloning efficiency of the differentiated cells to be less than one percent in some cases.

According to Wolf, et al., much more work has to be done in the field of primate embryonic stem cell research before effective application is undertaken. At present, very little is known regarding the differences among various cell lines. Better understanding would make it more feasible to establish stem cell lines to derive a primate line with more simplified growth medium and, in effect, use methods that would make the lines replicate faster. This is because at present, the variability among various stem cell lines is unknown; therefore, investigators from different centers working on different cell lines may not be able to compare results.

It is critical to start large numbers of embryonic stem cell lines to more completely characterize these lines as a resource for the scientific community. This way, scientific research in the field of nonhuman primate embryonic stem cells can progress so that potential medical benefits, including cures for ailments such as Parkinson's disease and multiple sclerosis, can be pursued.

**SEE ALSO:** Cells, Embryonic; Cells, Human; Cells, Monkey; Cells, Mouse (Embryonic); Oregon; Oregon Health & Science University; Stem Cells, Bush Ruling.

**BIBLIOGRAPHY.** Monya Baker, "Monkey Embryonic Stem Cells Cloned," *Nature Reports Stem Cells*, November 21, 2007, www.nature.com/stemcells (cited November 2007); J. A. Byrne, et al., "Producing Primate Embryonic Stem Cells by Somatic Cell Nuclear Transfer," *Nature* (v.450, 2007); D. P. Wolf, H. C. Kuo, F. Pau, and L. Lester, "Progress with Nonhuman Primate Embryonic Stem Cells," *Biology of Reproduction* (v.71, 2004).

Devin Edwin Shahverdian
Maricopa Integrated Health System

# North Carolina

**NORTH CAROLINA IS** well positioned to become a leader in stem cell research. The state's political establishment understands the importance of research for the growth of the state's educational and medical institutions in a competitive world. As early as 2005, the general assembly proposed that North Carolina become the first state in the southeastern United States to fund stem cell research, and thus join with states such as California and New Jersey in funding such endeavors. This proposal also included support for embryonic stem cell research, which is the most controversial aspect of the research.

The North Carolina General Assembly in 2006, through its Select Committee on Stem Cell Research, offered further research support, however, within the confines of ethical research guidelines. This approach in 2007 led to the Stem Cell Research Health and Wellness Act to Permit Stem Cell Research under Limited Circumstances and to Appropriate Funds to the Health and Wellness Trust Fund for Allocation as Stem Cell Research Grants. This legislation, which followed the 2006 Stem Cell Enhancement Act veto by President Bush, initially set aside a sum of $10 million to support stem cell research for 2007–08. However, even this modest level of funding remains problematic because of the pressures brought to bear by those who have severe reservations as to the ethical nature of embryonic research.

These reservations have meant that the North Carolina legislation comes with a number of restrictions that allow stem cells to be taken only from embryos drawn from ectopic pregnancy, miscarriage, and in vitro fertilization excesses. There are also prohibitions on reproductive cloning and possibly somatic cell nuclear transfer research; however, there is a lack of clarity on many of these points that confuses the overall research picture and its ultimate direction.

At the federal level, within the 110th Congress, North Carolina's Republican senators produced divided votes with regard to the Stem Cell Research Enactment Act of 2007 with Republican Senator Richard Burr voting for the legislation and Republican Senator Elizabeth Dole voting against the act in accordance with the administration's continuing position with regard to embryonic stem cell research. In the House, a similar mixed message was produced, with six votes for the legislation and seven against, with the Republican contingent generally voting against the proposition and the Democrats generally supporting the enhanced act. Of particular note, the previous North Carolina Senator John Edwards, during the 2004 election, when he was a vice presidential candidate, made it clear that a Kerry–Edwards administration would embrace stem cell funding to include embryonic stem cell research, and as a 2008 presidential candidate, Edwards maintained this position.

At present, most Democrats in Congress, and those in most state capitals, support embryonic stem cell research, but as an issue, the embryonic aspect of this research has split Republicans. Many politicians with conservative religious constituencies have maintained their distance from any research that involves embryos. However, some prominent Republicans, such as Nancy Reagan, whose husband, former Republican President Ronald Reagan, suffered from Alzheimer's disease, became a key supporter. Further, many national polls show that a majority of Americans have come to accept the need for funding stem cell research, including that using embryonic stem cells, and that this perhaps could in the short-term change the attitude of politicians who are worried about losing votes because of any perceived research support.

North Carolina, for all its research capacity, is a generally conservative southern state with a large religious component that finds embryonic stem cell research going a step too far. This has affected any legislation being proposed as well as the votes of some politicians. Many of these opposition groups fall within what the pro–stem cell campaigners call right wing, antiabortionist lobbying groups with a pro-life agenda. However, it is clear from church reactions, such as those witnessed in the proclamations of Catholic Bishop Michael F. Burbidge of Raleigh, that these concerns are complex and should not be dismissed as just backward or simply antiscientific. These groups argue caution and see many of the stem cell claims as propaganda. There is a lack of evidence that such research has resulted in any cures to date. In addition, progress, in their eyes, does not in itself constitute a moral justification for the destruction of embryos.

## RESEARCH UNIVERSITIES

North Carolina boasts the important Research Triangle, which helps put its universities in the forefront of scientific research both nationally and internationally. Therefore, the state's university system has maintained an active interest in research projects involving stem cells. As such, the University of North Carolina, Chapel Hill, was among those organizations that signed a 2004 petition to President Bush to relax U.S. policy restrictions on cell lines. In addition, the university introduced strict regulations in 2006 for maintaining the proper procedures for human embryonic stem cell research.

The award of a shared 2007 Nobel Prize in physiology/medicine to Professor Oliver Smithies of the University of North Carolina School of Medicine for his work with genes and cellular DNA modification in mice has increased the importance of the university's reputation in research. Many other departments within the university are researching applications and looking for ways in which stem cells can offer improvements in the treatment of illnesses; this starts with fundamental research, such as that involving the relationship between genes and blood vessel development.

In a similar manner, Duke University is engaged in stem cell research, investigating its many human health applications. In the case of the Duke Stem Cell Research Program, their interests are geared to bettering the clinical applications of stem cells in reducing human suffering. This effort could produce major improvement in cancer therapies. Other university activities, an example being Duke University's Bone Marrow and Stem Cell Transfer Program, provide further multidisciplinary approaches to cell therapies.

Given the important work being carried out in North Carolina's universities, the current debate over stem cell—and in particular embryonic stem cell research—is seen as an unfortunate diversion, and one that reflects political partisanship as much as ethical or scientific concerns. The recent discoveries involving the use of adult stem cells might offer a solution that could depoliticize the entire debate. Huntington F. Willard, director of Duke's Institute for Genome Sciences and Policy, sees the debate as a means of taking scientific research before the public, giving stem cell research a prominence that it might not otherwise have, which ultimately could end up changing public perceptions.

**SEE ALSO:** *Individual U.S. State Articles*; Biotechnology, History of; Clinical Trials Within U.S.: Batten Disease; Clinical Trials Within U.S.: Blind Process; Clinical Trials Within U.S.: Cancer; Clinical Trials Within U.S.: Heart Disease; Clinical Trials Within U.S.: Peripheral Vascular Disease; Clinical Trials Within U.S.: Skin Transplants (Burns); Clinical Trials Within U.S.: Spinal Cord Injury; Clinical Trials Within U.S.: Traumatic Brain Injury; Ethics; Federal Government Policies; Moral Status of Embryo; Special Interest/Lobby Groups; United States.

**BIBLIOGRAPHY.** Julie Clayton and Carina Dennis, *50 Years of DNA* (Palgrave-Macmillan, 2005); Cynthia B. Cohen, *Renewing the Stuff of Life: Stem Cells, Ethics and Public Policy* (Oxford University Press, 2007); James M. Humber and Robert F. Almeder, *Stem Cell Research* (Humana, 2004); "Research Triangle Partnership," *Business North Carolina* (v.24, 2004); Louis R. Wilson, *The Research Triangle of North Carolina: A Notable Achievement in University, Governmental and Industrial Cooperation* (Colonial, 1967).

THEODORE W. EVERSOLE
INDEPENDENT SCHOLAR

# North Dakota

**NORTH DAKOTA IS** a north central state of the United States that is bounded by Canada, Montana, South Dakota, and Minnesota. The state consists largely of rolling grasslands that have been converted into large-scale farms and cattle ranches. The total area of the state is 70,702 square miles, and most of the land is sparsely populated. Comparatively few large towns or cities have been established, and there have been many reported problems of rural poverty and, certainly before the widespread establishment of electronic media, isolation and its related phenomena.

The largest city in the state is Fargo; the centrally located capital is Bismarck. Although there are dangers in generalization, a significant proportion of the state's population originally hailed from northern European countries such as Germany, Norway, and Iceland. The proportions of people professing religious beliefs are high, with Lutheran and Catholic forms of Christianity being particularly prominent. A strong cooperative movement has to some extent enhanced the sense of self-reliance and independence that characterizes many North Dakotans. These characteristics tend to promote socially conservative values, although the state has a reputation for voting outside of party lines and in favor of the performance of individual officials and candidates.

North Dakota has banned the cloning of humans or human cells within its borders and extended this ban, in 2003, to outlaw embryonic stem cell research in the state on the basis that it destroys human life. Nevertheless, this decision has been challenged by the two Democratic senators, Byron Dorgan and Kent Conrad, who in 2006 voted in favor of two bills that contradicted the apparent will of President George W. Bush to prevent stem cell research on religious grounds. In advance of votes that passed to extend nonembryo stem cell research and to prevent fetal farming, Senator Dorgan observed that,

> I lost a beautiful daughter some years ago to heart disease. I wondered then and I wonder now and, I will wonder some long while, if there's anything that we could do to unlock the mystery of that devious killer.

There is a long history in the practice of ethics of all varieties that explores this dichotomy between impersonal macroscale ideologies and humanistic, personal microscale compassion.

Because the industrial and manufacturing base of the state is very low, there is little likelihood that private sector demands for reversing the overall ban will be very loud—indeed, the state offers few infrastructural advantages for attracting relevant high-tech firms even if there were the political will so to do. Similarly, tertiary-level educational institutions in the state are comparatively small and generally focused on location-specific issues, which tends to preclude the kind of scientific research that would be required to advance stem cell technology. However, the recent discovery that certain skin cells might be used in place of embryonic cells, hence avoiding the religious issues involved in using embryonic cells, offers some possibility for compromise ahead.

Nevertheless, as scientific research on embryonic cells is likely to be indicated for scientific purposes for several years irrespective of the success of the skin cell technique, it appears that North Dakota will not be at the forefront of research. However, should the anticipated benefits in due course materialize, then it will be less inconvenient for state citizens to take advantage of them. Various human interest stories portraying the benefits of stem cell technologies deriving from permitted uses already seem to be shaping public opinion, and it may be that this will inform future public policy.

**SEE ALSO:** *Individual U.S. State Articles*; Biotechnology, History of; Clinical Trials Within U.S.: Batten Disease; Clinical Trials Within U.S.: Blind Process; Clinical Trials Within U.S.: Cancer; Clinical Trials Within U.S.: Heart Disease; Clinical Trials Within U.S.: Peripheral Vascular Disease; Clinical Trials Within U.S.: Skin Transplants (Burns); Clinical Trials Within U.S.: Spinal Cord Injury; Clinical Trials Within U.S.: Traumatic Brain Injury; Ethics; Federal Government Policies; Moral Status of Embryo; Special Interest/Lobby Groups; United States.

**BIBLIOGRAPHY.** "Grand Forks Man Gets Heart Treatment Using His Own Stem Cells," *Bismarck Tribune* (July 31, 2006); "North Dakota Senators Support Embryonic Stem Cell Research," *Grand Forks Herald* (July 19, 2006); Christine Vestal, "States Vie for Stem-Cell Scientists," *Stateline* (January 15, 2008).

John Walsh
Shinawatra University

# Northwestern University

**NORTHWESTERN UNIVERSITY, FOUNDED** in 1855, is a private university in Illinois with an enrollment of approximately 13,000 students. The main university campus, including the Kellogg School of Management, the McCormick School of Engineering and Applied Science, and the Weinberg College of Arts and Sciences, is located in Evanston, Illinois, whereas several other professional schools, including the Feinberg School of Medicine (founded in 1859 and affiliated with Northwestern in 1870), are located in Chicago. The McGaw Medical Center, affiliated with the Feinberg School, is a consortium of hospitals in the Chicago area, including the Children's Memorial Hospital, Northwestern Memorial Hospital, the Rehabilitation Institute of Chicago, the Jesse Brown VA Medical Center, and the affiliated hospitals of Evanston Northwestern Healthcare.

Northwestern was among the first universities in the United States to embrace stem cell research and was the recipient of major grants to support that research. The university benefits from being located in Illinois, which was one of the first states to provide public funds for stem cell research. Northwestern faculty members are also engaged in studying ethical questions concerning research and therapeutics based on stem cells: This is one among many bioethical issues studied at Northwestern's Center for Bioethics, Science, and Society and in the degree-granting Medical Humanities and Bioethics Program. Northwestern has also played a major role in educating the public and other professionals about stem cell research through publications, sponsorship of public lectures and discussions, and dissemination of information through its Web site.

## GRANTS

In 2006 the state of Illinois awarded three Northwestern professors almost $3.5 million in grants for stem cell research; the funds came from the Illinois Regenerative Medicine Institute, which was established to support research into the medical application of stem cells. Mary J. C. Hendrix, Ph.D., a professor of pediatrics in the Feinberg School and president and scientific director of the Children's Memorial Research Center, received $2 million to determine the potential of human stem cells to reverse the progression of malignant tumors, muscular dystrophy, Parkinson's disease, brain injury, and epilepsy. Guillermo A. Ameer, Sc.D., assistant professor of biomedical engineering at the McCormick School and the Institute for Biotechnology in Medicine, received $870,000 to study stem cell–based vascular tissue engineering for the development of replacement blood vessels. Ziaozhong A. Wang, Ph.D., assistant professor of biochemistry, molecular biology, and cell biology at the Weinberg College, received $565,000 to study the genetic control of differentiation and pluripotency (ability to develop into different types of mature cells) in stem cells.

Northwestern was selected in 2006 by the National Institutes of Health as one of two Centers of Excellence in Transitional Stem Cell Research within the United States and was awarded a $2.6 million grant to further support its stem cell research. The purpose of the centers of excellence is to bring together experts from many scientific fields to investigate ways in which human stem cells may be used to treat human disorders, as well as to develop new technologies that advance the state of the art in using stem cells to treat particular diseases.

## RESEARCHERS

Northwestern's center is headed by John Kessler, who is also chair of the Department of Neurology and the Ken and Ruth Davee Professor of Stem Cell Biology in the Feinberg School. Coinvestigators on the center of excellence grant are Robert D. Goldman, chair of cell and molecular biology at the Feinberg School; Thomas Meade, professor of chemistry in the Weinberg College; James Hulyat, research assistant professor of materials science and engineering at the McCormick School; and Samuel Stupp, professor of materials science and engineering—chemistry in the Weinberg School. Laurie Zoloth, director of bioethics in the Center for Genetic Medicine and professor of medical ethics and humanities in the Feinberg School, is the ethical consultant for the grant.

The position of the Ken and Ruth Davee Professor of Stem Cell Biology at Northwestern was created in 2006, and the first (and continuing) recipient of that position was John Kessler, who is also the Benjamin and Virginia T. Boshes Professor of Neurology. Kessler's research focuses on the biology of embryonic stem cells and neural stem cells; one of his areas of focus is the exploration of how stem cells can be induced to transform themselves into neural stem cells, which could be used to regenerate the spinal cord after injury and brain cells after stroke. Kessler's life and research are the focus of a documentary film, *Terra Incognita: The Promise and Peril of Stem Cell Research*, which details his personal connection to stem cell research: After Kessler's daughter was paralyzed below the waist following a skiing accident, he shifted his laboratory's focus to spinal cord injury and regeneration.

## OTHER PROGRAMS

The roots of the Medical Humanities and Bioethics Program at Northwestern lie in a medical ethics course initiated in 1976–77 at the request of the medical students, who petitioned James Eckenhoff, M.D., who was then dean of the medical school, to institute such a course. The program expanded gradually: A second elective course was developed in the years 1977–80, and in 1980, ethics seminars were added as clinical activities during the third and fourth years of medical studies. By 1988, medical humanities and bioethics were joined in one program, and today the program grants a master's degree in medical arts and humanities, an M.D./M.A. degree, and a dual graduate degree with the Graduate Program in Genetic Counseling within the Center for Genetic Medicine. The Medical Humanities and Bioethics Program publishes *Atrium: The Report of the Northwestern Medical Humanities and Bioethics Program*. Issues of this publication are available from the program's Web site. The program also sponsors a weekly lecture series open to the general public and maintains a library of relevant links on its Web site.

The Center for Bioethics, Science, and Society at Northwestern is an interdisciplinary center intended to facilitate discussion of bioethical issues among professors and researchers working in different fields. Among its missions are assessing basic research carried out at Northwestern in the context of bioethics, examining the cultural and social framing of science, and understanding the nature, goals, and effects of science and technology. Stem cells and regenerative medicine is one of the major focuses of the center. Topics studied there include questions such as the moral status of the fetus, the question of whether there is a duty to heal people who are suffering, and the conflict between the moral action of healing and the destruction of blastocysts, which are the source of human embryonic stem cells.

Laurie Zoloth, Ph.D., is director of the Center for Bioethics, Science, and Society and director of bioethics for the Center for Genetic Medicine. Zoloth also holds several academic appointments, including professor of medical humanities and bioethics within the Feinberg School and professor of religion and professor in the program in Jewish Studies at the Weinberg College. Her research focuses on emerging issues in medical and research genetics, neuroscience, nanotechnology, ethical issues in stem cell research, and distributive justice in health care. She has also served on many monitoring and advisory boards on projects ranging from the National Institutes of Health Asia AIDS Vaccine Trials to the National Aeronautics and Space Administration Planetary Protection Advisory Committee. Zoloth has written or edited five books and serves on numerous editorial boards.

On April 6, 2002, Northwestern hosted a public outreach program on the Evanston campus that was intended to help students and the general public understand the issues involving human stem cell research and its potential effect on society. The program, titled "Human Stem Cell Research: Problems and Promises," was organized by the neurobiology and physiology departments. An archive of the expert panel discussion from this program, as well as related information regarding medical, ethical, and political issues surrounding stem cell research has been archived on the Web: Further information is available from the Northwestern Web site.

**SEE ALSO:** Illinois; United States.

**BIBLIOGRAPHY.** *Northwestern Magazine*, "An Extraordinary Potential to Heal," www.northwestern.edu (cited October 2007); Suzanne Holland, Karen Lebacqz, and Laurie Zoloth, eds., *Human Embryonic Stem Cell Debate: Science, Ethics, and Public Policy* (MIT Press, 2001); "Human Stem Cell Research: Problems and Promise," www.northwestern.edu/science-outreach (cited October 2007); *Terra Incognita: The Promise and Peril of Stem Cell Research*, documentary film by Maria Finitzo (Kartemquin Films, 2007).

Sarah Boslaugh
BJC HealthCare

# Nottebohm, Fernando

**FERNANDO NOTTEBOHM IS** the Dorothea L. Leonhardt Professor and director of the Laboratory of Animal Behavior at Rockefeller University in New York. Although he is primarily an animal researcher, his work on brain function since the 1980s has revolutionized the field of neurobiology and opened up new frontiers for researchers interested in stem cell biology.

A native of Argentina, Nottebohm received his doctoral degree from the University of California at Berkeley in 1966 and joined the Rockefeller faculty in 1967. He has spent most of his career studying songbirds, specifically, how they learn to sing. While studying chickadees in the early 1980s, he began to question one of the basic presumptions of neuroscience: That animals (including humans) are born with all the brain cells they will ever have, and if lost, those brain cells cannot be replaced.

To test his evolving theories, Nottebohm devised a way to observe changes in the brains of adult canaries by injecting individual brain cells with a radioactive hydrogen molecule called thymidine. The thymidine would remain attached to the cell, but more important, it would be present in any cell that divided from the original. At the end of the experiment, Nottebohm and his associates found that the canaries were not only producing new neural cells but were producing thousands of them per day.

The neurobiology community greeted Nottebohm's findings with skepticism. These results upended a century's worth of beliefs about the brain, and some wondered whether the function of a canary's brain could have any relevance to mammalian brains. However, researchers soon used Nottebohm's work to prove neurogenesis in mammals, and with that, they gained a whole new way of looking at the human brain and the potential usefulness of stem cells to help the brain heal itself from degenerative disease.

Nottebohm has coauthored more than 140 academic papers in his career and has been elected to the National Academy of Sciences. Among his many awards are the 2006 Franklin Institute Medal in Life Science, the 2005 Karl Spencer Lashley Award of the American Philosophical Society, and the 2004 Lewis S. Rosenstiel Award for Distinguished Work in the Basic Sciences.

**SEE ALSO:** Brain; Cells, Neural; Gage, Fred; New York; Rockefeller University.

**BIBLIOGRAPHY.** A. Alvarez-Buylla, J. R. Kirn, and F. Nottebohm, "Birth of Projection Neurons in Adult Avian Brain May Be Related to Perceptual or Motor Learning," *Science* (v.249, 1990); A. Alvarez-Buylla, M. Theelen, and F. Nottebohm, "Mapping of Radial Glia and of a New Cell Type in Adult Canary Brain," *Journal of Neuroscience* (v.8, 1988); A. Alvarez-Buylla and F. Nottebohm, "Migration of Young Neurons in Adult Avian Brain," *Nature* (v.335, 1988); A. Alvarez-Buylla, M. Theelen, and F. Nottebohm, "Proliferation 'Hot Spots' in Adult Avian Ventricular Zone Reveal Radial Cell Division," *Neuron* (v.5, 1990); W. Bleisch, C. Scharff, and F. Nottebohm, "Neural Cell Adhesion Molecule (N-CAM) Is Elevated in Adult Avian Slow Muscle Fibers with Multiple Terminals," *Proceedings of the National Academy of Sciences* (v.86, 1989); G. D. Burd and F. Nottebohm, "Ultrastructural Characterization of Synaptic Terminals Formed on Newly-Generated Neurons in a Song Control Nucleus of the Adult Canary Forebrain," *Journal of Comparative Neurology* (v.240, 1985); S. J. Clark, et al., "On Variables that Affect Estimates of the True Sizes and Densities of Radioactively Labeled Cell Nuclei," *Journal of Comparative Neurology* (v.301, 1990); F. Nottebohm, "Neuronal Replacement in Adulthood," *Annals of the New York Academy of Sciences* (v.457, 1985); F. Nottebohm, "From Bird Song to Neurogenesis," *Scientific American* (v.260/2, 1989); J. A. Paton, B. E. Oloughlin, and F. Nottebohm, "Cells Born in Adult Canary Forebrain Are Local Interneurons," *Journal of Neuroscience* (v.5, 1985); H. Williams, J. Cynx, and F. Nottebohm, "Timbre Control in Zebra Finch (*Taeniopygia guttata*) Song Syllables," *Journal of Comparative Psychology* (v.103, 1989).

Heather K. Michon
Independent Scholar

# Nuclear Reprogramming

**DIFFERENTIATED OR MATURE** cells of the body were once thought to be capable of giving rise to cells of the same type only. However, several distinct lines of research have shown that nuclei of mature cells can be "reprogrammed" to give rise to pluripotent cells—cells capable of generating the many different cells types of the body. Generating patient-specific pluripotent cells could greatly improve efforts to repair and replace organs and tissues by obviating the need for cell donors and circumventing the possibility of donor cell rejection.

## NUCLEAR TRANSFER

Somatic cell nuclear transfer is arguably the most well known and extensively studied approach to inducing nuclear reprogramming of mature/terminally differentiated cells. This approach involves removing the nucleus of an oocyte and replacing it with the nucleus of a somatic/differentiated cell. The newly formed cell is stimulated with either an electrical pulse or chemical initiators (i.e., strontium and ionomycin) to induce cell division. The dividing entity, now akin to an embryo, can be used in at least two different ways. First, the "embryo" can be implanted into a pseudopregnant animal and mature into a fully functional individual. This process is also known as reproductive cloning and has led to the generation of many types of animals (i.e., cat, cow, horse, mouse, pig, rabbit, and rat), beginning with Dolly the sheep.

Alternatively, the dividing entity can be propagated further in culture dishes (instead of being implanted into a pseudopregnant animal) to establish pluripotent cells that are genetically identical to the donor of the somatic cell. This process is also known as therapeutic cloning, as autologous pluripotent cells could provide an immune compatible source of cells for repair of damaged or diseased cells. To date, animal studies have shown that it is possible to establish pluripotent cells lines from somatic cells and that such lines are capable of tissue recovery in diseased animals. For example, pluripotent cells have been derived following nuclear transfers of mature lymphocytes or postmitotic olfactory neurons of mice. However, human pluripotent lines have not yet been established.

Nuclear reprogramming via somatic cell nuclear transfer is limited in several ways. First, the efficiency of successful cloning is low. For example, Dolly was the only lamb born out of 277 cloned embryos. This phenomenon has been attributed to incomplete or inappropriate reprogramming of the transferred nucleus. Second, this method requires obtaining oocytes, which for humans is limited by social and ethical concerns. Given the limitations of nuclear transfer, it is important to explore the mechanisms that drive nuclear reprogramming. In this way, alternative approaches to nuclear reprogramming will emerge to enhance the likelihood of success in human therapy.

## CELL FUSION

Cell fusion can also initiate nuclear reprogramming of a somatic cell. This approach involves stimulation of membrane fusion between adult somatic cells and embryonic stem (ES) cells via either polyethylene glycol or electropulse, although it can also occur spontaneously. The ES cell has the ability to reprogram the entire differentiated nucleus into its embryonic state. When fused cells are selected using appropriate antibiotics and are maintained under ES culture condition, a reprogrammed and pluripotent hybrid can be identified and propagated.

ES cell fusion circumvents the need to obtain human oocytes and therefore could be a potential alternative to obtain customized cells for clinical application. However, pluripotent hybrid cells are considered less useful therapeutically because of their abnormal number of chromosomes and the expression of nonautologous genes. Therefore, it is necessary to develop additional methods to remove or inactivate the chromosomal DNA originating from the ES nucleus after reprogramming is complete. A few attempts, such as eliminating ES specific chromosomes in hybrid cells, were reported and have increased enthusiasm for the therapeutic utility of this approach.

## SOLUBLE SIGNALING

The processes of nuclear transfer and cell fusion both expose a mature nucleus to the cytoplasmic milieu (and, in the case of fusion, potentially to the nucleus) of a pluripotent entity. To understand whether and to what extent soluble factors of the immature cell affect the nuclear reprogramming of the mature cell, somatic cells were cultured with cell extracts of ES cells or oocytes. Specifically, chemicals (i.e., SLO or digitonin) were used to permeabilize the cellular membrane of differentiated human cells, which were then incubated with cell extracts isolated from amphibian eggs or mammalian embryonic stem cells for up to one hour. Mature cells treated in this fashion were able to differentiate toward multiple cell lineages, indicating that nuclear reprogramming had occurred.

More recently, specific molecules required for reprogramming activities have been identified via immunodepletion. For example, Brg1, a protein involved in chromatin remodeling, was found necessary for reprogramming. As other such molecules are identified, it may be possible to eliminate the need of human oocytes by simply using cell extracts from ES cells or even recombinant proteins when molecules responsible for reprogramming are known or defined.

This approach also provides a good biochemical tool for scientists to pinpoint the molecules required for reprogramming. However, more studies are certainly required, as so far the reprogrammed cells obtained from this approach could not divide indefinitely and only show a transient reprogramming effect.

## GENE TRANSFER

Expression of factors essential for reprogramming might also be delivered via gene transfer. In recent studies, genes known to be upregulated in pluripotent cells (*Oct4*, *Sox2*, *c-Myc*, and *Klf4*) were delivered via retroviral transduction to terminally differentiated murine skin or fibroblast cells. Following gene transfer, the mature cells adopted ES-like phenotype and function.

Perhaps the most tantalizing implication of these results is that the reprogramming of a mature nucleus could be as simple as overexpressing a handful of genes. However, this method has only been successful with retroviral transduction. Because retroviral transduction results in the random insertion of new genes into the genome, it is possible that additional genes were activated or inhibited as a result of the transduction process. In addition, safety concerns would limit the use of retroviral gene transfer for the development of patient-specific pluripotent cells. Nevertheless, this experiment highlights the possibility that nuclear reprogramming could be controlled via gene transfer and thus provides an important stimulus to continue to uncover the mechanisms of nuclear reprogramming.

The discovery of the process of nuclear reprogramming overturned the long-standing dogma that development ends at the mature cell state and stimulated novel research in the area of regenerative medicine. To create and to maintain the plasticity of stem cells is of central importance for the advancement of stem cell biology and, ultimately, stem cell therapy because this process could lead to the generation of patient-specific multipotent stem cell reserves.

These reserves would alleviate the need to harvest tissue for autografts and corresponding donor site morbidity and would also circumvent the need for allograft donors and corresponding immunosuppression of the recipient. Unfortunately, our current understanding of nuclear reprogramming is limited and is, in most respects, phenomenological.

Thus, further dissection of this process at the molecular level is necessary to discern the spatial and temporal delivery of signals necessary to create and maintain pluripotency while avoiding tumorigenicity.

**SEE ALSO:** Cancer; Cloning; Differentiation, In Vitro and In Vivo; Egg Donation; Moral Status of Embryo; Viral Vectors: Lentivirus.

**BIBLIOGRAPHY.** Konrad Hochedlinger and Rudolf Jaenisch, "Nuclear Reprogramming and Pluripotency," *Nature* (v.441/7097, 2006); Masako Tada, et al., "Nuclear Reprogramming of Somatic Cells by In Vitro Hybridization with ES Cells," *Current Biology* (v.11/19, 2001); Kazutoshi Takahashi and Shinya Yamanaka, "Induction of Pluripotent Stem Cells from

Mouse Embryonic and Adult Fibroblast Cultures by Defined Factors," *Cell* (v.126/4, 2006); Christel K. Taranger, et al., "Induction of Dedifferentiation, Genomewide Transcriptional Programming, and Epigenetic Reprogramming by Extracts of Carcinoma and Embryonic Stem Cells," *Molecular Biology of the Cell* (v.16/12, 2005).

Ho-Pi Lin
Brenda M. Ogle
University of Wisconsin, Madison

# Nuclear Transfer, Altered

**THE FIRST STEM** cells were discovered in the early 1900s. Since then, stem cell research has mainly relied on three different sources for obtaining stem cells: embryonic cells, umbilical cord cells, and adult stem cells. For many years, murine embryonic stem cells have played a large part in helping us advance our understanding of many disease processes, including cancers. The abundance and ease of obtaining umbilical cord cells has also aided researchers.

Adult stem cells were used for the first time to produce a cloned mammal in 1995, when Dolly the sheep was born. However, it was not until 1998 that researchers took cells from human embryos and developed the first human embryonic stem cell lines. One of the first people to accomplish this feat was James Thomson at the University of Wisconsin.

After much consideration and discussion with ethicists regarding the morality of this matter, and taking into account that he would be using embryos that would otherwise have been discarded from fertility clinics, Thomson decided that the benefits of embryonic stem cell research outweighed the ethical issues that may be related to this type of research. He proceeded and was the first researcher to isolate cells from the inner cell mass of early embryos.

However, Thomson did not anticipate the intense surge in public debate regarding the controversial destruction of potential human life when embryonic stem cells are used. Similarly, in 1998, John Gearhart from Johns Hopkins University obtained stem cells from human fetal gonadal cells. In contrast to Thomson's procedure, which used in vitro human embryos, resulting in a great deal of controversy, Gearhart's method did not face as much antagonism, as the potential loss of human embryonic life apparently was not involved.

Many outspoken groups among the American public did not agree with embryonic stem cell research. Main concerns with regard to these issues included the destruction of human life (in the embryonic state) and the possibility of human cloning. Following these scientific breakthroughs, the major influencing factor in American stem cell research afterward remained the political leadership. A 1973 moratorium on federal funding for human embryo research was extended in 1998 by the U.S. Department of Health and Human Services.

Two years later, in 2000, President Bill Clinton allowed research funding for cells from aborted fetuses but not from human embryonic cells. Following Clinton's departure from presidential office, President George W. Bush, who held firm beliefs regarding the preservation of embryonic human life, was concerned about more human embryos being produced for the sole purpose of their destruction for research use. Thus, in 2001, a substantial delay was placed on U.S. embryonic

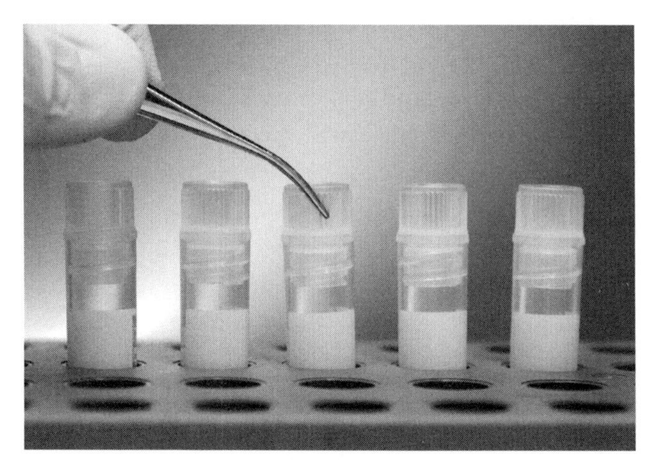

*Altered nuclear transfer holds promise for developing pluripotent cells without using functional human embryos.*

stem cell research when federal funding became limited only to the use of human embryonic stem cell lines derived before August 9, 2001, and disallowed taxpayer dollars from being used toward the destruction of human embryos.

## ALTERED NUCLEAR TRANSFER

Given these considerations, scientists have resorted to creative methods of devising human embryonic stem cells that do not involve the destruction of human life. One such method has been altered nuclear transfer (ANT). Unlike somatic nuclear transfer, in which the genetic material from a somatic cell is placed directly into an enucleated egg, in ANT, the genetic material of either or both the somatic cell and the egg would be altered before the somatic nucleus was placed into the recipient egg. The purpose of these alterations is to produce pluripotent cells that would lack the functionality of a human embryo in the hopes of alleviating the stem cell controversies.

One example of altered nuclear transfer is found in the mouse model, where suppression of the *Cdx2* gene in the somatic cell before placement into the egg produces pluripotent nonembryonic cells. A variation of this method is the suppression of the maternal messenger RNA of the *Cdx2* gene, as found in the egg, before the nuclear transfer. Another method is the overexpression of the gene *nanog* (found only the morula and the inner cell mass) in both the somatic cell and the egg for similar purposes.

This technique holds promise for developing pluripotent cells without the need for functional human embryos and has drawn support by many, including President Bush. Despite the support, ANT still faces scientific challenges before becoming a feasible procedure.

## INDUCED PLURIPOTENT STEM CELLS

Continuing the idea of nonembryonic cells, two separate research groups have since achieved similar discoveries. Based in Japan, Shinya Yamanaka and colleagues identified a set of four genes that are essential to the embryonic cell's pluripotent state. At approximately the same time, James Thomson's group in Wisconsin achieved the same discovery. These four crucial genes are: *c-myc*, *oct3/4*, *sox2*, and *klf4*. C-myc helps to loosen DNA chromatin, and the other three genes promote genetic regulation and pluripotency.

Although working separately, these two groups again published research in 2007 regarding their breakthrough discoveries that adult skin cells, when transfected to include the above four genes, could in fact produce pluripotent stem cells without the use of human eggs or embryos. With this method, no potential human life was lost, therefore possibly providing a solution to the qualms associated with human embryonic stem cell research. In essence, the potential exists for any cell in the body to be induced into stem cells by the addition of these genes while being provided with the proper cellular environment.

The cell lines derived through this method are referred to as induced pluripotent stem cells. Similar to transgenic issues faced in altered nuclear transfer, however, the risk of mutations, cancer, and infection remains and currently this is not feasible for actual therapeutic use. Nevertheless, with the genetic basis established and the ingenuity of this method confirmed, through cumulative knowledge gained from both ANT and induced pluripotent stem cells, scientists may now devise the next steps for stem cell research.

**SEE ALSO:** Johns Hopkins University; Induced Pluripotent Stem Cells; Nuclear Transfer, Somatic; Stem Cells, Bush Ruling; Thomson, James.

**BIBLIOGRAPHY.** K. Takahashi and S. Yamanaka, "Induction of Pluripotent Stem Cells from Mouse Embryonic and Adult Fibroblast Cultures by Defined Factors," *Cell* (v.126/4, 2006); J. Thomson, et al., "Induced Pluripotent Stem Cell Lines Derived from Human Somatic Cells," *Science* (v.318, 2007); Jeffrey M. Perkel, "Life Science Technologies—Beyond Somatic Cell Nuclear Transfer," *Science*, April 20, 2007, www.sciencemag.org (cited November 2007).

Susanna N. Chen
Western University of Health Sciences

# Nuclear Transfer, Somatic

**SOMATIC CELL NUCLEAR TRANSFER** (SCNT) is a process that was developed with the intent of producing immunologically compatible pluripotent embryonic cells that could be used for treating human diseases. Thus, SCNT was also termed *therapeutic cloning*. These pluripotent embryonic cells would be able to develop into any type of cell in the human body, and in addition, the technique used for these cells would address two important medical issues: immune system rejection and finding a genetically matching human donor.

The technique of SCNT involves the removal of the nucleus of an unfertilized egg cell (oocyte) and replacing it with the nucleus of a somatic cell. Somatic cells are nongermline cells that make up most cells in the body (e.g., cells found in bone, connective tissue, blood, skin, and internal organs). Ideally, the somatic cell would be obtained from the patient, so that adverse genetic and immunologic sequelae could be averted, thus also eliminating the need for finding a genetically compatible donor. These newly modified cells are then stimulated to divide, and stem cells are extracted five to six days afterward for research or potential therapeutic use.

At present, there is hope that SCNT may be used to treat diseases that are still incurable. Among these diseases are cancer, heart disease, sickle cell disease, psychiatric diseases, and many other medical conditions. SCNT also shows potential for addressing neurological conditions, such as Parkinson's disease, multiple sclerosis, amyotrophic lateral sclerosis, and various types of spinal cord injuries.

The idea of nuclear transfer has been present for many years, beginning with Hans Spemann of Germany, who performed the first such experiment using salamander embryos in the late 1920s and published his results in 1938 in his book *Embryonic Development and Induction*. Following him were Robert Briggs and Thomas King, who in 1952 cloned northern leopard frogs (*Rana pipiens*), using embryonic blastula nuclei, though by the end of their experiment, they had determined that it was impossible to produce clones from adult differentiated cells. It was Sir John Gurdon of Britain, who in the late 1950s and early 1960s further developed the technique using adult intestinal cells from *Xenopus laevis* tadpoles to clone 10 tadpoles, who then proved Briggs and Thomas' conclusion to be erroneous. Although some speculate whether Sir Gurdon's experiment was accurately performed, his work did open the way to scientific discussion regarding the ethics of cloning.

## DOLLY AND HER LEGACY

The current legacy of SCNT began with a group of scientists under the direction of Keith Campbell and Ian Wilmut at the Roslin Institute in Edinburgh, Scotland, in conjunction with the biotechnology firm Pharmaceutical Proteins Limited Therapeutics. This research group was the first to successfully clone a mammal using an adult cell. From the frozen udder of a deceased, six-year-old, pregnant Finn Dorset ewe, an adult sheep mammary cell was taken, allowing SCNT that included the application of an electric shock for the purpose of simulating the effect of a sperm, causing the newly transferred nucleus to fuse with the enucleated egg cytoplasm that had come from a Scottish Blackface ewe. The newly reconstructed embryonic cell was then placed in the reproductive tract of another surrogate ewe (also a Scottish Blackface sheep). After 276 similar attempts, of which only one was successful, and another 148 days of pregnancy, Dolly the Finn Dorset sheep was born on July 5, 1995. She was named after the mammiferous country singer Dolly Parton. Dolly the sheep died on February 14, 2003, via euthanasia, after suffering from ovine pulmonary adenocarcinoma, a common sheep lung cancer caused by the jaagsiekte sheep retrovirus.

The birth and survival of Dolly as the first cloned mammal has sparked many ethical debates in recent years, especially with regard to human cloning. Many have feared that stem cell research may be used in a similar fashion as in the production of Dolly the sheep, where the implantation of stem cells within a surrogate mother is involved, to produce the birth of a living organism. The basis of this fear is that this type of research would allow the development of human clones while giving humans unprecedented control in the production or destruction of potential human life. However, therapeutic cloning has been strongly supported by many parties of the scientific community, as well as much of the American people, for research into the treatment of a wide variety of diseases, and not for human cloning. To address these issues in the United States, in 2001, President George W. Bush restricted federal funding for stem cell research to research using only the human embryonic stem cell lines derived before August 9, 2001. According to President Bush, for these stem cell lines, "the life and death decision has already been made." As of this article, this debate has not been resolved in the United States, nor have there been actual reports of human cloning.

## APPLICATIONS

Research conducted after Dolly's birth has shown promise. An extension of the successful cloning of Dolly the sheep were the sheep Polly and Molly. These two ewes were produced via SCNT combined with recombinant DNA technology. Before being transferred into an enucleated egg, the donor nucleus was transfected with an additional gene for factor IX, which is deficient in hemophilia B patients. As a result of this transfection, livestock milk could potentially serve as a source of factor IX, which hemophilia B patients would otherwise have to receive via human blood transfusions. Similar transgenic "pharm" animals have been genetically engineered to produce other important substances, including alpha antitrypsin, human albumin, and antithrombin. In recent years, trial studies of therapeutic cloning use have also shown promise in heart tissue regeneration, diabetes treatment, nerve tissue regeneration, bone cancer, and liver cancer.

A non–health-related application of SCNT is the preservation of endangered species, commonly using interspecies SCNT, in which the enucleated egg is frequently from a bovine source regardless of the nuclear donor species. Among the list of endangered animals are the gaur, bucardo, Chinese giant panda, Sumatran tiger, African bongo antelope, and mouflon sheep. Some successful attempts at preserving endangered species include Noah the cloned gaur (born in 2001) and two gray wolves in Korea (born in 2005). However, most animals produced through this route have not survived very long.

Stem cell research persists as a potential method of alleviating numerous health conditions. The ethical issues involved have allowed scientists to develop other possible techniques of stem cell research, in which the destruction of human life may not be involved. Altered nuclear transfer is a technique that may detour away from the issue of the loss of human life altogether and that now provides hope for the many proponents of stem cell research.

**SEE ALSO:** Clinical Trials (Adults); Cloning; Mammary Stem Cells; Nuclear Transfer, Altered; Stem Cells, Bush Ruling.

**BIBLIOGRAPHY.** American Medical Association, "Report 5 of the Council of Scientific Affairs (A-03)," www.ama-assn.org (cited November 2007); International Society for Stem Cell Research, "Stem Cell Science," www.isscr.org (cited November 2007); I. Wilmut, et al., "Somatic Cell Nuclear Transfer," *Nature* (v.419, 2002).

Susanna N. Chen
Western University of Health Sciences

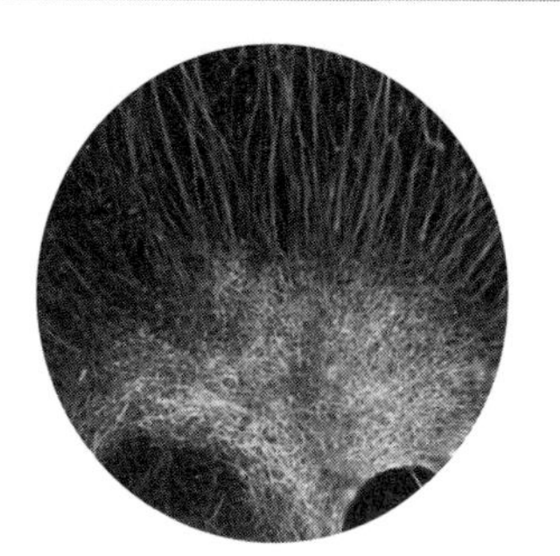

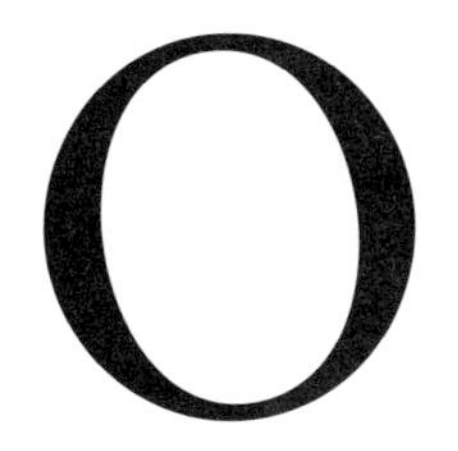

# Ohio

**OHIO CARRIES A** surprising history of stem cell and regenerative medicine research. Since 1980, it has managed to reconcile with its conservative nature by limiting research to nonembryonic cell lines, though current state legislation closely follows the views of President George W. Bush and forbids the use of embryonic or cadaveric fetal tissue for experimentation. With notable effort from former Governor Taft, the state has made even more headway with its recent development of the multi-institutional Center for Stem Cell and Regenerative Medicine.

State regulation regarding stem cell research was originally established in 1974 and has not been altered since then. Within the Ohio Revised Code, a single clause hidden in the depths of "Offenses against the Family" is used to carry the full weight of embryonic stem cell research legislation. Under section 2919.14(a), "No person shall experiment upon or sell the product of human conception which is aborted." Brief, yet succinct, this article is cited by the state to fully prohibit the use of any embryonic tissue with no stipulations for donations or excess embryos from in vitro fertilizations. Violation of this article is a misdemeanor of the first degree.

## STEM CELL RESEARCH

With §2919.14(a) being the only reference—albeit implied—to stem cell research, Ohio has become a thriving center devoted to regenerative medicine and adult stem cells. Home to multiple laudable academic institutions such as Case Western Reserve University (CWRU), the Ohio State University (OSU), the Cleveland Clinic Foundation (CCF), University Hospitals of Cleveland (UHC), University of Cincinnati, and Wright State University, Ohio is no stranger to biological research. Starting in 1980, oncologist Hillard M. Lazarus, M.D., treated a patient suffering from leukemia by performing the first Ohio bone marrow transplantation. Nine years later, Dr. Arnold Caplan and Dr. Stephen Haynesworth submitted and obtained patents for the use of mesenchymal stem cells in transplantation and gene therapy. They went on to found Osiris Therapeutics Inc., which is dedicated to developing treatments based on cells isolated from adult bone marrow.

Between 1996 and 2000, UHC experienced a boom in stem cell research, as it initiated three "first-in-the-nation" mesenchymal stem cell clinical trials and was also home to the first adult umbilical cord transplant, performed by Dr. Mary Laughlin. UHC was subsequently given a Stem

Cell Transplantation Center of Excellence award, in 2002, by the National Heart, Lung, and Blood Institute, and the National Cancer Institute, making it one of only 15 centers in the nation that participate in stem cell transplantation.

During that time, Ohio research found an ally in former Governor Robert Alphonso "Bob" Taft II, who was a strong proponent for expanding the boundaries of stem cell research during his two terms (1999–2007). Aside from his establishment of the "Third Frontier" program, his 2005 executive orders were a significant step for the stem cell legislation. Although they did ban the use of state funding to support embryonic tissue research and criminalized reproductive cloning (in keeping with federal laws), his orders placed no limitations on private initiatives for stem cell research. On the Ohio General Assembly's attempt to codify state policy on this matter, Taft vetoed a legislative ban on using state funds toward stem cell research, stating that it was too restrictive. With his support, Ohio was able to establish a statewide collaboration for stem cell exploration and regenerative medicine.

## CENTER FOR STEM CELL AND REGENERATIVE MEDICINE

Taft's greatest contribution to stem cell research in Ohio is his "Third Frontier" program. According to the former governor, Ohio's first and second frontiers were agriculture and manufacturing, respectively, and its third is to be knowledge and innovation. With approval from the state legislature, a $1.6 billion venture was formed to invest in research and technology and to create lucrative jobs. Of that money, $19.4 million went into a collaborative effort by researchers from CWRU, OSU, UHC, CCF, and Athersys Inc., to establish the Center for Stem Cell and Regenerative Medicine. The mission of the center was (and still is) to focus on combining the efforts of academia and industry to drive basic science research from "bench to bedside" to benefit patients suffering from disorders that can be cured by stem cell transplantation.

Since then, the center has received over $50 million in grants from the National Institutes of Health and the state of Ohio. The federal government has even seen fit to appropriate $4.5 million for the creation of the National Center of Regenerative Medicine in Ohio. To date, none of the grant money has been allowed to be used to study embryonic stem cells because of legislative restrictions, but there has been extensive investigation into adult stem cell possibilities. The center provides members of over 40 core facilities with access to nonembryonic multipotent progenitor cell types. These include adipose stem cells, mesenchymal stem cells, neural stem cells, and many others.

In the past five years, the center has seen incredible success in both the clinical and industrial worlds. With 27 ongoing U.S. Food and Drug Administration–approved clinical trials for the use of bone marrow stem cells toward treatments for disorders such as multiple myeloma, non-Hodgkin's lymphoma, chronic ischemia, and total coronary artery occlusion, the center provides an alternate hope for patients who are untreatable by existing methods.

Industry-wise, four new companies have been launched so far, based on work done by the center: Arteriocyte Inc., RegenRx Inc., Ohio BioGel, and Cell Targeting Inc. As joint ventures by individual institutional commercialization offices and BioEnterprise, these companies form a portion of the BioEnterprise Initiative. Arteriocyte Inc. is a research and development company focused on increasing blood flow via generation of new vasculature in ischemic diseases, whereas RegenRx Inc. directs its research toward increasing repair processes and restoration of function following a myocardial infarction. Ohio BioGel is a tissue-engineering corporation that develops organic scaffolds that encourage cartilage repair/replacement. Cell targeting develops biological markers that influence cell homing to increase the number of cells that successfully graft with target tissues.

With the success of these academic and industrial centers, Ohio has managed to avoid most of the controversy surrounding embryonic stem cells and has carried the momentum of its accomplished history forward to become a leader in regenerative medicine and nonembryonic stem cell research.

**SEE ALSO:** Case Western Reserve University; Federal Government Policies; National Institutes of Health.

**BIBLIOGRAPHY.** Center for Stem Cell and Regenerative Medicine, ora.ra.cwru.edu/stemcellcenter (cited October 2007); National Conference of State Legislatures, "State Embryonic and Fetal Research Laws," www.ncsl.org (cited September 2007); Ohio Revised Code, "Offenses against the Family," codes.ohio.gov/orc/2919 (cited September 2007).

PRISCILLA PANG
CASE WESTERN RESERVE UNIVERSITY

# Okano, Hideyuki

**HIDEYUKI OKANO IS** a Japanese scientist and currently one of the leaders in neural stem cell research. At present, he has an appointment as a professor in the Department of Physiology, Keio University School of Medicine, Japan. He graduated from the Keio University School of Medicine in 1983. He worked for Johns Hopkins University School of Medicine (1989–92), the Institute of Basic Medical Sciences in Tsukuba University, Japan (professor, 1994–97), and the Osaka University Graduate School of Medicine, Japan (professor, 1997–2001). Then he moved to Keio University in 2001.

Okano has published more than 180 scientific papers and given many lectures to audiences around the world. His writings can be found in publications such as *Cell*, *Science*, *Nature*, *Nature Medicine*, *Nature Neuroscience*, *Proceedings of the National Academy of Sciences*, *Journal of Neuroscience*, and *Stem Cells*. He has received lots of national and international awards including the *Stem Cells* Lead Reviewer Award from the journal *Stem Cells*. In addition, he has contributed to various journals as an editor, such as *Inflammation and Regeneration* (editor-in-chief, the official journal of the Japan Society of Inflammation and Regeneration), *Developmental Neuroscience*, *Gene to Cells*, *Stem Cells*, *Neuroscience Research*, and the *Journal of Neuroscience Research*. At present, he is a program member of the 21st Century Center of Excellence Program at the Graduate School of Medicine, Keio University, which is supported by the Japan Society of the Promotion of Science.

His current research interest is "development and regeneration of the central nervous system." He is studying the regulatory mechanisms of neural development and stem cell biology of the central nervous systems by focusing on development genetics of *Drosophila* and mammalian neural stem cells, the regulatory mechanism of mammalian brain development, the induction of particular neurons from embryonic stem cells, adult neurogenesis, and stem cell transplantation into the damaged brain and spinal cord. He is attempting to clarify the mechanism of formation of neurons and glia from the neural stem cells, with the goal of elucidating the basic mechanism of brain development and facilitating the development of new therapeutic strategies for the treatment of neurological diseases and injury.

Okano is noted for his serial studies about a neural RNA-binding protein *Musashi*, which has been broadly used as a specific marker for neural progenitor cells including neural stem cells in various organisms. In 1994 *Musashi* (MSI or Msi) was identified by a research group in the Johns Hopkins University School of Medicine (Makoto Nakamura, Hideyuki Okano, Julie A. Blendy, and Craig Montell) as the neural RNA-binding protein required for the asymmetric cell division of the sensory organ precursor cell of the *Drosophila melanogaster* adult external sensory organ. As the *Drosophila Musashi* mutant shows double bristle phenotype, the name *Musashi* was adapted, referring to a Japanese samurai warrior who lived about 400 years ago and originated a style of fighting that used two swords simultaneously, whereas typical samurai used only one sword.

The *Musashi* family is an evolutionarily conserved group of neural RNA-binding proteins that has representatives in *Drosophila, Caenorhabditis elegans*, *Halocynthia roretzi*, *Xenopus laevis*, mouse, and human. In mammals, the *Musashi* family is important for cell fate determination in the broader sense, playing roles in maintenance of the stem cell state, differentiation, and tumorigenesis. The mammalian homologue *Musashi1* is selectively expressed in neural progenitor cells, including neural stem cells. Outside the nervous system, *Musashi1* has also been recognized as a selective marker for intestinal stem or early lineage cells.

Recently, Okano published an interesting article in *Nature Medicine* showing that reactive astrocytes have a crucial role in wound healing and functional recovery, using mice with a selective deletion of the protein signal transducer and activator of transcription 3 (Stat3) or the protein suppressor of cytokine signaling 3 (Socs3), which is the negative feedback molecule of Stat3, under the control of the astrocyte-specific promoter-enhancer. Because the regenerative capability of the mammalian brain is poor, limited functional recovery occurs during the chronic phase of spinal cord injury. At the subacute phase of spinal cord injury, however, gradual functional recovery is observed to some extent in both rodents and humans (except in cases of complete paralysis). The mechanism behind this functional recovery remains unclear.

Okano used mice selectively deleted of Stat3 and Socs3 in astrocytes and demonstrated that the astrocytes with deleted Stat3 showed limited migration and resulted in markedly widespread infiltration of inflammatory cells, neural disruption, and demyelination, with severe motor deficits after contusive spinal cord injury. In contrast, rapid migration of reactive astrocytes to seclude inflammatory cells enhanced contraction of lesion area and made notable improvement in functional recovery in Soc3-knockdown mice. These results suggest that Stat3 is a key regulator of reactive astrocytes in the healing process after spinal cord injury, providing a potential target for intervention in the treatment of brain injury.

Okano also published another article in *Nature Medicine* showing that a natural product isolated from fungal fermentation promotes repair of injured spinal cords. Axons in the adult mammalian central nervous system exhibit little regeneration after injury, which has suggested that locally produced axonal growth inhibitors prevent central nervous system axonal regeneration. Semaphorin3A is a key inhibitor of axonal regeneration, and a small-molecule inhibitor of Semaphorin3A (SM-216289, isolated as a natural product from fungal fermentation), has been shown to promote brain repair in adult rats subjected to spinal cord transection. Treatment with a small-molecule inhibitor of Semaphorin3A caused increased regeneration of injured axons, Schwann cell–mediated myelination, enhanced angiogenesis, and decreased apoptotic cell death. These results suggested that Semaphorin3A is essential for the inhibition of axonal regeneration and may be able to be used for the treatment of spinal cord injury in humans.

**SEE ALSO:** Japan; Spinal Cord Injury.

**BIBLIOGRAPHY.** Martin Braddock, "Natural Product Promotes Repair of Injured Spinal Cord," *Expert Opinion* (v.6, 2007); Department of Physiology, Keio University School of Medicine, "Okano Lab Weblog," www.okano-lab.com (cited November 2007); Shinjiro Kaneko, et al., "A Selective Sema3A-Inhibitor Enhances Regenerative Responses and Functional Recovery of the Injured Spinal Cord," *Nature Medicine* (v.12/12, 2006); Keio University, "21st Century Center of Excellence (COE) Program, Basic Study and Clinical Application of Human Stem Cell Biology and Immunology: Approaches Based on the Development of Experimental Animal Models," www.coe-stemcell.keio.ac.jp (cited November 2007); Seiji Okada, et al., "Conditional Ablation of Stat3 or Socs3 Discloses a Dual Role for Reactive Astrocytes after Spinal Cord Injury," *Nature Medicine* (v.12/7, 2006).

Masatoshi Suzuki
University of Wisconsin, Madison

# Oklahoma

**EMBRYONIC STEM CELL** research is neither supported nor conducted in the state of Oklahoma. On July 18, 2006, both Oklahoma senators voted against a proposed bill (H.R.810) that would amend the Public Health Service Act to provide federal funding for research on human embryonic stem cells. These two Oklahoma senators were Tom Coburn and Jim Inhofe. The bill was nevertheless passed by the Senate but was later vetoed by President George W. Bush.

At Oklahoma University, coursework that touches on stem cell research typically uses the topic to generate discussions, rather than to teach about stem cell biology.

**SEE ALSO:** *Individual U.S. State Articles*; Biotechnology, History of; Clinical Trials Within U.S.: Batten Disease; Clinical Trials Within U.S.: Blind Process; Clinical Trials Within U.S.: Cancer; Clinical Trials Within U.S.: Heart Disease; Clinical Trials Within U.S.: Peripheral Vascular Disease; Clinical Trials Within U.S.: Skin Transplants (Burns); Clinical Trials Within U.S.: Spinal Cord Injury; Clinical Trials Within U.S.: Traumatic Brain Injury; Ethics; Federal Government Policies; Moral Status of Embryo; Special Interest/Lobby Groups; United States.

**BIBLIOGRAPHY.** M. Bellomo, *The Stem Cell Divide: The Facts, the Fiction, and the Fear Driving the Greatest Scientific, Political and Religious Debate of Our Time* (American Management Association, 2006); K. R. Monroe, R. Miller, and J. Tobis, eds., *Fundamentals of the Stem Cell Debate: The Scientific, Religious, Ethical, and Political Issues* (University of California Press, 2007); M. Ruse and C. A. Pynes, eds., *The Stem Cell Controversy: Debating the Issues (Contemporary Issues)* (Prometheus, 2006); C. Vestal, "States Take Sides on Stem Cell Research," www.stateline.org (cited January 2008).

Claudia Winograd
University of Illinois, Urbana-Champaign

# Oregon

**THE STATE OF** Oregon provides solid support of stem cell research. A chief site for stem cell research in Oregon is the Oregon Health & Science University (OHSU) in Portland. On the top floor of its Biomedical Research Building, the OHSU boasts its Oregon Stem Cell Center (OSCC). The mission of the OSCC is to conduct "basic and applied research in the field of stem cell biology with the long term goal to harness the properties of stem cells for regenerative medicine and cell therapy."

The OSCC was established on the first day of 2004 under the direction of Markus Grompe, M.D. It has three core labs directed by Philip Streeter, Ph.D. These core labs are for monoclonal antibody generation, cell sorting, and cell isolation; the purpose of these three core labs is to create specific, monoclonal antibodies for cell surface markers of individual tissue-type stem cells. These antibodies will aid in the sorting and isolation of specific stem cells that can then be engineered for therapeutic purposes. The OSCC has an advisory board, consisting of the OHSU vice president for research and three senior scientists at OHSU.

At the OSCC, Grompe's research focuses on pediatric diseases that can be treated with stem cell therapy, particularly metabolic liver diseases and Fanconi anemia, a DNA repair disease with recessive inheritance that can be caused by multiple mutations. Ultimately, Fanconi anemia leads to bone marrow failure and a propensity for squamous cell carcinoma. The risk of carcinoma remains even after successful blood stem cell transplantation therapy.

Streeter works to understand how to guide stem cells to differentiate into a particular tissue type. To begin these investigations, Streeter's laboratory team uses blood stem cells. To enhance the therapeutic potential of blood stem cell transplants against leukemia, the lab aims to induce a tumor-specific immune response in the patient before receipt of the stem cells, so as to create an environment in which the new, healthy cells can prosper.

The third faculty member at the OSCC is Soren Impey, Ph.D. Impey's lab investigates the molecular biology of stem cells and how genetic regulation affects a stem cell's differentiation, especially into neural cells. His work is supported by the National Institutes of Health.

The OSCC also has four affiliate faculty positions, held by William H. Fleming, M.D., Ph.D.; Brian Johnstone, Ph.D.; Shoukhrat Mitalipov, Ph.D.; and Melissa Hirose Wong, Ph.D. Fleming's laboratory focuses on factors involved in both blood stem cell differentiation and growth of new vasculature. This research could lead to novel therapeutics for blood vessel damage resulting from disease; in addition, as malignant tumors need angiogenesis to provide oxygen and nutrition, Fleming's work could lead to therapies that starve the tumor. Johnstone leads studies into the potential for mesenchymal stem cells to grow new cartilage in damaged joints and into harnessing the power of stem cells for tissue engineering.

Mitalipov is also the codirector of the Assisted Reproductive Technologies and Embryonic Stem Cell Core Laboratory at the Oregon National Primate Research Center of OHSU. His work therefore involves determining methods to guide the differentiation of human stem cells, using primates as a model organism.

As Wong's lab focuses on epithelial cell development, members also study the intestinal stem cell. Intestinal stem cells supply the constant turnover of cells lining the intestinal lumen; when damaged, severe intestinal problems ensue. Wong's team investigates the markers of intestinal stem cells in an effort to guide other stem cells into becoming new intestinal stem cells.

In July 2006, when the U.S. Senate convened to vote on a proposed bill (H.R.810) that would amend the Public Health Service Act and provide federal funding for research on human embryonic stem cells, both Oregon senators voted Yea. They were Republican Gordon Smith and Democrat Ron Wyden.

**SEE ALSO:** *Individual U.S. State Articles*; Biotechnology, History of; Clinical Trials Within U.S.: Batten Disease; Clinical Trials Within U.S.: Blind Process; Clinical Trials Within U.S.: Cancer; Clinical Trials Within U.S.: Heart Disease; Clinical Trials Within U.S.: Peripheral Vascular Disease; Clinical Trials Within U.S.: Skin Transplants (Burns); Clinical Trials Within U.S.: Spinal Cord Injury; Clinical Trials Within U.S.: Traumatic Brain Injury; Ethics; Federal Government Policies; Moral Status of Embryo; Special Interest/Lobby Groups; United States.

**BIBLIOGRAPHY.** M. Bellomo, *The Stem Cell Divide: The Facts, the Fiction, and the Fear Driving the Greatest Scientific, Political and Religious Debate of Our Time* (American Management Association, 2006); C. B. Cohen, *Renewing the Stuff of Life: Stem Cells, Ethics, and Public Policy* (Oxford University Press, 2007); C. Fox, *Cell of Cells: The Global Race to Capture and Control the Stem Cell* (Norton, 2007); K. R. Monroe, R. Miller, and J. Tobis, eds., *Fundamentals of the Stem Cell Debate: The Scientific, Religious, Ethical, and Political Issues* (University of California Press, 2007); M. Ruse and C. A. Pynes, eds., *The Stem Cell Controversy: Debating the Issues (Contemporary Issues)* (Prometheus, 2006).

Claudia Winograd
University of Illinois, Urbana-Champaign

# Oregon Health & Science University

**THE OREGON HEALTH** & Science University (OHSU) is a public university dedicated to healthcare and science research; most OHSU students are enrolled in graduate or professional degree programs or are engaged in postdoctoral studies. OHSU was formed in 1974 by combining the state dentistry, medicine, and nursing programs, and it adopted its current name in 2001 when it merged with the Oregon Graduate Institute of Science and Technology in Hillsboro, located 20 minutes from Portland. The main OHSU campus is in Portland, as are three hospitals affiliated with OHSU: the Oregon Health and Science University Hospital, the Doernbecher Children's Hospital, and the Portland Veterans Affairs Medical Center. A second OHSU campus, which is dedicated to graduate-level science and engineering education, is located in located in Hillsboro, the former location of the Oregon Graduate Institute of Science and Technology. In 2007 almost 2,000 students were enrolled in OHSU medical, dental, or nursing programs; almost 600 in science and engineering programs; and almost 200 in collaborative programs (primarily pharmacy). OHSU was also home to over 270 postdoctoral fellows, 590 interns and residents, and 120 clinical trainees.

## OREGON STEM CELL CENTER

The Oregon Stem Cell Center (OSCC), housed in the Biomedical Research Building on the OHSU medical campus in Portland, was created on January 1, 2004, to provide a hub for stem cell biology research at OHSU. Initial funding was provided by a three-year, $4.5 million grant from Oregon Opportunity, a $500 million fund supported by public and private dollars, which makes grants to promote biomedical and biosciences research. The focus of the OSCC, the first facility of its kind in the Pacific Northwest, is on adult stem cells and their use as therapies in human diseases, particularly diseases of the liver and pancreas. A priority of OSCC is rapid technology transfer from basic research in stem cell biology to preclinical trials in animal models, followed by human clinical trials.

The OSCC has three core laboratories, which also provide cell development and management services for research in other OSCC departments: a monoclonal antibody production core, a cell sorting core, and a cell isolation core. The center (as of 2007) was directed by Markus Grompe, M.D., professor in the departments of molecular and medical genetics and pediatrics at OHSU, and the core laboratories are directed by Philip Streeter, Ph.D., assistant professor in the Department of Medicine and a member of the OHSU Center for Hematologic Malignancies. The third faculty member affiliated with the OSCC is Soren Impey, Ph.D., assistant professor in the Department of Cell and Development Biology.

The OSCC intends to recruit three more faculty members over the next few years, with an emphasis on those who conduct basic research into stem cells, particularly nuclear reprogramming, cell fate plasticity, and stem cells of the lung, liver, pancreas, and intestine. In addition, four OHSU faculty members are currently affiliated with OSCC: William H. Fleming, M.D., Ph.D., associate professor of medicine; Brian Johnstone, Ph.D., adjunct professor in the Department of Orthopedics and Rehabilitation; Shoukhrat Mitalipov, Ph.D., assistant scientist and codirector of the Assisted Reproductive Technologies and Embryonic Stem Cell Core Laboratory at the Oregon National Primate Research Center (ONPRC); and Melissa Hirose Wong, Ph.D., assistant professor in the Department of Dermatology and assistant professor in the Department of Cell and Developmental Biology.

## OREGON NATIONAL PRIMATE RESEARCH CENTER

Stem cell research is also carried on at the ONPRC, in part because research on primate stem cells operates under fewer restrictions than research on human stem cells. ONPRC, which opened in 1962 and is today an institute of OHSU, is one of eight such centers supported by the National Institutes of Health. ONPRC is located on the OHSU West Campus in Beaverton, Oregon, about 12 miles west of downtown Portland, and is home to 60 doctoral-level scientists and 170 support and technical staff; many ONPRC scientists are also faculty members of the OHSU Medical School.

James Thomson, a former postdoctoral fellow at ONPRC, was the first person to isolate embryo stem cells from fertilized eggs in monkeys. Current ONPRC scientists use primate eggs fertilized in vitro to study cell differentiation and induce stem cells to become different types of mature cells. One advance in this field, made by ONPRC investigators Linda Lester, M.D.; Brian Nauert, Ph.D.; Don Wolf, Ph.D.; and Hung-Chih Kuo, Ph.D., was their success in inducing primate stem cells to become insulin-producing pancreatic cells in vitro; this breakthrough may ultimately lead to stem cell therapies for diabetes. Several ONPRC scientists, including Cynthia L. Bethea, Ph.D., are also part of international efforts to induce stem cells to become serotonin cells in vitro, which could lead to therapies for depression, and to induce stem cells to become dopamine-producing cells, which could be used to develop treatments for Parkinson's disease. Stem cell studies at the ONPRC are supported by the Assisted Reproductive Technologies and Embryonic Stem Cell Laboratory within ONPRC, which also provides services in stem cell biology and cell-based therapy for human diseases, as well as training in these fields, to scientists around the world.

The OSCC sponsors a seminar series throughout the year in which visiting scientists present the results of their research. A calendar of these events is available from the OSCC Web site. Basic information about stem cell research is also available from the OSCC Web site, as it has a collection of Web links to related sites.

**SEE ALSO:** Cells, Adult; Cells, Monkey; Non-Human Primate Embryonic Stem Cells; Oregon.

**BIBLIOGRAPHY.** "OHSU Primate Center Discovery Sheds Light into How Stem Cells Become Brain Cells," *Science Daily* (December 15, 2005); "OHSU Stem Cell Program Finds a Home," *Portland Business Journal* (March 23, 2004); Oregon Stem Cell Center, www.ohsu.edu/oscc (cited October 2007).

Sarah Boslaugh
BJC HealthCare

# Orkin, Stuart

**DR. STUART H. ORKIN** is the David G. Nathan Professor at the Department of Pediatrics at Harvard Medical School and is chairman of pediatric oncology at the Dana-Farber Cancer Institute at Harvard, as well as being investigator at the Department of Pediatrics at the Children's Hospital in Boston. There are currently 13 postdoctoral fellows, one graduate student, and one undergraduate working under Orkin at Harvard University.

Stuart H. Orkin was the younger son of Dr. Lazarus Allerton Orkin (1910–91) and Sylvia (née Holland). Lazarus Orkin was a graduate from New York University and former chief of urology at the Beth Israel Medical Center who taught at the Mount Sinai School of Medicine. He was also the author of *Trauma in the Ureter*, published in 1964, which became the standard work on the topic. Stuart Orkin decided to follow his father into medicine and gained his medical degree from Harvard University Medical School in 1971. After finishing his doctoral thesis, he then completed his postdoctoral research at the National Institutes of Health, working on clinical training in pediatrics and hematology and oncology at the Children's Hospital in Boston and the Dana Farber Cancer Institute.

Orkin was appointed a Howard Hughes Medical Institute investigator as well as being a member of the Institute of Medicine, the American Academy of Arts and Sciences, and the National Academy of Sciences. He has been a recipient of the Warren Alpert Foundation Prize and the Dameshek Award from the American Society of Hematology, as well as the 2005 Distinguished Research Award of the Association of American Medical Colleges. In 1998 he was the editor, with David G. Nathan, of the fifth edition of *Nathan and Oski's Hematology of Infancy and Childhood*, which was a revised edition of the work originally edited by Nathan and Frank A. Oski.

Orkin's research is in the area of stem cell biology. His research areas are in the development and function of the blood system, the relationship between cancer and stem cells, and the mechanisms responsible for self-renewal of stem cells. His laboratory studies gene regulation as it pertains to the properties and development of stem cells. This encompasses which gene is placed into a cell and which proteins control the formation and function of that cell's development, along with the gene into a particular type of cell.

Orkin's publications include "Gfi-1 Restricts Proliferation and Preserves Functional Integrity of Haematopoietic Stem Cells," coauthored with H. Hock, M. J. Hambleden, H. M. Rooke, J. W. Schindler, S. Saleque, and Y. Fujiwara, which was published in *Nature* in 2004; "The Placenta Is a Niche for Hematopoietic Stem Cells," coauthored with C. Gekas, F. Dieterlen-Lievre, and H. K.

Mikkola, and published in *Developmental Cell* in 2005; and "Developmental Stage-Selective Effect of Somatically Mutated Leukemogenic Transcription Factor GATA1," written with Z. Li, F. J. Godinho, J. H. Klusmann, M. Garriga-Canut, and C. Yu and published in *Nature Genetics* in 2005.

**SEE ALSO:** Cancer; Children's Hospital, Boston; Harvard University; Massachusetts.

**BIBLIOGRAPHY.** *American Men & Women of Science* (R. R. Bowker/Gale Group, 1994–2003); *Who's Who in Frontier Science and Technology. 1st ed., 1984–1985* (Marquis Who's Who, 1984); R. F. de Pooter, et al., "Notch Signaling Requires GATA-2 to Inhibit Myelopoiesis from Embryonic Stem Cells and Primary Hemopoietic Progenitors," *Journal of Immunology* (v.176/9, 2006); "Doctors Isolate a Human Gene, Allowing Birth-Defect Detection; Achievement Is Praised," *New York Times* (July 27, 1978); H. Hock, et al., "Tel/Etv6 Is an Essential and Selective Regulator of Adult Hematopoietic Stem Cell Survival," *Genes and Development* (v.18/19, 2004); Gina Kolata, "In the Rush Toward Gene Therapy—Some See a High Risk of Failure; the Field Is Driven by Nonmedical Concerns, Critics Say," *New York Times* (July 25, 1995); "Lazarus A. Orkin, Physician, 81," *New York Times* (July 26, 1991); Harold M. Schmeck, Jr., "The Promise of Gene Therapy: Gene Therapy," *New York Times* (November 10, 1985); Sheryl Gay Stolberg, "Panel Advises Resuming Gene Studies: U.S. Agency Halted Trials after Boy Fell Ill in French Experiment," *New York Times* (October 11, 2002); J. Wang, et al., "A Protein Interaction Network for Pluripotency of Embryonic Stem Cells," *Nature* (v.444, 2006).

Justin Corfield
Geelong Grammar School

# Osiris Therapeutics, Inc.

**OSIRIS THERAPEUTICS, INC.** (Osiris), is a private company founded to commercially develop therapeutic products using stem cells from adult bone marrow (mesenchymal stem cells, or MSCs), which have demonstrated the ability to repair various types of tissue within the human body and may be effective treatments for many diseases and conditions. Osiris uses proprietary stem cell technology to manufacture adult stem cells from donor marrow while maintaining their healthy, functioning state and preserving their multipotential characteristics (ability to give rise to other types of cells).

The management team for Osiris (as of October 2007) includes President and Chief Executive Officer C. Randal Mills, Ph.D.; Chief Operating Officer Harry E. Carmitchel, M.B.A.; Chief Financial Officer Carey J. Claiborne; and a five-member board of directors chaired by Peter Friedli. The lead investor in Osiris is Friedli Corporate Finance, a Swiss venture capital firm directed by Peter Friedli. Osiris has two facilities, in Baltimore, Maryland, and Columbia, Maryland, and is listed on the NASDAQ.

The roots of Osiris lie in the work of Dr. Arnold Caplan and colleagues from Case Western Reserve University in Cleveland, Ohio, who demonstrated that MSCs can engraft and selectively differentiate into different types of cells, depending on their tissue environment, and do not provoke an immune response, allowing the development and use of MSC products from unrelated donors. Osiris was founded in 1992 to develop the methodologies developed by Caplan to isolate and expand MSCs from donated bone marrow for therapeutic products; Caplan served as chief scientific officer of Osiris 1993–97.

The stem cells used at Osiris come from voluntary donations of bone marrow from healthy adults between the ages of 18 and 30 years who are screened and tested for transmissible diseases such as hepatitis and HIV.

The bone marrow is extracted from the donor by a physician, and samples are sent to Osiris, where they are tested for viability and appropriateness for Osiris products. Osiris technology for extracting and expanding MSCs from donor blood marrow is proprietary but can be described in general terms.

Less than 1 in 100,000 bone marrow cells is an MSC, so the first requirement in the Osiris process is to purify, isolate, and remove MSCs from the donor marrow. These MSCs are then expanded approximately 100-fold and harvested, packaged, and cryopreserved as an intermediate product. Following this, a second round of expansion on the intermediate product increases the cells by an additional 100-fold. Multiple levels of testing are used at each stage of this process to ensure quality and sterility, and all manufacturing is done in accordance with the Good Manufacturing Processes standards of the U.S. Food and Drug Administration (FDA).

MSC research at Osiris is organized into three main areas. In the autoimmune area, the focus is on providing support for bone marrow transplantation after chemotherapy or radiation to treat graft-versus-host disease (GVHD), a life-threatening complication that occurs in approximately 50 percent of all individuals receiving an allogenic hematopoietic stem cell transplant (i.e., when the transplanted cells are derived from another person). The focus of the cardiac program is on using MSCs to improve heart function following myocardial infarction (heart attack) and to prevent progression to congestive heart failure. The orthopedic applications area focuses on the use of MSCs to replace meniscal tissue after knee surgery, thus preventing arthritis of the knee from developing.

## PRODUCTS

Osiris currently has one product on the commercial market: Osteocel, a stem cell product used for the repair and replacement of bone. Osteocel provides several of the advantages of the procedure known as autograft, in which bone marrow is harvested from the individual who will receive it, without requiring the patient to submit to the discomfort and stress of that procedure. Stem cells contained in Osteocel are multipotential, meaning they can differentiate into different tissue types as needed, and have the major advantages of autograft: osteoconduction, osteoinduction, and osteogenesis.

Three Osiris products have completed or are currently being tested in FDA-approved clinical trials: Prochymal, Provacel, and Chondrogen. Prochymal is designated by the FDA as both an Orphan Drug and Fast-Track product and is being tested for two conditions: to prevent GVHD following allographic bone marrow transplants, and to treat Crohn's disease (regional enteritis). A phase 2 trial has been completed that tested the safety and efficacy of two dose levels of Prochymal in GVHD patients has been completed. Enrollment has been completed for a second phase 2 study to evaluate the safety and efficacy of Prochymal to prevent GVHD in persons aged from 6 months to 70 years who did not respond to steroids or at least one other therapy. A phase 2 trial testing the safety and efficacy of Prochymal to treat moderate-to-severe Crohn's disease has been completed, and results are available from the Osiris Web site; a phase 3 trial to evaluate Prochymal in treating Crohn's disease is currently enrolling patients.

A phase 1 clinical trial has been completed that tested the safety of Provacel, an MSC product designed to repair damaged heart tissue and administered through a standard intravenous line. Results of this trial, which enrolled 53 patients aged 21 to 85 years who had experienced their first heart attack no more than seven days previously and were in overall good health are available from the Osiris Web site.

A phase 1/2 clinical trial has been completed to test the safety and efficacy of Chondrogen, an MSC product that is injected into the knee of patients shortly after surgery for knee injury. The trial enrolled 55 patients between the ages of 18 and 60 years; all required surgery to remove meniscal tears or degeneration but were otherwise healthy and had no significant articular cartilage damage or degeneration.

Osiris has formed a partnership with Genzyme Corporation to develop Prochymal as a treatment for acute radiation sickness, a potential hazard of nuclear or radiological terrorism and other radiation emergencies that involve damage to DNA primarily in the gastrointestinal tract, skin, and bone marrow. Osiris has also formed a partnership with JCR Pharmaceutical Corporation to produce Prochymal in Japan, if and when it becomes commercially available, and has partnered with Boston Scientific Corporation to develop Provacel.

**SEE ALSO:** Clinical Trials (Adult Cells); Clinical Trials Within U.S.: Blind Process; Clinical Trials Within U.S.: Heart Disease; Maryland.

**BIBLIOGRAPHY.** S. Aggawar and M. F. Pittenger, "Human Mesenchymal Stem Cells Modulate Allogeneic Immune Cell Responses," *Blood* (v.105/4, 2004); Osiris Therapeutics Inc., www.osiristx.com (cited October 2007); M. F. Pittenger and B. J. Martin, "Mesenchymal Stem Cells and Their Potential as Cardiac Therapeutics," *Circulation Research* (v.95/1, 2004); Nicholas Wade, "Discovery Bolsters a Hope for Regeneration," *New York Times* (April 2, 1999).

Sarah Boslaugh
BJC HealthCare

# Ottawa Health Research Institute

**THE OTTAWA RESEARCH INSTITUTE** (OHRI)/ Institut de recherche en santé d'Ottawa is the research arm of the Ottawa Hospital and an affiliated research institute of the University of Ottawa. OHRI is a not-for-profit corporation, the purpose of which is to promote excellence in research, education, and innovation in healthcare. It is governed by a board of directors, which includes representatives from the Ottawa Hospital, Ottawa University, the Hospital Foundation, and the community. The board chair of OHRI as of 2007 was Jacquelin Holzman, and the chief executive officer and scientific director was Dr. Duncan Stewart. In 2007, OHRI employed over 1,350 staff members, received almost $80 million in funding (including $67.1 million in external grants), and had thousands of patients enrolled in clinical trials.

## MISSION

There are three facets to the OHRI mission: research, education, and patient care. Research at OHRI is aimed at the prevention, diagnosis, and treatment of disease, including basic, translation, clinical, population, and health services research. Education at OHRI includes teaching students at both the undergraduate and graduate levels, as well as training clinical research and postdoctoral research fellows.

Over 250 postdoctoral fellows and graduate students (pursuing a doctoral or Master's of Science degree) were working at OHRI as of 2007, and there are also programs for summer students and honors students. In addition, OHRI has several ongoing seminar programs, and additional seminars are offered through the University of Ottawa. The institute also disseminates information through news releases and its Web site. Innovation in patient care is the third focus of OHRI: this includes the development and testing of new therapeutic approaches and innovations in healthcare delivery.

OHRI is also committed to increasing the effect of basic research through technology transfer, and the OHRI Technology Transfer and Business Development Office was established to further this goal. The office works with OHRI researchers, companies, government departments, and other research institutes on issues such as licensing, investment, collaboration, and partnerships; information about intellectual property and the patenting process is available from the OHRI Web site.

## CORE RESEARCH PROGRAMS

OHRI has six core research programs: cancer therapeutics, chronic disease, clinical epidemiology, neuroscience, regenerative medicine, and vision. Stem cell research is involved in several of these areas; for instance, cancer stem cells and bone marrow stem cell transplantation are areas of research within the Cancer Therapeutics Program, the use of gene and stem cell therapy for retinal disease is studied within the Vision Program, and the use of transplanted neural stem cells in functional recovery is studied within the Neuroscience Program.

Stem cell research is also a central focus of some of the research on Parkinson's disease conducted with the Neuroscience Program, and OHRI spearheaded the foundation in 2004 of the Parkinson's Research Consortium, a collaboration among 11 Ottawa scientists engaged in the study of Parkinson's disease.

However, stem cell research is most central to the area of regenerative medicine, an emerging field that studies the repair and replacement of damaged cells and tissues. As of 2006, OHRI had 11 core scientists and a further 25 scientists and investigators working in the Regenerative Medicine Program; their fields include stem cell biology, molecular genetics and molecular biology, and applied sciences such as tissue engineering and transplantation. StemBase, the largest stem cell gene expression database in the world, was developed within the Regenerative Medicine Program under the direction of the bioinformatics expert Dr. Miguel Andrade. It contains data from samples accepted into the Stem Cell Genomics Project and may be accessed (after free registration) through the Internet. An online microarray analysis course, intended to aid researchers in using StemBase, is also freely available on the Internet.

Stem cell research at OHRI is centered within the Sprott Centre for Stem Cell Research, which officially opened in November 2006 with the goal of ensuring that Canadian scientists remain at the forefront of the field of stem cell research, which is a rapidly growing field within medicine. The vision for the Sprott Centre came from Dr. Ronald Worton of the OHRI, who worked in the Toronto labs, where stem cells were first discovered in the 1960s, and who led the team that discovered the gene responsible for Duchenne muscular dystrophy in 1986.

The Sprott Centre serves as the hub for a large group of stem cell and interdisciplinary medicine researchers at the OHRI, some of whom also hold appointments at the University of Ottawa or at the Ottawa Hospital; eventually, the center will house over 120 researchers and staff members. The center is named for Eric and Vizma Sprott, who donated $7 million toward the creation of a permanent endowment fund for scientific research. An additional $17.4 million in funding came from the Canada Foundation for Innovation, the Ontario Innovation Trust, the Kresge Foundation, the Ontario Research and Development Challenge Fund, Genome Canada, the Canadian Institutes of Health Research, and the Stem Cell Network.

The director (as of 2007) of the Sprott Centre was Dr. Michael Rudnicki, a professor of medicine at the University of Ottawa and a senior scientist at the center. His laboratory's research is focused on understanding the molecular mechanisms that regulate the determination, proliferation, and differentiation of stem cells during embryonic development and tissue regeneration, and he led the research team that discovered adult muscle stem cells. Rudnicki also leads the International Regulome Consortium and Canada's Stem Cell Network.

The International Regulome Consortium aims to discover how gene function is regulated in mammalian cells during development, knowledge of which will allow a new paradigm of medicine centered on the regeneration of diseased and dysfunctional tissues.

The Stem Cell Network, established in 2001, is a nonprofit corporation that serves as a catalyst for the translation of stem cell research into clinical applications, commercial products, and public policy and that also supports training the next generation of translational leaders and building capacity to further stem cell research and to transfer that knowledge to therapeutic care.

**SEE ALSO:** Canada; Canadian Stem Cell Network.

**BIBLIOGRAPHY.** The International Regulome Consortium, www.internationalregulomeconsortium.ca (cited October 2007); Ottawa Health Research Institute, www.ohri.ca (cited October 2007); StemBase, www.stembase.ca (cited October 2007).

Sarah Boslaugh
BJC HealthCare

# Oxford University

**THE UNIVERSITY OF OXFORD**, also known as Oxford University, is located in Oxford, England. It is the oldest English-speaking university, having records dating to the 13th century. The university is composed of 39 colleges and seven permanent private halls. Research on stem cell science is carried out within the scientific theme of Developmental and Stem Cell Biology within the Division of Medical Sciences (DMS), as well as the Sir William Dunn School of Pathology, a department within the DMS.

The DMS is the largest of Oxford's four academic divisions; the other three divisions are humanities; mathematical, physical, and life sciences; and social sciences. Within the DMS, there are numerous departments tailored to specific fields of the medical sciences. Additionally, there are research themes, including that of Developmental and Stem Cell Biology. Within other research themes, some scientific laboratories do carry out work related to stem cells and stem cell biology; however, the majority of the work on stem cells is carried out in the Dunn School of Pathology.

Spanning the research areas of immunology, cell biology and pathology, molecular biology, and molecular microbiology, scientists at the Dunn School work to understand genetic and other molecular mechanisms behind cell division and proliferation, including DNA replication, RNA transcription, and protein translation. Even when a particular laboratory does not focus directly on stem cells, the knowledge gained may be pivotal to understanding the maintenance, proliferation, and differentiation of stem cells. Some labs do work directly with stem cells; for example, Professor Paul Fairchild at the Dunn School is working to understand the immunological barriers to stem cell transplantation. Donated stem cells may be rejected by the immune system of the recipient; the Fairchild group works to avoid that rejection.

Especially considering that the United States has strict restrictions on public funding for stem cell research, the United Kingdom is taking advantage of its position to become a leader in international stem cell research. For this reason, Oxford University is actively seeking research fellows with expertise in stem cell biology. In 2005 Dr. Kenneth Fleming stated that key research areas for future fellows would include stem cell biology. In 2006 the Research Plan announced by the DMS included stem cell biology as a priority as well. Additionally, the ethics of stem cell biology are discussed in campus classes as well as at special events focusing on current scientific issues.

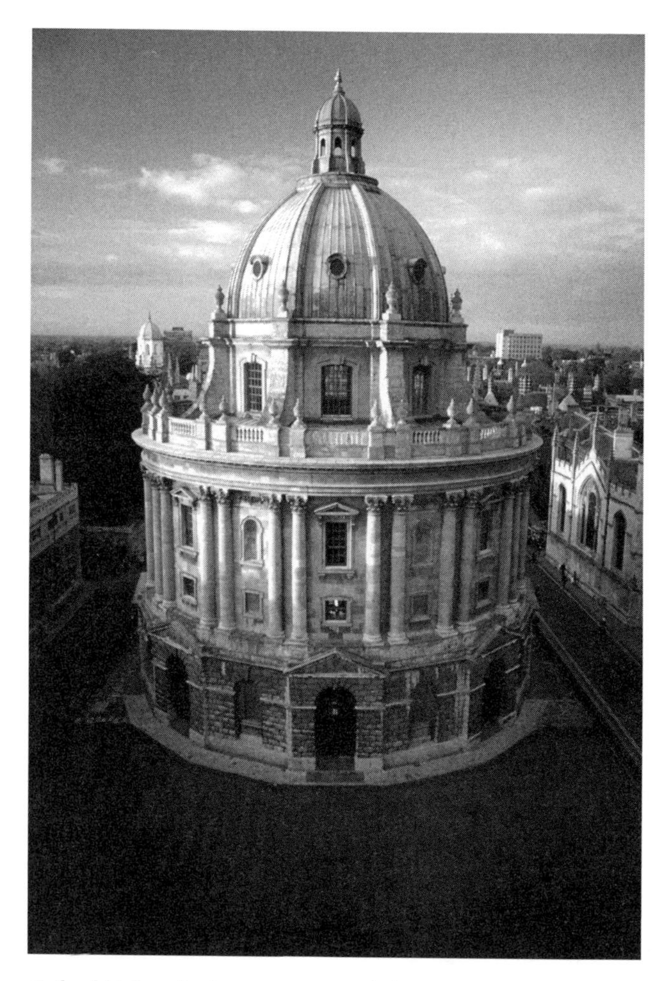

*Oxford University, home to some of the world's great libraries, like the Bodleian, is making stem cell research a priority.*

**SEE ALSO:** Cambridge University; European Consortium for Stem Cell Research—EuroStemCell; Human Embryonic Stem Cells; UK National Stem Cell Network; United Kingdom; University of Edinburgh.

**BIBLIOGRAPHY.** M. Bellomo, *The Stem Cell Divide: The Facts, the Fiction, and the Fear Driving the Greatest Scientific, Political and Religious Debate of Our Time* (AMACOM/American Management Association, 2006); C. B. Cohen, *Renewing the Stuff of Life: Stem Cells, Ethics, and Public Policy* (Oxford University Press, 2007); C. Fox, *Cell of Cells: The Global Race to Capture and Control the Stem Cell* (Norton, 2007); K. R. Monroe, R. Miller, and J. Tobis, eds., *Fundamentals of the Stem Cell Debate: The Scientific, Religious, Ethical, and Political Issues* (University of California Press, 2007).

Claudia Winograd
University of Illinois, Urbana-Champaign

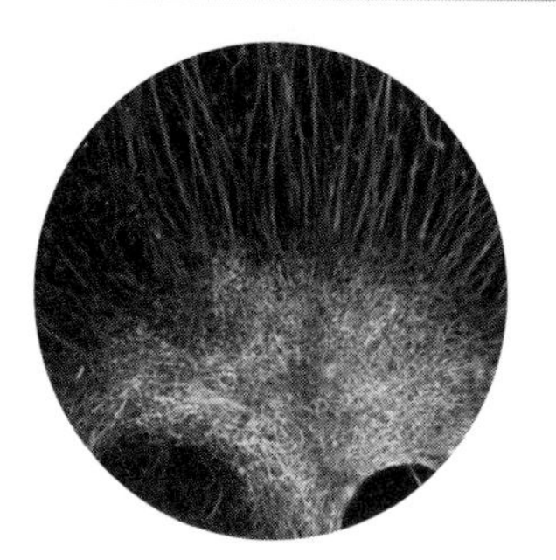

# P

## Pancreas

**THE PANCREAS IS** a small organ in the abdomen that produces and secretes substances to aid digestion, as well as hormones that regulate the balance of blood sugar (glucose) levels. Recently, scientists have begun to characterize the stem cell population in the pancreas, but little is yet understood. A common disease associated with the pancreas is diabetes mellitus type I (DMI), an autoimmune disorder where a person's immune system attacks and destroys his or her own pancreatic islet cells, which produce and secrete insulin.

Pancreatic secretions are categorized as exocrine and endocrine. Exocrine secretions are released into ducts that connect to other organs, while endocrine secretions are hormonal and enter the bloodstream directly. The pancreas secretes the enzymes trypsin and chymotrypsin via ducts into the small intestine to aid in protein digestion, as well as pancreatic amylase for starch breakdown and pancreatic lipase for fat digestion. In addition, the pancreas secretes important hormones including glucagon and insulin. Glucagon and insulin have counteractive effects on blood sugar—glucagon stimulates the breakdown of sugar stores in the liver, raising blood sugar; in contrast, insulin stimulates cells to take up glucose, thus lowering blood sugar levels. Further hormones released by the pancreas are gastrin, somatostatin, and pancreatic polypeptide which act on additional organs. Therefore, the pancreas and its secretions affect multiple organ systems.

As with other organs, the pancreas has specific cancers. Pancreatic cancer falls into two main categories. The first type is an adenocarcinoma, or cancer of the epithelial cells. Epithelial cells line the body, both on the outside with skin, and inside such as the lining of the gastrointestinal tract and blood vessels. Adenocarcinomas are the majority of pancreatic cancers. For these cancers, the prognosis is poor. The minority of pancreatic cancers are in other cells such as the  cells that produce insulin. These cancers generally have a better prognosis than adenocarcinomas.

A pancreatic disease with a potential stem cell-related cure is DMI. DMI has also been called juvenile onset diabetes, although this term is misleading because diabetes mellitus type II, also known as insulin-resistant diabetes, and sometimes adult onset diabetes, can also manifest in childhood. The result of both types of diabetes is an inability to control the levels of the sugar glucose in the blood, which can lead to devastating medical consequences. People with DMI have to take insulin shots several times daily; few people are able to have full pancreas transplants and in the case of a transplant 83 percent no longer need to take insulin. Although this transplant success rate is high, the availability of transplants is low compared to the prevalence of DMI. Given that only one cell type in the pancreas is affected in DMI, scientists believe it is possible to replace that cell type with stem cells and thereby cure DMI without the need for a full pancreatic transplant.

The first step is a better understanding of this cell type and how embryonic stem cells differentiate into cells. If researchers can determine the factors that induce development of the cells in an embryo, perhaps they can guide the differentiation of an embryonic stem cell into a pancreatic cell.

The cells are found in regions of the pancreas called islets of Langerhans; some evidence shows that perhaps the entire islets, which consist of glucagon-producing cells and insulin-producing cells, must be replaced and not only the cells, in order to provide an optimal insulin response to rising blood glucose.

Recently, a lab at the National Institute of Neurological Disorders and Stroke was able to isolate embryonic stem cells from a murine blastocyst, or embryo of approximately 80 cells. These stem cells were allowed to differentiate into pancreatic islet cells through a series of intricate cell culture steps.

Finally, they were introduced into a diabetic mouse where they continued to produce insulin. The success of this experiment, led by Dr. Ron McKay, brings hope that one day such transplants may be available for humans.

**SEE ALSO:** Cancer; Cells, Embryonic; Diabetes; Differentiation, In Vitro and In Vivo; Germ Layers (Mesoderm, Ectoderm, Endoderm); Gut Stem Cells; Liver.

**BIBLIOGRAPHY.** H. G. Beger, et al., *The Pancreas: An Integrated Textbook of Basic Science, Medicine and Surgery* (Wiley-Blackwell, 2008); H. G. Beger, S. Matsuno, and J. L. Cameron, *Diseases of the Pancreas: Current Surgical Therapy* (Springer, 2008); D. LeRoith, J. M. Olefsky, and S. I. Taylor, *Diabetes Mellitus: A Fundamental and Clinical Text* (Lippincott Williams & Wilkins, 2003); N. Lumelsky, et al., "Differentiation of Embryonic Stem Cells to Insulin-Secreting Structures Similar to Pancreatic Islets," *Science* (May 18, 2001); National Institutes of Health, Information on Diabetes and Stem Cells, http://stemcells.nih.gov/info/scireport/chapter7.asp (cited May 2008).

Claudia Winograd
University of Illinois, Urbana-Champaign

# Parkinson's Disease

**PARKINSON'S DISEASE (PD)** first described by James Parkinson in 1817, is a disorder of the central nervous system (CNS). It is marked by the presence of Lewy bodies (abnormal protein aggregates) and, more importantly, by a progressive loss of dopamine-producing neurons in the substantia nigra region of the brain. Although uncommon in people under age 40 years, the incidence of PD greatly increases with age, affecting approximately 1 percent of individuals older than 60 years.

As of yet, PD is incurable, and current therapies focus only on alleviating symptoms rather than on treating the underlying disease. However, because of the nature of its development, PD is a prime beneficiary candidate of stem cell research.

Traditionally, PD has been regarded as a motor system disorder, with four cardinal characteristics: resting tremor, muscular rigidity, bradykinesia (abnormally slow movements and difficulty initiating motion), and postural instability. Although nonmotor manifestations such as dementia and face recognition impairment are strongly associated with PD, diagnosis requires presence of these motor deficiencies.

## PATHOPHYSIOLOGY

It is believed that PD arises from a partial genetic predisposition, as it is more common in Caucasians than in Africans or Asians. This is supported by evidence that links the development of Parkinson's dementia with alterations in chromosome 4 at the gene that codes for the protein, alpha-synuclein.

Little is known about this protein, but major theories hold that overproduction or mutations of alpha-synuclein makes it more liable to gather into fiber clusters, forming Lewy bodies that are potentially toxic. These protein aggregations are also seen with dementia arising from other disorders such as Alzheimer's disease or diffuse Lewy body disease.

However, the change that appears to be most responsible for PD-induced motor deficits in patients is the deterioration of dopamine-producing neurons within the substantia nigra region of the brain. Insufficient amounts of dopamine, a chemical messenger of the CNS, results in diminished activation of the striatum—the control center for planning and modulation of movement. This causes problems with motor coordination. Research has shown that 70–80 percent of these neurons are lost before motor symptoms appear. In patients with PD, 9–13 percent of dopamine-producing neurons are lost every decade of life for reasons unknown, bringing the average age of diagnosis to 70.5 years.

## CURRENT THERAPIES

Because current therapies are still unable to halt the continual decline of dopamine-producing neurons, treatment methods focus on symptom improvement. The most common and effective approach is with oral administration of levodopa (or L-DOPA), an intermediate in dopamine synthesis. After L-DOPA crosses the blood–brain barrier (which dopamine cannot), it is converted to supplement the preexisting dopamine of the substantia nigra and putamen. Unfortunately, chronic administration, especially with higher doses, causes most patients to develop motor complications including dyskinesia (involuntary movements) and motor fluctuations. As a consequence, this renders levodopa an inappropriate agent for long-term treatment.

As other therapies similarly lose their efficacy, the need for a cure has opened the door to nonpharmacological remedies, including stem cell research. Of all advancements that have been made in potential treatments of PD, cell transplantation is the course that has shown the most promise of full recovery and restoration of functional capacity.

## CELL REPLACEMENT THERAPY

Because Parkinson's is cause by a relatively simple neuron deficit, stem cell research has been targeted toward cell replacement therapy. Under the basic principle of restoring dopamine-producing neurons via neural grafts, extensive studies have been done to bring this to fruition.

In 1987, after experiments with rodent and primate models showed that neural grafts could reinnervate the substantia nigra and striatum, clinical trials were initiated to see whether transplantation would be successful in the human brain. Approximately 350 patients received implants of tissue from human fetal mesencephalon, which contains an abundant amount of primary dopamine neurons. At the time, little was known about the viability of the neurons, the outcomes, and the problems associated with the usage of grafted neurons; 20 years later, answers are just now beginning to appear.

With the most successful cases, neuronal implants have shown survival of at least 10 years postoperation with little or no immunological rejection. Fortunate patients have even been able to withdraw from L-DOPA. For these patients, the integrated grafts have restored dopamine uptake levels as well as striatal activation and regulation, despite an ongoing disease process.

The functional integration of dopamine neuron grafts prove the efficacy of the cell replacement principle, but in reality, this clinical outcome is extremely inconsistent with respect to the percentage of cells that survive the grafting procedure and the amount of dopamine produced by the new neurons. In fact, average functional improvement of patients in the experiments only rises about 20 percent. Across the board, subjects achieve functioning levels less than or equal to that of patients undergoing deep brain stimulation, which carries a lower morbidity risk. To develop a practical, clinically competitive treatment, several issues are being addressed.

### GRAFT STANDARDIZATION

Grafting methods for the past 20 years have differed in everything from procurement process to tissue composition to implantation technique. To add even more variability, multiple donors are needed to create a graft large enough to carry some promise of efficacy. This, undoubtedly, plays an important role in determining survival, growth, and integration of the transplant. It is the hope of stem cell research that by inducing pluripotent cells to differentiate into dopaminergic neurons, dependency on existing (and oftentimes controversial) fetal tissue can be avoided. As stem cells can theoretically provide an endless source of quality-consistent neurons, standardization of the transplant tissue will enhance the reliability of the procedure and its results.

One promising study has shown that implantation of undifferentiated human neural stem cells (hNSCs) in Parkinsonian primate brains can restore functionality. Furthermore, the repair process not only reestablishes the gross anatomical structure of the organ but does so with appropriate proportions of neuron types. Guided by signals of the microenvironment of the damaged brain, uncommitted hNSCs are induced to differentiate into dopaminergic neurons, as well as other cells that mediate neuroprotection. As an interesting side note, hNSCs have also demonstrated a capacity to normalize alpha-synuclein aggregations, though the mechanism by which it does so remains unclear.

### PATIENT STANDARDIZATION

With standardization of transplant material, patients must likewise be evaluated for variables in their presentation of the disease. Specifically, the distribution of the damaged neurons should be taken into account before and after graft implantation. In earlier studies, patient selections overlooked the preoperative magnitude of the lesions, making it difficult to evaluate the extent of the graft incorporation. Similarly, it was also unknown whether continued postoperative degeneration of nongrafted regions would affect clinical response.

A review in 2005 investigated the dopamine uptake levels in pre- and postoperative graft and nongraft sites and concluded that patients experienced the worst functional outcome when there was a continued decrease in dopamine uptake in the ventral striatum (indicating progressive loss of dopaminergic neurons). Conversely, patients with little or no postoperative damage showed the best functional outcome.

Because the decline of dopaminergic cells in areas outside the nigrostriatal region seems to arise as PD progresses to a more severe state, it may be that implantation during earlier stages will exhibit a higher rate of success. This is mirrored in the survival of transplanted tissue, which survives and integrates better in younger patients. The reasons why this occurs have yet to be fully determined, but it is known that neural growth factors are expressed more in younger brains. Moreover, the older brain may simply respond less to an otherwise normal graft.

### GRAFT-INDUCED DYSKINESIAS

Progressive postoperative loss of dopaminergic neurons can also lead to graft-induced dyskinesias (GID). At the other extreme, overgrowth of the implant can also result in GID. In light of this, dyskinesias are thought to be caused by abnormal dopamine regulation that could potentially arise from an unsuitable graft composition with respect to the recipient tissue.

### IMMUNOSUPPRESSION THERAPY

The protocol for using immunosuppressants after implantation is undefined, as the brain is an immunologically privileged site with little intrinsic reactivity to foreign antigens. As such, patients can withdraw from immunosuppression therapy two to three years after transplantation, while the graft retains the ability to proliferate and integrate with the patient's tissue. In fact, elimination of immunosuppressants results in increased proliferation and dopamine uptake in the grafted regions. Not too surprisingly, the incidence of GIDs also increases in patients who have been taken off immunosuppression therapy. This is attributed to a potential dysregulation of dopamine production or uptake. An alternative hypothesis for the increase in GIDs is that discontinued immunosuppression paves the way for low-grade opportunistic inflammatory responses, which can manifest as dyskinesia.

## FUTURE DIRECTION OF RESEARCH

Supported by celebrities such as Muhammad Ali and Michael J. Fox, PD research has been given a great push in recent times. Though much has been elucidated regarding the mechanisms of a clinically successful transplantation treatment, cell replacement therapy must still contend with several issues. First, the implantation procedure must be tailored to each individual patient in terms of graft composition and severity of disease. Second, the use of uncommitted hNSCs must be studied under long-term conditions, with especial attention paid to potential side effects. Finally, the mechanisms of GIDs must be clarified and neutralized. If these matters can be solved, then there exists the very real possibility of an effective restoration of function to patients suffering from PD.

**SEE ALSO:** Michael J. Fox Foundation; Parkinson's Disease Foundation.

**BIBLIOGRAPHY.** Anders Bjorklund and Olle Lindvall, "Cell Therapy in Parkinson's Disease," *The American Society for Experimental NeuroTherapeutics* (v. 1/4, 2004); Yahya Choonara, Viness Pillay, and Neha Singh, "Advances in the Treatment of Parkinson's Disease," *Progress in Neurobiology* (v.81/1, 2007); Robert Hauser, "Parkinson Disease," www.emedicine.com/neuro/topic304.html (cited September 2007); Paula Piccini, et al., "Factors Affecting the Clinical Outcome after Neural Transplantation in Parkinson's Disease," *Brain* (v.128, 2006); D. Eugene Redmond Jr., et al., "Behavioral Improvement in a Primate Parkinson's Model Is Associated with Multiple Homeostatic Effects of Human Neural Stem Cells," *Proceedings of the National Academy of Sciences* (v.104/29, 2007).

Priscilla Pang
Case Western Reserve University

# Parkinson's Disease Foundation

**THE PARKINSON'S DISEASE** Foundation (PDF), founded in New York City in 1957, is a tax-exempt, charitable organization that supports research, education, and advocacy related to Parkinson's disease, a chronic and progressive disease that afflicts approximately 1 million Americans. The PDF annual budget is over $9 million, and the organization has corresponding relationships with over 100,000 members of the Parkinson's community.

PDF was founded by William Black, founder of the Chock Full o' Nuts Corporation; Black's immediate motivation was the plight of a business associate who was diagnosed with Parkinson's disease and found that there was little education or assistance available to help patients cope with the disease. PDF was originally located at the Columbia University Medical Center in New York City, where Black made major gifts to build a research building and to fund an endowment to support research. PDF today maintains a close relationship with Columbia but has expanded its activities nationally, and in 1999, it merged with the United Parkinson Foundation, an organization based in Chicago. Today, the head PDF office is in New York City, with a regional office in Chicago.

Since its founding in 1957, PDF has funded almost $70 million in research projects related to Parkinson's disease. Major ongoing center grants are provided to support multiyear research programs at the Columbia University Medical Center and the Cornell-Weill Medical Center, both in New York City, and the Rush University Medical Center in Chicago. Other research funds are disbursed through the International Grants Research

Program, which offers one-year grants to young scientists to allow them to collect baseline data required to apply for funding from governmental agencies such as the National Institutes of Health. Information and application materials for the International Grants Research program are available on the PDF Web site. PDF also funds postdoctoral programs and summer fellowships for students and recent graduates interested in studying Parkinson's disease.

PDF is governed by a board of directors with six officers and 17 directors. As of 2007, the chairman is Page Morton Black, widow of William Black; other officers include Scientific Director Stanley Fahn, M.D.; President Lewis P. Rowland, M.D.; and 17 other members of the board. A five-member scientific advisory conducts periodic reviews of research conducted at the research centers at Columbia University Medical Center, Cornell-Weill Medical Center, and Rush University Medical Center

PDF led the campaign to found Advancing Parkinson's Therapies (APT), an umbrella effort by PDF, the American Parkinson Disease Association, the Parkinson's Action Network, the Parkinsonian Alliance, the Michael J. Fox Foundation for Parkinson's Research, the National Parkinson Foundation, and WE MOVE (an international organization devoted to education and information dissemination regarding movement disorders). The goal of APT is to increase participation in clinical trials related to Parkinson's disease through greater public awareness: They publish a brochure twice yearly that contains information about open trials, and they maintain a Web site (www.pdtrails.org) that includes a continuously updated list of trials open for enrollment.

A major function of PDF is disseminating information about Parkinson's disease to patients and their families, healthcare providers, and the general public. The PDF Web site (www.pdf.org) is a readily accessible source of information and provides access to issues of the PDF quarterly newsletter and other educational publications about Parkinson's disease. Information about Parkinson's disease is also available through a toll-free telephone advice line (1-800-457-6676), staffed by healthcare workers and medical professionals, as well as the e-mail-based information service "Ask the Expert," accessible through the PDF Web site. Further educational efforts are conducted through the PDF annual symposiums; the 50th such symposium was held in New York City in October 2007, jointly sponsored with the Movement Disorder Society. The symposium program and a Webcast of the proceedings are available from the PDF Web site. PDF also sponsored the first-ever World Parkinson Congress in 2004, which brought together patients, caregivers, scientists, physicians, and other healthcare professionals in an effort to create a worldwide dialogue leading to improved treatment, prevention, and cure of Parkinson's disease.

PDF also acts as an advocate for patients with Parkinson's and their families, as well as scientists conducting research related to Parkinson's, and it is a major supporter of the Parkinson's Action Network, which acts as a public policy voice for the Parkinson's community. PDF also provides information and interpretation of scientific discoveries to the general news media, such as newspapers, television, and magazines.

Stem cell research is a recent and promising line of scientific inquiry for treating Parkinson's disease, and PDF has taken a leadership role in the promotion of studies involving stem cells. PDF was among the first organizations to become involved in New Yorkers for the Advancement of Medical Research (NYAMR), a coalition of 46 citizen's and patient's groups, university research centers, and biotech industry leaders formed in 2003 who advocate for state legislation supporting scientific research involving embryonic stem cells and other DNA therapies.

NYAMR has been successful in promoting the importance of stem cell research funding in the New York State legislature: In 2007, an appropriation of over $100 million for stem cell and regenerative medicine research funding was passed, and funding is expected to continue at the $50 million level for the next 10 years. Simultaneously with this appropriation, Eliot Spitzer, who was New York State governor at the time, established the Empire State Stem Cell Board, the

11 members (including Lewis P. Rowland, president of PDF) of which are charged to administer this funding and oversee ethical questions regarding stem cell research. Information about stem cell research and its relevance to Parkinson's disease is also available from the PDF newsletter and from the "News and Events" section of the PDF Web site.

**SEE ALSO:** New York; Parkinson's Disease; Special Interest/Lobby Groups; United States.

**BIBLIOGRAPHY.** New Yorkers for the Advancement of Medical Research, www.nyamr.org (cited October 2007); Mark Noble, "Stem Cells: Their Potential for Treating PD," *Parkinson's Disease Foundation News and Review*, www.pdf.org/publications/newsletters/spring05/spring_05-Newsletter.pdf (cited October 2007); Parkinson's Disease Foundation, www.pdf.org/ (cited October 2007); Parkinson's Disease Foundation, "PDF Today," www.pdf.org/AboutPDF/docs/PDF_Today.pdf (cited October 2007).

Sarah Boslaugh
BJC HealthCare

# Parthogenesis

**PARTHOGENESIS OR PARTHENOGENESIS** is the phenomenon that occurs in invertebrate organisms such as invertebrate arthropods and some vertebrate fish, including—rarely—sharks, by which an egg can develop into an adult organism without fertilization. Parthenogenesis can occur naturally or be induced by chemical or mechanical stimuli. These stimuli are believed to simulate the action of a sperm penetrating the ovum, which, even without the sequential addition of genetic material to combine with that of the ovum, can stimulate cell division and embryogenesis. Parthenogenesis rarely occurs in vertebrates under natural circumstances. When it is induced in organisms higher than arthropods, often the resulting development is retarded, incomplete, or otherwise abnormal.

Parthenogenesis is not the process by which hermaphroditic species self-fertilize. These species have both male and female sexual organs and can often fertilize their own eggs.

The word parthenogenesis is from Greek roots for *virgin birth*. *Partho-* or *partheno-* are roots for *virgin*, *maiden*, or *young girl*, and *genesis* is Greek for *birth* or *origin*. In insects such as ants and honeybees, unfertilized eggs mature via parthenogenesis to be drones. Fertilized eggs become females; a female then becomes a worker or develops into a new queen.

Charles Bonnet first described parthenogenesis in the 18th century in the insect aphid. Dr. Jacques Loeb, M.D., demonstrated parthenogenesis in 1900 with a frog oocyte that was stimulated to begin embryogenesis by a mere prick with a needle. Loeb also demonstrated that sea urchin eggs could be stimulated into parthenogenesis by chemical manipulation of their tank water. Several organisms have shown inducible parthenogenesis, but never the human. In 1936, Gregory Goodwin Pincus demonstrated mammalian parthenogenesis using rabbit eggs induced with temperature changes and chemical stimuli.

Parthenogenesis has been observed in lizards as large as Komodo dragons. If a female dragon has eggs that undergo parthenogenesis, the baby dragons will be male. These males could become adults that could then mate with their mother, thereby producing a new line of dragons. Parthenogenesis has been speculated to be one way in which a lone survivor female can repopulate a colony, or in which a stray female can start a new colony elsewhere.

Because parthenogenesis naturally occurs in females of species that lay multiple eggs, each egg will have slightly different genetic material as a result of natural changes that occur at the genetic level. Therefore, the offspring will not be genetically identical to each other but, rather, unique. Parthenogenesis is therefore not the same phenomenon as cloning.

Mammalian parthenogenesis often results in abnormal development because mammalian chromosomes have what is called imprinting. Imprinting is a phenomenon by which particular genes are shut off if they are maternally or paternally donated; therefore, only the paternal or maternal copies are expressed, respectively. If an egg from a female mammal is induced into parthenogenesis, this egg will have improper gene expression because it will not have the balancing genes from a male father.

Because of this technical complication, human parthenogenesis has not been an option for reproduction. If the technology were to be worked out, ethical concerns would still arise. Scientists are working, however, to exploit parthenogenesis as a way to propagate human embryonic stem cells.

**SEE ALSO:** Cells, Embryonic; United Kingdom.

**BIBLIOGRAPHY.** J. C. Avise, J. M. Quattro, and R. C. Vrijenhoek, *Evolutionary Biology* (Plenum, 1992); P. C. Watts, et al., "Parthenogenesis in Komodo Dragons," *Nature* (v.444, 2006); M. J. D. White, *Animal Cytology and Evolution* (Cambridge University Press, 1973).

Claudia Winograd
University of Illinois, Urbana-Champaign

# Pennsylvania

**PENNSYLVANIA IS NUMBER** two in the United States in state financial support of stem cell research. Pennsylvania follows only the State of California in state support. In the year 2001, the Commonwealth of Pennsylvania budgeted $2.3 million to support in-state stem cell research. The majority of that money, totaling $2 million, came from Pennsylvania's settlements with tobacco companies.

In early 2005, Pennsylvania Representatives and state lawmakers proposed an increase in state funding of stem cell research by developing a fund especially for this cause. Additionally, the proposal suggested a tristate collaboration between Pennsylvania, New Jersey, and Delaware to foster stem cell research.

In April 2005, the University of Pittsburgh Medical Center (UPMC) and the University of Nevada School of Medicine (UNSM) proposed to establish a joint academic medical center in downtown Las Vegas at Union Park. Faculty would come from both universities; however, while the UNSM would profit both financially and intellectually from the new medical center, most of the financial backing would come from UPMC. The purpose of the new medical center would be to incorporate stem cell biology with organ transplants.

The UPMC also collaborates with a transplant center in Palermo, Italy. The Mediterranean Institute for Transplantation and Advanced Specialized Therapies is run by the government of Italy but managed by the UPMC.

Other leading Pennsylvania institutions in the field of stem cell research and regenerative medicine include the McGowan Institute for Regenerative Medicine at the UPMC, the University of Pennsylvania, and Thomas Jefferson University.

At the McGowan Institute for Regenerative Medicine, numerous studies involve stem cell biology and their uses. For example, researchers are attempting to use a woman's own adipose, or fat cell, stem cells to create a breast implant to replace her breast if removed due to cancer. This research is conducted at the Adipose Stem Cell Center in the School of Medicine's Division of Plastic Surgery. Also at the McGowan Institute is Dr. Eric Lagasse, Pharm.D., Ph.D., conducting research into liver stem cells and the reparation of severe liver damage from liver disease.

Under the direction of Dr. Amit Patel, M.D., M.S., and in collaboration with other institutes, scientists at the UPMC showed that heart damage due to congestive heart failure could be turned around with adult stem cell therapy. The patient showed novel angiogenesis, or the growth of new vasculature. Another important study out of the McGowan Institute, led by Dr. Johnny Huard, Ph.D., showed that adult stem cells can divide and regenerate at a level comparable to embryonic stem cells. The results of both of these studies were announced in 2005.

At the University of Pennsylvania's Abramson Family Cancer Research Institute, scientists study stem cells extensively. The university also boasts a new Institute for Regenerative Medicine, established in 2007. The institute, directed by Drs. Jonathan Epstein, M.D., and Ralph Brinster, V.M.D., Ph.D., is dedicated to studying basic cell biology of stem cells and translating these insights into therapeutic technologies. Additionally, the institute aims to foster public discussion and debate about stem cells and the ethical issues surrounding them.

Dr. Epstein's laboratory examines neural crest cells and their development into multiple cell types including nervous tissue and bones, as a model for stem cell differentiation. Dr. Brinster's lab studies the spermatogonial stem cell and the subsequent development of sperm cells. He hopes to harness this process enough to be able to introduce genetic changes into progeny by altering the male sperm line. A far-reaching goal of this research could be to assist men harboring a genetic mutation in having healthy children. Additionally, the technique could be used to introduce paternally delivered mutations into research animals that would allow further studies into the function of the mutated gene.

In July 2006, when the United States Senate convened to vote on a proposed Bill (H.R.810) that would amend the Public Health Service Act and provide federal funding for research on human embryonic stem cells, the two Pennsylvania Senators voted against each other. Both Republicans, Rick Santorum voted Nay while Arlen Specter voted Yea. That May, Santorum and Specter worked together to release a proposal to increase funding for alternate sources of stem cells, such as adult stem cells.

**SEE ALSO:** *Individual U.S. State Articles*; Biotechnology, History of; Clinical Trials Within U.S.: Batten Disease; Clinical Trials Within U.S.: Blind Process; Clinical Trials Within U.S.: Cancer; Clinical Trials Within U.S.: Heart Disease; Clinical Trials Within U.S.: Peripheral Vascular Disease; Clinical Trials Within U.S.: Skin Transplants (Burns); Clinical Trials Within U.S.: Spinal Cord Injury; Clinical Trials Within U.S.: Traumatic Brain Injury; Ethics; Federal Government Policies; Moral Status of Embryo; Special Interest/Lobby Groups; United States.

**BIBLIOGRAPHY.** M. Bellomo, *The Stem Cell Divide: The Facts, the Fiction, and the Fear Driving the Greatest Scientific, Political and Religious Debate of Our Time* (AMACOM/American Management Association, 2006); C. B. Cohen, *Renewing the Stuff of Life: Stem Cells, Ethics, and Public Policy* (Oxford University Press, 2007); C. Fox, *Cell of Cells: The Global Race to Capture and Control the Stem Cell* (Norton, 2007); K. R. Monroe, R. Miller, and J. Tobis, eds., *Fundamentals of the Stem Cell Debate: The Scientific, Religious, Ethical, and Political Issues* (University of California Press, 2007); "UPMC Sees Stem-Cell Research in Vegas Plans," *Pittsburgh Business Times,* April 14, 2005, http://pittsburgh.bizjournals.com/pittsburgh/stories/2005/04/11/daily24.html (cited January 2008); M. Ruse and C. A. Pynes, eds., *The Stem Cell Controversy: Debating the Issues (Contemporary Issues)* (Prometheus Books, 2006); C. Vestal, "States Take Sides on Stem Cell Research," *Stateline.org*, January 31, 2008, http://www.stateline.org/live/details/story?contentId=276784 (cited January 2008).

Claudia Winograd
University of Illinois, Urbana-Champaign

# Pharmaceutical Industry

**PHARMACOLOGY HAS BEEN** practiced around the world since the first time a plant or other natural remedy was applied to a human ailment. Major modern pharmaceutical companies are the fruit of advances in the 20th century in biology, chemistry, genetics, manufacturing processes, technology, scientific advances and business practices. The advance have made modern pharmaceuticals products the great deliverer from disease.

The approximately 200 pharmaceutical companies around the world are commercial businesses that promote the discovery, development, and marketing of new medicines. Physicians who prescribe medicines and druggists at local drug stores are the end of their distribution system. Many are huge retail chains, others are owned by a single entrepreneur. The pharmaceutical companies are the makers of the drugs and other therapeutic products used in medical treatments. They make drugs that are sold under their brand names or as generics.

Before the 19th century most pharmacology was herbal or some inorganic mixtures. In the late 19th century advances in biology, chemistry, understanding of genetics, manufacturing processes as well as other inventions or scientific advance have made modern pharmaceutical's products what they are today. Most of the pharmaceutical companies developed from local drug stores in North America or Europe. Some were founded in the late 19th or early 20th century.

The modern pharmaceutical industry was born from several independent activities. With the discovery of the antibiotic effects of the mold from which penicillin is grown medicines such as penicillin, the sulfur drugs, insulin, or antibiotics became available in local drugstores. From this, small companies grew into mass market industrial giants.

Advances in dye chemistry in the 19th century by German chemists revealed that when certain microbes absorbed a particular dye, it killed them. The coal was the source of the new sulfur dyes which when combined with advances in germ theory enable synthetic drugs to be manufactured. The total pharmacopeia of medical practice was greatly enlarged. It has since grown into a global multibillion dollar giant. Germany, Switzerland, the United Kingdom, Italy, and the United States became major centers for the manufacture of drugs.

## NEW DRUG DEVELOPMENTS

In the 1950s and 1960s, a great many new drugs were developed. With a market in the tens of millions around the world heart medications or blood pressure drugs such as cortisone and thorazine extended the lives of millions.

Psychiatry was aided with a number of psychoactive drugs such as valium (diazepam) and other tranquilizers. They also ushered in a new era of drug abuse.

In the 1960s a tragic side effect was discovered in female users of thalidomide. Pregnant women who took the drug often gave birth to deformed children. The Declaration of Helsinki was issued in 1964 by the World Medical Association setting standards for the conducting of clinical trials. Pharmaceutical companies were expected to prove efficacy in the clinical trials that they conducted before marketing a drug.

The invention of "the pill" in the 1960s, which was the first of the oral contraceptives, enabled couples to plan their families. It also prevented unwanted pregnancies in those sexually active people who were unmarried.

Cancer drugs began to be developed in the 1970s. *Chemotherapy* became a familiar term for cancer treatments. Also in the 1970s, changes in patent laws opened the door to rapid expansion of the pharmaceutical industry. Small struggling biotechnology firms were bought by growing pharmaceutical companies. As they continued to grow they also bought smaller pharmaceutical corporations so that manufacturing became more concentrated. The effect was to create national pharmaceutical oligopolies in a small number of countries where drug manufacturing was concentrated.

In some cases the use of chemicals has often been a matter of trial and error, such as the famous case of the discovery of the effects of Viagra® which failed as a blood pressure medicine but succeeded as a treatment for erectile dysfunction.

Since the 1980s advances in the understanding of DNA (deoxyribonucleic acid) and the mapping of the human genome has been combined with computers to speed the development of new drugs. Studies of metabolic pathways and ways to manipulate them provided new ways to treat diseases. Growth in understanding of pathogens also opened the way for the development of more effective drugs. Instead of development by trial-and-error computers can be used to tests thousands of drugs on thousand of receptor sites on a relatively short period of time.

In the 1990s and the first decade of the 2000s, the challenges arose in the area of marketing of drugs through massive advertising. Other challenges were consumers seeking lower prices via new distribution system or mass purchase by health maintenance organizations (HMOs) or preferred provider organizations (PPOs), via internet sales, the lower cost of drugs from foreign countries, attacks by animal rights activists on laboratory animal studies or ever-changing government regulations. The growing consumption of drugs by Americans combined with the marketing by the pharmaceutical industry brought charges from some quarters of over merchandising to an overmedicated society.

Today, there are strong economic and political motivations to advance new drugs. The competition to develop new drugs is intense because the profits from breakthrough drugs can be enormous. In the United States and some other countries, they are heavily regulated. They are less regulated in many Third World countries. Government regulations seek to accomplish a number of goals. One is to protect the public from the modern-day equivalent of the numerous "snake oil salesmen" who traveled the United States in the 19th and early 20th century selling remedies that had little, if any, medical benefit other than the soothing effects of a combination of alcohol and opium. Quack remedies sold to innocent consumers as medical remedies are of dubious medical value making money for the salesmen, but providing little more than false hope for the consumer.

With advances in anatomy, biology, chemistry, toxicology, and the ability to manufacture drugs as well as advances in statistical science, it became possible to conduct clinical trials on drugs. The clinical trials seek to prove the effectiveness of a new drug, its toxicity, its side effects, the appropriate dosage levels, and other important considerations that ensure that the drug will minister to the health of the patient and not harm or kill them.

Today, the Food and Drug Administration (FDA) regulates pharmaceutical development in the United States. The FDA enforces standards set by the United States Pharmacopoeia. In Europe, the European Union's agency for regulating the development and application of pharmaceuticals is the European Medicines Agency (EMEA). It enforces the pharmaceutical standards set by the European Pharacopoeia. It also evaluates drugs developed in Africa and the Middle East. Regulatory agencies besides the FDA include the International Conference on Harmonisation of Technical Requirements for Registration of Pharmaceuticals for Human Use (ICH), the European Medicines Agency (EMEA), Ministry of Health, Labour and Welfare (Japan), Medicines and Healthcare products Regulatory Agency (MHRA), Central Drugs Standards Control Organisation (India) (CDSCO), and others. Pharmaceutical companies are less regulated in many Third World countries.

## LEADING COMPANIES

Leading pharmaceutical companies include Abbott, Astrazeneca, BASF, Bayer, Boehringer Ingelheim, Bristol-Myers-Squibb, CSL Behring, Eli Lilly, Ferring, Glaxosmithkline, Grunethal, Hoffmann-La-Roche, Johnson & Johnson, Merck, Novartis, Novo Nordisk, Nycomed, Organon, Pfizer, Sanofi-Aventis, Solvay Pharmaceuticals, Schering-Plough, UBC, and Wyeth. Most of these belong to industrial associations such as European Federation of Pharmaceutical Industries and Associations (EFPIA), European Pharmaceutical Market Research Association (EphMRA), International Federation of Pharmaceutical Manufacturers and Associations (IFPMA), Japan Pharmaceutical Manufacturers Association (JPMA), New York Health Products Council (NYHPC), Pharmaceutical Research and Manufacturers of America (PhRMA), Irish Pharmaceutical Healthcare Association (IPHA), or to other associations. The associations serve as clearing houses for matters of common concern or as lobby organizations for the industry. They promote the exchange of industry information and provide a forum for discussing matters of common concern.

Pharmaceutical companies engage in many charitable programs. Sometimes these include the donations of their products to treat diseases in Third World countries, such as River Blindness drugs donated by Merck to African countries or Pfizer's donation of AIDS drugs in South Africa. They also promote research or provide scholarships at universities or to hospitals.

Large corporations attract a variety of detractors. The pharmaceutical industry is no exception. In the litigious climate of the United States, successful tort actions can net attorneys who successfully sue pharmaceutical companies millions of dollars. Critics of the pharmaceutical industry often charge that the companies are extorting people by charging high prices, which have little to do with the cost and financial risk of research and development of the new drugs.

The role of pharmaceutical companies in the Third World has also been contested by critics, who charge that the companies conduct clinical trials without the same level of safeguards that exist in the United States. Some critics charge that the money spent on research and development is only spent on diseases that are the most likely to yield a higher reward. This criticism ignores the special rules that the FDA has to encourage the development of "orphan drugs." These are drugs that can be used to treat people who have a disease that affects fewer than 200,000 people. Companies that develop such drugs are rewarded with special tax reductions or other regulatory incentives.

Medicinal drugs are usually put into a dozen categories. Those used to treat humans are classified according to the way that they affect the human body. Or they can be classified by their chemical makeup, the disease they fight, by the effect they have on the heart or blood vessels, or by their effect on the nervous system.

Numerous new drugs have been developed since the 1950s that have been separated into prescription and nonprescription. However, the problem of drug abuse or excessive health claims by some companies for nonprescription vitamins or other products has forced closer supervision of some of these products.

Many observers of the pharmaceutical industry and futurists are predicting a bright future for the industry. Advances in stem cell research are expected to generate a huge new range of medicines that will cure a wide range of diseases or mitigate the effects of others. The changes will impact the practice of medicine which has for decades depended upon surgery or chemistry to accomplish its most important tasks.

Using stem cells, the pharmaceutical industry should be able to program biological material to accomplish a variety of tasks that have been impossible until now. These would include organ regeneration, and organ or nerve repairs.

The advent of stem cell technology and its application will mean that the industry will be more biotechnologically based. Instead of its own laboratories, it may turn to the army of academic researchers providing the intellectual resources for developing new therapies. It will also likely mean that a great many new companies will emerge or that spin-off companies will move into specializing in a new product. Biologists will play a much greater role in the development of a stem cell oriented pharmaceutical industry than has historically been the case.

**SEE ALSO:** Biotechnology, History of; Stem Cell Companies.

**BIBLIOGRAPHY.** Antonio Escohotado, *Brief History of Drugs: From the Stone Age to the Stoned Age* (Inner Traditions International, 1999); H. Winter Griffith, Stephen Moore, and Kevin Boesen, *Complete Guide to Prescription and Nonprescription Drugs 2006* (Perigee, 2005); Andre Jungmittag, G. Reger, and T. Reiss, *Changing Innovation in the Pharmaceutical Industry: Globalization and the New Ways of Drug Development* (Springer-Verlag, 2000); Melody Petersen, *Our Daily Meds: How the Pharmaceutical Companies Transformed Themselves into Slick Marketing Machines and Hooked the Nation on Prescription Drugs* (Farrar, Straus and Giroux, 2008); Lesley Richmond, Alison Turton, and Julie Stevenson. *Pharmaceutical Industry: A Guide to Historical Records* (Ashgate, 2003); Michael A. Santoro, *Ethics and the Pharmaceutical Industry* (Cambridge University Press, 2007); Glyn Stacey and John Davis, eds., *Medicines from Animal Cell Culture* (Wiley, 2007); Jane Williams and Lorraine Griffin, eds., *Insider's Guide to the World of Pharmaceutical Sales* (Principle, 2005).

Andrew J. Waskey
Dalton State College

# Plant Stem Cells

**STEM CELLS, WHICH** have an ability of self-renewal and potency to differentiate multiple types of cells, exist in plants as well as in animals, and play essential roles for the growth and development of both plants and animals. The most characterized stem cells in plants reside in growing tips of shoots (above-ground part of plants) and roots. Stem cells in shoot tips differentiate into the tissues that compose leaves and stems. In some circumstances these cells change their identity to produce flowers. Stem cells in root tips differentiate into various root structures. In woody plants, stem cells named cambial cells produce additional tissue that forms a thick trunk for support of shoot tissues (i.e. secondary growth).

There are several unique features of stem cells in plants compared with those in animals. First, plant stem cells in shoot and root tips maintain their pluripotency throughout the plant lifecycle. They thus continuously produce organs during the plant lifetime. Sometimes they keep their pluripotency for thousands of years in long-lived species such as *Sequoia sempervirens*. In contrast, animal stem cells lose their pluripotency during embryogenesis. Second, stem cells in plants produce most of the organs post-embryonically (i.e. after germination), while those in animals produce most organs embryonically. Third, plant cells are enclosed in thick cell walls and they are tightly connected to each other. They cannot move like animal cells. Therefore, plant stem cells develop most plant tissues and organs by "stacking" cells. Finally, plant stem cells are often reprogrammed from differentiated cells, to produce lateral buds or roots, or to compensate the loss of original stem cells. Thus, they contribute to lateral growth in addition to vertical growth of plants.

In spite of these developmental differences and the evolutionary distance, stem cells in plants and animals are maintained by a similar system called a stem cell niche. A stem cell niche is a cellular microenvironment providing intercellular signals that maintain stem cells. It consists of stem cells and organizing cells. In principle, the identity of stem cells is maintained by physical interaction with organizing cells. After cell division of a stem cell, one daughter cell maintains physical interaction with organizing cells and continues to be a stem cell. The other daughter cell, which lacks these physical interactions with organizing cells, loses its identity as a stem cell and starts to differentiate. This is called asymmetric division. The structures of stem cell niches in plants are described below.

## STEM CELL NICHE IN SHOOT TIP

Stem cells reside in a dome-shaped organ known as the shoot apical meristem, which is located at the growing tip of the shoot. Stem cells are maintained by an underlying organizing cell group named the organizing center. Around two-thirds of stem cells are not physically interacted with the organizing center, thus physical interaction with organizing cells is not prerequisite to maintain stem cell identity in plants. Stem cells divide into stem cells themselves and transit-amplifying cells by asymmetric division. Transit-amplifying cells are intermediate cells before cell differentiation, which retain dividing activity. They proliferate themselves in the meristem to accumulate enough cells to develop new organs.

The upper center region of the shoot apical meristem including the stem cell niche is the central zone, which is distinguished from other regions because of its slower rate of cell division. This slow cell division may reduce the possibility of mutations. Such mutations could be very detrimental as they can affect the large part of the shoot tissues including gametes (pollens and eggs), and can be transmitted into the next generation. In the peripheral zone, which is located around the central zone, cells divide more rapidly and initiate differentiation into several organs. In and below the peripheral zone, cells expand vertically, pushing the stem cell niche upward.

Components of the molecular mechanisms conferring stem cell maintenance in plants have been gradually revealed in the dicotyledonous model plant *Arabidopsis thaliana* (thale cress). Two genes, *Wuschel* (abbreviated as *WUS*) and *Clavata 3* (*CLV3*), play a key role. The *WUS* gene serves to keep the identity of an organizing center and thus maintains a stem cell population. Conversely, the *CLV3* gene prevents excess proliferation of stem cells. Both the positive factor, *WUS*, and the negative factor, *CLV3*, are required to maintain the proper size of the stem cell niche.

## STEM CELL NICHE IN ROOT TIP

The structure of stem cell niches in root tips differ from those in shoot tips. A few organizing cells are surrounded by several different types of stem cells. These organizing cells rarely divide, and have thus been called quiescent centers. Stem cells in root tips asymmetrically divide to produce stem cells themselves and differentiated root cells without forming transit-amplifying cells. On the distal (tip) side, stem cells produce a root cap that is continuously sloughed off and that serves to protect the stem cell niche. In the basal direction, stem cells differentiate into cell types that compose a typical root. Differentiated cells expand vertically to push the stem cell niche further in the soil, resulting in the elongation of roots.

Several genes function in stem cell maintenance in root tips in Arabidopsis. One of them, *Wushcel-related Homeobox 5* (*WOX5*), encodes a protein with similar structure to the WUS protein. Interestingly, the function of *WUS* and *WOX5* are exchangeable. *WOX5* can be a substitute for *WUS* in shoot tips and vice versa. This is the first example of a molecular mechanism shared between stem cell niches in shoot and root tips. Further analyses may reveal additional shared mechanisms.

## STEM CELL REPROGRAMMING OF DIFFERENTIATED CELLS

Certain differentiated cells are reprogrammed into stem cells in plants. In shoots, stem cell niches are formed from differentiated cells located in the base of leaves. They may grow out to form lateral buds or may be dormant. In roots, some differentiated cells, which are distant from the root tip, can dedifferentiate and begin vigorous cell division. A quiescence center and a stem cell niche then develop within the new cells, resulting in the formation of a lateral root. These lateral buds and roots build up the "tree structure" of the plant's architecture. Stem cell reprogramming also occurs when the primary stem cell niche is damaged. For example, after laser ablation of the organizing center or quiescent center, the stem cell niche is diminished. However, within a few days, surrounding cells dedifferentiate and a new stem cell niche is produced near the original position.

## POTENTIAL "TOTIPOTENCY" OF PLANT CELLS

Totipotency indicates the ability of cells to differentiate into any type of cells and to produce an entire organism. The word *totipotency* itself was introduced by Austrian botanist Gottlieb Haberlandt in 1902 to describe the developmental plasticity of plant cells. Plasticity of plant cells is well-known in gardens as well as laboratories. Many foliage plants can be easily propagated by cutting. A part of a plant, such as a leaf, stem or root, is cut, and put on soil or in water. After a while, new shoots and roots proliferate from the cutting surface. Totipotency of plant cells was first demonstrated using carrot cells in 1958 when an entire organism was produced from fully differentiated carrot cells. Now this is routinely done with many plant species. In such cases, the new plant is a genetically identical "clone" of original plant.

The process of creating clones from differentiated cells can be divided into two steps, dedifferentiation and redifferentiation. For both steps, the phytohormones (plant hormones), auxin and cytokinin, play essential roles. Auxin, a tryptophan derivative, and cytokinin, a purine derivative, typically work antagonistically, thus balance of the concentration is important to their function. Generally, when differentiated cells are incubated with high concentrations of both auxin and cytokinin, cells dedifferentiate and form a cell mass called *callus*. Callus can be easily maintained in tissue culture. Callus has totipotency and differentiates in response to hormone levels. It forms adventitious (developing in an unusual place) shoots when incubated with high concentration of cytokinin relative to auxin, and adventitious roots when the relative amounts of these hormones are reversed. By incubating callus in the appropriate manner, entire plants are propagated.

## PHYTOHORMONES

Auxin and cytokinin also play critical roles in stem cell maintenance and organ differentiation. Cytokinin contributes to stem cell maintenance in shoot tips. Additionally, genes that maintain stem cells in shoot tips (e.g., *WUS*) activate cytokinin synthesis and signal transduction.

In contrast, auxin functions in organ differentiation. Auxin suppresses the expression of genes that maintain stem cells in shoot tips. Conversely, in root tips, auxin plays an essential role in establishment and maintenance of stem cells. Auxin accumulation is a critical process to develop new stem cell niches in root tips. Revealing the relationship among genes, phytohormones, and stem cells is one of the hot topics in plant stem cell research. Straightforward analyses of intact stem cells as well as experiments using callus will give us new insights into this field.

## EPIGENETIC MECHANISMS

Plants and animals were evolutionarily divided when they were unicellular organisms. Thus, the similarity of stem cell niches is probably the result of evolutionary convergence. Likewise, no gene that functions in stem cell maintenance has been found to be conserved between plants and animals. However, broader mechanisms, such as the epigenetic mechanism, are recently found to be shared between them.

An epigenetic mechanism confers a stable maintenance of the gene expression/repression state through cell division. This is performed through chromatin remodeling (change of chromatin structure), and the remodeling occurs via chemical modifications of DNA and histones, which compose chromatin. Epigenetic regulation thus contributes to maintaining cell identity. For example, in stem cells, the genes involved in stem cell maintenance (e.g. *WUS*) must be stably expressed through cell division. Conversely, differentiated cells have to suppress those genes stably to keep their differentiated state. Such an epigenetic mechanism is required for stem cell maintenance and organ differentiation in both plants and animals. In addition, *Retinoblastoma*, a gene involved in epigenetic mechanism, was revealed to have similar functions in stem cell maintenance and organ differentiation in both plants and animals. Further studies are expected to reveal additional epigenetic mechanisms shared between plants and animals.

## CONCLUSION

Since plants are sessile, they have acquired a continuous and plastic developmental system to adjust to a varied surrounding environment. According to their unique features, there are several notable benefits to studying stem cells in plants. First, plant cells are fixed into cell walls, making it relatively easy to trace cell linage. Second, plants have plastic developmental systems. It is easy to study the mechanisms underlying both differentiation and dedifferentiation. In addition, the mutations in many genes involved in stem cell maintenance and organ differentiation do not cause severe phenotypes such as embryonic lethality. Therefore, genetic approaches can be used to study stem cells.

Finally, studies of stem cells in plants are free from ethical issues. People have a long history of propagating "clones" of plants in gardens. With these advantages, stem cells in plants can be studied from different points of view from those in animals. Recent advances in the studies of epigenetic mechanisms have opened up the possibility of adopting the mechanisms in plant stem cells for animal stem cells, and vice versa. Thus, it is important to clarify whether upcoming results of studies are common in both plants and animals or specific to either kingdom.

**SEE ALSO:** Cloning; Developmental Biology; Niche Self-Renewal; Nuclear Reprogramming; Tissue Culture.

**BIBLIOGRAPHY.** Mohan B. Singh and Prem L. Bhalla, "Plant Stem Cells Carve Their Own Niche," *Trends in Plant Science* (v.11, May 2006); Ben Scheres, "Stem-cell Niches: Nursery Rhymes across Kingdoms," *Nature Reviews Molecular Cell Biology* (v.8, May 2007); Brian E. Staveley, "Plant Development," *Department of Biology, Memorial University of Newfoundland*, www.mun.ca/biology/desmid/brian/BIOL3530/DB_Ch07/DBNPlant.html (cited May 2008); Wikipedia contributors, "Meristem," *Wikipedia, The Free Encyclopedia*, en.wikipedia.org/wiki/Meristem (cited May 2008); Peter von Sengbusch, "Meristems," *Botany Online: Cells and Tissues*, www.biologie.uni-hamburg.de/b-online/e04/04c.htm (cited May 2008).

Yosuke Tamada
University of Wisconsin, Madison

# Preimplantation Genetic Diagnosis

**PREIMPLANTATION GENETIC DIAGNOSIS** (PGD) is also known as genetic embryo screening. PGD is the testing of embryos using certain procedures prior to implantation within the uterus. PGD can also be performed on oocytes prior to fertilization. PGD is used as a testing option instead of prenatal genetic diagnosis that traditionally occurs after the fetus is in utero. PGD tests for genetic conditions that have the potential to cause the disease. The advantage of PGD is that the testing is performed prior to implantation. Embryos that are affected are identified and not implanted. PGD can only be used for women who are achieving pregnancy through in vitro fertilization (IVF). The main advantage is that it reduces selective termination of affected fetuses.

In PGD, polymerase chain reaction (PCR) is used to determine the sex of the embryo. This technology was first performed in 1967 by Dr. Robert Edwards who was able to determine the sex of rabbits. It would be decades later, in 1989, that Dr. Alan Handyside utilized PGD in couples who were carriers of the delta 508 gene in the cystic fibrosis transmembrane regulator gene. The couples had undergone IVF and the embryos were subsequently tested on the third day after fertilization. One woman had two embryos that were fertilized normally and were negative for the cystic fibrosis gene. That woman underwent an embryo transfer with the normal embryo and gave birth to a healthy female in 1990 who had no genetic (carrier or disease) abnormality. This early PGD proved that single-gene diseases could be identified prior to implantation, an important development for families with genetic abnormalities.

PGD can only be used for couples who are undergoing assisted reproductive technology (ART) and IVF. Proponents of PGD believe that PGD eliminates later elective terminations of pregnancies due to genetic conditions by eliminating the implantation of genetically mutated embryos. It can be used for couples who have a family history of a single gene monogenic disorder when the fetus will be at risk for inheriting a genetic disorder. The single-gene disorders include autosomal dominant, autosomal recessive, X-linked dominant traits, X-linked recessive traits, Y-linked, and mitochondrial disorders. Autosomal dominant, autosomal recessive, and X-linked abnormalities are commonly screened for with PGD.

PGD can also be utilized for screening for mitochondrial disorders, but this is rarely performed, although a few centers do perform the analysis. In these cases, PGD is used to test for reciprocal and Robertsonian translocations, or other abnormalities such as chromosomal inversions or deletions. The use of PGD has been used in detecting chromosomal translocations since 1996.

Autosomal dominant disorders involve the inheritance of only one mutated copy of the gene. Most individuals inherit the disorder from one parent and have a 50 percent risk of inheriting the gene. These disorders tend to have low penetrance, which means even if the gene is inherited, a small number will actually go on to develop the disease. Most people who inherit autosomal dominant diseases will not demonstrate symptoms until later in life. Examples of autosomal dominant diseases include Huntington's disease, neuroblastosis 1, Marfan's syndrome, and hereditary nonpolyosis colorectal cancer. Achondroplasia, the most common cause of dwarfism, is an autosomal dominant disorder. Multiple osteochondromatosis, on the other hand, is an autosomal dominant disorder with high penetrance that most commonly occurs in children.

Autosomal recessive disorders requires two copies of an affected gene, one from each parent.

Two parents that are carriers have a 25 percent of having a child with the inherited disorder. These same parents have a 50 percent chance of having a child who also carries the trait, and a 25 percent chance of having a child that is completely genetically negative for the disorder. Most people inherit the disorder from two unaffected parents. Many parents may be unaware of their carrier status, or may learn of their status, only after testing. If only one parent is affected, there is no chance the fetus will inherit the disease. Examples of autosomal recessive disorders include sickle cell disease, Tay-Sachs disease, cystic fibrosis, spinal muscular dystrophy, albinism, many types of glycogen storage diseases, and thalassemia.

X-linked dominant diseases occur when there is a mutation on the X chromosome. Few genetic disorders are transmitted through this type of mutation. Males are more likely to be affected. If a man is the carrier, his male children will not be affected, however female children would. If the woman is the carrier, she has a 50 percent chance of passing the disorder on to her children (either sex) with each pregnancy.

Aicardi syndrome is an X-linked dominant disorder that results in absence of the corpus callosum in the brain. It is a malformation syndrome that results in retina deformities, seizures, and spasms in females but is fatal in males. Other examples include hypophosphatemia and chokenflok syndrome.

X-linked recessive diseases occur when there is a mutation in the X chromosome. The father is hemizygous for the disorder while a female carrier is homozygous. An affected male will not pass any of the abnormal genetic material to a son, but will pass on one copy of the mutated gene to any female fetus. An affected mother will has a 50 percent chance of having an affected son and a 50 percent chance of having daughter inherit one copy of the mutated gene. In general, while mothers are the carriers and men are affected. Examples of X-linked recessive disorders include hemophilia A & B, Duchenne muscular dystrophy, color blindness, Fragile X syndrome, Rett syndrome, and muscular dystrophy androgenetic alopecia.

PGD has been be used to detect for aneuploidy since 1993, and is now the most common indication for using PGD. The average age of women undergoing IVF is 35 years old which in and of itself is a risk factor for a chromosomal disorder. Women with advanced maternal age or repeated failed IVF attempts are the most likely to undergo PGD. It is estimated that up to 30 percent of oocytes carry a chromosomal imbalance. Approximately one-third of all spontaneous abortions occur as a result of an aneuploidy. Proponents argue that the use of PGD can increase the success of IVF by the transfer of genetically healthy embryos.

The cost of PGD varies considerably but averages an additional $2,500 to $4,000. The procedure does involve removing cells from the developing embryo, which could result in damage to the embryo, most commonly a cessation of growth. This can result in having no embryos left to implant. The techniques used to perform PGD vary, and are based on the type of genetic abnormality testing being performed. The tests have been known to produce false positives in which a normal embryo is discarded or false negatives, when an embryo with an affected condition has been transferred, under the pretense that the embryo is genetically normal.

PGD has been at the center of great ethical debate since its inception in the early 1990s. In 2000, PGD was perfected to perform HLA testing. In 2001, the procedure was used to create the "perfect stem cell match" for a child who was terminally ill. In 2001, a woman underwent four IVF attempts with 30 embryos being tested that resulted in the pregnancy and birth of a sibling whose cord blood was used to treat a sibling with Fanconi anemia. The technique has also been used to produce a "treatment sibling" for children affected with b thalessemia and leukemia.

Other ethical concerns have been raised when parents want testing but do not want to know their own carrier status. Other issues have been raised with family balancing or sex selection has been performed. It is estimated that 9 percent of all procedures are now performed for sex selection purposes. In some countries, such as India, where it was being used to obtain the more desired male child, it is now illegal to perform PGD for this indication. In 1999, PGD was developed to screen for late-onset common disorders with hereditary predisposition. The debate about the testing for certain diseases, such as breast cancer (BRCA1 gene) which occurs when the individual is identified as being at higher risk to develop a life-threatening disease, but would possibly not ever develop the disease, has created considerable controversy. There is also great debate on using PGD to eliminate individuals with certain disabilities, such as deafness. Other ethical debate lies with the exclusive use of the technique which is limited to only those who can afford it.

In countries with socialized medicine, PGD is used much differently. For example, in the United Kingdom, PGD must be reviewed by expert reviewers who take into consideration the genetic condition, the seriousness of the condition, and make recommendations if the procedure should be approved.

In 2002, the number of babies born after PGD totaled 1,000 live births. The Preimplantation Genetic Diagnosis International Society was formed in 2002 to provide multidisciplinary research and education in the PGD arena and to advance the science of PGD.

Bob Lanza and colleagues recently developed a method to derive human embryonic stem cells from single cells isolated using PGD. This meant that the embryo did not need to be destroyed to generate a human embryonic stem cell line and has big ethical implications for the field. However, removing a single cell from a blastocyst is considered by some to "damage" the embryo and therefore carries its own ethical questions. Thus this method of deriving ES cells, while of great interest, does not address all of the ethical concerns.

**SEE ALSO:** Embryonic Stem Cells; Ethics: In Vitro Fertilization: Moral Status of Embryo.

**BIBLIOGRAPHY.** J. J. Marik, "Preimplantation Genetic Diagnosis," emedicine from WedMD, www.emedicine.com/MED/topic3520.htm (cited April 2008); Joyce C. Harper, Alan H. Handyside, and Delhanty Joy, *Preimplantation Genetic Diagnosis* (Wiley, 2001); Preimplantation Genetic Diagnosis International Society, www.pgdis.org (cited April 2008).

Michele R. Davidson
George Mason University

# Presidential Campaigns

**THE ISSUE OF** stem cell research, especially that involving embryonic stem cells, first surfaced as a presidential campaign issue, albeit on a very minor level, in 2000. In the presidential election in 2004, it became much more visible and was one of the topics discussed directly in national debates between the candidates.

The controversy over whether embryonic stem cell research should receive federal funding was elevated to the point at which a significant percentage of the American electorate knew about it, expressed opinions, and voted accordingly. The promise of a solution to diseases such as diabetes or Alzheimer's or the ability to repair spinal cord and similar injuries contrasted with what seemed to many others the creation of life only to destroy it, so as to harvest the material for effecting these cures.

In the end, however, its importance was outweighed by other considerations such as the war in Iraq and the economy. In 2008, it has formed part of the platforms of candidates from both parties, with some assigning it more importance than others. In this most recent election, however, the possibilities of using adult stem cells may have undercut some of the fierceness of the debate, which earlier centered on the use of embryonic stem cells.

Even if it is not a hot-button issue, stem cell research has been significant in at least two ways. First, it has been an instance of where scientific research has been of such potential importance to so many people that it has been discussed widely and become an issue and discussed as part of a national dialog as an integral part of presidential elections. Also, for those who study elections, it has provided an opportunity to see how an issue of moral, health, and scientific/technological interest can be used by presidential candidates and the parties and interests that support them. For other observers, it was an example of how scientific facts can be altered to help pursue a political agenda.

## PRESIDENTIAL ELECTION OF 2000

The issue of stem cell research was never debated or discussed with any frequency during either the primaries or the general election in 2000. Five years earlier, Congress had imposed a ban on any federal funding of any research that resulted in human embryos being destroyed. In 1999, the Clinton administration had ruled that the ban would not apply to stem cell research in which the embryos were destroyed, although the restriction on federal funding would stand. Republican candidate George W. Bush answered a questionnaire from the U.S. Conference of Catholic Bishops, and in response to one of the questions, he stated that taxpayer funds should not be used to support research that would result in the destruction of human embryos. That view was later repeated by a Bush spokesperson. The response from a spokesperson for the Gore campaign was that the vice president supported stem cell research to be able to make important new discoveries. Beyond this brief exchange of statements, however, stem cells as either a source for scientific research or the recipient of federal assistance were not mentioned.

Bush was inaugurated in 2001 and was soon engaged in what seems to have been very extensive research on stem cell research, especially the use of currently existing as well as future lines of embryonic stem cells. On August 9, 2001, he articulated his stem cell policy in a compromise statement that managed to draw the opposition of both pro– and anti–embryonic stem cell research advocates. Bush's policy stated that federal funding would be restricted to the embryonic stems cell lines that already existed. Beyond this, however, there would be no further federal funding for embryonic stem cell–based research. He did not ban funding on the original lines, nor did he ban embryonic stem cell research. Further, he stated that in the current year, the federal government was spending $250 million to fund stem cell research. The compromise was unacceptable to advocates for the use of embryonic stem cells. Pro-life groups, including the Catholic bishops who had sent the questionnaire to Bush in 2001, also opposed the decision, many of them feeling that they had been betrayed. Bush remained consistent in this view through the remainder of his first term, however.

## PRESIDENTIAL ELECTION OF 2004

In the presidential campaign of 2004, stem cell research would become a campaign issue, and although it did not, in the end, sway a significant number of voters, its visibility was much higher than four years earlier. Bush's policy regarding stem cells had become a rallying point for those in favor of research and expanded federal funding regardless of the source of the stem cells. Although the basis for opposing embryonic stem cell research was similar to that of opposing abortions, the lines were becoming, in at least some areas, less clear. Among Republicans in Congress, several had begun to favor embryonic research, including Republican Senate Majority leader Bill Frist of Tennessee (who is also a doctor).

In addition to this change in some Republican quarters, pleas for funding stem cell research came from what many considered the Republican Party's royalty, the Reagan family. In May 2004, Nancy Reagan, wife of the former president, stated her desire to see stem cell research funded, while speaking at a benefit for the Juvenile Diabetes Research Foundation. Two months later, her son Ron Reagan would address the Democratic National Convention, also asking for increased federal funding for stem cell research.

All of the major Democratic candidates for the 2004 nomination expressed support for the removal of restrictions on federal funding for embryonic stem cell research. Howard Dean, former governor of Vermont, a physician and, for a time, front-running candidate for the Democratic nomination, directly criticized President Bush's opposition to stem cell research. In January 2004, he criticized what he called Bush's bias against science and said that it should not be allowed to deprive Americans of cures for disease.

Other candidates agreed. Senator Joseph Lieberman of Connecticut expressed support for funding embryonic stem cell research. John Edwards, a Democratic Senator from North Carolina, who eventually became the Democratic Party's candidate for vice president, was a supporter, as was Massachusetts Senator John Kerry. All three were among the 58 Senators who in the summer of 2004 sent a letter to Bush asking him to ease the restrictions placed on funding stem cell research. As Democratic candidate for president, Kerry made the issue an important part of the Democratic health platform and also raised it as an issue in the general election campaign debates.

The Republican nominee, President Bush, had made his stance clear three years earlier and had not changed it in any respect.

As the debates progressed, it was noted by at least some observers that both candidates were often simplifying the issues, sometimes distorting the other's position or making claims that were either inaccurate of misleading. Kerry often criticized Bush's banning of stem cell research. Of course, that was not the case, as Bush's restrictions had applied only to federal funding of embryonic stem cell research. Funding for research based on adult stem cells was continued, and there was never a ban on the actual use of embryonic stem cells for research.

In one speech, Kerry claimed that there were 100 million Americans who could benefit from stem cell research. Although perhaps literally true, this figure, which came from the Coalition for the Advancement of Medical Research, included Americans suffering from a host of diseases and disabilities of varying severity such as Parkinson's disease, Alzheimer's disease, spinal cord injury, and so on.

In the second televised debate between the candidates, Bush made the claim that he was the first president to ever allow federal funding for stem cell research. In a sense this was true, but he was not the first president to attempt such funding: President Clinton had attempted to secure federal funding for stem cell research years before, but a Republican-dominated Congress had prevented his attempts.

As a sidebar to the national debate on embryonic stem cell research, there were also developments at the state level. In 2004, voters approved California's Proposition 71. The result was the approval of funding for stem cell research (to include embryonic stem cells) that would total $3 billion. Similar efforts have been approved in other states that may eventually render the question of federal funding moot.

The importance of stem cell research as an issue had increased dramatically since the last election. In a national survey taken in 2001, only 51 percent of the respondents understood that the major source of the controversy was that embryos were being destroyed to get stem cells. Three years later, debate and discussion in the years preceding the election, as well as the comments of the candidates, raised the awareness and intensified discussion at the national level. As national concern for healthcare issues grew (an issue in which Democrats were seen as consistently advocating), so did subsidiary aspects such as research.

According to a Pew Research Center poll conducted on October 20, 2004, 43 percent of all potential voters stated that stem cell research was a very important issue. In a follow-up postelection poll conducted by the same group taken on November 11, only 1 percent mentioned stem cell research as the reason why they chose a candidate. At the same time, studies showed that the general awareness surrounding the issues was fairly high, even though it was not a major factor.

Exit polls indicated that some voters had voted for Bush on the basis of moral values, which had included not only gay marriage but also abortion and stem cell research. Although the importance and even the accuracy of that exit poll was questioned, it at least seemed to be a validation for the idea that for some voters, embryonic stem cell research was bundled with other moral issues. In the end, however, other issues, primarily the "war on terror" and fighting in Afghanistan and Iraq, took priority.

Immediately after the election, the Bush administration dropped its efforts toward a U.N. treaty banning all human cloning. Thus, although the administration might have claimed victory on this issue domestically, on an international basis, it could not make its view prevail. At the same time, a Bush spokesperson was asked whether there would be any changes to the administration's stem-cell policy and answered that there would be no change.

## PRESIDENTIAL ELECTION OF 2008

Shortly after the 2004 election, it was predicted in at least one major newspaper (*The Boston Globe*) that although stem cell research had been an "asterisk" in the recent campaign, it could become a major campaign issue four years later. Although stem cell research and federal funding for it has not disappeared, it has become less important as a campaign issue. A survey published by *New England Journal of Medicine* in January 2008 seemed to support that contention. Although healthcare was very important domestic issue to potential voters, stem cell research represented only a small portion of the issue. The article did emphasize, however, that healthcare issues and support of stem cell research were more prevalent among Democratic than Republican voters. As 2008 wore on, however, even healthcare issues would diminish in importance compared to the question of the health of the economy.

Nevertheless, in 2008, Republican and Democratic candidates for the presidency staked out positions on federal funding for stem cell research, as well as the general issue of embryonic stem cell research. As was the case with so many issues among the Democratic contenders for the presidency, there was general agreement on the removal of restrictions on funding embryonic stem cell research. Among Republicans, there was more variety of opinion.

Fairly early in Senator Hillary Rodham Clinton's campaign (in June 2007), she criticized President Bush's veto of the Stem Cell Research Enhancement Act in 2005, which would have permitted working with a greater number of embryonic stem cell lines and allowing federal funding if certain conditions were met. Further, Senator Clinton stated that, as president, she would lift the ban on stem cell research, accusing Bush of having put ideology before science.

Senator Barack Obama's campaign included a similar stand, which would promote and support embryonic stem cell research as well as increasing the number of stem cell lines available for such research. While he was an Illinois state Senator in 2004, Obama had supported a state measure that became known as the Ronald Reagan Biomedical Research Act.

John Edwards's platform also included support for embryonic stem cell research, including federal funding, which he had supported as Democratic vice presidential candidate in 2004. When Edwards was a U.S. Senator from North Carolina, he, along with Clinton, had been among the signers of the August 2004 letter to President Bush asking him expand federal policy concerning embryonic stem cell research and to relax existing restrictions. Interestingly, another Senator who had signed that letter was John McCain, who would be running for the Republican nomination in 2008.

Among the Republican candidates, early front-runner Rudolph Giuliani stated his support of stem cell research and federal funding. His restrictions amounted to allowing stem cell research as long as the process was not creating life only to destroy it after, and assumed the ability to extract stem cells without destroying the embryo. Stem cell research, however, was a minor issue for a candidate whose strong suit until he dropped out after the Florida primary was the war on terror.

Mike Huckabee, former governor of Arkansas and a former Baptist minister, stated that he was completely opposed to embryonic stem cell research. Huckabee declared that Bush's decision to prevent federal funding for embryonic stem cell research had been correct. Although many pro-life advocates had criticized Bush for compromising by allowing funding for already-existing lines, Huckabee was supportive and mentioned in his campaigns that the promise of stem cell research from other cell types had validated Bush's actions.

During his candidacy, former Massachusetts governor Mitt Romney stated his opposition to embryonic stem cell research but struggled to remain convincing. Romney, it was pointed out, was stating positions as a presidential candidate that varied from those he had held as governor. His stance on abortion (which came to be conflated in the minds of many with embryonic stem cell research) was a significant case in point. In the 2008 primaries, Romney stated that he would outlaw cloning to create new stem cells but would allow the use of surplus embryos from in vitro fertilization.

Although the Republican nominee for president John McCain has opposed abortion, he has also still expressed some support for embryonic stem cell research, including federal funding. In 2006, McCain supported an increase to federal funding for stem cell research using embryos that had been created as part of fertility treatments and that would be discarded.

Once again, as had happened in 2004, although stem cell research and funding had been significant issues, they were to be eventually outweighed by other issues that were less abstract to the majority of voters. As 2008 progressed, the fifth anniversary of the Iraq war and the likelihood of a major economic recession preoccupied voters. When, and if, these issues are resolved and stem cells emerge as an issue for public debate, scientific advances may preempt the importance of whether embryos are the best method for stem cell research.

**SEE ALSO:** California; Cells, Sources of; Cloning; Congress; Dickey Amendment; Federal Government Policies; Reagan, Nancy; *Roe v. Wade*; Stem Cells, Bush Ruling.

**BIBLIOGRAPHY.** Jacques Berlinerblau, *Thumpin' It: the Use and Abuse of the Bible in Today's Presidential Politics* (Westminster John Knox, 2008); Robert J. Blendon, et al., "Health Care in the 2008 Presidential Primaries," *New England Journal of Medicine* (v.358, 2008); Peter Canellos, "Stem-Cell Vote Blurs Religion-Based Politics," *Boston Globe* (November 9, 2004); Cynthia B. Cohen, *Renewing the Stuff of Life: Stem Cells, Ethics, and Public Policy* (Oxford University Press, 2007); Eric Henley, "How the Presidential Candidates' Health Care Proposals Contrast," *Journal of Family Practice* (v.53/10, 2004); Kristen Renwick Monroe, Ronald B. Miller, and Jerome S. Tobis, eds., *Fundamentals of the Stem Cell Debate: The Scientific, Religious, Ethical, and Political Issues* (University of California Press, 2008); Dick Meyer, "Election 2004: How Did One Exit Poll Answer the Question of How Bush Won? Good Question," *Washington Post* (December 5, 2004); Narbara Norrander and Jan Norrander, "Stem Cell Research and the 2004 Election," in *A Matter of Faith? Religion in the 2004 Election* (Brookings Institution, 2007); Ted Peters, *The Stem Cell Debate* (Fortress, 2007).

Robert Stacy
Independent Scholar

# President's Council on Bioethics

**BIOETHICS COMPRISES THE** ethical issues involving the science of biology as it pertains to the practice of medicine. Bioethicists are concerned with a variety of ethical questions that involve relationships among the life sciences, biotechnology, medicine, politics, law, philosophy, and theology. The president of the United States is faced with multiple bioethical issues as technology in the bioscience and medical fields continues to evolve. The Office of the President of the United States frequently appoints specialized task forces made up of experts in particular fields to offer advice and guidance on complex issues. On November 28, 2001, President George W. Bush appointed a group of experts in the bioethical field to advise his administration. The Council on Bioethics was formed by an executive order, with members being directly appointed by the president himself. The chairperson is also directly named by the president. Although the group collaborates on issues, they do not have the ability to appoint their own leadership or to make any direct policy changes.

The council is charged with six tasks, as outlined by the executive order. The first task is to advise the president on bioethical issues that may emerge as a consequence of advances in biomedical science and technology. This includes but is not limited to inquiring about the human and moral significance of biomedical and technological advances in science, evaluating the political and ethical implications of these advances, building a foundation for national discussion of these topics, advancing public understanding of these issues, and identifying possible collaborating international partners in the bioscience field. The second task is to examine ethical issues related to specific advances, such as embryo and stem cell research, assisted reproduction, cloning, uses of knowledge and techniques derived from human genetics or the neurosciences, and end-of-life issues. The third task is to develop a thorough understanding of both the science and the moral implications of the biomedical advances being reviewed. It is recognized that members of the council may have differing views. Although the executive order states specifically that the members may have differing views, and in fact that a consensus on an issue was not the intended purpose of the council, there has been speculation that the views of two members led to their removal from the council. The dismissal of Dr. Elizabeth Blackburn and Dr. William F. May sparked widespread controversy and created speculation that members who did not agree with and support the views of President Bush were asked to resign. Dr. Janet Rowley, who also had conflicting views on several issues, has remained on the council.

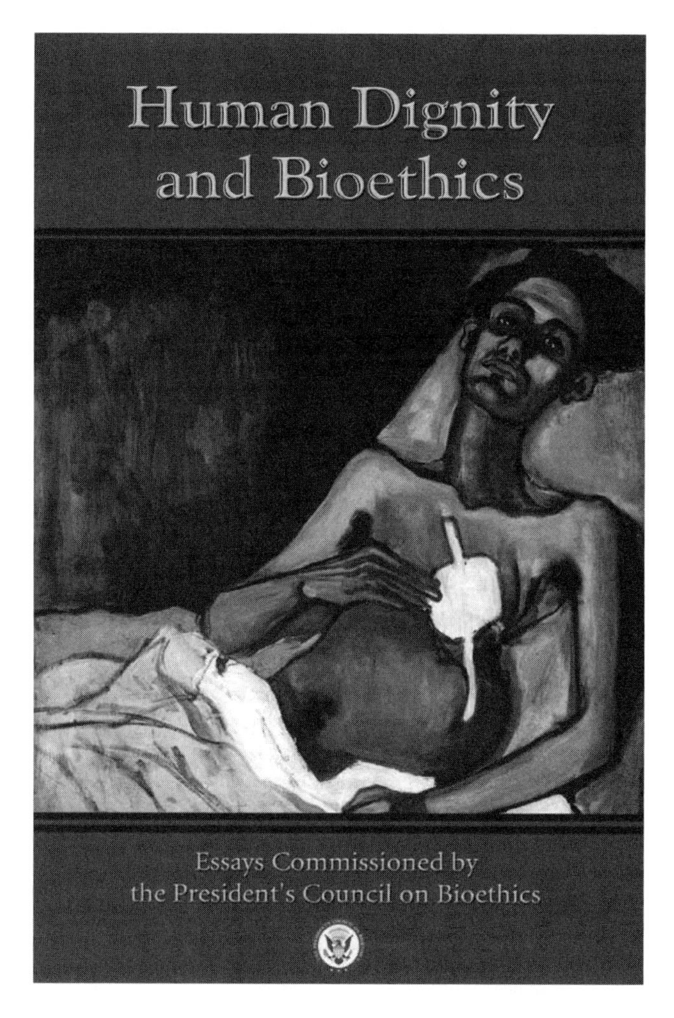


*The President's Council on Bioethics commissioned this report, which expresses various insights into the topic.*

Some skeptics have opposed the membership of the council, citing that the council is made up primarily of conservative scholars who are unlikely to truly engage in debate about these crucial ethical issues. Others have criticized the council for not being more active in studying broader-reaching social issues involving healthcare policy. Others have embraced the views of the council, especially religious groups. Certain topics have exploded into profound debate, including advances in fertility, aging, promotion of longevity, and treatment modalities that could cure genetic diseases. Both Blackburn and Rowley have publicly stated that the interpretations of the council have distorted the science. The council has conservative views about the use of embryonic stem cell research—a science that many scientific experts feel could yield enormous medical advances. There has been concern that the conservative views of the membership could impede open and honest dialogue within the council itself, thus diminishing the true intent and purpose of the council.

The council has undergone some changes in leadership since its inception in 2001. The original chairperson appointed in 2001 by President Bush was Dr. Leon R. Kass. Kass is a conservative who has well-known views that oppose human embryonic stem cell and cloning research. He also opposes all forms of intervention in the life cycle, specifically birth control and methods aimed at prolonging life. He also opposes interventions such as in vitro fertilization. Interestingly, one of his own grandchildren was conceived using this technology. Dr. Kass possesses both a medical degree from the University of Chicago and a doctorate from Harvard University. He is a current member of the President's Council on Bioethics, although his reign as chair ended in 2005. He maintains a teaching position at the University of Chicago and has authored multiple books.

The current chair is Edmund D. Pellegrino, M.D., who is also the president of Catholic University in Washington, D.C. Pellegrino is known for his willingness and ability to openly dialogue and exchange views in the field of medical ethics, along with his continued commitment and strong advocacy of the Roman Catholic tradition in medical ethics. He was the founder of the Center for Clinical Bioethics at Georgetown University and continues on the faculty there as professor emeritus of medicine and medical ethics. He is an avid researcher and has published more than 500 articles and chapters in the fields of medical science, physiology, and medical ethics. He has also authored 11 books.

In addition to the chair, the committee is made up of no more than 18 individuals who are appointed to the council for two-year terms. The council members are eligible for reappointment at the president's discretion. The 2001 executive order has been renewed in 2003, 2005, and 2007. The executive order that created the council must be renewed every two years or the council will be abolished. The board has had several members who have served their terms and no longer hold seats on the board. These include Elizabeth H. Blackburn, Ph.D. (2002–04); Stephen Carter, J.D. (2002); Francis Fukuyama, Ph.D. (2002–05); Mary Ann Glendon, J.D., M.Comp. L. (2002–05); William F. May, Ph.D. (2002–04); Michael J. Sandel, D.Phil. (2002–05); and James Q. Wilson, Ph.D. (2002–05). Current members include Edmund D. Pellegrino, M.D.; Ben Carson, M.D.; Rebecca S. Dresser, J.D., M.S.; Daniel W. Foster, M.D.; Michael S. Gazzaniga, Ph.D.; Robert P. George, J.D., D.Phil.; Alfonso Gómez-Lobo, D. Phil.; Leon R. Kass, M.D., Ph.D.; William B. Hurlbut, M.D.; Charles Krauthammer, M.D.; Peter Augustine Lawler, Ph.D.; Paul McHugh, M.D.; Gilbert C. Meilaender, Ph.D.; Janet D. Rowley, M.D.; and Diana J. Schaub, Ph.D. The current executive director is F. Daniel Davis, Ph.D.

The other responsibilities and roles of the council are quite clear. The order specifically states that members are not responsible for specific projects or advances or for devising and overseeing regulations for specific government agencies. It also states that the council may receive suggestions and recommendations from various government agencies. The final task of the council is to prioritize their analyses, taking into account the gravity and importance of varying advances, and to formulate recommendations as needed for the good of the public. The council needs to be aware of the importance that some advances may have and that many of these scientific advances may be time sensitive in nature.

The council has the authority under the executive order to create subcommittees, hold meetings, and conduct inquiries. They also can develop reports based on inquiries. The council receives administrative support from the Department of Health and Human Services, pending the availability of sufficient funds. The staff for the council has an executive director, who is appointed by the Secretary of Health and Human Services, in consultation with the chairperson. The council is a valuable asset to the president in providing recommendations about and evaluations of cutting-edge biomedical and technological advances.

**SEE ALSO:** Federal Government Policies.

**BIBLIOGRAPHY.** President's Council on Bioethics (U.S.), *Beyond Therapy: Biotechnology and the Pursuit of Happiness* (United States Government Printing Office, 2008); President's Council on Bioethics, *Human Dignity and Bioethics: Essays Commissioned* *by the President's Council on Bioethics* (United States Government Printing Office, 2008); President's Council on Bioethics, "Stem Cells, New Developments in Stem Cells Research," http://www.bioethics.gov/topics/stemcells_index.html (cited May 2008).

Michele R. Davidson
George Mason University

# Princeton University

**PRINCETON UNIVERSITY IS** a private coeducational research university located in Princeton, New Jersey. It is one of eight universities that belong to the Ivy League. Originally founded at Elizabeth, New Jersey, in 1746 as the College of New Jersey, it relocated to Princeton in 1756 and was renamed Princeton University in 1896. Princeton was the fourth institution of higher education in the United States to conduct classes. Princeton has never had any official religious affiliation, which is rare among American universities of its age. At one time, it had close ties to the Presbyterian Church, but today, it is nonsectarian and makes no religious demands on its students. The university has ties with the Institute for Advanced Study, Princeton Theological Seminary, and the Westminster Choir College of Rider University. Princeton has traditionally focused on undergraduate education and academic research, though in recent decades, it has increased its focus on graduate education and offers a large number of professional master's degrees and Ph.D. programs in a range of subjects.

The Department of Molecular Biology is a center for research in the life sciences at Princeton University. Housed mainly in four adjacent and connected buildings, it is home to 50 faculty and associated faculty, 120 graduate students, 130 postdoctoral fellows, 100 undergraduate majors, and 100 technical and administrative staff. The Commission on Science and Technology of the State of New Jersey received 71 complete applications for its $5 million Stem Cell Research Grant program, including proposals from private life science companies as well as New Jersey's research universities and nonprofit institutions. The Commission has awarded stem cell research grants to 17 scientists, including Tom Shenk and Kateri Moore of the Department of Molecular Biology. The grants from the New Jersey Commission on Science and Technology will further work in the field of stem cell advancements that began at Princeton more than 25 years ago. Two of the university's grant recipients, molecular biologists Ihor Lemischka and Kateri Moore, continue exploring the cutting edge of stem cell research. Collaborative efforts with electrical engineer Ron Weiss are attempting to program embryonic stem cells to "fix" disease. The third grant recipient, molecular biologist Thomas Shenk, will focus on producing stem cells from human umbilical cord blood.

Lemischka has been studying stem cells at Princeton for 20 years and has remained one of the world's leading innovators in the research since he was the first to show, in the 1980s, that a single blood-producing stem cell in bone marrow, known as a hematopoietic stem cell, could rebuild the entire blood system in a mouse whose blood system had been destroyed. Lemischka and colleagues, working in collaboration with scientists at the University of Pennsylvania led by G. Christian Overton, created a "library" of gene fragments from blood stem cells of mice. They also created a library of genes from a sample of mature blood cells that had been depleted of stem cells. They then "subtracted" the two libraries, removing the majority of commonly expressed "housekeeping" genes while enriching for those that are preferentially expressed in the immature stem cells. By analyzing the DNA sequences in the "subtracted" library using sophisticated computational techniques and comparing them to the sequences of many other genes and proteins, they were able to identify more than 2,000 genes that are likely to be active in stem cells. The approach is far more comprehensive than previous techniques, which typically involve finding an animal that has a stem cell disorder and looking for the gene mutation that causes it, or which focus on small numbers of genes previously identified in other systems. In addition to yielding a wealth of new genetic information, the research demonstrates an innovative approach to collecting, analyzing and presenting the data.

Kateri Moore brought her expertise in gene therapies and cell environments to Lemischka's lab in 1992. Moore's research group has been working with Lemischka for 16 years to contribute an understanding of the microenvironments where stem cells live and are nurtured.

Lemischka and Moore came together with Weiss after he wrote a paper on directed evolution published in the Proceedings of the National Academy of Sciences. The paper described analogies between building computer circuits and using nature to build similar natural connections. After years of breakthroughs identifying molecules that control stem cell function in mice, the logical next step for the biologists was to explore the engineering of stem cells.

**SEE ALSO:** New Jersey; Microenvironment and Immune Issues.

**BIBLIOGRAPHY.** Molecular Biology, Princeton University, www.molbio.princeton.edu (cited November 2007); NJCCC, www.njstemcell.org (cited November 2007); Science Daily, www.sciencedaily.com (cited November 2007).

Fernando Herrera
University of California, San Diego

# Prostate Tissue Stem Cells

**PROSTATE IS A** male sex accessory organ surrounding the urethra below the urinary bladder that is located in the pelvic floor. The prostate stores and secretes a clear, slightly alkaline fluid to form semen with spermatozoa during ejaculation. The prostate fluid helps maintain the activity and life span of sperm. Male hormone testosterone is required for development and proper function of prostate.

## ANATOMY OF THE PROSTATE

The human prostate is divided into the peripheral zone, the central zone and the transitional zone. Peripheral zone located in the peripheral part of the prostate gland and composes about 70 percent of the mass. Central zone constitutes the central part of the prostate gland that surrounds the ejaculatory ducts. Most of the prostatic cancer originates from the peripheral zone, and only a small proportion, less than one-third, arises from central zone. Transition zone is between central and peripheral zone and this region rarely causes prostate cancer.

## METHODS USED TO IDENTIFY PROSTATE TISSUE STEM CELLS

There are several commonly used methods to isolate and characterize prostate tissue stem cells. (1) Immunohistochemistry (IHC): This method uses antibodies specific to prostate stem cell markers that bind to prostate stem cells, followed by either chemical reaction or fluorescent dye to find the location of stem cells. The IHC is usually performed on fixed tissues sections. (2) Fluorescent-activated cell sorting (FACS) is the method of choice to isolate and enrich living prostate stem cells. Fluorescent-labeled antibody to cell surface marker is applied to prostate single-cell suspension, and then these cells are passed through a fine tube with a laser beam shining to cells. Cells that bind to fluorescent antibodies will be separated based on their fluorescent intensity and collected for further analysis. (3) Side population isolation. Prostate tissue stem cells can exclude Hoechst dye and other cells are stained with Hoechst. These cells that exclude Hoechst dye are called side population cells. Prostate stem cells can be enriched in side population. Prostate stem cells isolated by cell surface markers or side population exhibit the proliferation and differentiation potential that is expected for tissue specific stem cells by transplantation assay. (4) BrdU label retention identifies "slow cycling" prostate stem cells. Prostate stem cells are more quiescent and divide slower compared to non-stem cells, resulting in a prolonged preservation of the labeled DNA in prostate stem cells. Using this method, scientists find that the prostate stem cells are concentrated in certain regions of prostate.

Both in-dish sphere formation assay and in-animal transplantation assay are used to test prostate stem cell activity. The stem cells isolated using above methods need to be further confirmed for characteristic features of stem cells, such as enormous self-renew, proliferation, multipotent differentiation. These features can be evaluated by sphere formation assay in culture dish or transplant isolate stem cells to immunodeficiency mice to see whether isolated prostate stem cells can differentiate to prostate tissue when combined with prostate embryonic stromal cells. The embryonic stromal cells are needed to provide growth and differentiate factors for prostate development, and immunodeficiency mice are used to prevent immune rejection of transplanted tissue.

## PROPERTIES OF PROSTATE TISSUE STEM CELLS

Prostate tissue–specific stem cells are a minority population of early progenitor cells that typically remain quiescent until being activated to replenish tissue-specific cells that are lost because of injury, senescence, and/or apoptosis. Adult prostate stem cells are multipotent undifferentiated cells found in the tissue among differentiated cells. These stem cells can renew and can differentiate to yield the cell types in prostate. Early studies found that cells isolated from any part of the prostate can regenerate entire prostate gland, and the regenerative ability of prostate tissue taken from old mice is similar to that taken from young mice suggests the presence of prostate stem cells. Adult tissue–specific stem cells have been postulated to comprise a small fraction of cells in adult organ but provide the enormous proliferative reserve for self-renew and can differentiate to all cell types in a tissue. These tissue-specific stem cells exhibit an expanded potential for self-renewal and possess a broad repertoire of differentiation potential such that they can regenerate the diverse population of cells found in prostate. These long-lived slow-cycling prostate tissue stem cells are considered the prime target for neoplastic transformation and development of cancer, because they have the long life necessary for accumulating the multiple genetic or epigenetic changes required to escape growth control. These stem cells are also thought to confer the unique properties of therapy resistant and hormone independent that make the treatment of malignancies such as prostate cancer more difficult.

## THE RELATIONSHIP BETWEEN PROSTATE STEM CELLS AND PROSTATE CANCER

Prostate stem cell and tumor cells share features such as self-renewal capability, androgen independence, and telomerase expression. There are speculations that prostate cancer is developed from long-lived prostate stem cells that accumulate genetic and environment mutations. It is postulated that androgen-independent prostate cancer arises from a small fraction of cells within the tumor that are related to prostate tissue–specific stem cells—androgen-independent progenitor cells which have unlimited potential for self-renewal and serve as the precursor to all prostate epithelial cell lineages.

Prostate cancer is one of the leading causes of death in the United States and developed countries. Despite advances in diagnosis and treatment for localized prostate cancer, advanced prostate cancer remains a leading cause of death among men. Androgen deprivation is a mainstay of therapy for advanced disease, but most men ultimately develop recurrence of androgen-independent prostate cancer. The metastasis androgen-independent prostate cancer is the main cause of death for most patients. The unique biology of prostate stem cells holds promise as an avenue for new therapeutic approaches to advanced prostate cancer. However, this promise can only be realized when we understand the biology of the stem cell compartment. The studies of prostate stem cells will greatly advance the efforts to elucidate their role in normal prostate and will provide a staging ground for the role of stem cells in prostate cancer and other diseases.

**SEE ALSO:** Biotechnology, History of: Cancer; Fluorescence-Activated Cell Sorting.

**BIBLIOGRAPHY.** Nicole LeBrasseur, "Prostate Stem Cells Identified," *Journal of Cell Biology*, www.jcb.org (cited November 2007); Institute of Cancer Research, "Prostate Stem Cell Team," www.icr.ac.uk (cited November 2007); "Cancer Stem Cells Discovered by York Researchers," *Med India*, www.medindia.net (cited November 2007).

Daniel Xudong Shi
University of Wisconsin, Madison